REHABILITATION
in Spinal Cord Injuries

REHABILITATION
in SPINAL CORD INJURIES

Jacqueline Reznik & Joshua Simmons

Jacqueline E. Reznik
BAppSci, GradDip(Neurology), GradDip(Teach), MAPA, MCSP, PhD
Adjunct Senior Lecturer, James Cook University, Queensland, Australia
Associate Senior Lecturer, Curtin University, WA, Australia
Honorary Research Associate, Institute of Child Health, UCL/GOSH, London, UK

Joshua Simmons
BPhty
Director Digital Health Clinical Consultation Services
Clinical Lead Digital, Hospital Metro South, Queensland, Australia
Clinical Informatics, Metro South Health, Queensland, Australia
Former Clinical Team Leader Physiotherapy, Spinal Injuries
Queensland Spinal Cord Injury Service, Queensland, Australia

ELSEVIER

ELSEVIER

Elsevier Australia. ACN 001 002 357
(a division of Reed International Books Australia Pty Ltd)
Tower 1, 475 Victoria Avenue, Chatswood, NSW 2067

ISBN: 978-0-7295-4320-0

National Library of Australia Cataloguing-in-Publication Data

A catalogue record for this book is available from the National Library of Australia

---

Content Strategist: Melinda McEvoy
Content Project Manager: Shruti Raj
Edited by Margaret Trudgeon
Proofread by Tim Learner
Permissions Editing and Photo Research: Praveen Kumar
Cover and internal design by Lisa Petroff
Index by SPi Global
Typeset by Toppan Best-set Premedia Limited
Printed in China by 1010 Printing International Limited

Last digit is the print number: 9 8 7 6 5 4 3 2 1

DEDICATION

This book is dedicated with love to my friend and colleague Wilma Aniç (nee McPherson), whose love of life and exuberant personality allowed her to conquer all. What I learned from Wilma, in my early years as a physiotherapist at the Spinal Unit at Stoke Mandeville Hospital, allowed me to treat all my future patients with the care and understanding they needed.

Wilma's addition to the staff of the Physiotherapy Department at SMH by Ida Bromley taught us all the true meaning of rehabilitation.

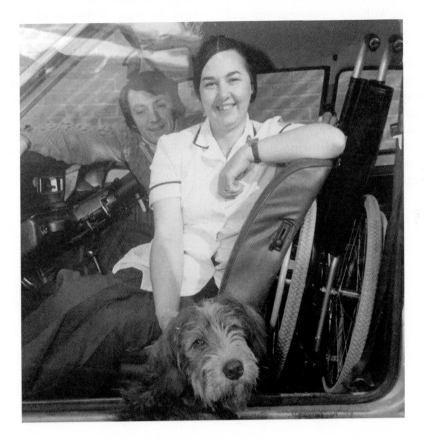

'Wee Jackie'
Wilma Aniç (nee McPherson) MCSP (1943–2019)

PREFACE

HOW THIS BOOK SHOULD BE USED

This book is not intended to be read 'cover to cover', but rather to be used as a handbook that allows easy access to the reader who is searching for specific answers to particular questions regarding the management of their patient(s) with a spinal cord injury (SCI). The book is divided into 21 chapters, beginning with the neuroanatomy and neurophysiology of the spinal cord. It endeavours to tell the story of the total rehabilitation of a patient with a traumatic SCI from the initial injury through to long-term living with the consequential neurological damage. The appendices included allow the reader easy access to commonly used assessments for the spinal cord injured person.

All chapters follow a general theme and have been written by experts in their fields. Some of the chapters are designed to give didactic instructions on treatments and interventions, others to furnish the treating therapist with new ideas and different approaches, while others are written by people with SCIs and give practical solutions to everyday problems. Each chapter is intended to be succinct and the reader is encouraged to read the Evidence-based practice points at the end of each chapter in order to gain an overview of the key messages associated with the topic. If further information is required, all chapters have a comprehensive bibliography.

The editors would like to note that the words 'patient, client, person/individual with a spinal cord injury' are used interchangeably throughout the text. The term is dependent upon the context in which it is used, for example, the stage of the rehabilitation journey (inpatient vs community) or the intention of the statement (e.g. health professional advice). However, each term is always used with the greatest respect intended.

FOREWORD

It gives me great pleasure to write a foreword for this book, which fills a need for a practical guide to the management of spinal cord injury (SCI). For centuries, this condition was considered 'an ailment not to be treated',[1] since it resulted in certain death, However, since the introduction of comprehensive care for people with SCI after World War II, and improvements in pre-hospital management and medical care, survivors now have a normal lifespan, and can expect to live a productive life.

While there is considerable international effort directed at new treatments for repair of the injured spinal cord, there has also been a transformation in the management of SCI. This book tracks the patient journey from pre-hospital and acute hospital management through to rehabilitation, and goes beyond hospital care to living in the community, including ageing with an SCI. Edited by two physiotherapists with substantial clinical experience in the field of spinal cord injury, this book includes contributions by an anatomist, a paramedic, medical practitioners, physiotherapists, occupational therapists and psychologists. Chapters on biomechanics, paediatric SCI, high cervical injuries and the tetraplegic upper limb are not typically addressed in other texts on this subject. The chapter on biomechanics provides an analysis of the biomechanical principles involved in basic tasks, such as bed mobility, sitting balance, transfers and pushing a wheelchair. One standout feature of the book is that three chapters have been written by people with lived experience of SCI, offering their welcome perspective on exercise and sport, sociological issues and the hazards of living with an SCI.

The material in this book is practical, each chapter including practice points, and it would be particularly useful for undergraduates and new graduates. However, more experienced graduates in medical and allied health disciplines may find this book helpful in refreshing or increasing their knowledge.

There will always be improvements in management strategies in the future, as well as advances in our understanding of the nature and consequences of SCI. However, this book provides new and important insights into current aspects of management of SCI, and can be highly recommended.

Mary P Galea AM PhD
Professorial Fellow
Department of Medicine
The University of Melbourne
Parkville, Victoria, Australia

ENDORSEMENT BY IDA BROMLEY FCSP

Congratulations to Jackie, my friend and colleague for many years for this interesting and informative book. All who work in this field of rehabilitation know that it is the patients who demolish their boundaries. We simply pass the information to the next generation.

Reference

1. Hughes, J.T., 1988. The Edwin Smith Papyrus; an analysis of the first case reports of spinal cord injuries. Paraplegia 26, 71–82.

CONTENTS

Contents

ABOUT THE EDITORS

Dr Jacqueline (Jackie) Reznik has a long clinical history in neurological, geriatric and paediatric physiotherapy, in addition to undergraduate and postgraduate teaching in neurosciences and neurological physiotherapy, both in Australia and internationally. She holds adjunct positions as Senior Lecturer in the Division of Tropical Health and Medicine at James Cook University, Townsville, Queensland, and as Research Associate at the Institute of Child Health, Great Ormond Street/ University College London, UK. Her main clinical and research interests lie in the investigation and treatment of the control of movement and function following neurological insult, both traumatic and non-traumatic. She has published numerous papers in these areas and is the author of a physiotherapy textbook *Pharmacology Handbook for Physiotherapists*.

Joshua (Josh) Simmons has been a physiotherapist for 20 years and has spent most of his professional life specialising in the management of spinal cord injury. He has worked across the continuum of SCI management, including acute management post-injury, facilitating transition back to the community and long-term follow-up. He was the Clinical Team Leader at the Spinal Injury Unit at Princess Alexandra Hospital as part of the Queensland Spinal Cord Injury Service (QSCIS) from 2005 to 2019.

Josh has served as an Executive Member of the Australia and New Zealand Spinal Cord Society (ANZSCoS), including roles as Secretary and Vice President. He is a member of the Australian and International Physiotherapy Networks and regularly lectures to undergraduate university students on the topic of SCI management.

Josh is currently a Clinical Lead and Director within the realm of Clinical Informatics, supporting clinicians in the transformation of clinical practice to a digital platform, including the utilisation of digital systems and technology to deliver safe, efficient patient-centred care supported by the best evidence.

CONTRIBUTORS

Helen Anscomb BSc(Hons), GradCertEd(TertTeach), PhD
Associate Professor, Head of Anatomy and Pathology, College of Medicine and Dentistry, James Cook University, Townsville, Queensland, Australia

Caroline Barmatz BPT, HT, MHA
Clinical Educator, Senior Lecturer Hydrotherapy, Researcher Hydrotherapy, Director of Hydrotherapy, Sheba Medical Center, Israel

David Berlowitz BAppSci(Phty), PostGradDipPhty(Research), PhD
Chair of Physiotherapy, University of Melbourne (Austin Health), Heidelberg, Victoria, Australia
Research Fellow, Institute for Breathing and Sleep, Austin Health, Heidelberg, Victoria, Australia
Physiotherapist, Victorian Respiratory Support Service, Austin Health, Heidelberg, Victoria, Australia

Iftah Biran MD
Director, In-patients Neuropsychiatry Section, Division of Neurology, Sourasky Medical Center, Tel Aviv, Israel

Vanesa Bochkezanian BPhysio, MAppSc, PhD
Lecturer Neurological Physiotherapy, Department of Exercise and Health Sciences, School of Health, Medical and Applied Sciences, Central Queensland University Australia, North Rockhampton, Queensland, Australia

Dan Buckingham BA(MassComm)
Acting CEO, Attitude Pictures Ltd, Auckland, New Zealand

Jennifer Dunn DipPhty, MPhil(Rehab), PhD
Research Fellow, Department of Orthopaedic Surgery and Musculoskeletal Medicine, University of Otago, Christchurch, New Zealand

Patrick Fok MDCM, PhD, FRCPC, DABEM
Assistant Professor, Department of Emergency Medicine, Dalhousie University, Halifax, Nova Scotia, Canada

Judah Goldstein PhD
Primary Care Paramedic, Emergency Health Services Nova Scotia, Canada
Research Coordinator, Assistant Professor, Dalhousie Department of Emergency Medicine, Division of Emergency Medical Services, Halifax, Nova Scotia, Canada

Emilie Gollan BEXSc, MPhty, MPhil
Clinical Team Leader Physiotherapy Spinal Injuries, Spinal Injuries Unit, Queensland Spinal Cord Injuries Service, Metro South Health, Queensland, Australia

Marnie Graco BPhty(Hons), MPH, PhD
Lead, Allied Health Research and Translation, Institute for Breathing and Sleep, Austin Health, Heidelberg, Victoria, Australia

Katie Hammond DipCounsel, DipCommServCoord, Cert IV Fitness
Peer Support Officer, Spinal Life Australia, South Brisbane, Queensland, Australia

Rafi J. Heruti MD, MPM&R, FECSM
Head, Sexual Therapy and Rehabilitation Clinic, and Director, Rehabilitation Division, Reuth Rehabilitation Hospital, Tel Aviv, Israel
Head, Human Sexuality Program, Sackler Faculty of Medicine, Tel Aviv University, Tel Aviv, Israel

Col Mackereth DipLifeCoach, DipCommServCoord
Peer Support Officer, Spinal Life Australia, South Brisbane, Queensland, Australia

Shailendra Maharaj BPhty(Hons)
Physiotherapist Advanced (Rehabilitation), Queensland Paediatric Rehabilitation Service, Queensland Children's Hospital, South Brisbane, Queensland, Australia

Daniela Mazor PhD(Social Work)
Sex therapy, Reuth Rehabilitation Hospital, Tel Aviv, Israel
Academic Director, Sexuality for People with Disabilities, EDNM and University of Haifa, Israel

Camila Quel de Oliveira BPhty(Hons), PhD
Lecturer, Physiotherapy, Graduate School of Health, University of Technology Sydney, NSW, Australia
Clinical and Research Advisor, NeuroMoves, Spinal Cord Injuries Australia, NSW, Australia.

Jacqueline E. Reznik BAppSci, GradDip(Neurology), GradDip(Teach), MAPA, MCSP, PhD
Adjunct Senior Lecturer, James Cook University, Queensland, Australia
Associate Senior Lecturer, Curtin University, Western Australia
Honorary Research Associate, Institute of Child Health, UCL/GOSH, London, UK

Jacqueline Ross BAppSc(Phty), GradDipNeuroscience
Senior Clinician Physiotherapist, Victorian Spinal Cord Service, Tracheostomy Review and Management Service (TRAMS), Austin Health, Heidelberg, Victoria, Australia

Boaz Shamir MSc, BPT
Director Steps – Rehabilitation in Motion, Department of Neurological Rehabilitation, The Chaim Sheba Medical Center, Tel Hashomer, Israel

Joshua Simmons BPhty
Director Digital Health Clinical Consultation Services, Clinical Lead Digital Hospital Metro South, Clinical Informatics, Metro South Health, Queensland, Australia
Former Clinical Team Leader Physiotherapy Spinal Injuries, Queensland Spinal Cord Injury Service, Queensland, Australia

Jonathan Tang BPhty(Hons)
Sydney Medical School, Faculty of Medicine and Health, The University of Sydney, Royal North Shore Hospital, St Leonards, NSW, Australia

Nicola Thomas BPhty
Advanced Physiotherapist, Physiotherapy Department, Children's Health Queensland Hospital and Health Service, Queensland Children's Hospital, South Brisbane, Queensland, Australia

Oren Tirosh BEd(PhysEd), MSc(Rehab Therapy), PhD(Human Movement)
Senior Lecturer in Biomechanics, Director Health Science Honours, School of Health Sciences, Swinburne University of Technology, Melbourne, Australia

Greg Ungerer BPhty
Manager, Transitional Rehabilitation Program, Queensland Spinal Cord Injuries Service, Princess Alexandra Hospital, Metro South Health, Brisbane, Queensland, Australia

Arik D. Vamosh BSc(SpeechComm)
Travel Consultant for persons with mobility impairments
FITA judge, Paralympic Games (1994–2009)

Julie Vaughan-Graham GradDipPT, MSc, PhD
Post-Doctoral Fellow and Adjunct Lecturer, Department of Physical Therapy, Faculty of Medicine, University of Toronto, Ontario, Canada

Kate Walker BBus(HR), BSc(OT)(Hons)
Occupational Therapist, Upshot Occupational
Therapy, Newcastle, NSW, Australia

Johanna Wangdell OT, PhD
Senior Occupational Therapist, Centre for Advanced
Reconstruction of Extremities, Sahlgrenska University
Hospital, Clinical Sciences, Dept of Orthopaedics,
University of Gothenburg, Gothenburg, Sweden

Tiffany Wilson BPhty, GradCert(Clin Rehab)
Senior Physiotherapist, Queensland Spinal Cord
Injuries Service, Princess Alexandra Hospital, Brisbane,
Queensland, Australia

Anthony Wright BSc(Hons), MPhty, PhD
Professor, School of Physiotherapy and Exercise
Science, Curtin University, Perth, WA, Australia

REVIEWERS

Dinesh Palipana LLB, MD
Lecturer, Griffith University, Gold Coast University Hospital, Menzies Health Institute of Queensland, The Hopkins Centre for Rehabilitation, Queensland, Australia

Benjamin Weeks BPhty(Hons), BExSc, GCertHEd, PhD
Program Director, Master of Physiotherapy; Senior Lecturer, Physiotherapy
School of Allied Health Sciences, Gold Coast Campus, Griffith University, Queensland, Australia

ACKNOWLEDGEMENTS

The authors of Chapter 2, 'From the field to the emergency department and beyond', would like to acknowledge the support received from a number of people: Ms Katie McLean (Librarian, Nova Scotia Health Authority) provided assistance with a literature search; Ms Jennifer Greene (Advanced Care Paramedic, Paramedic Knowledge Translation Coordinator, Dalhousie Department of Emergency Medicine, Division of EMS, Prehospital Evidence-based Practice (PEP) program coordinator) helped with the literature search and article identification. We would like to thank Ms Sue Macleod (Physiotherapist, NSHA Rehabilitation Hospital) for helpful comments on this chapter. We would like to thank Ms Samantha Lamplugh (Advanced Care Paramedic, Emergency Health Services) for editorial support; Ms. Melissa MacDougall provided support in locating articles. Finally, we would like to thank the PEP Team for their continued work in locating and critically appraising EMS research. The PEP website informed our writing of this chapter.

The authors of Chapter 4, 'Early hospital management of the patient with a spinal cord injury', would like to acknowledge QSCIS physiotherapy staff: Beth Baird, Carey Bayliss, Lucy Maugham, Greg Ungerer, Brooke Wadsworth, Jennifer Campbell, Emilie Gollan, Khanh Nguyen, Tiffany Goss.

The author of Chapter 10 'Hydrotherapy' would like to acknowledge Omer Shenar, hydrotherapist, for his helpful comments on this chapter and for allowing the use of his personal photographs to enhance the manuscript.

The authors of Chapter 12, 'Overview of sexual function and changes post-SCI' would like to acknowledge Ms Shelly Varod for her help with this chapter.

The authors of Chapter 18, 'Common complications of spinal cord injury' would like to acknowledge the expert advice received on the writing of this section from Denise Goodwin and Catherine Byrne.

CHAPTER 1
Introduction to spinal cord injury

Helen Anscomb

1. OVERVIEW OF THE ANATOMY AND PHYSIOLOGY OF THE SPINAL CORD

INTRODUCTION AND OVERVIEW

The spinal cord is a component of the human central nervous system (CNS), which includes the brain and spinal cord. The brain is complex and has many diverse functions, such as consciousness, thought, imagination, creativity, attention, executive functions, language, emotional experience, learning and memory. Additionally, it modulates and regulates the functions of the organ systems, the endocrine system and motor control.

The spinal cord is, in many ways, a more straightforward part of the CNS. The structure of the spinal cord is much simpler, and it displays a uniform organisation throughout its length. The processing within the spinal cord, however, is complex and it serves extremely important functions: it receives much of the sensory information we have about the world around us, carries all of the motor information that supplies our voluntary muscles and it serves as a conduit for the longitudinal flow of information to and from the brain.

Sensory receptors outside of the CNS act as transducers that change in response to physical and chemical stimuli in our internal and external environments. These stimuli produce nerve impulses that are sent directly to the spinal cord, which performs the initial processing of inputs. These sensations are then sent to the brain, which can interpret our sensations and provide us with meaning. Some of this input directs the voluntary control of our body movements, the signals for which come directly from the neurons of the spinal cord.

DEVELOPMENT FROM THE NERVOUS SYSTEM

A brief overview of the development of the nervous system and an understanding of these processes aids

1

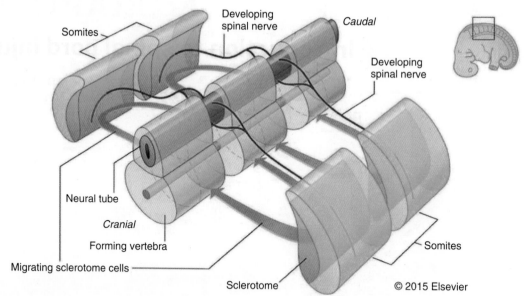

Figure 1.1 Developing spinal cord.
The developing spinal cord/neural tube (derived from endoderm) and somites (derived from mesoderm). This image illustrates the relationship between the developing spinal cord, the spinal nerves and the somites.
Source: Drake, R., Vogl, W., et al., 2014. Gray's anatomy for students, 3rd edn. Elsevier.

in understanding the adult structure and organisation of the spinal cord (Fig. 1.1).

In early embryo development, three germ layers are formed which subsequently give rise to the tissues and structures of the human body. These are: the ectoderm, endoderm and mesoderm. The ectoderm gives rise to the nervous system (and epidermis of the skin) and these tissues become integrated early in life with the other germ layers and their structures. The endoderm develops into the internal organs (viscera) of the body and the mesoderm gives rise to somites. Somites are segmental structures that develop into bone, skeletal muscle and the dermis of the skin (from which many receptors for sensations are developed).

Innervation to the structures derived from somites is through the somatic division of the nervous system, while the innervation of the structures derived from the endoderm is through the visceral part of the nervous system (Fig. 1.2).

The early development of the nervous system originates from a simple tube of ectodermal tissue, termed the neural tube. This begins through a process termed neurulation that occurs at around the third week of gestation. Neurulation commences through the thickening of a longitudinally oriented (from rostral to caudal) band of ectodermal tissue. This thickening is the neural plate, which develops due to the presence of the notochord, a rod-like structure that lies beneath the neural plate. The notochord is an important primary inductor in the early embryo, which is known to initiate and control the process of neural tube development and which, if damaged, can lead to spinal cord and CNS defects (such as spina bifida).

Following development of the initial neural plate, a midline groove appears on the plate and the plate folds inwards, creating a deepening groove with neural folds at the outer edges. This folding continues until the neural folds meet in the midline

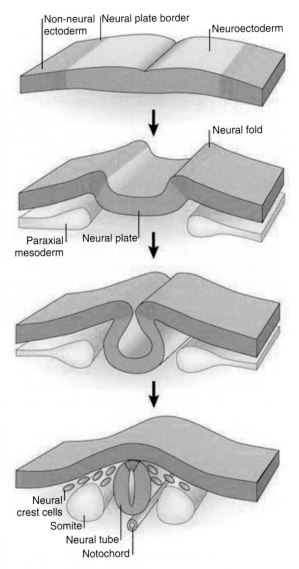

Non-neural ectoderm | Neural plate border | Neuroectoderm

Neural fold

Paraxial mesoderm | Neural plate

Neural crest cells
Somite
Neural tube
Notochord

Figure 1.2 The development of the neural tube from endoderm.

The formation of the neural plate (under the influence of the notochord), and folding of the plate to create the neural tube, sitting beside paraxial mesoderm that forms the somites.

Source: Gammill, L.S., Bronner-Fraser, M., 2003. Neural crest specification: migrating into genomics. Nature Reviews Neuroscience 4, 795–805.

and fuse to create a hollow neural tube towards the end of the third week. The rostral end of the neural tube undergoes a complex and expansive process of development to form the human brain, while the remaining neural tube develops into the spinal cord. The neural tube becomes isolated from the other developing tissues of the human embryo in early development, following closure of the neural pores at either end, to allow the developing neurons of the nervous system to form complex and diverse connections and protecting and isolating them from damage.

THE BLOOD-SPINAL CORD BARRIER (BSCB)

Capillaries in the CNS have a unique structure, being formed by a continuous layer of non-fenestrated endothelial cells linked by tight junctions that have extensive contacts with pericytes, astrocytes, microglia and neurons.[1] Unlike the blood vessels in other organs, CNS blood vessels do not allow the passive leakage of plasma proteins or the entry of immune cells from the blood into the nervous tissue, a structural feature commonly referred to as the blood–brain barrier (BBB), which also exists in the spinal cord. The maintenance of a functional blood–spinal cord barrier (BSCB) is essential to the regulation of the microenvironment in the nervous tissues of the CNS and prevents the exposure of neurons to potentially toxic blood-borne molecules such as fibrinogen and haemoglobin.[2]

The vitally important homeostatic and protective functions of the BSCB in keeping toxic metabolites, peripheral immune cells and other inflammatory substances excluded from the CNS are demonstrated following traumatic injury to the spinal cord. Upon injury, this protective barrier is completely disrupted, the cell membrane and glycocalyx of endothelial cells is damaged and the tight junctions between cells are lost. This leads to the breakdown of the BSCB, widespread vascular permeability and an inflammatory response.[3] Additionally, it is now understood that BSCB breakdown and inflammation are both widespread in neurological diseases and are hallmarks of conditions such as stroke,[4] epilepsy[5] and multiple sclerosis.[6] This demonstrates the importance of the BSCB in maintaining the CNS microenvironment for normal physiological processing.

CELLS OF THE CNS AND SPINAL CORD

Neurons

Neurons are the excitable cells of the nervous system and are located both centrally and peripherally. A wide variation in neuronal structure (morphology) is found in the CNS and spinal cord, allowing specificity to function (i.e. sensory neurons are structured differently to motor neurons); however, the basic components of all neurons include a cell body (soma), dendrites, an axon and a synaptic terminal (Fig. 1.3).

Glial cells

Glia were regarded for some time as 'extra' or additional cellular components of the nervous system, whose presence was predominantly related to providing structural support or scaffolding for neurons. This view can be understood when considering the role of some glial cells (Schwann cells and oligodendrocytes) in the formation of myelin and the association of these cells in structural support of axonal processes. The functions of glial cells in the nervous system are now recognised as being significant for normal functioning, and not just structural support. In addition, the glial cells act to provide first-line defence (immune functions) for the CNS due to the separation of the brain and spinal cord from the systemic circulation. This barrier limits the effects of the systemic immune system on injured and damaged regions of the CNS. In other tissues, following damage and injury to cells, a localised inflammatory response is initiated that will remove damaged tissue and begin repair. This process is initiated through a vascular response, in which increased blood flow and specific white blood cells (immune cells) are sent directly to the site of injury. In the CNS, this cannot happen due to the BSCB. Instead, under the influence of the systemic circulation (and blood-based signalling molecules, such as cytokines), the glial cells of the CNS are

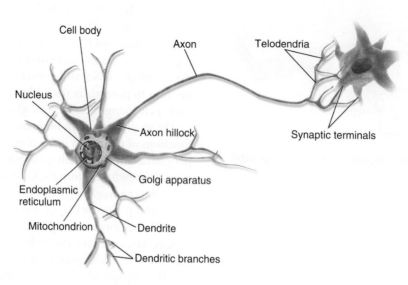

Figure 1.3 The structure of a neuron.
Source: Bruce Blaus C.C. BY 3.0

activated to perform immune-like functions such as phagocytosis.

The 3-part (tripartite) synapse

The term 'tripartite synapse' refers to the theory that synaptic physiology and cellular communication at synapses are dependent upon the activity of three components: the presynaptic neuron, the post-synaptic neuron and an astrocyte.[7] This concept of glial cells playing an active role in synaptic functions, by responding to and regulating synaptic activity,[8] was first proposed due to the observation of bi-directional communication between astrocytes and neurons at the synapse.[9,10] The study of neuron–glial interactions (especially astrocytes) is a rapidly expanding field that challenges the traditional understanding of nervous system physiology, that CNS function results exclusively from neuronal activity/excitability.

An understanding that astrocytes function to assist synaptic physiology is important, given the involvement of glial cells in the inflammatory and repair processes that follow CNS injury. It is most likely that altered and maladaptive functioning within the CNS following injury is the result of altered activity in the neuron–glia network that impacts on both neuronal and glial functioning and disrupts normal physiological processing.

Astrocytes were once considered to be non-excitable cells due to the fact that they do not show electrical excitability as neurons do. However, it has now been firmly established through numerous studies performed in cultured cells, isolated cells and through *in vivo* studies,[11] that astrocytes do exhibit excitability. Unlike neurons, astrocyte excitability occurs through elevated levels of calcium ions (Ca^{2+}) in the cytoplasm. This elevated Ca^{2+} is able to act as a cellular signal.[12] The Ca^{2+} elevations of astrocytes can occur both spontaneously and in response to neurotransmission.[13]

Importantly, the Ca^{2+} responses observed in astrocytes are not simply the result of an excess or overspill of neurotransmitter release at the synapse. Indeed, astrocytes have been shown to selectively respond to different neurotransmitters (i.e. glutamate and acetylcholine [ACh]), and they are even able to discriminate between different pathways that use the same neurotransmitter. When the astrocytic Ca^{2+} signals produced by different synaptic terminals are analysed in detail, there is evidence that astrocytes are able to integrate synaptic information in the same way neurons do.[13] In summary, there is clear evidence to support the idea that astrocytes are active cellular processors of synaptic information and contribute an important role to the functioning of the synapse (Fig. 1.4).[7]

Astrocytes (or astroglia) are star-shaped glial cells which are now considered to be active players in CNS

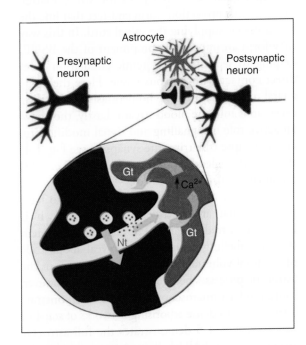

Figure 1.4 The tripartite synapse.

Scheme of the tripartite synapse. Cartoon representing the transfer of information between neuronal elements and astrocyte at the tripartite synapse. Astrocytes respond with Ca^{2+} elevations to neurotransmitters (Nt) released during synaptic activity and, in turn, control neuronal excitability and synaptic transmission through the Ca^{2+}-dependent release of gliotransmitters (Gt).

Source: Perea, G., Navarrete, M., et al., 2009. Tripartite synapses: astrocytes process and control synaptic information. Trends in Neuroscience 32:421–431.

function. They contribute to the maintenance of the BSCB, undertake multiple homeostatic mechanisms (mainly relating to neurotransmitter and ion levels) and support synaptic physiology.

There are two major types of astrocytes: fibrous astrocytes, which are found in white matter, and proteoplasmic astrocytes, which are located in the central grey matter of the spinal cord. An additional third type of astrocyte is the Müller cell, found in the retina of the eye. The astrocyte's main function is to support and nurture neurons. They do this through a variety of activities. In the grey matter they take up and recycle excess neurotransmitters from the synapse and maintain ion homeostasis around the neuron to help regulate excitability. In the white matter, their star-like projections form end-feet that line the blood vessels supplying the spinal cord. In this way they form an important component of the BSCB, helping to separate the systemic circulation from direct contact with nervous tissue. Here they play a vital role in maintaining homeostasis by shuttling excess ions into the blood stream. Lastly, they have an active role in signalling and signal modification at the synapse (the tripartite synapse – see Fig. 1.4) through the release of 'gliotransmitters' (i.e. ATP, glutamate, serine).

The largest astrocytes have been shown to have processes that are up to 1 mm in length. It is believed that traditional glial fibrillary acidic protein (GFAP) labelling is only able to reveal about 15% of the total volume of these cells, with most of the astrocytic processes being GFAP-negative. However, more modern microscopy techniques demonstrate astrocytes with dense arborising networks of star-like processes. Fig. 1.5 demonstrates the full astrocyte structure with GFAP labelling. Astrocytes in human parietal cortex are identified in the image using GFAP labelling.[14]

Oligodendrocytes

Oligodendrocytes have multiple branching processes that wrap around axons to provide an insulating and protective layer of myelin within the CNS. One oligodendrocyte can myelinate multiple axons, and axons are myelinated by numerous consecutive oligodendrocytes, each forming a segment of the myelin sheath. As such, oligodendrocytes are present in enormous numbers within the CNS, far exceeding those of astrocytes. Gaps in the myelin sheath, called nodes of Ranvier, occur at regular intervals to allow saltatory propagation of action potentials for neural transmission (Fig. 1.6).

Microglia

Microglia are the smallest of the glial cells and are the immune cells resident within the CNS, having derived from the monocyte–macrophage cell lineage in development. These cells act as specialised phagocytes removing cellular debris and damaged cells. Due to being immune cells they are activated through the release of inflammatory molecules such as cytokines (pro-inflammatory cell signals) and become recruited to areas of neuronal damage. In addition to responding to inflammatory signals, they can function as immune effector cells, secreting cytokines themselves, contributing to the inflammatory cascade and even impacting on neuronal function.

Ependymal cells

The fourth type of CNS glial cell is the ependymal cell, a type of epithelial cell that lines the ventricles of the brain and the central canal of the spinal cord. They separate the cerebrospinal fluid (CSF) from the nervous tissue and function as part of the choroid plexus (along with the pia mater), which secretes the CSF.

SPINAL CORD STRUCTURE

The spinal cord sits within the intervertebral canal of the bony spinal column. It is a long, cylindrical and segmented structure with a consistent organisation throughout its course. It is a direct continuation of the brainstem and does not descend lower than the lumbar vertebrae in the adult. It receives sensory inputs from the limbs, trunk and many internal organs, and contains the somatic motor tracts that

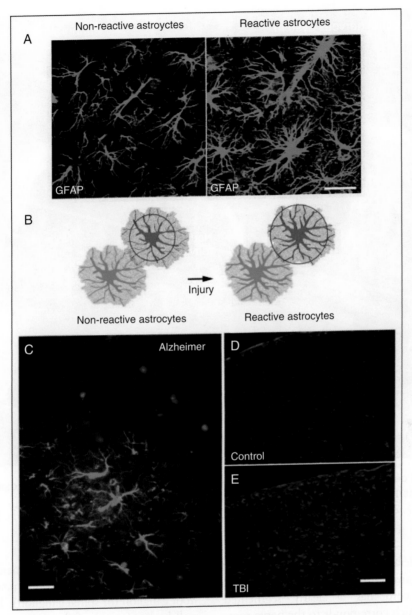

Figure 1.5 Reactive astrocytes show an upregulation of the IF protein GFAP and hypertrophy of cellular processes, but stay within their tiled domains.

Source: Hol, E.M., Pekney, M., 2015. Glial fibrillary acidic protein (GFAP) and the astrocyte intermediate filament system in diseases of the central nervous system. Current Opinion in Cell Biology, 32, 121–130.

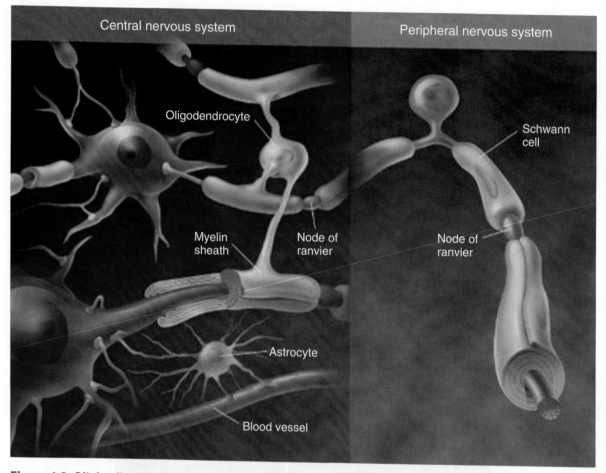

Figure 1.6 Glial cells. Myelinating glia form the electrical insulation on axons that is essential for high-speed transmission of impulses through nerve fibres (axons).
Source: Fields, R.D., 2012. Glial cells. In Ramachandran VS Encyclopedia of human behavior, 2nd edn. Elsevier.

innervate the skeletal muscles and the visceral efferent fibres to the organs, smooth muscles and glands.

The spinal cord has a clearly segmented organisation, which corresponds to the nerve roots attached to it. Posteriorly (dorsally), a continuous series of rootlets containing sensory axons enter the spinal cord. Anteriorly (ventrally), a continuous series of rootlets containing motor axons leave from the spinal cord. These sensory and motor axons merge together to form the spinal nerves, which are a part of the peripheral nervous system (PNS). Lying in

the posterior root is an enlargement, just proximal to the formation of the spinal nerve – the dorsal root ganglion (or spinal ganglion). This contains the cell bodies (soma) of the sensory nerve fibres (the pseudo/unipolar neurons) (Fig. 1.7).

Along the length of the spinal cord are two regional swellings, the cervical enlargement and the lumbosacral enlargement. These represent areas of increased neuron numbers due to the motor supply to the upper limb (cervical enlargement), and lower limb (lumbosacral enlargement). At its caudal end, the spinal cord is tapered into the conus medullaris and ends in the filum terminale, which is a thickening of the covering meningeal tissues (pia mater) that anchors the spinal cord to the sacral bones of the pelvis. At its rostral end, the spinal cord begins at the level of the foramen magnum of the skull.

The spinal nerves of the PNS emerging from the spinal cord are generally named according to the intervertebral foramina through which they exit. However, the segments of the spinal cord giving rise to these nerves are not at the same level, with most spinal nerves originating more rostrally from the spinal cord than the intervertebral foramina through which they exit. This is due to the differences in growth rate between the tissues of the spinal cord and vertebrae which take effect from approximately the third month of fetal life. The vertebral column, developed from mesoderm, grows more rapidly than the nervous tissue of the spinal cord, developed from ectoderm. In response to this, the anterior and posterior roots of the lower spinal nerves increase in length as they travel further to exit through the appropriate intervertebral foramen. The lumbosacral nerve roots (represented in blue in Fig. 1.8) are the longest and form the cauda equina of the spinal cord. At birth, the spinal cord therefore terminates at approximately the level of L3, with the adult spinal cord terminating at the L1/L2 level due to similar growth differences in these tissues occurring postnatally.

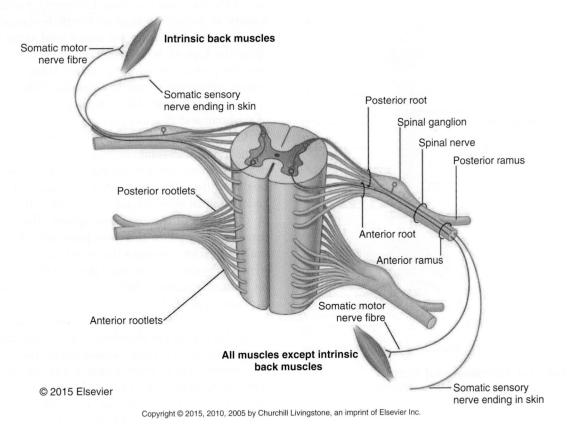

© 2015 Elsevier

Copyright © 2015, 2010, 2005 by Churchill Livingstone, an imprint of Elsevier Inc.

Figure 1.7 The spinal cord.
Source: Drake, R., Vogel, A.W., et al., 2014. Gray's anatomy for students, 3rd edn. Elsevier.

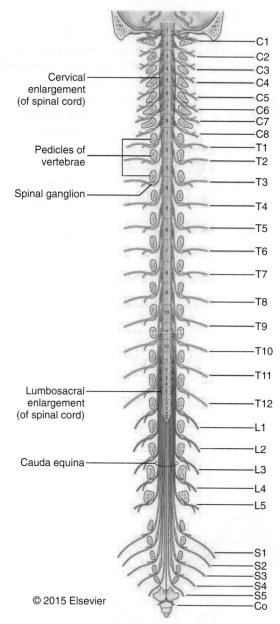

Cervical enlargement (of spinal cord)

Pedicles of vertebrae

Spinal ganglion

Lumbosacral enlargement (of spinal cord)

Cauda equina

C1
C2
C3
C4
C5
C6
C7
C8
T1
T2
T3
T4
T5
T6
T7
T8
T9
T10
T11
T12
L1
L2
L3
L4
L5
S1
S2
S3
S4
S5
Co

© 2015 Elsevier

Figure 1.8 The spinal cord in situ.
Source: Drake, Vogel, A.W., et al., 2014. Gray's anatomy for students, 3rd edn. Elsevier.

Grey and white matter

The spinal cord is marked on its external surface by longitudinal fissures and sulci that are related to the positioning of white matter fibre tracts and the location of entry and exit points for nerve rootlets to the internal grey matter. The external white matter is where the ascending and descending fibre tracts (columns or funiculi) are located. There are three columns of white matter: anterior, posterior and lateral. The internal grey matter is where neurons are located according to their functions, forming motor (ventral), sensory (dorsal) and autonomic (lateral) horns.

The spinal cord has a left and right side, which mirror each other (Fig. 1.9). The left side of the spinal cord receives and sends information from/to the left side of the body and vice versa. Ultimately, whether sensory or motor information travels ipsilaterally or contralaterally within the spinal cord depends upon the type of information being carried and thus the pathway in which it travels. However, all sensory information from the right side of the body is processed at a cortical level in the left hemisphere of the brain and all sensory input from the left side of the body is sent to the right hemisphere of the brain. Similarly, all voluntary motor information sent to produce movement in the right side of the body originates from the cortex of the left hemisphere, and movement in the left side of the body is directed by the cortex of the right hemisphere. The exact details regarding how this takes place and whether the information crosses in the spinal cord or brain stem will be discussed in more detail in the section on sensory systems, which examines the specific pathways (pp. 12–14).

Anteriorly, there is a prominent anterior median fissure that can be seen the whole length of the spinal cord. In this fissure, in the subarachnoid space, sits the anterior spinal artery, which is a major blood supply to the spinal cord. Deep within the fissure and anterior artery sits the anterior white commissure, which is a location for the decussation (crossing from left to right) of a number of sensory and motor fibre paths. Between the anterior median fissure and

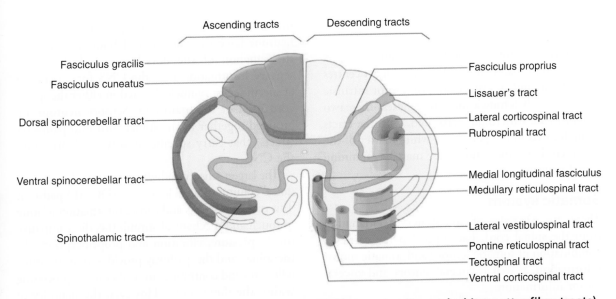

Figure 1.9 Cross-section of spinal cord (demonstrating the grey matter and white matter fibre tracts).
Ascending and descending tracts of the spinal cord. All ascending and descending tracts are present bilaterally. In this image, ascending tracts are emphasised on the left side and descending tracts are emphasised on the right side. In addition, the location of Lissauer's tract and the fasciculus proprius (which contain both ascending and descending fibres) are shown.
Source: Crossman, A., Neary, D., 2015. Neuroanatomy: An illustrated colour text. 5th edn. Churchill Livingstone, Fig. 8.15.

the exit point of the ventral (motor) rootlets sits the anterior column. This column contains a number of ascending and descending fibre tracts, the most prominent of which is the *anterior corticospinal pathway*.

Posteriorly, a posterior median sulcus can be identified on the external surface of the spinal cord. Sitting on both the left and the right sides of the spinal cord, between the posterior median sulcus and the entry point of the dorsal (sensory) rootlets, lies the posterior column. This column contains the large sensory fibre tracts of the *dorsal column–medial lemniscus (DCML) pathway*. In the upper part of the spinal cord (the cervical and upper thoracic regions), this column contains two tracts (or fasciculi): the *fasciculus gracilis* (medially) and the *fasciculus cuneatus* (laterally). These carry somatic sensory information from the lower trunk and limbs and the upper trunk and limbs, respectively.

Therefore, in the lower spinal cord only the fasciculus gracilis is present. The sensory information carried by these fibre tracts to the brainstem includes fine (discriminative) touch, vibration and proprioception from muscles and joints.

Laterally, sitting between the ventral (motor) and dorsal (sensory) rootlets of the spinal cord, lies the lateral column. This is the largest white matter column of the spinal cord and contains both ascending and descending fibre tracts, including the *spinocerebellar* (sensory), *spinothalamic* (sensory) and the *lateral corticospinal* (motor) *pathways*.

The clinical presentation of spinal cord injuries (SCI) is dependent upon the severity and location of injury, since the long white matter tracts of the spinal cord are arranged somatotopically as they interconnect the brain with the autonomic and peripheral nervous systems.

SPINAL CORD: SYSTEMS

The spinal cord functions both as a conduit for tracts that send information to and from the higher centres in the brain and as a processing centre for intrinsic functions, such as muscle tone and reflexes. These two functions are structurally separated, with the tracts being located in the peripheral white matter of the spinal cord and the central grey matter containing spinal neurons.

Somatic system

There are 31 pairs of spinal nerves emanating from the spinal cord. Each spinal nerve carries a combination of somatic sensory and somatic motor information, as well as visceral sensory and visceral motor information.

Each segment of the spinal cord and associated spinal nerve supplies a specific area of the skin, forming a *dermatome*. There is overlap between dermatome areas, yet they can be identified on a dermatome map, which is useful clinically for identifying where there has been damage to the spinal cord. Similarly, the anterior spinal roots and the associated segment of the spinal cord provide motor control to a predetermined group of muscle fibres, which forms a *myotome*. Each skeletal (somatic) muscle of body is innervated by several spinal nerves and this is represented on a myotome map. Thus, a myotome map provides information about the types of movements that will be affected by damage to the spinal cord and/or spinal nerves (Fig. 1.10).

Sensory systems

There are three sensory (ascending) pathways in the spinal cord: the dorsal column, the spinothalamic and the spinocerebellar pathways. All of these pathways carry inputs from the somatic (body) tissues, relating to the sensory modalities of touch, pain, temperature and proprioception (Fig. 1.11).

Sensory neurons are structured to have their dendrites associated with specialised receptors that respond to specific stimuli. This information is then carried into the CNS and the spinal cord through the sensory component of the spinal nerve. Sensory neurons have their soma (cell bodies) located in the ganglion of the dorsal root and they send sensory information into the CNS for processing at specific sensory nuclei located in either the spinal cord itself or the brainstem. Sensory neurons are grouped together in the spinal cord into pathways (tracts) that carry specific sensory modalities into the CNS.

The largest sensory pathway of the spinal cord is the dorsal column–medial lemniscus (DCML) pathway. This pathway detects and carries information relating to touch and mechanical stimuli (i.e. discriminative touch, pressure, vibration and proprioception). In the spinal cord this pathway provides input to spinal reflex arcs and contributes to further input processing within the dorsal horn. However, the majority of inputs form the posterior column of spinal cord white matter, composed of two tracts (or fasciculi): the *fasciculus gracilis* (medially) and the *fasciculus cuneatus* (laterally). Information travelling in this sensory pathway is carried ipsilaterally within the spinal cord, only crossing to the opposite side of the CNS after synapsing in the medulla oblongata at the nucleus gracilis or nucleus cuneatus. This information is then processed by the sensory centres of the brain.

In the lateral white matter column of the spinal cord are two more sensory (ascending) spinal pathways: the spinothalamic pathway (also referred to as the anterolateral pathway) and the spinocerebellar pathway. The *spinothalamic pathway* detects and carries information relating to non-discriminative touch, pain and temperature. This information is sent to the thalamus and therefore this pathway is vital in mediating conscious awareness of pain and temperature. Within the spinal cord, fibres carrying spinothalamic information travel only a short distance before synapsing in the superficial laminae or in the nucleus proprius of the dorsal horn. Following this, fibres are carried in the white matter of the spinal cord on the opposite side (contralateral) to the origin of the input (i.e. pain and temperature from the left side of the body is carried in the right

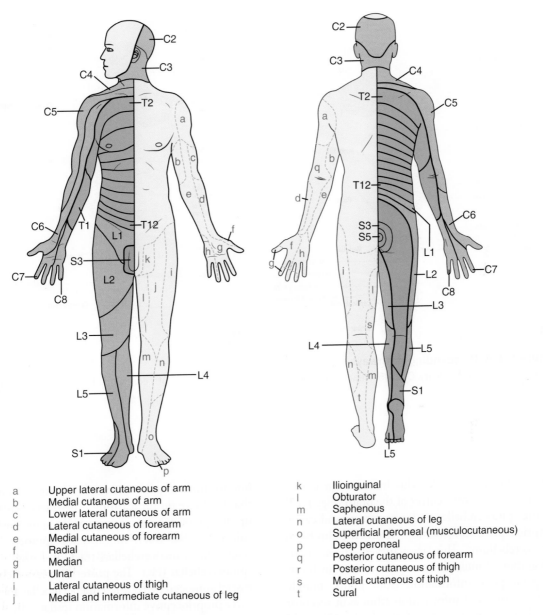

a	Upper lateral cutaneous of arm	k	Ilioinguinal
b	Medial cutaneous of arm	l	Obturator
c	Lower lateral cutaneous of arm	m	Saphenous
d	Lateral cutaneous of forearm	n	Lateral cutaneous of leg
e	Medial cutaneous of forearm	o	Superficial peroneal (musculocutaneous)
f	Radial	p	Deep peroneal
g	Median	q	Posterior cutaneous of forearm
h	Ulnar	r	Posterior cutaneous of thigh
i	Lateral cutaneous of thigh	s	Medial cutaneous of thigh
j	Medial and intermediate cutaneous of leg	t	Sural

Figure 1.10 Dermatome and myotome maps.

Source: Crossman, A., Neary D., 2015. Neuroanatomy: An illustrated colour text, 5th edn. Churchill Livingstone. Fig 3.14, p. 43.

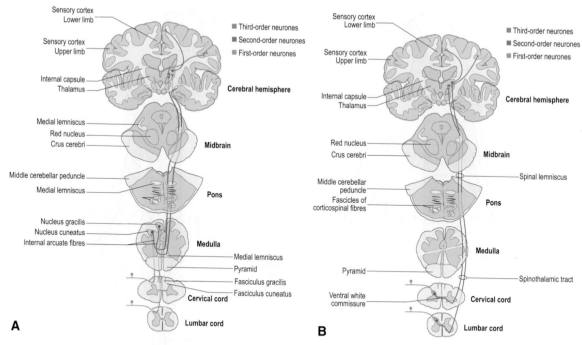

Figure 1.11 A, B ascending pathways.
Source: Crossman, A., Neary, D. 2015. Neuroanatomy: An illustrated colour text, 5th edn. Churchill Livingstone. Figs 8.16, 8.17.

side of the spinal cord). This information is then taken to the sensory centres of the brain (Fig. 1.12).

The spinocerebellar pathway detects and carries proprioceptive information from the limbs to the cerebellum. This is achieved through the integration of multiple sensory modalities, including proprioceptive information from joints, muscles and tendons and information from skin receptors which sense movement of the body. Once this information enters the spinal cord through the dorsal root there are a number of tracts that direct these sensations to the cerebellum, all of which contribute to the spinocerebellar pathway. In this way, the spinocerebellar pathway not only provides input to the cerebellum regarding body positioning, it also contributes important information for the

fine-tuning and adjustment of ongoing movements that facilitate motor learning. The tracts that make up the spinocerebellar pathway include the posterior spinocerebellar tract, the anterior spinocerebellar tract, the cuneocerebellar tract and the rostral spinocerebellar tract. The posterior spinocerebellar, rostral spinocerebellar and cuneocerebellar tracts all carry proprioceptive information ipsilaterally within the spinal cord, and the anterior spinocerebellar tract carries proprioceptive information contralaterally within the spinal cord. This pathway does not take this proprioceptive information to the sensory centres of the brain.

The typical clinical presentations that reflect the implications associated with damage of the pathways are discussed in Chapter 11.

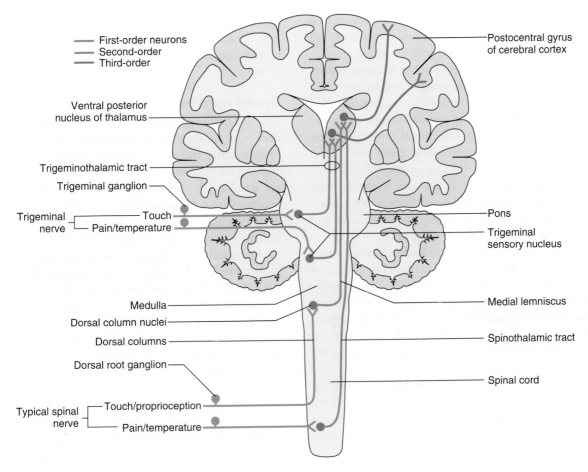

Figure 1.12 Sensory pathways

Source: Crossman, A., Neary D. 2015. *Neuroanatomy: An illustrated colour text*, 5th edn. Churchill Livingstone. Fig 1.28, p. 20.

Motor systems

Human movement is generated by the combined activity of multiple neuronal circuits that collect, integrate and feed back neural information to produce precisely timed and sequenced skeletal muscle contractions. Research over many years has demonstrated that the motor control system consists of multiple, interconnected levels of organisation, often referred to as hierarchical levels. Together, these levels of motor control are able to produce a vast array of movements, ranging from repetitive routine movements, such as walking, to more specialised movements as, for example, playing a musical instrument.

In all movements there are three main component systems that must interconnect to produce the desired output, whether it be a simple reflex or a sophisticated movement pattern. However, the input of each of these systems can be varied, which gives rise to the diversity and range of movements possible.

The first motor system involves neurons confined to the spinal cord, which are essential for producing rhythmic and patterned motor activity.[15] This system includes the diverse range of spinal interneurons that interconnect within the spinal cord to produce and support activities for movement execution.

The second motor system involves interconnections between the local spinal circuits and higher CNS centres in the brainstem and cerebral cortex. This includes many ascending and descending pathways (Fig. 1.13), allowing bi-directional communication and interaction between the local spinal circuits and the higher CNS control and command centres.[16] These supraspinal centres (located in the cerebral cortex, basal ganglia and cerebellum, among other locations) are involved in selection, initiation and activation of motor action programs.

Lastly, there are the sensory feedback systems that constantly monitor the consequences of motor action and initiate adjustments.[17] Sensory feedback circuits provide important input to the spinal cord relating to external inputs and from specific body regions (i.e. proprioception is somatotopically processed) and thus contribute to the coordinating and sequencing of motor outputs.

These three separate and yet highly interconnected systems of motor control are responsible for both the diversity and the specificity seen in motor behaviour.[18] The ability of these systems to operate individually and collectively, depending upon the task, create a huge challenge in the understanding of the connectivity and functions of the motor system.

Spinal cord neurons

Research on the physiological characteristics of spinal cord neurons, their functional output and their role in generating and regulating movement, has been evolving for more than a century. Unfortunately, there are significantly different profiles of activity from neurons within the spinal cord across different species of mammals, which has added to this challenge. The human motor systems of the CNS (both within the brain and within the spinal cord), are among the most complex of all species both structurally and functionally. The human brain has significant regions of cortex involved in the decision-making, planning and patterning for movement, and humans are capable of very precise, controlled and coordinated movements as a result of this system.

The motor cortex, along with other brain areas such as the midbrain, hindbrain, cerebellum and basal ganglia, are involved in decision-making and planning for movement initiation. However, the quality of movement produced relies heavily on the

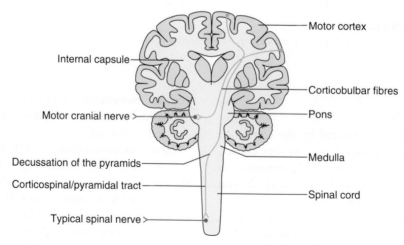

Figure 1.13 Motor pathways
Source: Crossman, A., Neary D., 2015. Neuroanatomy: An illustrated colour text, 5th edn. Churchill Livingstone. Fig 1.29, p. 21.

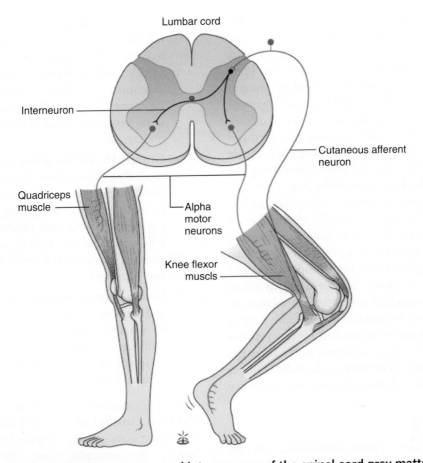

Figure 1.14 **An example of motor neurons and interneurons of the spinal cord grey matter.**
Source: Crossman, A., Neary, D., 2015. Neuroanatomy: An illustrated colour text, 5th edn. Churchill Livingstone. Fig. 8.14.

translation of descending inputs and the feedback from the periphery by spinal motoneurons (such as the γ motor neurons) and interneurons that form multiple spinal neural networks.

Motor neurons

Motor neurons whose cell bodies are located in the cortex of the brain are referred to as upper motor neurons (UMNs), and those motor neurons whose cell bodies are located in the spinal cord are termed lower motor neurons (LMNs). LMNs for the somatic (skeletal) motor system are located in the ventral (anterior) horn of the spinal cord grey matter, as

are a number of regulatory and modulatory motor interneurons (Fig. 1.14).

α-motor neurons are large multipolar neurons that directly innervate skeletal muscle fibres. The α-motor neuron and the muscle fibres it innervates are together referred to as the **motor unit**. When the α-motor neuron is activated, those fibres it supplies will contract. There are many different sized motor units throughout the human body, allowing different muscles and body regions to display varying degrees of movement strength, control and dexterity. The powerful postural muscles of the body motor units are large, allowing strong muscle contractions to be produced easily, generating enough force for whole-body movement and preventing muscle fatigue. In other regions of the body, motor units are small allowing for more precise control of body movements and increasing dexterity of movement. α-motor neurons of the ventral horn are organised into three distinct groupings (motor nuclei): medial, central and lateral. These groups are arranged topographically, with those innervating distal muscle groups located laterally and those innervating the proximal muscles located medially (Fig. 1.15).

γ-motor neurons are smaller multipolar neurons that innervate the muscle spindles of the skeletal muscles. Muscle spindles provide important, ongoing proprioceptive input to the CNS from the skeletal muscle and are structured from modified skeletal muscle fibres. The muscle spindle needs to adjust as the skeletal muscle is contracted or relaxed, in order to continue to provide proprioceptive input and this adjustment is controlled by the γ-motor neurons. γ-motor neurons receive input from the brainstem and play an important role in determining muscle tone, as well as generating proprioceptive inputs.

Interneurons

Interneurons are local circuit neurons that function to interconnect descending inputs to motor neurons and modulate inputs within the spinal circuits. Interneurons are multifunctional and their role at any given time is context-dependent. Interneurons can perform different roles in multiple spinal reflex pathways, can function within multiple networks and have an important role to play in the generation and modulation of rhythmic movements.[19]

- **Group 1a interneurons** function to produce reciprocal inhibition of agonist and antagonist muscles in neural pathways. They are inhibitory interneurons (glycinergic) that inhibit the activity of antagonist motor neurons and thus allow movements to be produced due to the inhibition of the antagonist muscle.
- **Renshaw cells** are inhibitory interneurons (mostly glycinergic, some GABAergic) that mediate recurrent inhibition. Recurrent inhibition means that these interneurons act to inhibit the α-motor neuron of the agonist muscle. While Renshaw cells have been demonstrated to have important modulatory functions, the exact role of recurrent inhibition in movement patterns in humans is not fully understood.
- **Group 1b interneurons** are involved in mediating information about muscle tension from Golgi tendon organs. They function to mediate information relating to active and passive muscle tension, producing a reflexive self-regulation of muscle action that is essential to the spinal control of movement and locomotion.
- **Group 2 interneurons** exert both inhibitory and excitatory actions on motor neurons by working through multiple pathways. A significant contribution of these interneurons in spinal circuits is the coordination of the contractions of stretched muscles.

A large number of other interneurons have also been classified and studied for their roles in movement circuits (see Chapter 18 for a detailed review); for example, those that interconnect circuits across the two sides of the spinal cord (**commissural interneurons**) and those that interconnect spinal cord sections longitudinally (**propriospinal interneurons**). The varied and context-dependent functions of interneurons in spinal motor circuits are important for both normal physiological functioning and potentially for motor recovery after spinal cord injury. Interneurons exhibit a high level of plasticity, allowing local circuits to adapt following injury and those that interconnect circuits longitudinally (propriospinal interneurons) have been identified as key players in the formation of detours or relays in the injured spinal cord.[20] Their role in promoting functional recovery and their increased resistance to injury and degeneration[21] means that these local circuit neurons and their functions following SCI warrant further research.

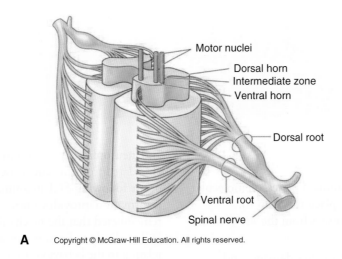

Motor nuclei
Dorsal horn
Intermediate zone
Ventral horn
Dorsal root
Ventral root
Spinal nerve

A

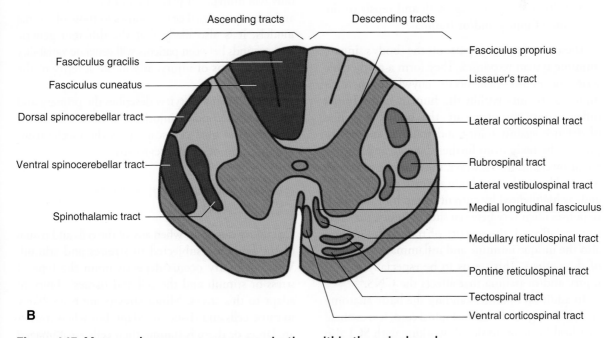

Ascending tracts   Descending tracts

Fasciculus gracilis
Fasciculus cuneatus
Dorsal spinocerebellar tract
Ventral spinocerebellar tract
Spinothalamic tract

Fasciculus proprius
Lissauer's tract
Lateral corticospinal tract
Rubrospinal tract
Lateral vestibulospinal tract
Medial longitudinal fasciculus
Medullary reticulospinal tract
Pontine reticulospinal tract
Tectospinal tract
Ventral corticospinal tract

B

Figure 1.15 **Motor and sensory neuron organisation within the spinal cord.**
Source: A. Martin, J.H., 2012. Neuroanatomy text and atlas, 4th edn. McGraw-Hill, New York.

2. PATHOPHYSIOLOGY OF SPINAL CORD INJURY

INTRODUCTION

Following SCIs and trauma a series of molecular and cellular events take place that aim to:

- remove damaged tissues from the site of injury and/or trauma
- reduce or prevent further damage, and
- initiate structural regrowth and repair to the site of injury and/or trauma.

These events are a part of the body's innate immune system responses. They form a predictable series of events that occur anywhere there is injury or trauma within the human body. Initial inflammatory responses are the body's first line of defence against injury and trauma, and act to protect the body from further damage and initiate repair mechanisms. However, the immune responses initiated by the human body are extremely complex and, as highlighted by current research in this field, responses often vary between sites of injury, the body systems affected, the severity of trauma/injury and also the unique immune and inflammatory profiles of the patient. This seems to be especially true of injury and/or trauma that affects the CNS.[22, 23]

In addition to understanding the basic anatomy and physiology of the normal spinal cord, it is essential that healthcare professionals working with SCI also appreciate the mechanisms of pathophysiology underlying SCI. A good understanding of the cellular and molecular mechanisms following SCI will assist healthcare professionals to provide management strategies that will not compromise regeneration or neuroplasticity.

Most of our understanding of the extrinsic and intrinsic factors that block axonal regeneration and neuroplasticity is founded on the knowledge elucidated from the course of molecular events that occur following SCI in animal models. While this information provides great insights, it should be remembered that the mechanisms at play in human SCI are likely to be more complex, particularly those relating to the behaviour of the immune system. Not only will humans display variations in inflammatory and subsequent glial cell responses to those of animal models, it is also likely that the different genetic backgrounds between patients will generate variability in mechanisms of injury, as will the severity of the injury itself.

The following overview describes the primary and subsequent secondary injuries that contribute to the formation of glial cell scars, plus the mechanisms of inhibition of axonal regrowth.

OVERVIEW OF INJURY AND CELL DEATH

Cell injury can occur when any of the cells and tissues of the body are subjected to stresses and stimuli. Whether injury occurs depends upon the type of stress or stimuli and the cell and tissues' ability to adapt to this stress. Minor stresses are more likely to cause cells and tissues to adapt, but when stresses are larger or there is trauma then cells are damaged beyond adaptation and repair.

When cell injury does occur, there are processes that activate a mechanism designed to eliminate the damage caused and aid in the repair and healing of those tissues affected (**acute inflammatory response**). This response and its consequences will vary according to the tissues and sites injured, the severity of the injury and the ability of the individual (and the tissue) to repair adequately. However, an understanding of these events, their basic mechanisms and potential outcomes is essential for understanding the basic mechanisms of tissue injury, repair and the inflammatory processes that occur to facilitate these activities.

Inflammation, mediated through the body's immune system, helps to clear injury and infection, removes noxious stimuli that can cause cell damage (including necrotic debris) and initiates the repair mechanisms of tissues. However, the inflammatory reaction and the repair processes that follow can themselves cause harm by impacting on normal tissue structure and function (**chronic inflammatory response**) (Fig. 1.16).

SPINAL CORD INJURIES

Primary injury

The vast majority of injuries to the spinal cord are caused by contusive forces, in which the force of impact rapidly displaces the cord without there being

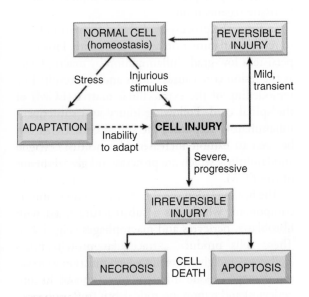

Figure 1.16 Cellular inflammatory process.
Source: Kumar, V., Abbas, A., et al., 2012. Robbins and Cotran: pathologic basis of disease, 8th edn. Saunders Elsevier.

external trauma. This means that physical trauma to the cord is usually brief (taking place most commonly during a motor vehicle collision or fall and due to impact forces); however, significant tissue damage and remodelling occurs immediately and continues for a number of weeks post-injury. Tissue remodelling following injury has even been shown to persist throughout the remainder of a person's life.

During the primary injury phase, the force of physical impact will cause an area of tissue damage due to neuronal and glial necrosis. Necrosis is a disordered (non-programmed) and pathological cell death in which cells will swell and may rupture, stimulating an inflammatory response by the body. The area of necrotic damage will generally expand from a central focal point and generate an area of damaged and disrupted tissue, referred to as a lesion. In the early stages of injury there will also be death of neurons and glial cells through apoptosis. In contrast to necrosis, apoptosis is a regulated and controlled form of cell death; it elicits a much less potent inflammatory signal than necrosis and does not create injury to surrounding cells.

Twenty-four hours post-injury, glial cell apoptosis is seen to continue, but neuronal apoptosis is significantly reduced.[24] Apoptosis is seen to continue in some glial cells for a number of days post-injury and there will also be shearing and degeneration of ascending and descending axons along the lesion site. Axons severed in these areas and separated from their soma will undergo Wallerian degeneration, along with their associated myelin sheaths. Axonal dieback in the area of injury is due to aggressive macrophage (phagocytic immune cells) activity. Macrophages access the spinal cord from the systemic circulation as a result of blood vessel rupture due to contusive force and breakdown of the blood–spinal cord barrier (BSCB). Oedema (swelling due to increased fluid) and bleeding into the region of injury can also cause further injury due to compression. Additionally, oedema causes disruption of the homeostatic balance of localised ions and neurotransmitters, causing further damage to neurons through excitotoxicity.

The body's immediate response to these events and haemorrhage within the spinal cord is vasospasm (contraction/restriction of blood vessels). This leads to ischaemia, which particularly affects neurons, but which can also lead to oxidative stress (hypoxia) for glia, causing glial apoptosis.[25] The lesion following primary injury therefore contains red blood cells, cellular debris (such as necrotic and apoptotic cells, myelin and subcellular components). The BSCB will remain damaged following SCI, and the haemorrhage, oedema and cellular debris will all contribute to the initiation of secondary injury.

Inflammation and secondary injury

Primary injury in SCI leads to a prolonged secondary injury cascade through innate inflammatory responses (chronic inflammation). This can last for weeks and will itself lead to the formation of a glial scar due to the tissue repair mechanisms initiated through the inflammatory response. Secondary injury leads to an expansion in the tissue damage of the initial lesion as a result of inflammatory-induced apoptosis and further damage to neuronal axons beyond that which will have occurred as a direct result of the initial injury.[26] The degree of inflammation and subsequent secondary injury will relate to the level of immune cell 'reactivity' that occurs following injury, as the body launches an immune response to halt cell and tissue necrosis and aims to initiate tissue repair and structural stability in the spinal cord. The inflammatory response will be initiated by cell signals (alarmins), which are usually cell-bound proteins released during necrosis and apoptosis.[27] These alarmins will act to awaken the immune system within the CNS and stimulate inflammation, which acts as a cascade of events recruiting the activities of both resident immune cells of the CNS (microglia) and infiltrating immune cells from the systemic circulation (leukocytes). Ultimately these immune cells and other cells of CNS that become 'reactive' or activated will aid in controlling the inflammatory response through the development of the glial scar. This scar is an example of the tissue regeneration that is stimulated in the body by inflammation.

The structure, formation and cells of the glial scar are discussed below.

Glial scar

Major cellular contributors to the formation of the glial scar include:

- microglia
- astrocytes
- oligodendrocytes and their progenitors
- fibroblasts/pericytes.

Additionally, and depending upon the degree of damage to the BSCB, peripherally-derived leukocytes and ependymal cells can contribute to formation of the scar.

Primary injury to the spinal cord causes an influx of inflammatory cells and the resident glial cells, including astrocytes and oligodendrocyte progenitor cells, become activated to undergo structural and physiological modification. These changes enable the cells to proliferate in number and migrate to the site of the lesion with the purpose of initiating an inflammatory response (secondary injury) leading to tissue regeneration.

In time, the process of glial scar formation helps to resolve inflammation at the lesion site. However, persistent low-grade inflammation by macrophages at the lesion core causes gliosis and this results in a remodelling of the extracellular matrix (ECM) of the spinal cord. Following injury and subsequent inflammatory responses the spinal cord ECM can be seen to exhibit increased fibronectin, collagen and laminin – which are proteins and glycoproteins of the ECM.

The healing lesion site thus forms a central fibrotic component, which has a substructure filled with fibroblasts, pericytes and macrophages (Fig. 1.17). These cells produce extracellular protein fibres (collagens) and glycoproteins which function to repair the damaged tissue infrastructure (fibroblasts and pericytes) and remove necrotic debris (macrophages). The glial cells located here include reactive astrocytes, oligodendrocyte precursors with a small number of microglia (Fig. 1.18).

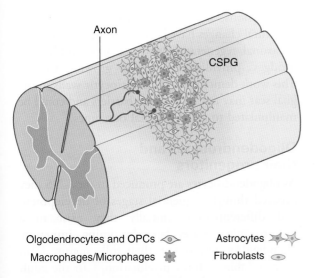

Figure 1.17 The mature glial scar.
A mature glial scar, demonstrating the cellular contributors and their organisation. The lesion core is occupied by microglia/macrophages and fibroblasts (the fibrotic core), astrocytes form a wall around this core and are joined by oligodendrocytes and OPCs (oligodendrocyte pregenitor cells). The region contains high levels of CSPGs (chondroitin sulfate proteoglycans) and axonal growth in the region is inhibited.

Microglia

During normal CNS functioning the microglia function to remove debris and act as a first-line defence against injury and pathogens. They are the CNS's resident macrophages, but are largely inactive. This is referred to as an M2-like phenotype. Following injury, they become rapidly activated, proliferate, alter their morphology, migrate to the site of the lesion and become M1-like in their behaviour. In their M1-like form they act as active macrophages, migrating to the site of injury in large numbers to clear cellular debris from the injury site, presumably with the aim of limiting the lesion. However, in this way the microglia contribute to further loss of neurons by phagocytosing any damaged cells before they can repair and/or regenerate and by releasing cytokines and pro-inflammatory signals that activate more astrocytes within the region. This triggers a cascade response in the tissue and is a trigger for secondary injury. As time passes and the glial scar forms, microglia eventually return to their original M2-like form as a result of feedback from astrocytes.[27]

Astrocytes

Astrocytes are known to display a wide heterogeneity and can exhibit plasticity. Different regions of the

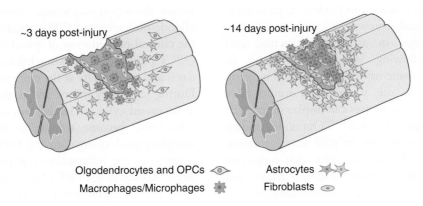

Figure 1.18 The development of the glial scar.
The developing glial scar, demonstrating the cellular activity at around 3 days post-injury (left image) and around 14 days post-injury (right image).

CNS display different populations of resident astrocytes,[28] and it has even been demonstrated that neurons can influence their local astrocytic populations, adjusting subtypes and their functions to better serve the neurons of a particular region.[29] Astrocytes are, however, bound to specific regions and although they proliferate and migrate to lesion sites, they are largely incapable of long-distance migration. For this reason, the exact site of injury to the spinal cord will lead to differential astrocytic responses and this can also influence axonal regeneration.

In a post-injury inflammatory environment, astrocytes change and become 'reactive'. This consists predominantly of a structural change and hypertrophy of the astrocytes (increase in cell size) rather than large amounts of proliferation (increased cell numbers). These alterations in the astrocytes lead to the formation of a rigid, densely bundled structure comprised of reactive or 'scar' astrocytes that surround and sit adjacent to the inflammatory core of the lesion. This behaviour of astrocytes is often described as reactive astrocyte 'wall building'. The astrocytes undergo intracellular adaptations, including the increased production of cytoskeletal decorating proteins such as glial fibrillary acidic protein (GFAP), which assists in forming a rigid margin or 'wall' of astrocytes around the lesion core. Reactive astrocytes in these wall regions also secrete a number of ECM proteins that create an inhibitory growth environment around the lesion, preventing axonal growth and regrowth.

While changes in astrocytic structure and functioning following SCI typically result in near-irreversible tissue remodelling and wall building around the lesion site, some recent studies have demonstrated that astrocytes can display differential and dynamic responses to SCI.[28–31] Our understanding of the role of astrocytes in glial scar formation is evolving to take into account that astrocytes respond plastically to different environments and will therefore respond differently depending on their age, cellular lineage (where they are derived from) and the extent of the inflammatory environment they are in. In some environments, especially very

small lesions, astrocyte reactivity and subsequent structural changes have been demonstrated to assist in axonal regeneration and act as scaffolding or 'bridges', providing support for growing axons.[30] This work demonstrates that astrocytic walls in the glial scar may not be absolute barriers and could be manipulated to aid functional outcomes.[31]

Oligodendrocytes and their progenitors

As oligodendrocytes are produced in the CNS they proceed though sequential stages of development and differentiation. Initially they exist in a pre-progenitor state, later becoming immature oligodendrocytes, and in their fully mature form they are able to form myelination.[32] In the adult spinal cord, oligodendrocyte progenitor cells (OPCs) are constantly undergoing proliferation in order to maintain progenitor cell numbers, allow the development of mature cells and support and maintain myelination.[33]

Immediately following impact and primary injury to the spinal cord there is apoptosis of both mature oligodendrocytes and OPCs, causing a depletion of myelination in and around the lesion site. The loss of oligodendrocytes can continue for a number of weeks post-injury, with a loss of cells both rostrally and caudally to the injury site along degenerating axon tracts. This creates a loss of myelination within the region of a lesion. These changes in the oligodendrocytes and OPCs possibly account for the clinical presentation of spinal shock. However, OPCs proliferate following injury (peaking at 5 days) and accumulate at the epicentre of the lesion. During secondary injury, and under the influence of increased cytokine levels from other active glial cells, OPCs become 'reactive' as well. This causes morphological changes to the OPCs and further potentiates the inflammatory response as reactive oligodendrocytes and OPCs can in turn activate other glial cells and also secrete proteases that increase the permeability of the BSCB. An important behaviour of activated oligodendrocytes and their progenitor cells at lesion sites is the structural relationship that they form with axonal endings and growth cones. The functional effects of this anatomical relationship between the activated oligodendrocytes and axons is highly debated; however, there seem to be a number of possible explanations for this association. It has been suggested that the OPCs entrap and stabilise retracting axonal endings, perhaps protecting them from further regeneration and injury in the inflammatory environment.[34]

Oligodendrocyte function (myelination) is compromised following SCI, indicating that the glial scar is an environment that not only inhibits regenerative growth, but also remyelination of axons.[33]

Fibroblasts, pericytes and fibrotic component of the glial scar

Fibroblasts are the primary connective tissue cells of the body. They secrete protein fibres (collagen is the most abundant fibre type) and maintain the components of the extracellular matrix (ECM) to provide structure to tissues. They are only produced in the CNS following injury, or due to invasion when there is damage to the BSCB barrier. Recently, pericytes have also been shown to contribute to the formation of the fibrotic scar following CNS injury.[35] Pericytes normally surround and support the blood vessels of the CNS, functioning to maintain the BSCB barrier, aiding in the control of blood flow and supporting other homeostatic mechanisms of the CNS. However, when there is injury and/or disruption of the BSCB barrier, pericytes have been shown to leave their location at the BSCB barrier and migrate to the lesion core, becoming a source of proliferating fibroblasts. Additionally, some studies of contusive SCI have linked the increase in fibroblasts at the lesion core to the invasion and infiltration of peripheral leukocytes.[36]

Overall, fibroblasts aid in the contraction of the lesion and are essential in subsequent wound healing following injury. The fibrotic scarring process provides structural stability to the CNS tissues following widespread cell death and damage; however, it also contributes to the inhibition of axon regeneration due to the secretion and deposition by fibroblasts of factors that have been shown to limit regeneration of axons and inhibit neuronal plasticity that could aid functional recovery.

Lastly, chondroitin sulfate proteoglycans (CSPGs) play an inhibitory role within the mature glial scar, limiting axonal regrowth within the region of the healed lesion. CSPGs are a protein of the ECM that is produced and fills the lesion site following wound healing. CSPGs are upregulated following traumatic CNS injury and are secreted by both fibroblasts and reactive glial cells. This allows the astrocytic 'wall' surrounding the lesion core to block axonal regrowth both anatomically and physiologically. The high CSPG content of the ECM within and surrounding the glial scar hinders plasticity and actively prevents axonal regeneration.[37,38] Consequently, the physiological processes of the CNS in the removal of cellular debris, inflammation, wound healing and structural repair act to prevent the neural repair required for functional recovery following spinal cord injury.

Spasticity

Spasticity is classically defined as a velocity-dependent increase in the tonic stretch reflex (muscle tone). It presents clinically with exaggerated tendon jerks, clonus and spasms, resulting from the hyperexcitability of the stretch reflex.[39] Spasticity is a syndrome that results from lesion of both pyramidal (corticospinal) and non-pyramidal motor pathways, with pathophysiology varying depending upon the site of lesion. A highly prevalent medical condition following traumatic SCI, it develops in as many as 71% of affected individuals.[40]

Following SCI, a highly specific pattern of spasticity develops and it is therefore believed that the mechanisms underlying spinal spasticity are different from those seen following cortical damage (i.e. stroke or traumatic brain injury [TBI]). Spinal spasticity (spasticity following SCI) is thought to be the result of neural mechanisms, as opposed to cortical spasticity, which is believed to occur as a result of altered muscle contractile properties. Spasticity that leads to pain, spasms and contractures is a debilitating secondary complication of SCI. In addition to muscle hypertonus, spinal spasticity can involve hyperreflexia, clonus, clasp-knife responses, long-lasting cutaneous reflexes and muscle spasms evoked by brief non-noxious cutaneous stimuli.[41]

Spinal spasticity develops gradually over several months following injury. Immediately after SCI, the spinal cord becomes areflexic (spinal shock), during which time there is a loss of tendon reflexes below the level of the lesion, flaccid muscle tone and muscle paralysis. Weeks later, various reflexes such as the flexor withdrawal reflex, tendon reflex and the Babinski sign appear. For individuals with incomplete SCI, spasticity may interfere with the functional control of any residual voluntary motor control, compromising rehabilitation efforts.[41]

Mechanisms underlying spinal spasticity

The detailed pathogenesis of spasticity following SCI remains uncertain. The increased excitability of the stretch reflex in patients with spasticity has directed research efforts towards investigating the

spinal mechanisms modulating the excitability of this reflex (Fig. 1.19) and the potential alteration in its excitability after SCI (Table 1.1).

In Fig. 1.19, the excitatory interneurons (A) are represented by open circles and excitatory synapses by V-shaped bars. Inhibitory interneurons and inhibitory synapses are represented by filled circles. The pathways illustrated are the following:

1. The Ia-afferent fibres from two antagonistic muscles, their excitatory monosynaptic connection with the homonymous motoneuron (orange), and their inhibitory disynaptic reciprocal connection with the heteronymous motoneuron (blue).
2. The Ia-afferent inputs with their presynaptic inhibitory interneuron (PS, blue synapse).
3. Group II afferents with their polysynaptic connections to the α-motoneuron through propriospinal neurons (PO, yellow).
4. The γ-motoneurons innervating intrafusal muscle fibres (green).
5. The α-motoneurons innervating extrafusal muscle fibres (red).

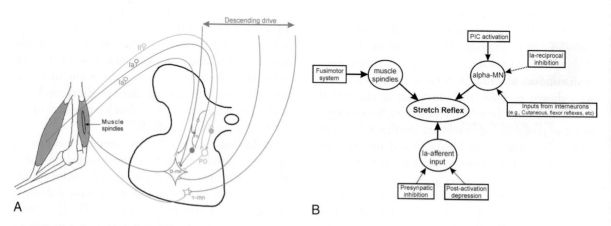

Figure 1.19 Schematic and block diagrams illustrating the main spinal circuits involved in the control of movement and the alteration in their excitability during spasticity.

Key: PIC = persistent inward current; mn = motoneuron.

Source: Elbasiouny, S.M., Moroz, D., et al., 2010. Management of spasticity after spinal cord injury: current techniques and future directions. Neurorehabilitation and Neural Repair 24 (1), 23–33.

In part (B) of Fig. 1.19, the block diagram summarises the alteration in excitability of spinal mechanisms contributing to the exaggerated reflexes in spasticity. Solid arrows indicate increased input and dotted arrows indicate reduced input after chronic SCI.

In summary, the pathogenesis of spasticity resulting from SCI is multifactorial and extends beyond the stretch reflex to include alterations in the excitability of motor neurons and interneurons of spinal circuits, Spinal spasticity is distinct from that seen following cortical injuries with presentation and pathogenesis being dependent upon the type, site and duration of injury. An understanding of this is critical for the successful design of rehabilitation programs.

Table 1.1 The most likely mechanisms thought to contribute to spinal spasticity

Mechanism	Involvement in spasticity	Significance for spasticity
Enhancement in the excitability of motoneurons	Most likely	High
Enhancement in the excitability of interneurons	Most likely	High
Axonal sprouting	Likely	High
Reduction in presynaptic inhibition	Likely	Moderate
Reduction in postactivation depression	Likely	Uncertain
Reduction in Ia-reciprocal inhibition	Likely	Unclear
Fusimotor hyperexcitability	Unlikely	None

Source: Elbasiouny, S.M., Moroz, D., et al., 2010. Management of spasticity after spinal cord injury: current techniques and future directions. Neurorehabilitation and Neural Repair 24(1):23–33.

Evidence-based practice points

- There is a progressive sequence of events that occurs following SCI (Fig. 1.20). The stages of this process vary in their length and exact timing, depending upon the location, type and severity of injury incurred, but ultimately lead to the development of a glial scar at the injury site.
- The recovery and repair mechanisms that occur at a cellular level in the spinal cord focus on structural repair to the area of injury. This involves the activation of local glial cells, which first remove cellular debris via phagocytosis and then assist in the reformation and reconfiguration of the ECM.
- The involvement of glial cells in this process, along with systemic inflammatory responses, control the spread of damage and potentially act to limit the loss of function that occurs through traumatic injury.

Continued

Evidence-based practice points—cont'd

- The fibrotic content of the remaining glial scar limits functional recovery following SCI due to the inhibition it exerts over axonal regrowth and regeneration. However, the plasticity of the CNS neurons and the heterogeneity of glial cell responses provide potential therapeutic avenues for further study.

- Spasticity resulting from SCI is multifactorial, extends beyond the stretch reflex and has a presentation distinct from that seen following damage to the motor cortex. Clinical presentation is also influenced by the type, site and time since injury.

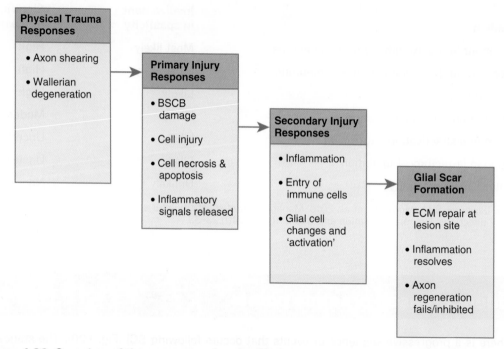

Figure 1.20 Overview of the sequence of pathophysiological events following SCI. The glial scar limits functional CNS recovery following SCI.

These progressive stages vary in length and timing depending upon severity of injury, but ultimately lead to the development of an axon-inhibitory structure called the glial scar. The glial scar limits functional CNS recovery following SCI.

Source: Tran, A.P., Warren, P.M., et al., 2018. The biology of regeneration failure and success after spinal cord injury. Physiological Reviews 98 (2), 881–917.

SUMMARY

The complex circuitry of the spinal cord allows for functions that include receiving and processing sensory information, generating and regulating movement of skeletal muscles, autonomic output and relaying signals to and from the higher brain and brainstem centres.

Following traumatic SCI, a complex and distinctive pathophysiology occurs, an inflammatory response is initiated and ultimately there is development and maturation of a glial scar (gliosis). This biological cascade of events not only creates a post-injury environment that is resistant to cellular recovery and repair, but which also acts to reduce cellular plasticity. This typically results in poor or absent functional recovery and maladaptive plasticity, giving rise to symptoms that require ongoing clinical treatment and management.

Clinical presentation of SCI, along with subsequent recovery and management, are dependent upon many factors. These include not only the severity and location of injury, but also the unique physiology of the individual and complex interactions between neurons, glia, immune cells and fibroblasts.

References

1. Winkler, E.A., Bell, R.D., et al., 2011. Central nervous system pericytes in health and disease. Nat. Neurosci. 14 (11), 1398–1405.

2. Zlokovic, B.V., 2008. The blood–brain barrier in health and chronic neurodegenerative disorders. Neuron 57 (2), 178–201.

3. Mautes, A.E., Weinzierl, M.R., et al., 2000. Vascular events after spinal cord injury: contribution to secondary pathogenesis. Phys. Ther. 80 (7), 673–687.

4. Sakuma, R., Kawahara, M., et al., 2016. Brain pericytes serve as microglia-generating multipotent vascular stem cells following ischemic stroke. J. Neuroinflammation 13 (1).

5. Klement, W., Garbelli, R., et al., 2018. Seizure progression and inflammatory mediators promote pericytosis and pericyte-microglia clustering at the cerebrovasculature. Neurobiol. Dis. 113, 70–81.

6. Dendrou, C.A., Fugger, L., et al., 2015. Immunopathology of multiple sclerosis. Nat. Rev. Immunol. 15 (9), 545–558.

7. Perea, G., Navarrete, M., et al., 2009. Tripartite synapses: astrocytes process and control synaptic information. Trends Neurosci. 32 (8), 421–431.

8. Araque, A., Parpura, V., et al., 1999. Tripartite synapses: glia, the unacknowledged partner. Trends Neurosci. 22 (5), 208–215.

9. Seifert, G., Steinhäuser, C., 2001. Ionotropic glutamate receptors in astrocytes. Prog. Brain Res. 132, 287–299.

10. Sontheimer, H., 1994. Voltage-dependent ion channels in glial cells. Glia 11 (2), 156–172.

11. Nimmerjahn, A., Kirchhoff, F., et al., 2004. Sulforhodamine 101 as a specific marker of astroglia in the neocortex in vivo. Nat. Methods 1 (1), 31–37.

12. Perea, G., Araque, A., 2005. Glial calcium signaling and neuron–glia communication. Cell Calcium 38 (3–4 SPEC. ISS.), 375–382.

13. Perea, G., Araque, A., 2005. Properties of synaptically evoked astrocyte calcium signal reveal synaptic information processing by astrocytes. J. Neurosci. 25 (9), 2192–2203.

14. Hol, E.M., Pekney, M., 2015. Glial fibrillary acidic protein (GFAP) and the astrocyte intermediate filament system in diseases of the central nervous system. Curr. Opin. Cell Biol. 32, 121–130.

15. Kiehn, O., 2011. Development and functional organization of spinal locomotor circuits. Curr. Opin. Neurobiol. 21 (1), 100–109.

16. Grillner, S., Hellgren, J., et al., 2005. Mechanisms for selection of basic motor programs – Roles for the striatum and pallidum. Trends Neurosci. 28 (7), 364–370.

17. Rossignol, S., Dubuc, R., et al., 2006. Dynamic sensorimotor interactions in locomotion. Physiol. Rev. 86 (1), 89–154.

18. Arber, S., 2012. Motor circuits in action: specification, connectivity, and function. Neuron 74 (6), 975–989.

19. Côté, M.P., Murray, L.M., et al., 2018. Spinal control of locomotion: individual neurons, their circuits and functions. Front. Physiol. 9, JUN.

20. Benthall, K.N., Hough, R.A., et al., 2017. Descending propriospinal neurons mediate restoration of locomotor

function following spinal cord injury. J. Neurophysiol. 117 (1), 215–229.

21. Conta, A.C., Stelzner, D.J., 2004. Differential vulnerability of propriospinal tract neurons to spinal cord contusion injury. J. Comp. Neurol. 479 (4), 347–359.

22. Blume, J., Douglas, S.D., et al., 2011. Immune suppression and immune activation in depression. Brain Behav. Immun. 25 (2), 221–229.

23. Baune, B.T., Camara, M.L., et al., 2012. Tumour necrosis factor – ALPHA mediated mechanisms of cognitive dysfunction. Transl. Neurosci. 3 (3), 263–277.

24. Liu, X.Z., Xu, X.M., et al., 1997. Neuronal and glial apoptosis after traumatic spinal cord injury. J. Neurosci. 17 (14), 5395.

25. Hausmann, O.N., 2003. Post-traumatic inflammation following spinal cord injury. Spinal Cord 41 (7), 369–378.

26. Fitch, M.T., Doller, C., et al., 1999. Cellular and molecular mechanisms of glial scarring and progressive cavitation: in vivo and in vitro analysis of inflammation-induced secondary injury after CNS trauma. J. Neurosci. 19 (19), 8182–8198.

27. Gadani, S.P., Walsh, J.T., et al., 2015. Dealing with danger in the CNS: the response of the immune system to injury. Neuron 87 (1), 47–62.

28. Norden, D.M., Muccigrosso, M.M., et al., 2015. Microglial priming and enhanced reactivity to secondary insult in aging, and traumatic CNS injury, and neurodegenerative disease. Neuropharmacology 96 (PA), 29–41.

29. Emsley, J.G., Macklis, J.D., 2006. Astroglial heterogeneity closely reflects the neuronal-defined anatomy of the adult murine CNS. Neuron Glia Biol. 2 (3), 175–186.

30. Farmer, W.T., Abrahamsson, T., et al., 2016. Neurons diversify astrocytes in the adult brain through sonic hedgehog signaling. Science 351 (6275), 849–854.

31. Jin, Y., Dougherty, S.E., et al., 2016. Regrowth of serotonin axons in the adult mouse brain following injury. Neuron 91 (4), 748–762.

32. White, R.E., Jakeman, L.B., 2008. Don't fence me in: harnessing the beneficial roles of astrocytes for spinal cord repair. Restor. Neurol. Neurosci. 26 (2–3), 197–214.

33. Baumann, N., Pham-Dinh, D., 2001. Biology of oligodendrocyte and myelin in the mammalian central nervous system. Physiol. Rev. 81 (2), 871–927.

34. Barnabé-Heider, F., Göritz, C., et al., 2010. Origin of new glial cells in intact and injured adult spinal cord. Cell Stem Cell 7 (4), 470–482.

35. Göritz, C., Dias, D.O., et al., 2011. A pericyte origin of spinal cord scar tissue. Science 333 (6039), 238–242.

36. Zhu, Y., Soderblom, C., et al., 2015. Hematogenous macrophage depletion reduces the fibrotic scar and increases axonal growth after spinal cord injury. Neurobiol. Dis. 74, 114–125.

37. Quraishe, S., Forbes, L.H., et al., 2018. The extracellular environment of the CNS: influence on plasticity, sprouting, and axonal regeneration after spinal cord injury. Neural Plast. 2018.

38. Tran, A.P., Warren, P.M., et al., 2018. The biology of regeneration failure and success after spinal cord injury. Physiol. Rev. 98 (2), 881–917.

39. Lance, J.W., 1980. Pathophysiology of spasticity and clinical experience with baclofen. Spasticity: Disordered Motor Control 185–203.

40. Mills, P.B., Holtz, K.A., et al., 2018. Early predictors of developing problematic spasticity following traumatic spinal cord injury: a prospective cohort study. J. Spinal Cord Med. October. doi: doi.org/10.1080/10790268.2018.1527082.

41. Elbasiouny, S.M., Moroz, D., et al., 2010. Management of spasticity after spinal cord injury: current techniques and future directions. Neurorehabil. Neural Repair 24 (1), 23–33.

CHAPTER 2

From the field to the emergency department and beyond

Judah Goldstein and Patrick Fok

INTRODUCTION

Emergency medical services (EMS) and emergency departments (ED) are the first points of contact within the healthcare system for patients with acute spinal cord injury (SCI). The care received within the first few hours of injury can have lasting implications. Historically, those who sustained an SCI often experienced poor outcomes and high mortality rates, but this is changing, particularly in high income countries. This improvement can be attributed to a number of factors, including updated emergency response systems, improved patient handling and transport and early hospital care.[1] Early recognition of SCI and the prevention of further neurological injury are critical during this early phase. EMS clinicians are able to mitigate neurological deterioration by providing timely evidence-based care and expeditious transport to the most appropriate healthcare facility. Upon arrival at a hospital, the goal of emergency medicine is to initiate early definitive care.

EMS/ED clinicians focus on providing life-saving interventions, thereby reducing further risk of secondary SCI by preventing advancement of neurological damage. Rehabilitation clinicians should understand the role and nature of this care. This chapter will focus on the burden of SCI and the acute care provided in the EMS and ED settings within the first few hours of injury.

EPIDEMIOLOGY OF SPINAL CORD INJURY

The causes of SCI are generally classified into one of two categories: traumatic spinal cord injury (TSCI) and non-traumatic SCI (NTSCI). Trauma can subsequently be classified as either blunt trauma SCI or penetrating trauma SCI.

Blunt trauma mechanisms can be isolated or multisystem. Multisystem trauma involves more than one body system (e.g. nervous, skeletal and cardiovascular system involvement), whereas isolated trauma may only affect one body system (e.g. central nervous system). The risk of cervical spine injury in blunt trauma is highest for certain injury mechanisms, such as axial load injury (odds ratio [OR] 7.3, 95% confidence intervals [CI] 5.1–10.4), falls (OR 2.1, 95% CI 1.6–2.7), diving incidents (OR 12.0, 95% CI 6.0–24.1) and non-traffic motor vehicle collisions (e.g. all-terrain vehicles) (OR 2.8, 95% CI 1.1–7.0)[2,3] (Table 2.1). Motor vehicle collision types that involve high speed, head-on collision, rollover collision or when seatbelts are not worn also increase the risk of cervical spine injury.[2]

Table 2.1 Common modes of traumatic SCI

Mode of SCI	OR (95% CI)/n (%)
Falls	2.1 (1.6–2.7)/1981 (25.29)
Diving incidents	12.0 (6.0–24.1)/366 (4.67)
Non-traffic motor vehicle collisions (e.g. all-terrain vehicles)	2.8 (1.1–7.0)/140 (1.79)
Traffic motor vehicle collisions	2465 (31.47)
Animal-related (e.g. horseback riding)	54 (0.69)
Violence (blunt)	60 (0.77)
Sports (rugby)	82 (1.05)
Violence (penetrating trauma – gunshot wound, stabbing injury)	816 (10.42)

Sources: Thompson, W.L., Stiell, I.G., et al., 2009. Association of injury mechanism with the risk of cervical spine fractures. Canadian Journal of Emergency Medicine 11 (1), 14–22; Chen, Y., Tang, Y., et al., 2013. Causes of spinal cord injury. Topics in Spinal Cord Injury Rehabilitation 19 (1), 1–8.

Common trauma mechanisms of injury are displayed in Figure 2.1. Non-traumatic causes are wide-ranging and include vascular disorders, infectious conditions, spinal canal stenosis, disc herniation, myelopathy and cancer.[1,3]

Common injury causes vary by country, region and age.[4] Adequate surveillance of injury mechanisms can inform injury prevention activities and policy to address modes of injury common in a particular system. The highest prevalence of SCI is associated with high-risk activities, with motor vehicle collisions (MVCs) and falls being the most common. Even so, seemingly rare incidents can happen during a wide variety of everyday activities including diving into the surf, horseriding, playing rugby league or rugby union.

Incidence and prevalence of TSCI

The global incidence and prevalence of TSCI varies widely due to challenges with data collection and reporting. To clarify, incidence is the rate of new, or newly diagnosed, cases of the disease, while prevalence is the actual number of cases alive with the disease, either during a period of time (period prevalence) or at a particular date in time (point prevalence). A recent systematic review estimated the global incidence to range from eight individuals per million population in Spain, to a high of 246 people per million inhabitants in Taiwan Province of China.[5] Globally, this means that between 250,000 and 500,000 individuals acquire an SCI each year.[1] Considering the Australian and New Zealand context specifically, the incidence rate varied from 10 to 77 individuals with traumatic SCI per million inhabitants per year.[5] Most studies suggest TSCI rates are increasing; however, regional studies have also shown a decreasing incidence in Canada, Taiwan Province of China and Australia.[5] In most countries, the incidence of acute TSCI is highest in the young (ages 15–34 years) (Fig. 2.2). In contrast, NTSCI is most prevalent in older adults.[3]

The reported prevalence of TSCI varies substantially, with estimates from 50 to 4187 cases per million population worldwide[4,5] and in Australia the observed rate is 681 people per million population.[1,6] Variation in incidence and prevalence is observed between countries (Fig. 2.2). This observed variation between countries may be due to methodological differences in reporting and in country-specific differences such as socioeconomic factors, public policy and the healthcare system.[5] In developed countries, the incidence of TSCI has been declining since the early 1980s due to legislative changes for motor vehicle manufacturing and compulsory seatbelt laws, random breath-testing and educational programs. An opposite trend is observed in developing countries where infrastructure is insufficient.[4]

Incidence and prevalence of NTSCI

The incidence and prevalence of NTSCI are less well described. Ageing may be the primary driver

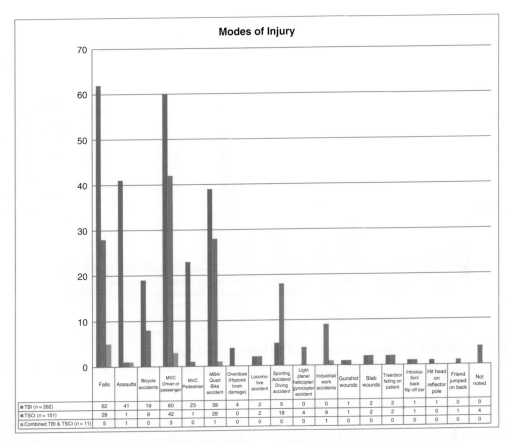

	Falls	Assaults	Bicycle accidents	MVC Driver or passenger	MVC Pedestrian	MBA/Quad Bike accident	Overdose (Hypoxic brain damage)	Locomotive accident	Sporting Accident/Diving accident	Light plane/helicopter/gyrocopter accident	Industrial/work accidents	Gunshot wounds	Stab wounds	Tree/door falling on patient	Intoxication/on back	Hit head on reflector pole	Friend jumped on back	Not noted
TBI (n = 262)	62	41	19	60	23	39	4	2	5	0	0	1	2	2	1	1	0	0
TSCI (n = 151)	28	1	8	42	1	28	0	2	18	4	9	1	2	2	1	0	1	4
Combined TBI & TSCI (n = 11)	5	1	0	3	0	1	0	0	0	0	1	0	0	0	0	0	0	0

Figure 2.1 Numbers of patients with TBI and TSCI according to the mode of injury.
TBI Traumatic Brain Injury; TSCI Traumatic Spinal Cord Injury; MVC motor vehicle collision; MBA Motorbike accident; *n* = number of patients; *statistically significant difference

Source: Reznik, J.E., Biros, E., et al., 2014. Prevalence and risk factors of neurogenic heterotopic ossification in traumatic spinal cord and traumatic brain injured patients admitted to specialised units in Australia. Journal of Musculoskeletal and Neuronal Interactions 14 (1), 19–28.

for increasing NTSCI incidence and prevalence worldwide.[1,3] While TSCI is found most often in young males,[7] NTSCI is notably higher in older adults and women. During 2015–16, 398 new cases of SCI were reported to the Australian Spinal Cord Injury Register (ASCIR) with 145 of these resulting from non-traumatic causes.[8] This translates to about 26 cases per million adults per year, with the most common causes being tumours, degenerative and vascular illnesses.[9] Prevalence estimates of NTSCI for Australia are 455 per million population.[1,3]

EPIDEMIOLOGY OF EMERGENCY RESPONSES FOR POTENTIAL SCI

Paramedics frequently respond to trauma-related incidents with the majority classified as minor trauma. Otier and colleagues[10] conducted a retrospective cohort study of all adult patients with a potential TSCI who were cared for by Ambulance Victoria paramedics. Falls, traffic collisions, violence and sport-related incidents were the leading cause of potential TSCI in Victoria, Australia (Table 2.1).[10]

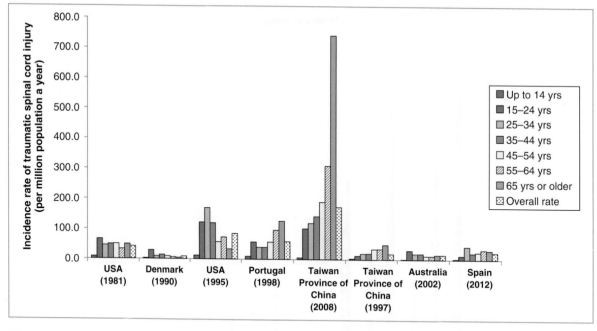

Figure 2.2 Variation in incidence rate of TSCI by country and age.

Source: Furlan, J.C., Sakakibara, B.M., et al., 2013. Global incidence and prevalence of traumatic spinal cord injury. The Canadian Journal of Neurological Sciences 40 (4), 456–464.

Close to one-third of potential patients with SCI were transported to a major trauma service.[10] This study demonstrated that paramedics frequently respond to patients with potential SCI. Using predefined rules to identify patients who meet spinal immobilisation criteria, paramedics can provide appropriate care to those most at risk and facilitate rapid and direct transport to major trauma facilities. Otier and colleagues provide a robust description of the burden of TSCI in one state within Australia.[10] Of note, in those patients who suffer blunt trauma, only 2% will suffer a SCI.[2,11] Cervical spine clearance rules and their application by paramedics will be described in this chapter. With the application of these rules, fewer patients are now being immobilised unnecessarily.

Individual and societal consequences of SCI

The consequences of SCI are vast, having an impact at both the individual level and the societal level (see Chapters 16, 21 and 22). Traumatic SCI is often associated with preventable causes, such as MVCs, falls and violence.[1,12]

Sustaining an SCI affects the patient's ability to function, depending on the severity of the injury. The functional issues can include basic activities of daily living (ADL), negatively affecting their quality of life, and can cause significant financial burden to communities, family and the affected individual.[9,13] The SCI can result in the patient's decreased ability to obtain income, increased homecare needs, hospital/medical bills, ADL accommodation, equipment and home adjustment.

Victims of multisystem trauma are now surviving with catastrophic injuries for much longer due to advances in early emergency care. This has wide-ranging implications for rehabilitation needs and the patient's ability to engage in rehabilitation (e.g. a patient with an upper extremity injury, traumatic brain injury and SCI will have substantially different needs to a patient with an isolated SCI).

These topics will be presented in greater depth in later chapters.

Compared to multisystem trauma survivors without SCI, higher rates of sepsis and multi-organ failure are observed post-cervical SCI, but prognosis is favourable with appropriate care.[14]

Finally, caring for patients with chronic SCI in the EMS/ED setting can be challenging.[15] This is a group that frequents the ED for care and due to the nature of their SCI can present without the typical features of other common illnesses. For example, they can present with autonomic dysreflexia, vascular issues (venous thromboembolism), respiratory complications (pneumonia), gastrointestinal and urological complications or integumentary complications (e.g. pressure injuries).[15] Many of these concerning pathologies will be explored in subsequent chapters.

SCI MANAGEMENT BY EMS

As mentioned earlier, paramedics are often the first point of contact with the healthcare system for patients with acute SCI. For this reason, it is imperative that paramedics have the best available evidence to guide care. Since 1998, the Prehospital Evidence-based Practice (PEP) program, based at Dalhousie University Department of Emergency Medicine, Division of EMS, Canada, has been appraising the research evidence on EMS interventions.[16–18] PEP is an evidence repository for EMS clinicians and medical directors which can be used to inform the writing of clinical practice guidelines and protocols. It can also be a resource for other allied health professionals, including physiotherapists, to understand the evidence for out-of-hospital interventions or in the design of regionalised systems of care.

The PEP database and website are organised by nature of complaint (e.g. trauma) and clinical presentation (e.g. spinal injury) as the main categories, with EMS interventions (e.g. cervical spine clearance, long spinal immobilisation devices) listed as sub-categories under each condition. EMS interventions include assessments (e.g. Cervical spine clearance rules), treatments (e.g. steroids, long spinal immobilisation devices) and dispositions (e.g. transport direct to trauma centre). Primary research is listed under each associated intervention. Included research is critically appraised and assigned a level of evidence and direction of evidence. Each intervention is then plotted on an evidence matrix table (Fig. 2.3). The full PEP methodology has been previously published.[16]

Clinical interventions supported by research, as evaluated by PEP include: in-line stabilisation for intubation, C-spine clearance decision rules, scoop stretchers and self-extrication. Further research on steroid and spinal precaution use is required. A number of interventions may be harmful, based upon the critically appraised research: long spinal immobilisation devices[19] and immobilisation in penetrating trauma.[20,21]

INITIAL ASSESSMENT AND MANAGEMENT OVERVIEW

There have been major changes in prehospital SCI care over the past ten years. Significant advancements have been made in understanding how best to assess the cervical spine (C-spine), provide spinal motion restriction (SMR) and in transport decision-making. These changes have led to: 1) fewer patients suffering additional harm by improper handling; and 2) reduced mortality. The paramedic approach to care is to first correct problems with ventilation and/or circulation while protecting patients from further injury. Earlier practice was to stabilise the spinal column from the head to below the buttocks.[22] Following stabilisation, patients are transported to trauma centres specialising in spinal care, if available.

In the past, there were few protocols for selective spinal immobilisation and little belief that paramedics could discriminate between injured patients with no SCI and those with unstable SCI requiring careful handling.[23] The result was that most patients underwent spinal immobilisation. This led to many patients being immobilised without SCI, causing

Recommendation		RECOMMENDATION FOR INTERVENTION			
		SUPPORTIVE (Green)	**NEUTRAL (Yellow)**	**AGAINST (Red)**	**NOT YET GRADED (White)**
STRENGTH OF EVIDENCE FOR INTERVENTION	1 (strong evidence exists)	• In-line stabilisation for intubation	• Steroid	• Long spinal immobilisation devices	• Hypertonic saline
	2 (fair evidence exists)	• C-spine clearance • Scoop stretcher • Self-extrication	• Short extrication devices (ex: KED)	• Cervical collar • Immobilisation in penetrating trauma	
	3 (weak evidence exists)	• Leave helmet in place	• Spinal precautions		

Figure 2.3 The PEP evidence matrix for spinal injury.

Source: Carter, A.J.E., Jensen, J.L., et al., 2018. State of the evidence for the emergency medical services (EMS) care: the evolution and current methodology of the Prehospital Evidence-based Practice (PEP) program. Healthcare Policy 14 (1), 57–70.

harm in some cases and undue distress for many trauma victims.

As paramedics become more integrated into the healthcare system, there is increasing recognition of the value brought by the paramedic's initial assessment and documentation of on-scene findings.[2] The paramedic Patient Care Report (PCR) is a valuable source of information for the physiotherapist who is providing post-injury care. Physiotherapists should be aware that paramedics frequently document important information about the trauma including time of injury, details about the scene, forces involved and mechanisms of injury (vehicle speeds, heights of falls, nature of fall; and for penetrating trauma, velocity and size of bullets or blades). This information may help the therapist understand the extent of tissue injury and care needs beyond the obvious SCI.

Neurological examination

Upon ED arrival, an initial neurological assessment is conducted that can inform further in-hospital care. A complete neurological examination performed in the ED should document motor and sensory function at each spinal level. American Association of Neurological Surgeons and the Congress of Neurological Surgeons suggest use of the International Standards for Neurological Classification of Spinal Cord Injury (ISNCSCI), an evaluation developed by the American Spinal Injury Association (ASIA) and endorsed by the International Spinal Cord Society (ISCOS), for assessment of neurological deficits.[24] The ASIA Impairment Scale (AIS) was developed by ASIA and implemented in 1992, replacing the physiological injury-based Frankel method. The ISNCSCI uses AIS to classify neurological injuries:

A = Complete – No sensory of motor function to S4–5 segments

B = Sensory Incomplete – Sensory, but no motor function preserved below neurological level and S4–5 segments

C = Motor Incomplete – less than half of key muscles function below neurologic level with muscle grade strength ≥ 3

D = Motor Incomplete – half or more of key muscles function below neurological level with muscle grade strength ≥ 3

E = Normal – sensation and motor are normal in all segments.

The use of the ISNCSCI for physiotherapists will be discussed further in Chapter 4.

Choices of imaging and medical interventions performed in the ED will be discussed in more detail below.

Initial management

Initial management of patients with suspected spinal trauma mirrors that of an undifferentiated trauma patient. Advanced Trauma Life Support (ATLS) principles guide the initial assessment and stabilising interventions.[25] The approach to the trauma patient is divided into two separate parts: the primary and secondary survey. The primary survey addresses the so-called 'ABCs' (Airway, Breathing and Circulation) to assess for and treat immediate life-threatening injuries, while the secondary survey is a thorough examination for all traumatic injuries. Although a neurological examination is part of the primary survey, this is usually abbreviated to an assessment of Glasgow Coma Scale (GCS), pupil size and reactivity and gross movement of each extremity. Assessment for SCI can be deferred to the secondary survey, as stabilisation of the patient takes priority. Nevertheless, in patients where the trauma mechanism could be compatible with a spinal injury, the treatment team remains cognisant of this possible injury and takes precautions to minimise spinal movement. Use of hard, long spinal boards in the EMS/ED settings had been standard care until recent literature showed that their use increases patient morbidity, specifically to pressure injuries, respiratory compromise, increased intracranial pressure and increased pain, leading to unnecessary imaging.[26] Given that a majority of immobilised patients do not have spinal injuries, with even fewer having unstable spinal injuries,[27] spinal boards are now considered solely extrication devices, and not suitable for transportation in the EMS/ED setting. Use of the spinal board has, for the most part, been abandoned, as recommended by the American College of Emergency Physicians and National Association of EMS Physicians.[28–30] Current methods for spinal motion restriction will be discussed later in this chapter.

Cervical spine clinical decision instruments

Clinical decision rules have been developed to assist clinicians in identifying patients who are at a low risk for cervical spine injuries, and can safely avoid imaging. Two commonly used rules are the National Emergency X-Radiography Utilisation Study (NEXUS) Low-risk Criteria (NLC) and the Canadian C-spine (cervical-spine) rules (CCR). Hoffman and colleagues[31] developed and validated the first clinical decision instrument, the NLC. Patients must meet all five criteria to be considered sufficiently low-risk for cervical spine injury to forgo cervical spine imaging: No midline cervical tenderness, no focal neurological deficit, normal alertness, no intoxication and no painful, distracting injury (Table 2.2). The decision instrument has a 99.6% sensitivity and 99.9% negative predictive value for clinically significant cervical spine injury.[31] Independently, Stiell and colleagues (2001)[32] developed and validated a separate clinical decision instrument to identify the same population of low-risk patient, the CCR.[32–34] Unlike the NEXUS Low-risk Criteria, the CCR were more complicated with different criteria. Specifically, CCR has a three-step instrument in which the patient is assessed for the absence of high-risk features, the presence of a low-risk feature and ability for lateral head rotation; the inability to clear any of the three steps mandates radiological imaging (Table 2.2). The advantages of the CCR are the ability to clear a patient despite midline C-spine tenderness and the absence of subjective criteria as opposed to the NLC (i.e. 'painful, distracting injury'). In a head-to-head comparison between the NLC and CCR, the latter was shown to be more sensitive and specific than the former (Fig. 2.4).[35]

There is currently moderate quality evidence that supports the use of CCRs in the EMS setting, according to the PEP website.[18] It is recommended that a C-spine rule be applied as early as possible. In the event that the rule cannot be applied, patients should have spinal motion restricted.[36]

Table 2.2 Comparison of the Canadian C-spine rule criteria with the NEXUS Low-risk Criteria (NLC)

Canadian C-spine rule (consider imaging as pre-algorithm)	NEXUS Low-risk Criteria (NLC) (consider imaging if one criteria is present)
Any high risk factor (age, dangerous mechanism, paraesthesia in extremities)? **If yes, consider imaging**	Focal neurological deficit
Any low-risk factor allowing safe assessment of range of motion (simple rear end MVC, sitting position in ED, ambulatory at any time, delayed onset neck pain, absence of mid-line C-spine tenderness)? **If no, consider imaging**	Midline spinal tenderness
Able to actively rotate the neck? **If unable, consider imaging**	Altered level of consciousness
	Intoxication
	Distracting injury present

Sources: Hoffman, J.R., Mower, W.R., et al., 2000. Validity of a set of clinical criteria to rule out injury to the cervical spine in patients with blunt trauma. National Emergency X-Radiography Utilization Study Group. N Engl J Med. 343 (2), 94–99; Stiell, I.G., Wells, G.A., et al., 2001. The Canadian C-spine rule for radiography in alert and stable trauma patients. JAMA 286 (15), 1841–1848.

Patient extrication and spinal motion restriction

Patient extrication and handling are important considerations for paramedics determining whether there is the potential for SCI. There is lower quality evidence demonstrating that self-extrication may reduce cervical motion when feasible.[37,38] Furthermore, a recent case study identified harm due to immobilisation in a patient with ankylosing spondylitis.[39] This case suggests that spinal immobilisation should be avoided in cases of ambulatory patient without clear indication for immobilisation.[39] Partial self-immobilisation by SMR could be superior to traditional full spinal immobilisation.[40]

A major change for many EMS agencies has been the move away from long spinal immobilisation devices. In Australia, spinal immobilisation devices are now used only for extrication (e.g. moving patients from enclosed spaces, such as wrecked vehicles, collapsed buildings or other challenging situations). In many other EMS systems, spinal immobilisation for suspected spinal injury was synonymous with the mandatory use of the long

spine board during extrication and transport to the ED.[18] Early biomechanical research in healthy volunteers demonstrated that spinal immobilisation with the board and collar improved immobilisation, but this immobilisation led to increased discomfort, tissue interface pressures, development of pressure ulcers and airway complications.[36] Unstable SCI can progress to severe neurological injuries when excessive movement of the injured spine is not controlled. True spinal immobilisation is a challenge in the prehospital setting, therefore the term SMR has been adopted. Contemporary biomechanical research has demonstrated that current techniques used to limit spinal motion do not provide true spinal immobilisation, but rather provide SMR.[42] SMR most likely achieves the same benefit as spinal immobilisation and can be realised with other modalities, including scoop stretchers, vacuum splints, and ambulance cot, provided the patient can be safely secured.[40,41]

Removal of extrication devices (e.g. long spine board) should be performed by EMS personnel if enough resources are available once in the transport

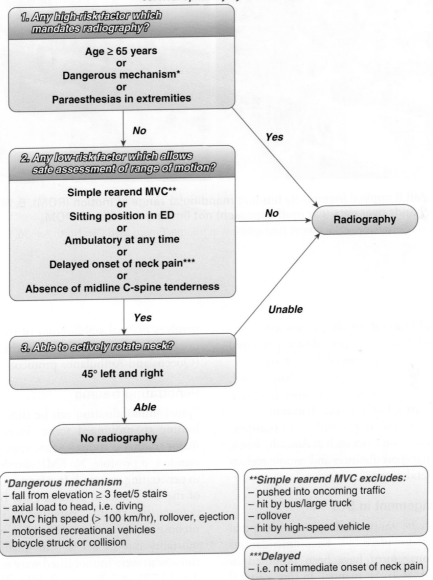

Figure 2.4 The Canadian C-Spine Rule.
Key: MVC = motor vehicle collision; ED = emergency department.
Source: © Ottawa Health Research Institute, Emergency Medicine Research

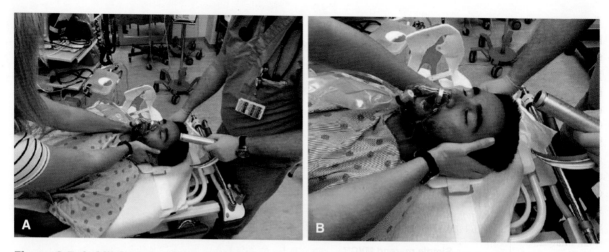

Figure 2.5 A, MILS applied incorrectly limiting mandibular range of motion (ROM). B, MILS applied correctly with hands over ears (ear muff approach) not limiting mandibular ROM.
Source: Kovacs, G., Sowers, N., 2018. Airway management in trauma. Emerg Med Clin North Am 36, 61–84.

vehicle or upon ED arrival. Finally, patients with TSCI should be expeditiously transported to a specialised trauma centre within 24 hours of time of injury.[36,42] While transport by air platform is faster than ground, no difference in neurological outcomes has been found between ground or helicopter transport as long as spinal precautions are respected.[43,44] Air transport may be favoured in countries such as Australia where there are long transport distances and remote regions with difficult land access.

Airway management in SCI

Intubation can be more challenging with spinal immobilisation in place.[36,45] Recommendations for airway management have been proposed in the context of SCI: 1) manual in-line cervical spine stabilisation (MILS) should be used;[46] 2) EMS providers should not rely on cervical collars alone; and 3) indirect methods of intubation may be preferred if available.[36,47] No worsening of neurological status after airway management was observed using MILS in several studies.[35] MILS involves manual stabilisation of the cervical spine usually prior to application of the cervical collar (Queensland Ambulance protocol) (Fig. 2.5).[48]

Penetrating trauma

Spinal immobilisation can be time intensive, thus leading to prolonged scene times. The goal for major trauma is to limit scene time to less than 10 minutes, if possible. No SMR should be performed in penetrating trauma.[49] In a large secondary analysis of the US National Trauma Data Bank of 45,284 penetrating trauma patients, 4.3% underwent prehospital spine immobilisation with an overall mortality rate of 8.1%.[19] In unadjusted analysis, those who were immobilised were twice as likely to die (14.7% vs 7.2%; $p < 0.001$). This relationship remained using multiple logistic regression to control for confounders.[19] Although there were limitations with the analysis (e.g. inability to control for scene times), this provided evidence that spinal immobilisation in the context of penetrating trauma may be harmful.

Emergency department management
Radiological screening for cervical spine injury

Plain film radiography had been the standard of care for screening patients for C-spine injury who were unable to be clinically cleared by either NLC or CCR. Three views were obtained – anterior–posterior, lateral and open-mouth odontoid views. With the advancement of computed tomography (CT) scans, this modality has emerged as the imaging modality of choice for trauma patients. Multiple studies have shown CT to have superior sensitivity for cervical spine injury compared to plain radiography.[50,51] A meta-analysis demonstrated that plain film radiography had a grouped sensitivity of 52% versus CT at 98%.[52] The US-based Eastern Association of Surgeons in Trauma (EAST) has since changed its guidelines to recommend CT over plain film radiography as the screening modality for cervical spine injury.[53] There has been inconsistent management of patients with a negative CT, but persistent cervical spine tenderness. For example, some patients are discharged with a hard collar for comfort, only when not sleeping, while other are discharged with a collar for use at all times. The American-based Western Trauma Association has prospectively demonstrated that in the absence of a neurological deficit, an alert patient can be cleared for significant cervical spine injury with a negative technically-adequate CT scan.[54] In non-alert patients, EAST guidelines now conditionally support removal of cervical collars in obtunded, unexaminable patients following a high-quality CT as a result of a meta-analysis demonstrating no missed unstable cervical spine injuries.[55] A similar diagnostic approach has been adopted by Trauma Victoria's Spinal Trauma Guideline.[6]

Medical management
Haemodynamic support

Patients with a SCI can present with life-threatening haemodynamic instability due to neurogenic shock, especially if the injury is above the T4 level. However, in the setting of trauma, other injury, such as intra-abdominal or thoracic injury, must be ruled out as the cause of hypotension. Neurogenic shock is caused by disruption of the sympathetic chain, resulting in unopposed vagal tone. This results in vasodilatation of blood vessels, resulting in pooling of blood in the peripheral circulation. This is compounded by the presence of bradycardia, resulting in decreased cardiac output. Neurogenic shock is a haemodynamic alteration in physiology and should not be confused with 'spinal shock'. Spinal shock is a neurological transient flaccid paralysis and loss of reflexes below the level of spinal cord injury, lasting from 30 minutes to 6 weeks post-injury (see Chapter 4 for further detail on spinal shock).

Initial management of the hypotensive trauma patient is volume resuscitation with intravenous fluids and blood. In neurogenic shock, vasopressors, such as noradrenaline or adrenaline are also required to restore vascular tone and cardiac output for a goal mean arterial pressure (MAP) of 85–90 mmHg. This ensures sufficient spinal cord perfusion to prevent secondary injury.[57]

Steroid use

The benefit of steroids immediately post-injury remains a highly debated topic. The original National Acute Spinal Cord Injury Study (NASCIS) I showed no beneficial influence in neurological recovery with high-dose methylprednisolone (MP) administration.[58] The subsequent NASCIS II study demonstrated no neurological benefit of higher dose MP administration after SCI, but post-hoc analysis found significant neurological improvement to patients treated with MP if administered within 8 hours of injury.[59,60] As multiple retrospective studies thereafter had shown conflicting results on the benefit of MP within the 8-hour window, a prospective, double-blind, randomised study was conducted. NASCIS III compared functional outcomes after a 24-hour vs 48-hour course of MP. Only after post-hoc analysis was a benefit shown for 48-hour MP administration within 3–8 hours of injury.[59] The same studies have documented significant complications due to steroid administration, including sepsis, pneumonia, gastrointestinal bleed, hyperglycaemia requiring inclusion administration and mortality independent of injury severity.[61–63] Due to the limited power of these studies and high morbidity associated with steroids, steroid administration for spinal injury is not recommended by many medical societies, including the American Association of Neurological Surgeons, Congress of Neurological Surgeons[61] and the Neurosurgical Society of Australasia.[63] The Canadian Association of Emergency Physicians (CAEP) released a position statement, endorsed by the Association of Academic Emergency Medicine, which lists steroids in acute spinal injury as a treatment option, not standard care.[60,64]

Deep vein thrombosis prophylaxis

Venous thromboembolism (VTE), comprising both deep vein thrombosis (DVT) and pulmonary embolism (PE), are common in the acute SCI population, with incidence of DVT and PE reported to be as high as 67% and 18% respectively, despite chemical prophylaxis.[65] Accordingly, the American Association of Neurological Surgeons/Congress of Neurological Surgeons list VTE prophylaxis within 72 hours as a Level 1 recommendation.[66] The timing of prophylaxis initiation has remained unclear, as premature initiation may cause haemorrhagic complications. Recently, the Transforming Research And Clinical Knowledge in SCIs (TRACK SCI) study has shown that VTE prophylaxis with subcutaneous enoxaparin within 24 hours of SCI is safe, with 0% rate adverse bleed events.[67] For patients undergoing operative management, enoxaparin was withheld for 24 hours postoperatively.

SPECIAL TOPICS IN ACUTE SPINAL CORD INJURY

Geriatric trauma

Few studies have examined the impact of EMS care on the older SCI patient. The primary mechanism of injury observed most often in this population is a fall from standing height.[68] In addition, patient outcomes are often worse in this population. For example, mortality rates in older adults with SCI were 46.9%

compared with 4.9% in younger adults.[68,69] Even so, those who do survive can fare well and can benefit from aggressive care, provided this approach aligns with the patient's own goals of care.

EMS clinicians require clarity on the value of SMR and selective spinal immobilisation in older adults. A recent paper by Underbrink and colleagues (2018)[70] aimed to evaluate immobilisation methods of older adults with confirmed C-spine injury following the implementation of a new spinal precautions protocol. They conducted a retrospective, observational study of older adult trauma patients with cervical spine injury before and after protocol implementation. Multivariate logistic regression was used to calculate the odds ratio of in-hospital mortality/hospice placement. Of the 7737 injured older adults, only 237 (1.6%) had a confirmed C-spine fracture or cervical cord injury.[70] Full spinal immobilisation decreased by 31.3% following protocol implementation. No change in mortality outcomes was observed. The authors concluded that prehospital choice of immobilisation method did not affect the incidence of neurological deficit, mortality or disposition.[70] This research suggests that SMR may not be inferior to full spinal immobilisation in this population. Consideration for the potential to reduce harms such as pressure ulcers and deconditioning should also be examined. Of note, there was a lower than expected use of full spinal immobilisation prior to protocol implementation, which the authors suggested may be due to EMS clinicians being hesitant to immobilise patients with complex pathologies (e.g. heart failure, chronic obstructive pulmonary disease [COPD]) or that they may not recognise the seriousness of the injury with seemingly benign mechanisms of injury.

Paediatric trauma

Similar to geriatrics, there is a paucity of research on SCI management in paediatric populations.[71] SCI in children is rare (see Chapter 14 for further details). Even so, devastating, long-lasting effects for the injured child are possible if care is not optimal. Younger children are more likely to experience upper

C-spine injury with high mortality rates (33%), whereas older children more commonly experience lower C-spine injury.[72] Blunt trauma (e.g. MVCs) are a common cause of SCI in paediatrics.[71] Traditional care for children often included spinal immobilisation using a spinal board and rigid cervical collar. There is some evidence that spinal immobilisation is associated with worse pain and higher rates of imaging.[73] For this reason, SMR can be considered for children as well. The application of a cervical collar is recommended for children with a complaint of neck pain, torticollis, neurological deficit, altered mental status or involvement in a high-risk MVC, high impact diving injury or with substantial torso injury.[42,73,74] Other recommendations include minimising the time on backboards, as with adults, and using padding under the shoulders to avoid excessive cervical spine flexion.[42,72]

Evidence-based practice points

- The incidence of SCI is low compared to the large volume of trauma patients attended to by emergency medical services (EMS).
- Physiotherapists can access important information on mechanism of injury from paramedic assessment documentation. This is an important resource that could inform future care delivery.
- Spinal motion restriction is preferred over spinal immobilisation.
- Manual in-line cervical spine stabilisation should be used and indirect intubation is preferred, if available.
- Patients with penetrating trauma should not undergo spinal immobilisation.
- EMS and ED clinicians can apply C-spine clearance rules to determine who would benefit from imaging.
- Steroids are not recommended for traumatic spinal cord injury.

SUMMARY

The initial emergency care provided to patients with SCI can have long-lasting implications for the patient and their rehabilitation. It is important for physiotherapists to understand the nature of care provided, and potential effects of this care, while also being aware of how the paramedic incident documentation might inform the therapist's rehabilitation of their clients. Having an awareness of the care provided in the initial phases will help a physiotherapist to better understand the overall clinical presentation. The EMS and ED management of the spinal cord-injured patient has changed significantly in the past decade. In particular, the routine use of long spine boards in extrication and transport has been replaced by the judicious use of the device and SMR guidelines for transport. These improvements in care have been associated with reductions in mortality and morbidity. This change in practice has also meant less imaging for those unlikely to have an SCI. It is important that rehabilitation clinicians are aware of the initial EMS/ED management of the patient with acute SCI to better understand the overall clinical presentation and prognosis.

References

1. World Health Organization, 2013. International perspectives on spinal cord injury. The International Spinal Cord Society. 1–250. http://apps.who.int/iris/bitstream/handle/10665/94190/9789241564663_eng.pdf;jsessionid=6AAE1AC5DA5F4C01897A965E6FC0E508?sequence=1.

2. Thompson, W.L., Stiell, I.G., et al., 2009. Association of injury mechanism with the risk of cervical spine fractures. CJEM 11 (1), 14–22.

3. New, P.W., Farry, A., et al., 2013. Prevalence of non-traumatic spinal cord injury in Victoria, Australia. Spinal Cord 51, 99–102.

4. Lee, B.B., Cripps, R.A., et al., 2014. The global map for traumatic spinal cord injury epidemiology: update 2011, global incidence rate. Spinal Cord 52, 110–116.

5. Furlan, J.C., Sakakibara, B.M., et al., 2013. Global incidence and prevalence of traumatic spinal cord injury. Can. J. Neurol. Sci. 40 (4), 456–464.

6. O'Connor, P.J., 2005. Forecasting of spinal cord injury annual case numbers in Australia. Arch. Phys. Med. Rehabil. 86 (1), 48–51.

7. Otier, A.O., Smith, K., et al., 2014. The prehospital management of suspected spinal cord injury: an update. Prehosp. Disaster Med. 29 (4), 399–402.

8. Tovell, A., 2019. Spinal cord injury, Australia, 2015–16. Injury research and statistics series no. 122. Cat. No. INJCAT 202. Canberra: AIHW. www.aihw.gov.au/reports/injury/spinal-cord-injury-australia-2015-16/contents/table-of-contents.

9. New, P.W., Cripps, R.A., et al., 2014. Global maps of non-traumatic spinal cord injury epidemiology: towards a living data repository. Spinal Cord 52, 97–109.

10. Otier, A.O., Smith, K., et al., 2016. The epidemiology of pre-hospital spinal cord injuries in Victoria, Australia: a six year retrospective cohort study. Inj. Epidemiol. 3, 25.

11. Crosby, E.T., 2006. Airway management in adults after cervical spine trauma. Anesthesiology 104, 1293–1318.

12. Umana, E., Khan, K., et al., 2018. Epidemiology and characteristics of cervical spine injury in patients presenting to a regional emergency department. Cureus 10 (2), e2179.

13. Pickett, G.E., Campos-Benitez, M., et al., 2006. Epidemiology of traumatic spinal cord injury in Canada. Spine 31 (7), 799–805.

14. Kamp, O., Jansen, O., et al., 2018. Cervical spinal cord injury shows markedly lower than predicted mortality (>72 hours after multiple trauma) from sepsis and multiple organ failure. J. Intensive Care Med. [epub ahead of print]. doi: dx.doi.org/10.1177/0885066617753356.

15. Kupfer, M., Kucer, B.T., et al., 2018. Persons with chronic spinal cord injuries in the emergency department: a review of a unique population. J. Emerg. Med. 55 (2), 206–212.

16. Carter, A.J.E., Jensen, J.L., et al., 2018. State of the evidence for the emergency medical services (EMS) care: the evolution and current methodology of the prehospital evidence-based practice (PEP) program. Healthc. Policy 14 (1), 57–70.

17. Prehospital Evidence-Based Practice (PEP) Program [Internet], 2018. Halifax, NS: Dalhousie University – Division of Emergency Medical Services. https://emspep.cdha.nshealth.ca/Default.aspx. (Accessed 28 August 2018).

18. Greene, J., Cook, J., et al., 2017. Challenging the dogma of spinal immobilization and other evidence from the Prehospital Evidence-based Practice (PEP) program. Ambul. Today 14 (4), 17–21.

19. Hemmes, B., Brink, P.R., et al., 2014. Effects of unconsciousness during spinal immobilization on tissue-interface pressures: a randomized controlled trial comparing a standard rigid spineboard with a newly developed soft-layered long spineboard. Injury 45 (11), 1741–1746. Medline.

20. Haut, E.R., Kalish, B.T., et al., 2010. Spine immobilization in penetrating trauma: more harm than good? J. Trauma 68, 115–121.

21. Otier, A., Smith, K., et al., 2015. Should suspected cervical spinal cord injury be immobilised?: a systematic review. Injury 46, 528–535. Medline.

22. Somers, M.F., 2001. Spinal Cord Injury: Functional Rehabilitation. Prentice-Hall, Inc., Upper Saddle River, New Jersey.

23. Burton, J.H., Harmon, N.R., et al., 2005. EMS provider findings and interventions with a statewide EMS spine-assessment protocol. Prehosp. Emerg. Care 9 (3), 303–309.

24. American Spinal Injury Association, 2018. Retrieved 28 August 2018 from: http://asia-spinalinjury.org/wp-content/uploads/2016/02/International_Stds_Diagram_Worksheet.pdf.

25. Trauma ACOSCO, 2012. Advanced Trauma Life Support: ATLS Student Course Manual. American College of Surgeons.

26. Tello, R.R., Braude, D., et al., 2014. Outcome of trauma patients immobilized by emergency department staff, but not by emergency medical services providers: a quality assurance initiative. Prehosp. Emerg. Care 18 (4), 544–549.

27. Clemency, B.M., Bart, J.A., et al., 2015. Patients immobilized with a long spine board rarely have unstable thoracolumbar injuries. Prehosp. Emerg. Care 20 (2), 266–272.

28. Connor, D., Greaves, I., et al. On behalf of the consensus group, Faculty of Pre-Hospital Care, 2013. Pre-hospital spinal immobilisation: an initial consensus statement. Emerg. Med. J. 30 (12), 1067–1069. doi:10.1136/emermed-2013-203207.

29. American College of Emergency Physicians, 2015. EMS Management of patients with potential spinal injury. Ann. Emerg. Med. 66 (4), 445.

30. White, C.C., IV, Domeier, R.M., et al. the Standards and Clinical Practice Committee, National Association of EMS Physicians, 2014. EMS spinal precautions and the use of the long backboard – resource document to the position statement of the National Association of EMS Physicians and the American College of Surgeons Committee on trauma. Prehosp. Emerg. Care 18 (2), 306–314.

31. Hoffman, J.R., Mower, W.R., et al., 2000. Validity of a set of clinical criteria to rule out injury to the cervical spine in patients with blunt trauma. National Emergency X-Radiography Utilization Study Group. N. Engl. J. Med. 343 (2), 94–99.

32. Stiell, I.G., Wells, G.A., et al., 2001. The Canadian C-spine rule for radiography in alert and stable trauma patients. JAMA 286 (15), 1841–1848.

33. Canadian CT Head and C-Spine (CCC) Study Group, 2002. Canadian C-Spine Rule study for alert and stable trauma patients: I. Background and rationale. CJEM 4 (2), 84–90.

34. Canadian CT Head and C-Spine (CCC) Study Group, 2002. Canadian C-Spine Rule study for alert and stable trauma patients: II. Study objectives and methodology. CJEM 4 (3), 185–193.

35. Stiell, I.G., Clement, C.M., et al., 2003. The Canadian C-spine rule versus the NEXUS low-risk criteria in patients with trauma. N. Engl. J. Med. 349 (26), 2510–2518.

36. Ahn, H., Singh, J., et al., 2011. Pre-hospital care management of a potential spinal cord injured patient: a systematic review of the literature and evidence-based guidelines. J. Neurotrauma 28, 1341–1361.

37. Dixon, M., O'Halloran, J., et al., 2015. Confirmation of suboptimal protocols in spinal immobilisation. Emerg. Med. J. 32 (12), 939–945.

38. Engsberg, J.R., Standeven, J.W., et al., 2013. Cervical spine motion during extrication. J. Emerg. Med. 44 (1), 122–127.

39. Maarouf, A., McQuown, C.M., et al., 2017. Iatrogenic spinal cord injury in a trauma patient with ankylosing spondylitis. Prehosp. Emerg. Care 21 (3), 390–394.

40. Swartz, E.E., Tucker, W.S., et al., 2018. Prehospital cervical spine motion: immobilization versus spine motion restriction. Prehosp. Emerg. Care 22 (5), 630–636.

41. Fischer, P.E., Perina, D.G., et al., 2018. Spinal motion restriction in the trauma patient – a joint position statement. Prehosp. Emerg. Care 22 (6), 659–661.

42. Theodore, N., Aarabi, B., et al., 2013. Transportation of patients with acute traumatic cervical spine injuries. Neurosurgery 72 (11), 35–39.

43. Foster, N.A., Elfenbein, D.M., et al., 2014. Comparison of helicopter versus ground transport for the interfacility transport of isolated spinal injury. Spine J. 14 (7), 1147–1154. doi:10.1016/j.spinee.2013.07.478.

44. Fleming, J., Hutton, C.F., et al., 2016. Spinal cord injuries and helicopter emergency medical services, 6,929 Patients: a Multicenter Analysis. Air Med. J. 35 (1), 33–42.

45. Ollerton, J.E., Parr, M.J.A., et al., 2006. Potential cervical spine injury and difficult airway management for emergency intubation of trauma adults in the emergency department – a systematic review. Emerg. Med. J. 23, 3–11.

46. Kovacs, G., Sowers, N., 2018. Airway management in trauma. Emerg. Med. Clin. North Am. 36, 61–84.

47. Maruyama, K., Yamada, T., et al., 2008. Randomized cross-over comparison of cervical spine motion with AirWay Scope or Macintosh laryngoscope with in-line stabilization: a video-fluoroscopic study. Br. J. Anaesth. 101 (4), 563–567.

48. Queensland Ambulance protocol. Retrrieved on 28 August 2018 from: https://www.ambulance.qld.gov.au/docs/clinical/cpp/CPP_Manual%20inline%20stabilisation.pdf.

49. Velopulos, C.G., Shihab, H.M., et al., 2018. Prehospital spine immobilization/spinal motion restriction in penetrating trauma: a practice management guideline from the Eastern Association for the Surgery of Trauma (EAST). J. Trauma Acute Care Surg. 84 (5), 736–744.

50. Mathen, R., Inaba, K., et al., 2007. Prospective evaluation of multislice computed tomography versus plain radiographic cervical spine clearance in trauma patients. J. Trauma 62 (6), 1427–1431.

51. Schenarts, P.J., Diaz, J., et al., 2001. Prospective comparison of admission computed tomographic scan and plain films of the upper cervical spine in trauma patients with altered mental status. J. Trauma 51 (4), 663–668, discussion 668–669.

52. Holmes, J.F., Akkinepalli, R., 2005. Computed tomography versus plain radiography to screen for cervical spine injury: a meta-analysis. J. Trauma 58 (5), 902–905.

53. Como, J.J., Diaz, J.J., et al., 2009. Practice management guidelines for identification of cervical spine injuries following trauma: update from the Eastern Association for the Surgery of Trauma practice management guidelines committee. J. Trauma 67 (3), 651–659.

54. Inaba, K., Byerly, S., et al., 2016. Cervical spinal clearance: a prospective Western Trauma Association Multi-institutional Trial. J. Trauma Acute Care Surg. 81 (6), 1122–1130.

55. Patel, M.B., Humble, S.S., et al., 2015. Cervical spine collar clearance in the obtunded adult blunt trauma patient. J. Trauma Acute Care Surg. 78 (2), 430–441.

56. Trauma Victoria's Spinal Trauma Guideline (ver 1.0 – 25/09/14). https://trauma.reach.vic.gov.au/sites/default/files/Spinal%20Trauma%20Guideline_Ver1.0_25092014_complete.pdf. (Accessed 8 January 2019).

57. Ryken, T.C., Hurlbert, R.J., et al., 2013. The acute cardiopulmonary management of patients with cervical spinal cord injuries. Neurosurgery 72 (3), 84–92.

58. Bracken, M.B., Collins, W.F., et al., 1984. Efficacy of methylprednisolone in acute spinal cord injury. JAMA 251, 45–52.

59. Matsumoto, T., Tamaki, T., et al., 2001. Early complications of high-dose methylprednisolone sodium succinate treatment in the follow-up of acute cervical spinal cord injury. Spine 26 (4), 426–430.

60. Canadian Association of Emergency Physicians, 2003. Steroids in acute spinal cord injury. CJEM 5 (1), 7–9.

61. Hurlbert, R.J., Hadley, M.N., et al., 2013. Pharmacological therapy for acute spinal cord injury. Neurosurgery 72 (8), 93–105.

62. Hurlbert, R.J., 2000. Methylprednisolone for acute spinal cord injury: an inappropriate standard of care. J. Neurosurg. 93 (1 Suppl.), 1–7.

63. Neurosurgical Society of Australasia, www.surgeons.org/media/425936/pos_2009-9-14_management_of_acute_neurotrauma_in_rural_and_remote_locations.pdf. (Accessed 8 January 2019).

64. Hugenholtz, H., 2003. Methylprednisolone for acute spinal cord injury: not a standard of care. CMAJ 168 (9), 1145–1146.

65. Spinal Cord Injury Thromboprophylaxis Investigators, 2003. Prevention of venous thromboembolism in the acute treatment phase after spinal cord injury: a randomized, multicenter trial comparing low-dose heparin plus intermittent pneumatic compression with enoxaparin. J. Trauma 54 (6), 1116–1124, discussion 1125–1126.

66. Dhall, S.S., Hadley, M.N., et al., 2013. Deep venous thrombosis and thromboembolism in patients with cervical spinal cord injuries. Neurosurgery 72 (3), 244–254.

67. DiGiorgio, A.M., Tsolinas, R., et al., 2017. Safety and effectiveness of early chemical deep venous thrombosis prophylaxis after spinal cord injury: pilot prospective data. Neurosurg. Focus 43 (5), E21–E24.

68. Christie, S.D., Cowie, R., 2017. Disorders of the spinal cord and nerve root. In Brocklehurst's Textbook of Geriatric Medicine and Gerontology. Fillit H, Rockwood K, Young J. 538–544.

69. Furlan, J.C., Bracken, M.B., et al., 2010. Is age a key determinant of mortality and neurological outcome after acute spinal cord injury? Neurobiol. Aging 31 (3), 434–446.

70. Underbrink, L., Dalton, A., et al., 2018. New immobilzation guidelines change EMS critical thinking in older adults with spine trauma. Prehosp. Emerg. Care 22, 637–644.

71. Copley, P.C., Tilliridou, V., et al., 2019. Management of cervical spine trauma in children. Eur. J. Trauma Emerg. Surg. 45 (5), 777–789.

72. Patel, J.C., Tepas, J.J., et al., 2001. Pediatric cervical spine injuries: defining the disease. J. Pediatr. Surg. 36 (2), 373–376.

73. Leonard, J.C., Mao, J., et al., 2012. Potential adverse effects of spinal immobilization in children. Prehosp. Emerg. Care 16 (4), 513–518.

74. Leonard, J.C., Jaffe, D.M., et al., 2015. Age-related differences in factors associated with cervical spine injuries in children. Acad. Emerg. Med. 22 (4), 441–446.

CHAPTER 3

The shifting paradigm

Camila Quel De Oliveira

INTRODUCTION: COMPENSATION VERSUS RECOVERY

Traditionally, physiotherapy or physical-based rehabilitation after spinal cord injuries (SCIs) employ interventions to achieve mobility and independence by teaching strategies to compensate for the loss of movement in the paralysed or partially paralysed body parts.[1] These strategies are focused on using the remaining available function in those parts of the body above the site of injury. These strategies include strengthening of the preserved musculature, task-specific training of bed mobility and transfers by using leverage and momentum, early prescription of orthotic devices and environmental adaptations based on the level of injury and training of wheelchair skills for locomotion. Although these strategies lead to increased independence and mobility, they do not take into consideration the body parts below the site of injury nor the potential of the spinal cord to undergo plastic changes after injury, which could lead to re-innervation of those muscles paralysed post-trauma. Hence, this does not explore the individual's full potential of recovery after injury.

It is well known that the non-use of those body parts below the level of injury can lead to health-related complications, such as muscle atrophy and contractures, reduced bone mineral density, pressure injuries, reduced peripheral circulation and, ultimately, increased risk of cardio-metabolic diseases.[2] These complications can impact upon health, increase the number of hospitalisations and reduce the lifespan after SCI (see Chapter 15 for information on ageing with an SCI). Furthermore, it has been demonstrated that deprivation from sensory and motor stimulation to the limbs can result in negative plasticity in the brain, with reduction of the areas of representation in the sensorimotor cortex.[3]

Over the past 30 years, new findings have shown that the spinal cord is not only a conduit that transports information from the brain to the periphery and vice-versa, but it also has the capacity to interpret the sensory stimulation coming from the periphery to enable movement (see Chapters 1 and 4). This occurs because of a complex network of interneurons, called central pattern generators, present at different levels of the spinal cord; these are responsible for the control of complex movements, such as reaching and walking. Furthermore, it has been found that, similarly to the brain, the spinal cord can undergo plastic changes in response to appropriate sensory cues and intense, repetitive practice.[4]

Based on this new knowledge, novel therapies have emerged, aimed at maximising recovery after SCI. This group of therapies is collectively known as activity-based therapies (ABTs) and are based on the activity-dependent plasticity of the SCI, which involves changes in the neuromuscular system driven by repetitive activity below the level of lesion.[5] By activating the body parts below the level of injury, ABTs also aim to avoid or delay the onset of secondary complications from non-use, promoting a healthier life for people with SCI.

TRADITIONAL REHABILITATION AFTER SPINAL CORD INJURIES

Individuals with SCI experience a permanent and devastating injury that affects many body systems and profoundly impacts upon quality of life and the ability to participate in the community. The most obvious impairments are paralysis of muscles and loss of sensation below the site of injury, but an SCI also affects the autonomic nervous system, resulting in impaired control of bowel, bladder, respiratory, cardiovascular and sexual function (see Chapters 4, 12, 16 and 18).[6] Those impairments reduce the individual's mobility, independence, ability to work and engage in social activities and psychological wellbeing,[7] frequently involving the immediate family, the community and society at large.

Regardless of the level or severity of injury, a period of spontaneous recovery occurs due to endogenous repair processes that involve reduction of swelling and inflammation, intact or lesioned axon collateral sprouting, synaptic rearrangements and spontaneous remyelination (see Chapter 1 for further details on these pathophysiological processes).[8] Although these processes lead to significant improvements in the acute and subacute phases (12–18 months post-injury),[9] they are insufficient to promote complete neural and functional recovery, resulting in permanent impairments and disability. Therefore, physical interventions, such as exercise and physiotherapy, play an important role in enhancing physical performance, functional activities and promoting independence after SCI.

Conventionally, the management of a person with SCI involves the determination of the person's neurological level of injury and associated functional capacity (see Chapter 4). A problem list of activity limitations and prescription for therapies can then be produced, with the overall goal of having the patient achieve their maximum functional potential, according to the overall level and severity of neurological injury.[1,10] SCI leads to impairments in many body systems and its management is complex, requiring a multidisciplinary approach, including many healthcare professionals, in addition to non-government organisations and government services.[7]

Traditional rehabilitation, or the compensatory model, is based on the concept that the spinal cord is a 'hard-wired', non-malleable and irreparable system. Although this model enables the individual to recover mobility and function, it does not remediate the disability. Furthermore, it guides clinical decision-making based solely on expected functional outcomes according to the level and severity of SCI,[11] which may distract clinicians from fully exploring further functional gains that may be possible.

Another limitation of the compensatory model is that by neglecting the paralysed areas, the deleterious effects of non-use and immobilisation are more likely to be realised. Paralysis and reduced mobility often lead to a sedentary lifestyle. Physical deconditioning contributes to the decreased level of independence and health-related functional status.[12] Because of the reduced physical capacity, people with SCI are more susceptible to cardiovascular diseases, such as obesity, diabetes, dyslipidaemia and hypertension.[13] Other secondary complications are late-life renal diseases, musculoskeletal injuries, pain and osteoporosis (see Chapter 15 for further details).[14] Therefore, physical rehabilitation after SCI not only needs to maximise functional independence, but must also focus on maintenance of optimum health and fitness by incorporating the areas below the level of injury.[2]

Even though compensation is the predominant basis of SCI rehabilitation, little is known about what specific activities and interventions comprise the rehabilitation process. There is limited evidence supporting the efficacy and the contribution of each intervention for the final outcomes of rehabilitation. Rehabilitation typically involves the simultaneous application of multiple treatments by multiple team members, with individual team members having considerable professional discretion as to what interventions to apply.[15]

Exercise therapy is often employed to improve muscle strength, regulate tone and augment muscle length and joint mobility. Moreover, increased fitness, reduction of pain and prevention of cardio-metabolic conditions are priorities. Retraining of motor tasks, such as hand and arm function, bed mobility, transfers and wheelchair use, standing and walking are frequent goals during in-patient rehabilitation (see Chapters 4 and 6 for specific retraining activities).[16] A systematic review conducted by Harvey and colleagues[17] concluded that out of the 22 most commonly administered physical therapy interventions for people with SCI, only four were clearly effective. The interventions that were proven to be effective were: fitness training, hand function, wheelchair skills training and transcutaneous electrical nerve stimulation (TENS) (see Chapter 7). The strength of the evidence was not high for any of those interventions. This demonstrates that new and effective interventions focused on neuro-recovery are required to improve rehabilitation outcomes and reduce the burden of living with an SCI.

High volumes of training (i.e. frequency and duration) have been shown to promote motor learning and skill acquisition for people with neurological conditions,[18] and therefore facilitate neuroplastic changes. However, there is no consensus in the literature about the optimal timing, intensity and duration of therapies after SCI. The volume of conventional physical interventions is usually low and varies among hospitals and countries, according to the funding available and healthcare policies.[15]

A multicentre study conducted across Netherlands, Australia and Norway revealed that the time (in minutes) spent during each exercise session was less than one hour. Australia had the longest session duration among the countries surveyed, with each lasting 43 minutes. Furthermore, the mean weekly time spent in physical therapy across the three countries was 5.4 hours,[19] demonstrating that exercise and physiotherapy are delivered at very low doses that may not be sufficient to promote changes in the nervous system that could lead to recovery after injury.

THE ACTIVITY-DEPENDENT PLASTICITY OF THE SPINAL CORD

As discussed earlier, physical rehabilitation after SCI has been based on the premise that the spinal cord is incapable or has a very limited capacity to repair itself after injury.[11] Hence, it is focused on teaching patients compensatory strategies because recovery is often considered an unrealistic goal. However, advances in neuroscience research have shown that a high level of functional recovery can be achieved even years after SCI (see Chapter 1 for further details on the neuropathological and recovery processes).[20]

Historically, the role of the spinal cord has been described as a bundle of axons that transmit information from the periphery to the brain and vice-versa, with the brain being the centre of control for movement and sensation. The role of the spinal cord on the control of movement was described as restricted to reflex activity. Spinal reflexes were described as rapid, stereotyped, automatic responses to specific stimuli to preserve homeostasis by making rapid adjustments in the function of organs and organ systems, the idea being that they were triggered by a single input that always produced the same motor response.[21] This hierarchical model, which has been proven to be not entirely correct, has substantially underestimated the spinal cord's ability to control postural and complex motor tasks such as locomotion[22] and reaching.[23]

Central pattern generators

There is extensive evidence, dating back more than 100 years, that the spinal cord has a network of interneurons that can generate an automatic cyclic motor output that enables stepping. Those circuits, called central pattern generators (CPGs), are present in the spinal cord of all mammals, including humans.[24] More recently, research has shown that those neural circuits are more sophisticated than it was initially believed and can actually use ensembles of sensory information to generate appropriate motor responses without input from supraspinal centres. This property of the spinal cord shows a level of automaticity, which is the ability of the neural circuitry of the spinal cord to interpret complex sensory information in its context and to make appropriate decisions about how the motor behaviour will be elicited. The automaticity of motor control in the spinal cord relies on the CPG's responses to sensory input during postural and complex motor tasks, such as locomotion, in both animals and humans.[25]

Studies with animals and humans have shown that effective standing and walking occurs with considerable precision and discrimination without conscious thought, which demonstrates the sophisticated level of automaticity of the spinal cord.[26] This suggests that there is significant potential for sensorimotor recovery if the CPGs or their residual components are functionally optimised following SCI.[27] Studies with mammals proved that the lumbosacral spinal cord can regain the ability to generate weight-bearing locomotion after a complete spinal cord transection when the correct sensory stimuli are given and when exposure to repetitive training occurs. When spinal rats and cats were provided with support on trunk and manually assisted loading and stepping over a treadmill, they were able to generate hind-limb stepping response. Furthermore, the animals were able to adjust their cadence and step length according to the treadmill speed. All of this was achieved in the absence of suprasegmental input.[28] This phenomenon of appropriately responding to sensory inputs illustrates the capacity of the neural network at the level of the spinal cord to integrate incoming information, interpret it and respond with a motor output.

The same strategies have been applied to humans after SCI, based on the growing evidence that suggests that the human spinal networks have similar neuronal properties to animals. The presence of CPGs and the ability of the spinal cord to relearn when provided with sensory information related to a specific motor task has been reported in humans.[24] The human spinal cord has the capacity of integrating and interpreting complex sensory signals to produce functional motor output and to adapt to repetitive training.[29] Moreover, it has been postulated that plasticity and motor learning in the spinal cord are a result of the association of specific sensory inputs with repetitive performance of a motor task.[25]

This new knowledge on the role and plasticity of the spinal networks when applied to activity and training following injury can lead to important functional recovery. Translational research has shown that intensive training and sensory cues are key factors to yielding the activity-dependent plasticity in the spinal cord. Training and exercise appear to play an important role in enabling spinal plasticity by inducing changes at the cellular and molecular levels. In addition, proprioceptive and cutaneous feedback are necessary to reprogram the spared circuits by rebalancing changes in excitatory and inhibitory input, as well as promoting the reconfiguration of the spinal reflexes and interneuron networks (CPGs). The repeated activation of the CPGs via sensory stimuli would seem to be the mechanism underlying the plasticity in the spinal cord that leads to recovery after injury.[22,25] The physiological mechanisms behind spinal cord plasticity are possibly related to changes in the cerebral cortex, growth of new axonal branches, remodelling of synapses, changes in neuronal excitability and modulation of neurotransmitters in the spinal cord.[30]

It has been suggested that the type and intensity of motor training and sensory stimulation provided following the injury may to some extent influence the degree of motor recovery.[31] As such, repetitive physical training can be critical for promoting changes to the spinal networks that will result in functional recovery. There is evidence demonstrating the capacity of the human spinal cord to respond to inputs and adapt after injury. This plasticity can be induced by physical activity, thus leading to sensorimotor recovery after injury.[32] Therefore, physical interventions aimed to optimise the neuroplasticity mechanisms of the spinal cord should be implemented as a rehabilitation tool to promote and maximise functional recovery after SCI.[27]

THE RECOVERY MODEL: ACTIVITY-BASED THERAPIES (ABTS)

In contrast to the traditional compensatory approach, activity-based interventions aim to optimise the recovery of the nervous system. These interventions are based on the activity-dependent recovery principle that the spinal cord is plastic and can learn after injury. This new model of rehabilitation is described as activity-based therapies (ABTs).[27] ABT is used as an umbrella term to describe interventions that are targeted mainly at the paralysed and partially paralysed body parts with the aim of maximising recovery. The activation of the central nervous system through intense task-specific practice is the foundation for therapeutic interventions that target recovery.[5]

Exercise targeted at the body parts below the SCI has promoted neuroplastic changes at cellular and biochemical levels in animal models[33] and has led to cortical changes in humans with incomplete injuries.[34,35] Besides preserving muscle mass and restoring motor and sensory function, exercise can induce synaptic plasticity by increasing the concentration of neurotrophic factors and the number of regenerating neurons.[32] This exercise-induced plasticity and the emerging concepts that the spinal cord has the capacity to undergo plastic changes and to control complex movements provides the theoretical foundation for ABT interventions.

Backus and colleagues[36] defined ABT as:

> any intervention that specifically uses tools and interventions to improve muscle activation or sensory function below the level of injury in the spinal cord, and does not rely on compensatory

mechanisms for improving function after SCI. Such an approach includes interventions that combine intensive active movement with one or more of the following: facilitation techniques (use of tactile or vibratory stimulation); electrical stimulation applied to muscles or nerves (surface or indwelling); body-weight supported locomotor training (manual or robotic); use of upper extremity robotics; or massed practice training.

ABT interventions aim to retrain the nervous system, and therefore require high-intensity practice, involving a high number of repetitions and high frequency.[11,27] ABT performed for 1.5 to 5 hours per day at a frequency of three to five times per week produced benefits in people with chronic SCI that included improved lower limb muscle strength, balance, mobility, increased gait speed, symmetry and endurance.[37]

Another key principle of ABT is the use of sensory cues as a rehabilitation tool. While the compensatory model often ignores the body parts below the level of injury with respect to sensory information, ABT interventions rely on providing a myriad of sensory stimuli to promote neuromuscular activation. Any orthotic device prescribed after SCI to stabilise the paralysed areas for function can restrict possible movement in the joints, possibly leading to reduced proprioceptive and cutaneous feedback. Furthermore, traditional exercise prescription can be limited to the wheelchair or positions with no or minimal load bearing to the paralysed areas, limiting the sensory input to those areas. ABT interventions aim to maximise the sensory cues to the nervous system via manual guidance, weight-bearing, appropriate kinematics of the desired movement and proprioceptive input to tendons and muscles.

Traditional physiotherapy techniques that rely on providing sensory input to facilitate movement, such as proprioceptive neuromuscular facilitation (PNF), use of vibration and cutaneous tactile stimulation with different textures, when applied to the body parts below injury, can provide important sensory cues to the spinal cord and facilitate movement. Furthermore, exercising in sensory enriched environments, such as in a hydrotherapy pool (see Chapter 10), may also be an important cutaneous stimulus to facilitate movement. Sensory cues have an important role in changing the physiological state of the spinal circuitry. Following an upper motor neuron spinal injury (above the lumbosacral levels), the feedback loop between afferent and efferent nerves (arc reflex) remains intact and able to generate a motor output in response to sensory stimuli.[38] However, the injury decreases the central state of excitability of the spinal cord, hindering a more complex motor response. Task-specific sensory cues have been shown to increase the central state of excitability of the spinal cord, enabling voluntary movement even in those with severe injuries.[39] The central state of excitability of the spinal cord seems to be a critical factor in recovery of movement after SCI. The activity-dependent plasticity in the spinal cord can be driven by neuromuscular activation below the injury, using task-specific sensory cues. The 'retrained' nervous system, then, must adapt in the home and community for functional integration. The level of success is dependent on the spinal networks maintaining the appropriate central state of excitability for the desired task.[4,5]

There is growing evidence in both adults and children that the use of regular and intense ABT directed at activating the paralysed extremities can promote neurological improvements.[40,41] Inherently, ABT is a cluster of previously used evidence-based interventions developed to target impairments above and below the site of SCI to reduce the impact of disability and increase activity and participation levels.[42] So far, this novel intervention has shown greater benefits if applied during the early phases following injury and for individuals with incomplete injuries (see Chapter 11).[36]

Individuals with SCI who have completed in-hospital rehabilitation programs and transitioned back to the community have shown increased interest in being involved in this type of therapy. The costs and the time commitments of participation in ABT programs are high, raising concerns from the medical and allied-health community about creating unrealistic expectations for recovery and delaying return to a productive community life. Additionally, the benefits of increased physical rehabilitation for some patients, particularly those with motor complete injuries (ISNCSCI A and B), remains unproven.

In recent years, there has been an increase in the numbers of incomplete SCIs worldwide when compared to complete injuries.[43] Various factors have collaborated to this shift and include better understanding of the injury mechanisms that lead to improved on-site care from the paramedical teams; increased awareness and education of the population on how to act and assist the victim after trauma; implementation of protocols for early intervention and better management of patients in acute care (see Chapter 2). Acute medical management of people with SCI currently focuses on minimising further neurological damage to the spinal cord and optimise recovery (see Chapter 4 for further detail). Neuroprotective strategies such as early spinal decompression, pharmacological interventions and intra-operative temperature management[44] have been successful in reducing the secondary neuronal damage due to vascular mechanisms, inflammatory response and apoptosis, hence minimising the damage to the spinal cord (see Chapter 1 for further explanation).[45]

Post-mortem research on humans post-injury has demonstrated that the spinal cord is rarely completely severed following blunt trauma, with central nervous tissue connectivity being preserved in over 50% of the injuries classified as clinically complete.[46] The term 'discomplete' refers to the group of patients that present with clinically undetectable motor or sensory function below the site of injury, but have some intact axonal pathways that have been spared from damage. However, those connections are not strong enough to produce movement or sensation. Residual subclinical motor control[47] and sensory function[48] were observed in clinically complete SCI. Hence, there is a potential for those partially preserved pathways to be targeted with ABT interventions to maximise recovery, even in people diagnosed as complete SCI.

To date, the most frequently investigated ABT intervention has been locomotor training (LT) (see Chapter 9). While there is substantial proof to support the benefits of LT on recovery of standing, walking and balance for people with motor incomplete SCI,[40,49] its effectiveness for people with motor complete injuries and its possible benefits in areas unrelated to ambulatory capacity remains unclear. ABT interventions focused on the upper limb, such as neuromuscular electrical stimulation, robotics and massed practice, have proven to be successful in improving upper limb strength, mobility, independence and hand function (see Chapter 17 for further details on rehabilitation of the upper limb).[50]

A secondary aim of ABT interventions is to delay and prevent secondary health complications that result from an SCI, such as deleterious changes in muscle, bone and circulation. The maintenance of optimum health by targeting systems below the level of injury seems to be essential for improvements in glucose and fat metabolism, muscle and bone composition.[2] ABT interventions, such as functional electrical stimulation (FES) (see Chapter 7) and body-weight supported treadmill training, demonstrated improvement in cardiorespiratory and vascular function, which may attenuate the risk of

cardiovascular diseases.[51] However, when applied in a multimodal combination or at lower intensities, ABT interventions did not promote changes in body composition, nor metabolic profile.[52]

ABT strategies, such as FES, load bearing and sensory stimulation of the paralysed extremities, can be easily incorporated in rehabilitation settings without increasing costs or the burden to the therapists. More costly strategies such as LT could be incorporated in in-patient and outpatient settings as block-therapy (high-frequency and intensity for a set amount of weeks) or as an adjunct to current rehabilitation strategies (low-frequency, but throughout the whole rehabilitation), thus minimising the financial burden to the health system and to the person with SCI.

Overall, ABT seems to be a promising rehabilitation strategy to maximise neurological recovery, even years after injury, and to offset the rapid ageing, the physical deterioration and secondary complications associated with SCI. However, further research is needed to investigate its effects on independence, quality of life, social participation and functional outcomes rather then walking ability and changes in the ISNCSCI motor score. Table 3.1 outlines the main differences between compensatory therapy and ABT.

Table 3.1 Main differences between the compensatory and the recovery models

	Conventional therapy	Activity-based therapy
Aim	Activation of the nervous system above the level of injury	Activation of the nervous system above and below the level of injury
Principles	Spinal cord is a 'hard-wired' structure	Spinal cord is 'smart' and has the ability to learn
Goals	Achieve optimal functional capacity according to the level and severity of injury. Compensate for loss of function.	Promote recovery regardless of the level or severity of injury. Restore lost function
Intensity	Low: 1–2 hours per day	High: 1.5 to 5 hours per day
Training strategies	Task-specific (non-patterned movements)	Task-specific and patterned activity above and below the level of lesion
Adaptive devices	Early prescription of adaptive devices to allow for mobility and independence (i.e. wheelchair, lower limb orthosis)	Prescribed when recovery is not achieved. Least restrictive device is recommended

ACTIVITY-BASED THERAPIES MODALITIES

Functional electrical stimulation (FES)

FES consists of an electrical current applied to the skin that elicits involuntary muscle contractions (see Chapter 7). It has largely been used in other populations to increase muscle strength. When applied to the muscles affected by the SCI, FES is considered to be an ABT modality and has been widely investigated. In individuals with SCI, FES aims to recruit the paralysed or partially paralysed muscles or to provide sensory stimulation to the nerves enabling voluntary movement. FES has been shown to improve voluntary strength of muscles directly affected by SCI[53] and improve function and independence during activities of daily living.[54] The technique has been used to promote cycling and stepping, aiming to stimulate the CPG and elicit neural plasticity.[55] FES has also been found to lead to cardiovascular and haemodynamic benefits, reverse muscle atrophy,[56] increase bone mass, reduce spasticity and neurogenic pain, prevent pressure sores and improve psychosocial outcomes such as self-image and depression for people with complete and incomplete injuries.[57]

Weight-bearing

Weight-bearing on the paralysed or partially paralysed limbs is another component of ABT interventions (see Chapter 6). Few studies to date have investigated the effects of loading the extremities for people with SCI. Benefits related to improved bowel and bladder function, bone mineral density,[58] decreased number of pressure injuries, improved joint range of motion, prevention of muscle contractures, enhanced autonomic and cardiovascular function[59] and effects on spasticity,[60] motor function and quality of life have all been reported.[61]

ABT incorporates exercises in positions that allow weight-bearing through lower limbs, whole-body coordination exercises and task-specific training in positions where the trunk must work against gravity. Therefore, ABT can contribute to increased strength

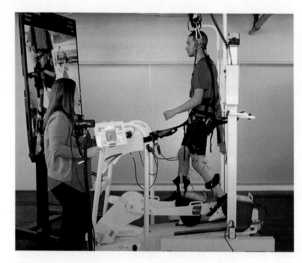

Figure 3.1 FES-assisted stepping. Device: RT 600.
Source: © Restorative Therapies

and control of trunk musculature, which contributes to better posture, general mobility and independence.

Patients train in positions such as: four-point kneeling, kneeling, standing with partial or full body weight while performing active-assisted exercises; resistance training; and neuromuscular electrical stimulation, balance and coordination tasks. All of the exercises are performed out of the wheelchair, incorporating whole-body movements.

It should be highlighted that exercising in standing is important, even when standing is not a functional goal, due to the benefits described above. Furthermore, exercise in standing can improve trunk control, which may translate to better posture and balance when sitting[62] or pushing a wheelchair.

Robotics

Robot-assisted training is a novel rehabilitation strategy for people with neurological conditions. In SCI, robotics can be applied to the affected body regions to allow for intensive functional training (massed practice), offering a high volume of training without continuous involvement of a therapist.

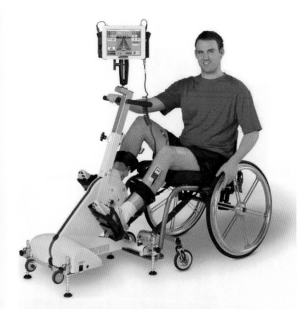

Figure 3.2 FES-assisted cycling, paraplegia. Device RT 300.

Source: © Restorative Therapies

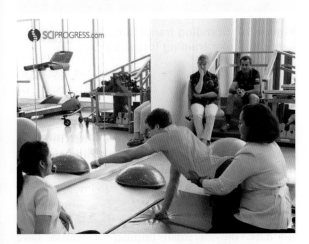

Figure 3.3 Load bearing to upper and lower limbs to increase trunk activation. T3 paraplegia.

Source: © SCI Progress.com

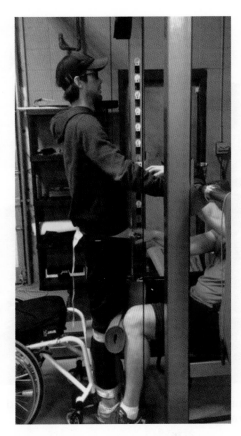

Figure 3.4 Upper limb strengthening in standing. C7 incomplete tetraplegia.

Preliminary evidence has shown that robot-assisted exercise therapy in people with SCI is safe, and reduces the need for therapist supervision (available robotic locomotor training devices for the lower limbs are discussed in Chapter 9).[63]

Evidence acquired while investigating the effects of robotic training for the lower limbs in people with SCI has demonstrated increased independence and endurance during walking,[64] reduction of pain perception and spasticity, improved sensation (proprioception, temperature, vibration and pressure), increased electrical activity at muscular and cortical level, improvements in sitting posture, intestinal, cardiorespiratory, metabolic, physiological and psychological functions.[65] Similarly, positive

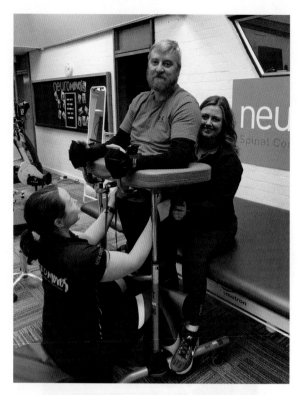

Figure 3.5 Standing with walking frame and therapist support. Complete tetraplegia.

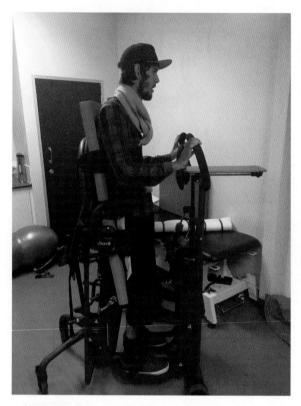

Figure 3.7 Standing frame that allows for cardiovascular training (cross trainer). C6 tetraplegia.

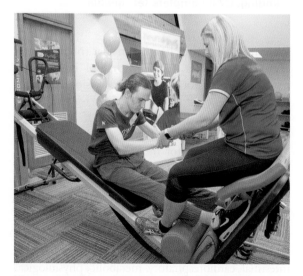

Figure 3.6 Partial load bearing. Paraplegia.

results have been found when robotic training has been applied to the upper limbs. Improvements in range of motion, sensation, muscle strength, arm and hand function and functional independence have been described.[63]

Research considerations of ABT in SCI

To date, only a small number of studies have investigated the effects of multimodal ABT interventions for people with chronic SCI, as they are currently delivered in most community-based centres. Hence, there is a gap between the literature and clinical practice.

The current literature is heavily focused on applying ABT interventions that improve ISNCSCI

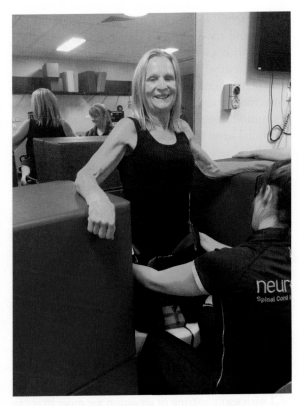

Figure 3.8 Assisted standing. Tetraplegia.

individuals. In addition, exercising in standing may have effects on psychological outcomes, promoting greater quality of life and wellbeing.[60,61] Future qualitative studies should investigate not only the effects of a multimodal ABT exercise program on outcomes related to physical abilities, but also its impact on psychological wellbeing, quality of life and community participation.

Another downfall of current studies is that trials often fail to deliver ABT at high duration and high frequencies of four to five times per week, as recommended in order to achieve activity-dependent plasticity in the spinal cord. Research has shown that 60 to 100 ABT sessions are necessary to promote neurological recovery in individuals with chronic SCI.[40] Future studies aimed at assessing neurological recovery after SCI should have longer and higher intensity training protocols.

ABT programs worldwide

In Europe, the UK and the United States, ABT interventions are often incorporated into management plans throughout the acute and subacute spinal cord rehabilitation hospitals and outpatient clinics. Those interventions are delivered mostly at high intensity to maximise rehabilitation outcomes and reduce length of stay. In Australia, ABT has yet to become entrenched as a routine practice within the acute spinal cord rehabilitation hospitals. However, there is a growing number of subacute and outpatient clinics beginning to incorporate ABT as the basis of their intervention philosophy.

This shifting paradigm has seen a number of ABT programs gain popularity as they provide an avenue for patients with SCIs and healthcare providers to explore the health benefits and the possible neurological and functional benefits post-SCI. The first enterprise to really embrace this concept in Australia was NeuroMoves (formerly known as Walk On). NeuroMoves was established in 2008 by Spinal Cord Injuries Australia (SCIA), a non-government consumer association for people with SCI, in response to requests from people with SCI to participate in an ABT programs after their

scores as a measure of neurological recovery. However, strategies to effectively measure and monitor the overall impact of SCI on people's lives and the holistic effects of interventions have been poorly explored. Future studies in ABT should use the World Health Organization International Classification of Functioning, Disability and Health (WHO–ICF) as a theoretical framework to choose outcome variables in all three ICF domains (1 function of the body structure; 2 activities; and 3 participation).[66]

Most studies in ABT assessed outcomes related to lower limb mobility such as walking, standing and balance. However, ABT involves the practice of intense exercise, performed out of the wheelchair, in various body positions, mostly against gravity, which can improve trunk control and posture,[62] increasing functional capacity of wheelchair-bound

discharge from hospital. In Australia, there are now several other programs, such as Making Strides and The Next Step, that also offer outpatient ABT-based programs. All these programs design individually tailored exercise regimens, prescribed by exercise physiologists and physiotherapists, to improve exercise and functional abilities post-discharge from SCI rehabilitation hospitals.

NEUROMODULATION

Neuromodulation is the most recent addition to the list of potential treatments to reduce the impairments and impact of an SCI. It consists of applying gentle electrical currents to stimulate the remaining circuits below the point of injury, allowing those circuits to receive and act upon messages coming from the brain. To achieve this, a stimulation device is implanted into the epidural surface of the spinal cord, delivering electrical pulses. The electrical impulses have also been successfully applied to the spinal cord transcutaneously, avoiding the need for surgical intervention.[67]

The electrical current applied to the spinal cord reactivates the neuron networks that were silent after injury by raising the level of excitability of the spinal circuitry,[68] hence enabling movement and facilitating activity-dependent re-organisation of the spinal neuronal network via the propriospinal network.[39] As described by the pioneer in this technique, Professor Reggie Edgerton, 'the stimulator acts as a hearing aid for the spinal cord; without it, the spinal cord cannot hear the messages coming from the brain'.[39]

Repetitive exercise and intensive training have been shown to be crucial in enabling movement and leading to functional improvements in association with neuromodulation. Recent studies using epidural stimulation in people with motor complete injury have demonstrated latent voluntary control below the level of injury that resulted in recovery of walking. Participants with complete chronic thoracic injuries (AIS A) received epidural stimulation to the lumbosacral spinal cord associated with intense locomotor training for 24 to 85 weeks, and have regained the ability to walk over ground with a walking frame or the ability to stand independently.[68,69]

When applied to the cervical spinal of individuals with motor complete tetraplegia (ISNCSCI B), neuromodulation has been shown to improve volitional hand strength, coordination and accuracy as well as increase independence in functional tasks such as drinking from a cup, dressing, grooming, transferring and mobility in bed. Those benefits persisted even when the stimulation was removed.[23] Studies have also demonstrated that epidural stimulation applied to the lumbosacral spine led to improvements in autonomic function, resulting in enhanced temperature control, bowel, bladder and sexual function.[70-72] Improvements in cardiovascular function and blood pressure control have also been reported.[73] Those benefits may be attributed to the activation of the interneural networks in the spinal cord by the electrical stimulation through the dorsal nerve roots and by direct stimulation of the parenchyma of the spinal cord. As such, people with SCI with some sparing of sensation are more likely to be suitable candidates for this type of intervention.[74]

Another promising application of neuromodulation is in association with stem cells. The electrical stimulation applied to the spinal cord can maintain and increase the activity of the neuron circuitry. Appropriate neural activity is a prerequisite for stem cells to improve function in the damaged central nervous system. Neural activity is critical for avoiding cell death, improving blood circulation and maintaining the health of neurons. It is also important for regulation of brain-derived neurotrophic factor (BDNF), which is essential for plasticity and recovery.[75] Furthermore, electrical stimulation has been shown to facilitate neural stem cells to migrate directionally and differentiate into neurons ex-vivo, paving the way for regenerative medicine for CNS disorders in vivo.[75] Although the association of electrical stimulation and stem cells seems promising for recovery after SCI, further studies are needed to demonstrate its efficacy in humans.

Evidence-based practice points

- In the light of new knowledge on the plasticity of the spinal cord, treatment of individuals with SCIs is moving away from compensation techniques and towards recovery techniques.
- These techniques are built upon ABTs, which facilitate activation of the nervous system above and below the level of injury.
- ABTs incorporate whole-body exercises, targeted to improve function to the body parts above and below the site of injury.
- Neurological recovery has been seen in individuals with motor incomplete injuries following ABT interventions, mainly after locomotor training. However, improved mobility (balance in sitting) and general health benefits have also been reported in complete injuries.
- ABT requires intensive practice, which is not always feasible in hospital and outpatient settings.
- Advances in technology (robotics and neuromodulation) are promising strategies to promote recovery and minimise the burden of disability for those living with an SCI.

SUMMARY

The field of rehabilitation after SCI is rapidly evolving. New advances in surgical interventions, cell therapy and neuromodulation are giving hope to people living with an SCI. Exercise will play an even more important role in restoring function after those new interventions are applied. Physiotherapists will then be responsible for harnessing the potential of these therapies via intensive rehabilitation involving the paralysed body parts below the site of injury. Focusing on compensatory strategies, targeting only the preserved body parts after injury and establishing patients' outcomes according to their level of injury will soon be an outdated approach.

It is worth noting that physical rehabilitation after SCI needs to move beyond the goal of maximising independence to focus on maintenance of optimum health and fitness, as well as maintenance of system function below the level of injury.[2] This would reduce the secondary complication of paralysis and give individuals better opportunities to benefit from those emerging treatment strategies.

If emerging technologies can be effectively associated with intensive physical therapy to induce activity-dependent plasticity in the spinal cord and remodelling of injured tissues, regenerative rehabilitation therapies may soon dramatically improve outcomes and participation for people with SCI.[75]

References

1. Brown, J.M., Deriso, D.M., et al., 2012. From contemporary rehabilitation to restorative neurology. Clin. Neurol. Neurosurg. 114 (5), 471–474.

2. Galea, M.P., 2012. Spinal cord injury and physical activity: preservation of the body. Spinal Cord 50 (5), 344–351.

3. Nudo, R.J., Milliken, G.W., et al., 1996. Use-dependent alterations of movement representations in primary motor cortex of adult squirrel monkeys. J. Neurosci. 16 (2), 785–807.

4. Edgerton, V.R., Tillakaratne, N.J., et al., 2004. Plasticity of the spinal neural circuitry after injury. Annu. Rev. Neurosci. 27, 145–167.

5. Behrman, A.L., Ardolino, E.M., et al., 2017. Activity-based therapy: from basic science to clinical application for recovery

after spinal cord injury. J. Neurol. Phys. Ther. 41 (Suppl. 3 Supplement, IV STEP Special Issue), S39–S45.

6. Nandoe Tewarie, R.D., Hurtado, A., et al., 2010. A clinical perspective of spinal cord injury. Neurorehabilitation 27 (2), 129–139.

7. Harvey, L.A., 2016. Physiotherapy rehabilitation for people with spinal cord injuries. J. Physiother. 62 (1), 4–11.

8. Onifer, S.M., Smith, G.M., et al., 2011. Plasticity after spinal cord injury: relevance to recovery and approaches to facilitate it. Neurother. 8 (2), 283–293.

9. Burns, A.S., Marino, R.J., et al., 2012. Clinical diagnosis and prognosis following spinal cord injury. Handb. Clin. Neurol. 109, 47–62.

10. Sipski, M.L., Richards, J.S., 2006. Spinal cord injury rehabilitation. Am. J. Phys. Med. Rehabil. 85 (4), 310–342.

11. Behrman, A.L., Bowden, M.G., et al., 2006. Neuroplasticity after spinal cord injury and training: an emerging paradigm shift in rehabilitation and walking recovery. Phys. Ther. 86 (10), 1406–1425.

12. Haisma, J.A., Post, M.W., et al., 2008. Functional independence and health-related functional status following spinal cord injury: a prospective study of the association with physical capacity. J. Rehabil. Med. 40 (10), 812–818.

13. Bauman, W.A., Spungen, A.M., 2000. Metabolic changes in persons after spinal cord injury. Phys. Med. Rehabil. Clin. N. Am. 11 (1), 109–140.

14. Bauman, W.A., Spungen, A.M., 2001. Body composition in aging: adverse changes in able-bodied persons and in those with spinal cord injury. Top. Spinal Cord Inj. Rehabil. 6 (3), 22–36.

15. Burns, A.S., Marino, R.J., et al., 2017. Type and timing of rehabilitation following acute and subacute spinal cord injury: a systematic review. Global Spine J. 7, 175S–194S.

16. Harvey, L.A., Lin, C.W., et al., 2009. The effectiveness of physical interventions for people with spinal cord injuries: a systematic review. Spinal Cord 47 (3), 184–195.

17. Harvey, L.A., Glinsky, J.V., et al., 2016. The effectiveness of 22 commonly administered physiotherapy interventions for people with spinal cord injury: a systematic review. Spinal Cord 54 (11), 914–923.

18. Waddell, K.J., Birkenmeier, R.L., et al., 2014. Feasibility of high-repetition, task-specific training for individuals with upper-extremity paresis. Am. J. Occup. Ther. 68 (4), 444–453.

19. Van Langeveld, S.A., Post, M.W., et al., 2011. Comparing content of therapy for people with a spinal cord injury in postacute inpatient rehabilitation in Australia, Norway, and the Netherlands. Phys. Ther. 91 (2), 210–223.

20. Kirshblum, S.C., O'Connor, K.C., 2000. Levels of spinal cord injury and predictors of neurologic recovery. Phys. Med. Rehabil. Clin. N. Am. 11 (1), 1–27.

21. Martini, F.H., Nath, J.L., et al., 2012. Fundamentals of Anatomy and Physiology, ninth ed. Pearson, United States.

22. Roy, R.R., Harkema, S.J., et al., 2012. Basic concepts of activity-based interventions for improved recovery of motor function after spinal cord injury. Arch. Phys. Med. Rehabil. 93 (9), 1487–1497.

23. Lu, D.C., Edgerton, V.R., et al., 2016. Engaging cervical spinal cord networks to reenable volitional control of hand function in tetraplegic patients. Neurorehabil. Neural Repair 30 (10), 951–962.

24. Dimitrijevic, M.R., Gerasimenko, Y., et al., 1998. Evidence for a spinal central pattern generator in humans. In: Kiehn, O., HarrisWarrick, R.M., et al. (Eds.), Neuronal Mechanisms for Generating Locomotor Activity. Annals of the New York Academy of Sciences, New York. pp. 360–376.

25. Edgerton, V.R., Roy, R.R., 2009. Activity-dependent plasticity of spinal locomotion: implications for sensory processing. Exerc. Sport Sci. Rev. 37 (4), 171–178.

26. Barriere, G., Leblond, H., et al., 2008. Prominent role of the spinal central pattern generator in the recovery of locomotion after partial spinal cord injuries. J. Neurosci. 28 (15), 3976–3987.

27. Edgerton, V.R., Kim, S.J., et al., 2006. Rehabilitative therapies after spinal cord injury. J. Neurotrauma 23 (3–4), 560–570.

28. Barbeau, H., Fung, J., et al., 2002. A review of the adaptability and recovery of locomotion after spinal cord injury. In: McKerracher, L., Doucet, G., et al. (Eds.), Spinal Cord Trauma: Regeneration, Neural Repair and Functional Recovery. Progress in Brain Research. 137. Elsevier Science Bv, Amsterdam, pp. 9–25.

29. Harkema, S.J., 2001. Neural plasticity after human spinal cord injury: application of locomotor training to the rehabilitation of walking. Neuroscientist 7 (5), 455–468.

30. Fouad, K., Tse, A., 2008. Adaptive changes in the injured spinal cord and their role in promoting functional recovery. Neurol. Res. 30 (1), 17–27.

31. Fouad, K., Krajacic, A., et al., 2011. Spinal cord injury and plasticity: opportunities and challenges. Brain Res. Bull. 84 (4–5), 337–342.

32. Sandrow-Feinberg, H.R., Houle, J.D., 2015. Exercise after spinal cord injury as an agent for neuroprotection, regeneration and rehabilitation. Brain Res. 1619, 12–21.

33. Tillakaratne, N.J., Guu, J.J., et al., 2010. Functional recovery of stepping in rats after a complete neonatal spinal cord transection is not due to regrowth across the lesion site. Neuroscience 166 (1), 23–33.

34. Beekhuizen, K.S., Field-Fote, E.C., 2005. Massed practice versus massed practice with stimulation: effects on upper extremity function and cortical plasticity in individuals with incomplete cervical spinal cord injury. Neurorehabil. Neural Repair 19 (1), 33–45.

35. Chisholm, A.E., Peters, S., et al., 2015. Short-term cortical plasticity associated with feedback-error learning after locomotor training in a patient with incomplete spinal cord injury. Phys. Ther. 95 (2), 257–266.

36. Backus, D., Apple, D., et al., n.d. Systematic review of activity-based interventions to improve neurological outcomes after SCI January 1998 – March 2009. In: Disability research right to know. www.bu.edu/drrk/research-syntheses/spinal-cord-injuries/activity-based-interventions.

37. Fritz, S., Merlo-Rains, A., et al., 2011. An intensive intervention for improving gait, balance, and mobility in individuals with chronic incomplete spinal cord injury: a pilot study of activity tolerance and benefits. Arch. Phys. Med. Rehabil. 92 (11), 1776–1784.

38. Edgerton, V.R., Courtine, G., et al., 2008. Training locomotor networks. Brain Res. Rev. 57 (1), 241–254.

39. Angeli, C.A., Edgerton, V.R., et al., 2014. Altering spinal cord excitability enables voluntary movements after chronic complete paralysis in humans. Brain 137, 1394–1409.

40. Harkema, S.J., Schmidt-Read, M., et al., 2012. Balance and ambulation improvements in individuals with chronic incomplete spinal cord injury using locomotor training-based rehabilitation. Arch. Phys. Med. Rehabil. 93 (9), 1508–1517.

41. Fox, E.J., Tester, N.J., et al., 2010. Ongoing walking recovery 2 years after locomotor training in a child with severe incomplete spinal cord injury. Phys. Ther. 90 (5), 793–802.

42. Padula, N., Costa, M., et al., 2015. Long-term effects of an intensive interventional training program based on activities for individuals with spinal cord injury: a pilot study. Physiother. Theory Pract. 31 (8), 568–574.

43. National Spinal Cord Injury Statistical Center, 2015. Facts and Figures at a Glance. University of Alabama, Birmingham.

44. Kraft, J., Karpenko, A., et al., 2016. Intraoperative targeted temperature management in acute brain and spinal cord injury. Curr. Neurol. Neurosci. Rep. 16 (2), 18.

45. Wilson, J.R., Fehlings, M.G., 2012. Management strategies to optimize clinical outcomes after acute traumatic spinal cord injury: integration of medical and surgical approaches. J. Neurosurg. Sci. 56 (1), 1–11.

46. Kakulas, B.A., 1999. A review of the neuropathology of human spinal cord injury with emphasis on special features. J. Spinal Cord Med. 22 (2), 119–124.

47. McKay, W.B., Lim, H.K., et al., 2004. Clinical neurophysiological assessment of residual motor control in post-spinal cord injury paralysis. Neurorehabil. Neural Repair 18 (3), 144–153.

48. Wrigley, P.J., Siddall, P.J., et al., 2018. New evidence for preserved somatosensory pathways in complete spinal cord injury: a fMRI study. Hum. Brain Mapp. 39 (1), 588–598.

49. Hicks, A., Adams, M., et al., 2005. Long-term body-weight-supported treadmill training and subsequent follow-up in persons with chronic SCI: effects on functional walking ability and measures of subjective well-being. Spinal Cord 43 (5), 291–298.

50. Lu, X., Battistuzzo, C.R., et al., 2015. Effects of training on upper limb function after cervical spinal cord injury: a systematic review. Clin. Rehabil. 29 (1), 3–13.

51. Backus, D., Apple, D., et al., 2011. Health-related outcomes after lower extremity and walking activity-based interventions for persons with spinal cord injury: a research synthesis. Top. Spinal Cord Inj. Rehabil. 16, 73.

52. Astorino, T.A., Harness, E.T., et al., 2015. Chronic activity-based therapy does not improve body composition, insulin-like growth factor-I, adiponectin, or myostatin in persons with spinal cord injury. J. Spinal Cord Med. 38 (5), 615–625.

53. Aravind, N., Harvey, L.A., et al., 2019. Physiotherapy interventions for increasing muscle strength in people with spinal cord injuries: a systematic review. Spinal Cord. 57 (6), 449–460.

54. Popovic, M., Kapadia, N., et al., 2014. Improving voluntary upper limb function in individuals with chronic incomplete spinal cord injury. J. Spinal Cord Med. 37 (5), 637.

55. Griffin, L., Decker, M.J., et al., 2009. Functional electrical stimulation cycling improves body composition, metabolic and neural factors in persons with spinal cord injury. J. Electromyogr. Kinesiol. 19 (4), 614–622.

56. Bochkezanian, V., Newton, R.U., et al., 2018. Effects of neuromuscular electrical stimulation in people with spinal cord injury. Med. Sci. Sports Exerc. 50 (9), 1733–1739.

57. Hamzaid, N., Davis, G., 2009. Health and fitness benefits of functional electrical stimulation-evoked leg exercise for spinal cord-injured individuals: a position review. Top. Spinal Cord Inj. Rehabil. 14 (4), 88–121.

58. Can, A., Dosoglu, M.S., et al., 2007. Effect of axial loading on bone mineral density in patients with traumatic spinal cord injury. Ulus. Travma Acil Cerrahi Derg. 13 (2), 101–105.

59. Soyupek, F., Savas, S., et al., 2009. Effects of body weight supported treadmill training on cardiac and pulmonary functions in the patients with incomplete spinal cord injury. J. Back Musculoskelet. Rehabil. 22 (4), 213–218.

60. Adams, M.M., Hicks, A.L., 2011. Comparison of the effects of body-weight-supported treadmill training and tilt-table standing on spasticity in individuals with chronic spinal cord injury. J. Spinal Cord Med. 34 (5), 488–494.

61. Semerjian, T.Z., Montague, S.M., et al., 2005. Enhancement of quality of life and body satisfaction through the use of adapted exercise devices for individuals with spinal cord injuries. Top. Spinal Cord Inj. Rehabil. 11 (2), 95–108.

62. Quel de Oliviera, C., Middleton, J., et al., 2019. Activity-based therapy in a community setting for independence, mobility, and sitting balance for people with spinal cord injuries. J. Cent. Nerv. Syst. Dis. 11, 1–9.

63. Singh, H., Unger, J., et al., 2018. Robot-assisted upper extremity rehabilitation for cervical spinal cord injuries: a systematic scoping review. Disabil Rehabil-Assist Technol. 13 (7), 704–715.

64. Cheung, E.Y.Y., Ng, T.K.W., et al., 2017. Robot-assisted training for people with spinal cord injury: a meta-analysis. Arch. Phys. Med. Rehabil. 98 (11), 2320–2331.

65. Holanda, L.J., Silva, P.M.M., et al., 2017. Robotic assisted gait as a tool for rehabilitation of individuals with spinal cord injury: a systematic review. J. NeuroEng. Rehabil. 14, 7.

66. Escorpizo, R., Bemis-Dougherty, A., 2015. Introduction to special issue: a review of the international classification of functioning, disability and health and physical therapy over the years. Physiother. Res. Int. 20 (4), 200–209.

67. Gerasimenko, Y., Gorodnichev, R., et al., 2015. Transcutaneous electrical spinal-cord stimulation in humans. Ann. Phys. Rehabil. Med. 58 (4), 225–231.

68. Gill, M.L., Grahn, P.J., et al., 2018. Neuromodulation of lumbosacral spinal networks enables independent stepping after complete paraplegia (p. 1677). Nat. Med. 24 (12), 1677–1682.

69. Angeli, C.A., Boakye, M., et al., 2018. Recovery of overground walking after chronic motor complete spinal cord injury. N. Engl. J. Med. 379 (13), 1244–1250.

70. Walter, M., Lee, A.H.X., et al., 2018. Epidural spinal cord stimulation acutely modulates lower urinary tract and bowel function following spinal cord injury: a case report. Front. Physiol. 9, 7.

71. Herrity, A.N., Williams, C.S., et al., 2018. Lumbosacral spinal cord epidural stimulation improves voiding function after human spinal cord injury. Sci. Rep. 8, 11.

72. Pettigrew, R.I., Heetderks, W.J., et al., 2017. Epidural spinal stimulation to improve bladder, bowel, and sexual function in individuals with spinal cord injuries: a framework for clinical research. IEEE Trans. Biomed. Eng. 64 (2), 253–262.

73. Harkema, S.J., Ditterline, B.L., et al., 2018. Epidural spinal cord stimulation training and sustained recovery of cardiovascular function in individuals with chronic cervical spinal cord injury. JAMA Neurol. 75 (12), 1569–1571.

74. Galea, M.P., Dunlop, S.A., et al., 2018. SCIPA full-on: a randomized controlled trial comparing intensive whole-body exercise and upper body exercise after spinal cord injury. Neurorehabil. Neural Repair 32 (6–7), 557–567.

75. Moritz, C.T., Ambrosio, F., 2017. Regenerative rehabilitation: combining stem cell therapies and activity-dependent stimulation. Pediatr. Phys. Ther. 29 (3), S10–S15.

CHAPTER 4

Early hospital management

Joshua Simmons

INTRODUCTION

Spinal cord injury (SCI) rehabilitation should be a patient-centred and goal-orientated process with input from the whole treating team, including the patient and their support network. Within this context, the aim of physiotherapy for patients with a spinal cord lesion is to optimise quality of life by enhancing their physical capabilities.

The role of physiotherapy is to maximise the ability of every patient post-injury. This involves helping them to be as independent as possible and return to their desired activities of daily living. While physiotherapy techniques in isolation are unable to elicit or facilitate neurological recovery, they are well equipped to assist in maximising neurological potential.[1]

ASSESSMENT FRAMEWORK

Using the International Classification of Functioning, Disability and Health (ICF) as a starting point, an effective physiotherapy program for people with a spinal cord lesion should include:

- assessment of key impairments and their severity, activity limitations and participation restrictions

- setting jointly agreed goals to address these limitations and restrictions
- identifying, developing and administering treatments
- measuring outcomes and success.

While physiotherapy interventions are most effective in the management of impairments that are directly or indirectly related to physical impairments involving motor and sensory loss, it is paramount that physiotherapy management be holistic and targeted towards managing the individual rather than the condition.

Box 4.1 presents a framework that allows clinicians to consider a holistic approach to physiotherapy management of patients with an SCI.

Using this framework, we can explore a program of physiotherapy management that begins as soon as possible following admission of a patient to the Spinal Injuries Unit (SIU).

RELEVANT HISTORY

Before commencing a subjective assessment, it is recommended the physiotherapist review relevant information as shown in Box 4.2, either from the

Box 4.1 Framework for holistic approach to patients with SCI

- Relevant history
- Respiratory assessment and management
- Neurological assessment (ISNCSCI)
  - Sensation (including proprioception)
  - Muscle strength (including other relevant muscles not included in the ISNCSCI)
- Skin condition
- Muscle tone and spasm
- Joint range of motion
- Strength and fitness training
- Balance
- Posture
- Functional skills, including bed mobility, transfers etc.
- Mobility, including wheelchair, walking etc.
- Assessment of equipment needs and prescription, including wheelchairs, cushions, exercise equipment, walking aids etc.
- Education provision
- Discharge planning

ISNCSCI: International Standards for Neurological Classification of Spinal Cord Injury

Box 4.2 Patient history

1. Personal details
2. History and mechanism of injury (flexion vs extension injury, involvement of water)
3. Type of injury and orthopaedic injury management (surgical vs conservative)
4. Other associated injuries (fractures, contusions, implications for respiratory function)
5. Past medical and surgical history
6. Social history
7. Radiology investigations (X-ray, CT, MRI, ultrasound)
8. Medications (pain relief, chest therapy and muscle relaxants)
9. Turning regimen (standard regimen is 2 hrs on each side and 4 hrs on back, which may be varied due to pressure care requirements)

The following information should be noted when first observing the patient:

- Type of bed used
- Type of traction or immobilisation
- Type of catheter used
- Presence of anti-embolism stockings and pneumatic compression devices
- Presence of nasogastric tube
- Conscious state, febrile etc.

medical record/chart or other relevant patient care documentation.

Conservative management

Individuals suffering an SCI are traditionally managed either via a conservative approach involving a prolonged period of bed rest, or via surgical intervention. There is much debate about the benefits of each treatment method, including neurological recovery, functional outcomes and the overall healthcare cost. While there is a trend towards surgical intervention using the advances of medical imaging and anaesthetic techniques, there is evidence to suggest that there is little or no long-term benefit compared to the conservative approach.[2]

Patients managed conservatively will be typically managed on an Engrit™ bed, or similar, which allows the implementation of a turning regimen without compromising the required spinal precautions that may be required. The bed is effectively divided into three sections which facilitates the ability to place the patient in alternative side-lying positions or in a supine position for pressure injury relief without having to physically roll or move the patient.

The Engrit bed also has the ability to be tipped slightly into either a Trendelenburg or reverse Trendelenburg position for blood pressure management, if approved by the medical staff (Fig. 4.1).

In addition, cervical injuries may be managed with any combination of skull tongs and traction with sandbags next to the head to prevent movement, Philadelphia collar or soft collar (Fig. 4.2).

Conversely, thoracic and lumbar injuries are usually managed without any additional devices and are restricted to a flat, supine position.

For all levels of injury, it is advisable to provide additional pressure relief by placing two pillows under the lower legs, lengthways, to ensure that the heels remain free of pressure.

Surgical management

Cervical injuries are commonly managed using surgical techniques that involve decompression with or without fusion. Depending on the surgeon, patients will often be provided with a soft collar postoperatively to be worn when mobilising for the purposes of pain management (Fig. 4.3).

Lumbar injuries that are managed surgically may have an intercostal catheter (ICC) inserted postoperatively, depending on surgical approach. This needs to be considered when performing any respiratory or range of motion (ROM) exercises.

Patients managed surgically will probably return from theatre on a standard hospital bed. Surgeons will give mobilisation instructions/restrictions after reviewing the patient postoperatively, as well as whether any collars or braces are required. An X-ray to check the alignment may be required prior to mobilisation or sitting the patient out of bed. It is important to ensure that appropriate documentation on the medical chart from the medical team is completed and verified prior to mobilisation.

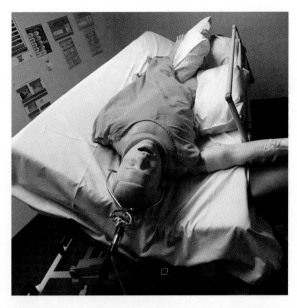

Figure 4.1 Engrit bed being used for pressure relief.

When approaching the postoperative management of a patient with an SCI it is important to consider the soft tissue damage also present at the injury/surgery site. It is easy to focus on the vertebral body injuries that have contributed to the SCI without developing an appropriate management plan for the ligamentous and muscle damage that has also been sustained, either through the initial injury or from the surgical technique. This is particularly important as the patient starts to mobilise and the core antigravity and stability muscles are required to support the vertebral column.

Similar precautionary care should be considered regarding the care of the whole nervous system. Due to the initial trauma to the spinal cord, the whole nervous system is effectively in a 'heightened state of vulnerability' and must be treated with caution. (See Chapter 1 for further detail on the pathological processes following injury.) With the trend for early surgical intervention, there is a risk to assume that the nervous system has also been 'fixed', which can subsequently lead to the potential implications of overstretching the neural structures

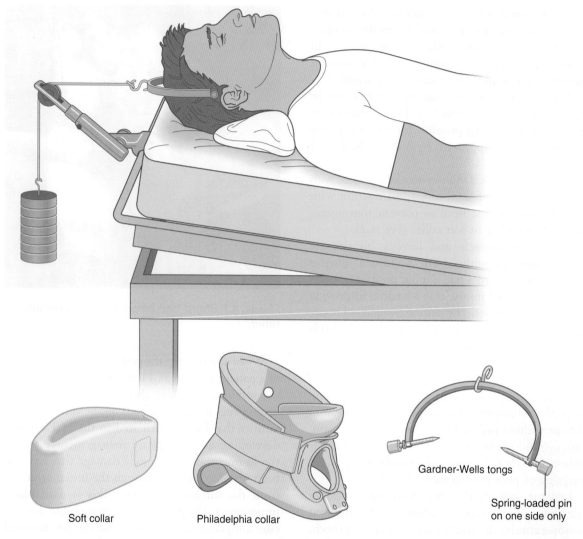

Soft collar

Philadelphia collar

Gardner-Wells tongs

Spring-loaded pin
on one side only

Figure 4.2 Skull tongs for cervical traction Philadelphia collar and soft collar.

being ignored when positioning the patient or performing passive movements. It is important to be aware of the potential for the swelling around the neural structures, which can develop cord tethering and adhesions of the neural tissue. As such, it is advisable to avoid overstretching neural structures (i.e. straight leg raise, prolonged long sitting with knees in full extension, upper limb neural tension positions with cervical rotation) and be aware of any symptoms of neural tension and/or the presence of autonomic dysreflexia (AD), which may suggest presence of a noxious stimulus.

Autonomic dysreflexia

Autonomic dysreflexia occurs when a noxious afferent stimulus arises somewhere in the body below the level of the spinal cord lesion, resulting in a sympathetic response, including reflex hypertension and an altered heart rate.

The symptoms of AD can be mild or severe and can include elevated blood pressure (BP) (up to 300/220 mmHg), a characteristic pounding headache, blurred vision, and a blotchy red rash on the neck and upper chest. If left untreated, AD can result in strokes, seizures and death.

To try and accommodate the sympathetic response, a variety of parasympathetic reactions take place above the level of SCI that are facilitated by the baroreceptors in the aortic arch when they sense a rise in BP. This includes compensatory bradycardia (via the vagus nerve), dilatation of blood vessels, which leads to a blotchy rash (Fig. 4.3), and profuse sweating above the level of injury.[3]

Most people with SCI who are prone to AD will have knowledge of the symptoms, its likely causes and potential remedies. In the first instance, where possible, a cause for the noxious stimulus should be identified. Often, people who experience AD also carry medication (e.g. nitroglycerine or glyceryl trinitrate), which can be taken to temporarily relieve symptoms while the cause can be determined. This could be as simple as emptying an over-distended bladder (which can occur if catheter tubing is kinked) or loosening tight straps/clothing. The person with AD should not be permitted to lie down, as this could cause a further increase in intra-cranial pressure; instead they should be placed in an upright position. If symptoms do not resolve quickly with simple measures, emergency medical treatment should be sought (Fig. 4.4). (See Online resources at end of chapter for further information on how to manage AD.)

RESPIRATORY ASSESSMENT AND MANAGEMENT

In the words of renowned physiotherapist Mary Massery, 'If you can't breathe – you can't function!' As such, the priority is always respiratory management. In the acute phase, patients with SCI are particularly at risk of developing a chest infection due to inadequate ventilation and/or retained secretions. It is therefore paramount that a thorough respiratory assessment is completed as soon as possible.

Respiratory assessment

Initially the focus should be directed on understanding if the patient is experiencing any difficulties associated with breathing (shortness of breath, cough, sputum, etc). This can be achieved through subjective questioning and paying close attention to how the patient is able to express themselves. Observation of voice control, their ability to talk in sentences, speech volume and whether they can take a deep breath without triggering any bronchospasm will provide valuable information about their respiratory capacity and focus the objective element

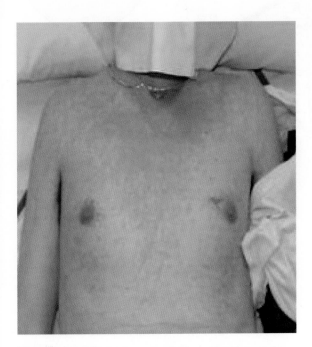

Figure 4.3 Clinical presentation of autonomic dysreflexia.

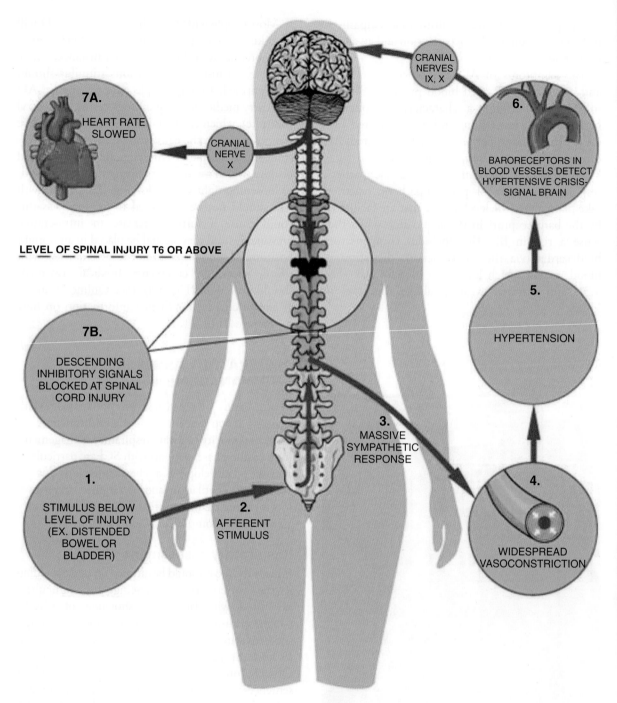

Figure 4.4 Autonomic dysreflexia.

Source: Ontario Neurotrauma Foundation. Autosomal dysreflexia. Caring for persons with spinal cord injury, e-learning resource for family physicians. www.rnoh.nhs.uk/our-services/spinal-cord-injury-centre/medical-management-advice/autonomic-dysreflexia

of the assessment on quantifying their respiratory function.

A detailed objective respiratory assessment should include a review of:

- respiratory musculature (diaphragm, intercostals, accessory, abdominals)
- respiratory rate
- auscultation and palpation
- breathing pattern
- voice (ability to shout)
- effectiveness and quality of cough
- sputum (colour, thickness, amount)
- investigations – X-ray and arterial blood gases (ABG) reports
- respiratory function tests (tidal volumes, FVC [forced vital capacity], FEV_1 [forced expiratory volume in 1 second]).

Ideally, the therapist should observe the patient both laterally and from the end of the bed, both at rest and while talking. It is important to make a note of epigastric rise, anterior/posterior movement, lateral flare, intercostal recession, upper chest movement and any paradoxical breathing (i.e. where the chest contracts during inhalation and expands during exhalation – the opposite of how it should move).

Physiotherapists need to be aware of the following factors when developing an appropriate respiratory management plan:

- pre-existing respiratory disease (e.g. chronic obstructive airways disease (COAD), asthma, smoking history)
- associated chest injuries (e.g. fractured ribs/sternum, pneumothorax/contusions)
- aspiration (particularly if sea water or sand are involved as they create a recurrent irritation of the airways leading to chronic secretion production)
- drowsiness from analgesia/sleep deprivation/increased CO_2 retention will contribute to a lower respiratory drive and breathing is likely to be more shallow (see Chapter 18 on sleep apnoea)
- disruption of the sympathetic nervous system leading to:
  - blockage of nasal passages (Guttman's sign), which has implications for non-invasive ventilation options
  - altered cardiac function leading to increased risk of pulmonary oedema
  - decreased blood pressure and thermoregulation (Fig. 4.5).

The risk of respiratory failure is directly associated with the level of injury as the diaphragm and other respiratory muscles fatigue. Respiratory fatigue most commonly occurs in the first 24–72 hours post-injury. During this time the pulmonary compliance deteriorates rapidly as lung expansion is decreased, leading to lower levels of pulmonary surfactant production. The flow-on effect is an accumulation of secretions, atelectasis, impaired aeration, infection and pneumonia.[4]

Respiratory complications are the most common cause of morbidity and mortality in acute SCI. Eighty per cent of deaths in cervical SCI are secondary to pulmonary dysfunction, with pneumonia the cause in 50%. A large multi-centre study showed that 67% of acutely injured SCI patients experienced severe respiratory complications during acute rehabilitation.[5]

Damage to the cervical spine interrupts sympathetic nerve supply to the lungs, which originate from the upper 6 thoracic ganglia. The parasympathetic innervation arising from vagal nuclei of brainstem remains intact, which means that cervical and high thoracic SCI may have increased resting airway tone, resulting in airway hyperactivity, shortness of breath, wheezing and excessive respiratory secretions.[4]

Surgical intervention that uses an anterior fusion approach may be associated with increased sputum production for 24–48 hours postoperatively due to swelling, which places pressure on the recurrent laryngeal nerve.

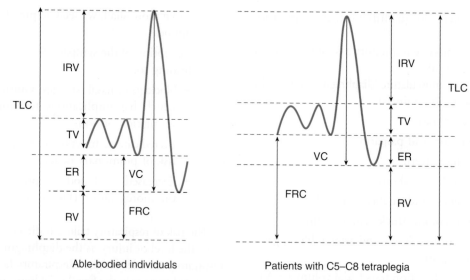

Able-bodied individuals   Patients with C5–C8 tetraplegia

Figure 4.5 Impact of SCI on respiratory function.

Respiratory management

Respiratory physiotherapy with spinal patients should be focused on prevention (see Chapter 16 on the respiratory management of high cervical SCI). A respiratory infection for a tetraplegic SCI patient can be life threatening, requiring extremely vigorous and regular physiotherapy.

Respiratory complications are primarily related to three possible issues – reduced inspiratory volume (inability to take a deep breath); reduced expiratory capacity (inability to clear secretions); or respiratory fatigue.

Reduced inspiratory volume

- Related to the lack of lateral expansion, paralysis of inspiratory muscles, and immobility.

- Best managed by placing the patient in the optimal position for ventilation and providing positive pressure ventilation via intermittent positive pressure breathing (IPPB), biphasic positive airway pressure (BiPAP), manual hyperinflations or a cough assist machine.

- Supine is the optimal position to begin with, as this allows the diaphragm to operate in

a gravity-eliminated position and maintain its natural dome-shaped resting position. The higher or more upright a patient sits, the greater the mechanical disadvantage the diaphragm is placed in, as the abdominal viscera will move anteriorly and inferiorly, pulling the diaphragm into a flattened, inefficient inner range position.

- IPPB devices are often used routinely in an acute setting as a prophylactic measure unless contraindicated (i.e. 2–4 hourly). Most patients enjoy using IPPB once they are used to it as it gives them assistance to receive larger lung volumes of air, and enables them to be more familiar with the device in the event of respiratory distress. However, evidence suggests there are no short- or long-term improvements in function, lung compliance or the work of breathing in patients with a recent SCI (and without acute respiratory failure) when using IPPB.[6] The literature suggests that it should be used to enhance secretion clearance when respiratory tract infections occur, with respect to the high cost and patient discomfort associated with IPPB.[6]

If an IPPPB is unavailable, it is possible to utilise the patient's own effort by using deep inhalation/holds, straws, bubbles or an incentive spirometry device.

- While there is a lack of evidence to support the use of incentive spirometry in the management of surgical patients,[7] it can be useful for the patient to monitor their own respiratory progress. A staff/family member may be required to hold the item for the patient.

- To complement these interventions, manual techniques such as palpation, stretch facilitation and rib spring can promote improved inspiratory function and mobilise secretions to clear for increased volume.

Reduced expiratory capacity

- Related to a combination of inhalation insufficiency and a lack of force from the expiratory abdominal muscles, resulting in an inability to expel air quickly.

- Best managed by providing assistance with inhalation and forced exhalation by using active cycle of breathing techniques (ACBT) or positive pressure breathing support, appropriate positioning to facilitate secretion drainage and removal, huff or assisted cough.

- If there are problems with sputum retention and/or collapse it will be advantageous to use side-lying positions.

- In this case, it is best to treat a patient just before and again just after a turn, as a change in position will often aid the mobilisation and expectoration of sputum.
  - The use of manual techniques such as vibes, percussion, assisted cough +/−. Cough assist machine will assist in mobilising the secretions to a point where they can be expectorated effectively and efficiently.

- Most acute SCI patients will not be able to tolerate vigorous vibrations, percussion and tipping. However, as the patient begins to settle down and if the removal of secretions continues to be a problem, gentle percussion and tipping the bed (with doctor's approval) may be useful.

- In the early stages, vibration with IPPB is often very effective. This requires two people, but is much less fatiguing and more beneficial for the patient. A third person may be required to brace the shoulders if the vibrations are vigorous and the patient had not had internal fixation and is being managed in traction or a cervical collar.

Respiratory fatigue

- Related to the overall increased work of breathing due to neurological insult to both inspiratory and expiratory muscles.

- Best managed by decreasing the effort to breathe via appropriate positioning, providing inspiratory assistance via non-invasive ventilation through IPPB, BiPAP, continuous positive airway pressure (CPAP) and clearing any obstructions to allow optimal breathing.

- At some point it is relevant to consider a transfer to the intensive care unit (ICU) to allow the patient to be intubated and sedated so that they can rest.

- Signs of deterioration include drowsiness and lack of concentration, slurring of speech, decreased ability to cooperate with coughing, altered respiratory rate, decreased respiratory function tests (RFT)/FVC, decreased air entry on auscultation, increased production of sputum +/− colour change.

- Patients who have diaphragm involvement and need longer-term ventilation will be transferred back to the SIU on the ventilator where an assessment will be completed to determine an appropriate plan for weaning and decannulation. (See Chapter 16 for more information on high cervical lesions.)

Assisted coughing

High level SCI patients (tetraplegia and high-level paraplegia) who have abdominal and intercostal muscle paralysis will be unable to cough effectively.

All patients must be taught to cough with manual assistance. If they develop a respiratory infection, they will be sick and exhausted and it is not the right time to be teaching them how to cough. It is imperative to teach this cough from Day 1 and continue it as an integral part of physiotherapy. The physiotherapist will assist the cough by replacing the work of the abdominals by creating pressure underneath the working diaphragm. It takes very little time once mastered, and is the most effective way to keep the chest clear.

An assisted cough can be combined with IPPB or a cough assist machine for increased effectiveness. Manual compression (assisted cough) and insufflation by positive pressure improves cough effectiveness with a significant increase in peak cough flow rate compared to an unassisted method.[6]

There are several methods for performing an assisted cough, which can involve between one and three people. An additional person is required to brace the shoulders of cervical injured patients to prevent movement at the fracture site. Nursing staff will need to be shown how to continue with assisted coughing when the physiotherapist is not available.

Methods of assisted coughing

One-person abdominal thrust – This technique is best used when attempting to perform an assisted cough with someone lying on their back or positioned one-quarter turn from supine. Initially, palpate the xiphoid process (at the base of the sternum) and follow the rib cage until it starts to move laterally and posteriorly until the point approximately halfway between the xiphoid and the navel is located. Hands can then be placed in one of the following positions:

- the heel of both hands on the abdomen, inferior to the patient's sternum at the halfway point between navel and xiphoid, as described above (care should be taken not to place any pressure over the xiphoid process) (Fig. 4.6)

or

- one hand inferior to the sternum to thrust, while the other arm is across the anterior rib cage or other hand placed laterally on the ribs.

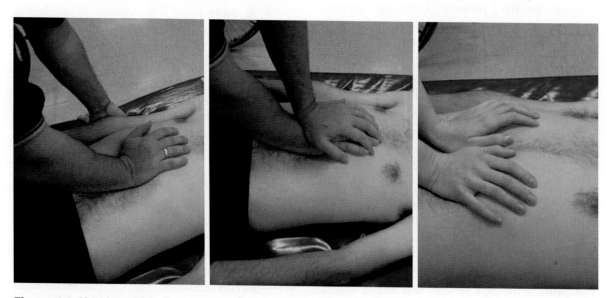

Figure 4.6 Hand position for one-person assisted cough.

Explain to the patient what is about to be done:

- Place hands in the preferred position.
- Follow the natural inspiratory and expiratory movements of the patient for 2–3 breaths.
- On the third breath out, perform a forceful upward thrust as an adjunct to the function of the diaphragm (the movement is posterior and superior – 'in and up').
- Ensure that each 'cough' includes several thrusts to mimic a 'normal' cough.

Alternatively, place both hands on the lower rib cage and squeeze the lower rib cage 'up and in' as the patient tries to cough. This technique is a little more difficult to master, but is potentially more comfortable for the patient as it does not place direct pressure on the abdominal wall.

With all techniques described, the therapist's hands should mimic the non-functioning abdominal muscle with the pressure delivered evenly and firmly.

An assisted cough is most effective if the physiotherapist uses their own body weight using a stride stance and keeping elbows straight. At times it may be appropriate to kneel on the bed or stand on a stool, depending on the type of bed in which the patient is being managed.

The sound of the cough is the best guide as to the amount of force required. It is better to start with a small cough and work up so as not to alarm the patient. The cough must not be as forceful or violent as to cause pain or movement at the fracture site, but must be sufficiently effective to deliver sputum to the mouth. Each patient is different, and several attempts may be required to establish the appropriate timing.

Pressure on the abdominal wall alone must be avoided, as the patient may have a paralytic ileus or other unknown internal damage.

These techniques can be modified to be performed when the patient is sitting in their chair; however, it is important to position the chair up against a wall and ensure that brakes are applied if possible to stabilise the chair.

Two-person abdominal thrust (with thoracic brace)
– Each person positions themselves on either side

of the patient and one therapist provides vibrations and applies a stabilising downward pressure on the thoracic cage to ensure all expiratory force is directed up towards the glottis and not lost in the chest wall. The second therapist uses both hands to give pressure on the diaphragm (Fig. 4.7).

This method may be needed if the patient is particularly large, there is a copious amount of sputum, the sputum is very tenacious, the patient is becoming exhausted or the therapists require an opportunity to rest.

When treating an acute respiratory infection, it is advisable, where possible, for therapists to treat in pairs to prevent the development of overuse injuries of the neck, shoulder and wrist.

Key points to note about assisted coughing

- An assisted cough should be considered an emergency technique to clear an airway and is something that has been adapted for use as a treatment technique.
- An additional person is required for all techniques described to brace the shoulders of all patients with unstable acute cervical or upper thoracic injuries.
- A mechanical cough assist device should be used if prolonged treatment is indicated.

Cough assist machine (In-Exsufflator)

The Cough Assist™ is used to allow expectoration of secretions when a cough is ineffective. This machine can be used in conjunction with an abdominal thrust to further improve a cough. The machine allows a higher flow and volume of air to be expelled quickly (FEV_1) to simulate a cough.

The machine delivers positive airway pressure followed by a quick change to negative pressure. The contraindications for its use are the same as for IPPB (Fig. 4.8).

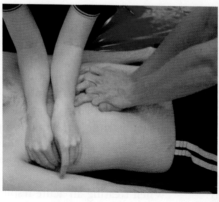

Figure 4.7 Hand position for two-person assisted cough with thoracic brace.

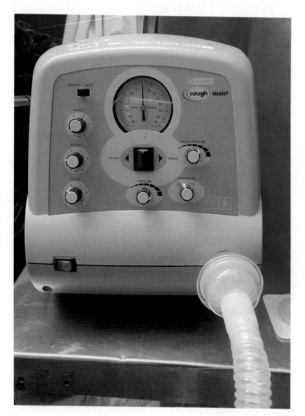

Figure 4.8 Cough Assist™.

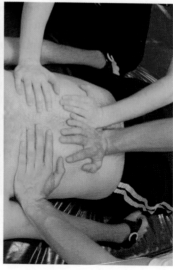

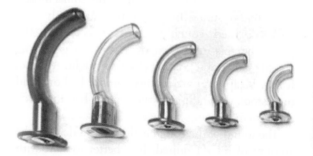

Figure 4.9 A range of Guedel airways.

Suction

A Guedel airway may be used if assisted coughing is not sufficient (Fig. 4.9). It is an unpleasant and traumatic experience to the patient and is to be avoided if possible. Pharyngeal suction may also result in bradycardia due to vagal nerve stimulation. Therefore, it is essential that the medical staff are aware and they may stand by with norephedrine or similar.

Abdominal binder

An abdominal binder is an elastic strap applied around the patient's abdomen. It provides support to the abdominal contents and encourages improvement in cardiac output in patients lacking adequate abdominal muscle activation/support (injury above T12). It significantly increases FVC and maximum expiratory pressure in sitting.[6] It improves inspiratory pressures, vital capacity (VC), maximal expiratory flow rate or maximal expiratory pressures and voice in patients with cervical SCI.[8]

Consequently, patients with thoracic SCIs are encouraged to wear their abdominal binder when mobilising to prevent shortness of breath and reduce the presence of orthostatic hypotension. There is also an argument that wearing an abdominal binder will assist with reducing energy consumption and preventing fatigue by minimising the effort directed towards breathing and maintaining posture (Fig. 4.10).[9]

It is advisable to provide the patient with two binders, one for showering (if patient is using a shower commode) and one for during the day.

NEUROLOGICAL ASSESSMENT

Before commencing an initial neurological assessment, it is beneficial to start with passive movements and general handling of the patient's limbs, as this assists in gaining the confidence and relaxation of the patient. It can also serve to relieve any pain and stiffness related to a prolonged period of travel prior to admission or any extended period of restricted movement.

Passive handling of the limbs while conducting the subjective assessment also allows the therapist to obtain a 'feel' for the patient and pre-empt some of the potential objective findings. It is important to be honest with the patient and explain the purpose of conducting a neurological assessment, emphasising that this has no bearing on their overall prognosis and will simply provide a summary of where they are at a point in time. Emphasis should be placed on ensuring that the patient is truthful in the sensory assessment and gives their best effort in the motor assessments. The sensory assessment is effectively a subjective examination and, while it is possible to detect inconsistencies, it is important to build on establishing rapport between clinician and patient.

The standardised neurological assessment for acute traumatic spinal cord injuries is the International Standards for Neurological Classification of Spinal Cord Injury (ISNCSCI) (see Appendix 1). It is an examination that was developed by the American Spinal Injuries Association (ASIA) to score the motor and sensory impairment and severity of an SCI. It provides a standardised language that allows all clinicians to describe the level of neurological activity available and objectively describes if there is a complete block of messages travelling from the

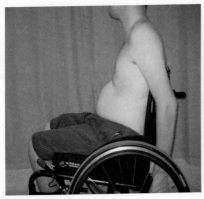 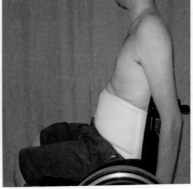

Figure 4.10 Abdominal binder.
Source: Ross, J., Wadsworth, B., 2016. Cardiorespiratory management of special populations. In Main E, Denehy L. (Eds). Cardiorespiratory physiotherapy: adults and paediatrics, 5th edn. Elsevier Health Sciences.

Box 4.3 ASIA Impairment Scale (AIS)

AIS A – Sensory and motor complete injury

- No sensory or motor function is preserved in the sacral segments S4–5.

AIS B – Sensory Incomplete Injury

- Sensory but not motor function is preserved below the neurological level and includes the sacral segments S4–5 (light touch or pinprick at S4–5 or deep anal pressure) AND no motor function is preserved more than three levels below the motor level on either side of the body.

AIS C – Motor incomplete injury

- Motor function is preserved at the most caudal sacral segments for voluntary anal contraction (VAC) OR the patient meets the criteria for sensory incomplete status (sensory function preserved at the most caudal sacral segments (S4–5) by light touch, pinprick or deep anal pressure), and has some sparing of motor function more than three levels below the ipsilateral motor level on either side of the body. (This includes key or non-key muscle functions to determine motor incomplete status.)
- For AIS C – less than half of key muscle functions below the single neurological level have a muscle grade ≥ 3.

AIS D – Motor incomplete injury

- Motor incomplete status as defined above for AIS C, with at least half (half or more) of key muscle functions below the single NLI having a muscle grade ≥ 3.

AIS E – Normal

- If sensation and motor function as tested with the ISNCSCI are graded as normal in all segments, and the patient had prior deficits, then the AIS grade is E. Someone without an initial SCI does not receive an AIS grade.

Source: ASIA

---

start of the spinal cord (brain) to the end of the spinal cord (S4/5 dermatome). Box 4.3 explains the scale used in the ISNCSC.

It is recommended that an ISNCSCI assessment is completed on admission to the emergency department prior to any surgical intervention. This will allow the establishment of a reference point to determine if there are any adverse outcomes or neurological deterioration postoperatively. A formal ISNCSCI is also often performed on admission and discharge from the acute rehabilitation setting to measure patient progress and provide reference points to quantify or qualify any neurological change.

The ISNCSCI effectively provides the therapist with the greatest insight into the neurological damage suffered by the patient by assessing three primary 'pathways' within the spinal cord (for further detail on pathways, see Chapter 1):

1. Dorsal columns – an ascending pathway that runs up the posterior aspect of the cord, crossing at the brainstem; carries light touch messages.
2. Spinothalamic tracts – an ascending pathway that runs up the lateral aspect of the cord, crossing at the spinal cord level; carries pain (and temperature) messages.
3. Corticospinal tracts – a descending pathway that runs down the anterior aspect of the cord, crossing mostly at the brainstem; carries motor messages.

Sensory assessment

The sensory aspect of the ISNCSCI assesses light touch and pain (pinprick) sensation. All dermatomes from C2 to S4/5 are assessed and given with scores as follows:

2 = Normal
1 = Abnormal – may be diminished or hypersensitive
0 = Absent
UTA = Unable to assess (e.g. due to braces, plasters, burns, drains).

The key elements of the light touch sensory assessment are as follows:

- Use a teased-out cotton bud or similar and perform a single, small sweep over the key point.
- Use the patient's face as a reference point. It is not possible to compare side to side due to the nature of SCI and, as such, cranial nerves are used.
- The intent is to determine if the patient can accurately discriminate the difference between touching vs not touching
- The suggested verbal cue is 'Am I touching?'

- If the patient can determine the difference between touching and not touching, then they score at least 1.
- If the stimulus on the face feels the same as the dermatome, then it is considered normal/ intact and they score a 2.
- If it feels different, then the dermatome is considered impaired and the score remains as 1.
- If the patient is unable to accurately discriminate the difference, then the dermatome is scored as a 0 (absent) (Fig. 4.11).

For further detailed information pertaining to the standardised sensory and motor assessments for the ISNCSCI see Online resources at end of chapter.

The key elements of the pinprick sensory assessment are as follows:

- Use a Neurotip™ with a sharp metal spike at one end and a plastic-coated tip at the other end.
- The patient's face is used as a reference point.
- The intent is to determine if the patient can accurately discriminate the difference between pain and deep pressure.

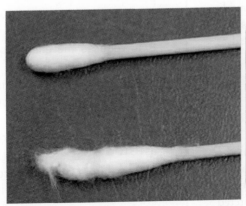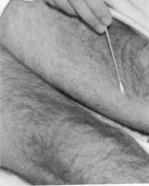

Figure 4.11 Q-Tip with end teased out being used to assess light touch at L3.

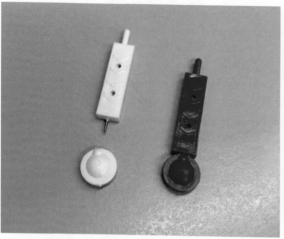
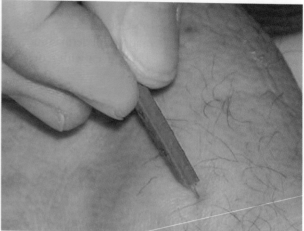

Figure 4.12 Neurotip™ being used to assess pinprick.

- The suggested verbal cue is 'Sharp or blunt?'
- If the patient can determine the difference between sharp and blunt, then they score at least 1.
- If the sharp stimulus on the face feels the same as the sharp stimulus on the dermatome, then it is considered normal/intact and they score a 2.
- If the sharp stimulus feels different, then the dermatome is considered impaired and the score remains as 1.
- If the patient is unable to accurately discriminate the difference between sharp and blunt, then the dermatome is scored as a 0 (absent) (Fig. 4.12).

Based on this information, the therapist can determine the sensory level, which is referred to as the most caudal segment with normal light touch and pinprick sensation.

The accuracy of the sensory component of the ISNCSCI has been shown to be highly dependent upon the experience of the assessing therapist and the results obtained should therefore be interpreted with caution.[10]

Key points to remember when completing the sensory assessment

- Allow enough time for patient to respond.
- Provide the patient with enough stimulus to provide a response.
- Do not give clues, such as leaning on the bed to touch the opposite limb.
- Accumulated touches can generate a false positive.
- If in doubt about the accuracy of the response, repeat the test × 10 (a score of 8/10 reduces the chance of guessing to < 5%).
- Always complete one side of the body before moving to the other side (to ensure accurate documentation).
- If abnormal at C2 = score the patient as 'C1'.
- If normal from C2–S5 = document 'INT' to indicate that the sensation is intact.

Motor assessment

The ISNCSCI requires the therapist to assess ten key muscles – five from the upper limb and five from the lower limb. According to the standards, each of the key muscles identified were selected based on the following criteria:

- 1 muscle per segment
- functional significance
- accessible and easily isolated in supine
- innervation from at least two spinal segments.

While the standardised assessment is conducted in supine postion to allow for any spinal precautions or conservative management plans, in the event of inconclusive information the therapist should consider modified assessments to ascertain the true level of function to develop an appropriate management plan.

The key muscles are graded from 0–5 using a traditional manual muscle testing scale. To achieve a full grade, the available passive range must equal the active range assessed for grades 0–3. The ISNCSCI requires that all grade 4 and 5 muscle assessments are performed as a static muscle test. It can be argued that a static muscle test is more informative of the muscle/tendon integrity than the functional strength, therefore it is recommended to also separately conduct a through-range muscle assessment of the key muscles at a later point (Table 4.1).

Based on the assessment recorded, the motor level is identified, which is described as the lowest key muscle that has a grade of at least 3, providing all the key muscles above are normal (i.e. grade 5/5). If the segment does not have a testable muscle (i.e. C1–4, T2–L1, S2), then the sensory assessment is referred to as an indicator of whether that level is 'normal'.

Zones of partial preservation (ZPP)

The zones of partial preservation refer to the myotomes and dermatomes (see Chapter 1 for further explanation) below the neurological level that remain partially innervated in an AIS A (complete injury). (Note that the definition of the Zone of

> ### Key points to remember when completing the motor assessment
>
> - Start with grade 3 position for the upper limb key muscles.
> - Test flickers of the upper limb key muscles in the grade 2 position.
> - Test flickers of the lower limb key muscles in grade 3 position (except plantar flexors, which should be tested in the grade 2 position).
> - If using a plus and minus scale, record the lowest whole grade on the recording chart (i.e. 3–/5 is recorded as a 2/5 and 2+/5 is recorded as 2/5).
> - In the event of pain or orthopaedic precautions preventing an accurate assessment, the muscle grade documented on the recording chart should be the predicted value to ensure that any improvement over time can be attributed to neurological recovery instead of resolution of pain or removal of precautions. For example:
>   - when grading acute admissions (unstable fractures), resistance can sometimes be contraindicated which requires the therapist to grade the movement based on the quality of the movement as to whether it is normal.

Partial Preservation was changed in 2019 and now can be used in some cases of incomplete injuries.) It refers to the lowest segment with some sensory and/or motor function. The segment is recorded on the classification sheet for sensory and motor function bilaterally.

While this classification system provides a standardised method of describing neurological activity post SCI, correct determination of motor

Table 4.1 ISNCSCI key muscles and static muscle test positions

Level	Muscle group	Grade 4 and 5 test position
C5	Elbow flexors	90° elbow flexion
C6	Wrist extensors	Full wrist extension
C7	Elbow extensors	45° elbow flexion
C8	Finger flexors	Full finger flexion
T1	Finger abductors	Full finger abduction in grade 3 position
L2	Hip flexors	90° hip flexion
L3	Knee extensors	15° knee flexion
L4	Ankle dorsi flexors	Full dorsi flexion
L5	Toe extensors	Full toe extension (in dorsi flexion)
S1	Ankle plantar flexors	Full plantar flexion

Neurological level

The neurological level refers to the lowest segment with normal sensory and motor function on both sides. Normal sensory refers to the lowest segment with normal pin prick and light touch sensation. Normal motor function refers to the lowest key muscle that has a grade of at least 3/5, provided that all the key muscles represented by segments above that level are judged to be normal (5/5).

levels and the differentiation between AIS B and AIS C/D are the most difficult concepts to grasp for clinicians. As such, training is strongly recommended to improve classification skills for clinical practice.[11] Support for interpretation of the results and classification of the AIS is available from their website (see Online resources at end of chapter).

Aside from the standardised assessment provided by the ISNCSCI, it is important to assess all the other relevant muscles, including the shoulder, forearm, fingers etc. in the upper limb and hip extensors, knee flexors, ankle inversion/eversion and toes etc. in the lower limb. In order to understand the full functional capacity of the neurological system and to gain a more accurate indication of functional ability, it is also important to conduct a through-range assessment of these muscles (as well as the key muscles in the ISNCSCI).

When performing muscle tests, positioning and the amount of resistance permitted may be limited if the patient is still considered unstable (e.g. acute stage). Please clarify any restrictions or precautions with the treating medical team.

Key points to remember when performing any muscle tests

- Always observe and, where possible, palpate the muscle being assessed.
- The only way to accurately assess if a muscle is working is to be able to see and palpate the muscle. If the muscle cannot be seen or palpated, it cannot be tested (e.g. inter-scapular muscles) and is documented as *unable to assess* (UTA).
- Be sure to isolate the muscle being assessed by stabilising the proximal joints and be aware of any trick movements:
  - triceps – shoulder external rotation, shoulder abduction and extension
  - finger flexors – wrist extension.
- Poor proximal stability may affect accuracy.
- Be ready to palpate and distinguish the smallest flicker of movement – often very easily fatigued and not repeatable.

RANGE OF MOTION

The available range of motion (ROM) of all joints in both the upper and the lower limbs should be assessed and an appropriate management plan, using the techniques described below, developed to maintain or regain range as appropriate.

Passive movements

Passive movements are traditionally performed with the purpose of maintaining good circulation (including preventing the development of venous thromboembolism [VTE]), maintaining joint and soft tissue range and thereby reducing the risk of pressure injuries. It is important to be sensitive to soft tissue and joint limits as the patient is unable to feel overstretching or rough movement.

Historically it was believed that passive movements should be performed to all affected limbs using a set routine of 10–20 repetitions twice daily for the first 6 weeks or until the patient mobilised, as this was the period of greatest risk of VTE, and after that, joint range and good circulation would be maintained through mobilisation.

However, there is little or only a slight increase in arterial and skin blood flow following treatment with passive leg movements and no difference in blood flow between 5 and 30 repetitions of passive movements, which indicates the efficacy of passive movements for VTE prevention is doubtful in acute SCI patients.[12]

Furthermore, there are some studies that suggest there is little benefit associated with stretching and passive movements following SCI to improve ROM, reduce pain, reduce spasticity and improve function.[13,14] The studies concluded that regular stretch does not produce a clinically important change in joint mobility, pain, spasticity or activity limitation, has little or no short- or long-term effect on joint mobility and no statistically significant immediate or long-term effects on spasticity.[13,14] In addition, stretch applied on a regular daily basis for less than 3 months provides little or no added benefit over and above usual care of patients

with SCI, and there is only a small benefit of passive movements when applied for 6 months, making it unclear whether this benefit is clinically worthwhile.[14]

These studies wisely caution any therapist to consider the impact of overservicing or overtreating their patient. Therefore, it is probably more important to ensure that the clinical reasoning associated with the maintenance of range of motion is focused on the effectiveness of the intervention being provided in the context of the nature and the aim of the intervention. For example, if the primary focus is on maintaining range, then the patient who presents with an upper motor neuron injury characterised by spasticity may require more frequent or regular review, compared with the patient who presents with an areflexic lower motor neuron injury.

Consequently, regular reassessment of range of motion is the best measure of the appropriate level of intervention required and passive movements are continued by the therapist until the patient can do these themselves or the movement patterns are incorporated into the daily routine of functional tasks, such as dressing and hygiene.

Upper limb

The upper limbs must have full ROM for maximum independence. Any restrictions need to be investigated to determine if the cause is related to pain, stiffness, associated injuries, positioning, spasticity or a pre-existing problem. It is particularly important to review shoulder range, elbow extension and wrist extension, as any restrictions may have implications on long-term functional abilities and care requirements.

Full shoulder range of motion is essential for people with tetraplegia. Those in cervical traction can be taken through full range (the sandbag on the side being ranged can be removed), provided there is no neck movement. The orthopaedic surgeons will give specific instructions if this is not appropriate.

Similarly, if the patient is being ventilated, consider switching the circuit to the other side or having the nurse provide manual hyperventilation while stretching the limb on the ventilator side.

Sustained stretch positions can also be utilised to maintain shoulder range. The following principles should be employed for positioning:

- Avoid direct pressure on the shoulder.
- Provide support to the upper limb at all points.
- When the patient is supine, position the upper limb in abduction and external rotation on a regular basis.
- Avoid pulling on the arm when positioning the upper limb to prevent subluxation.
- Remember that preventing pain is a primary goal of positioning (Figs 4.13 and 4.14).

A tailored upper limb passive movement regimen can assist in the management of the following:

1. *Shoulder pain*: one of the most common problems for the tetraplegic patient and

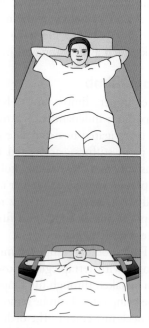

Shoulder stretch (sunbather)

Shoulder stretch (crucifix)

Figure 4.13 Sustained upper limb stretch positions.

Source: Physiotherapyexercises.com

usually related to referred pain from the fracture site, pain from associated shoulder trauma, pain from poor or prolonged positioning and pain from unopposed pull of the traction. Furthermore, there is evidence that exercise can be used to manage shoulder pain in a number of situations for tetraplegic patients.[15]

2. *Decreased range of movement*: the limitations often observed are shoulder flexion and external rotation, elbow extension, pronation and wrist extension. The main reasons for tight joints are the unopposed action of innervated muscles, pain and inadequate passive movements. Full range must be obtained as soon as possible, as limited range can significantly restrict functional ability. Gentle regular passive movements are the most effective means of prevention, together with constant attention to positioning. Plastic airbag type splints may be of use in stretching tight elbows, as are gentle resisted exercises in the later stages.

3. *Spasticity*: lower cervical lesions are more likely to present with a flexor-type pattern of spasticity in the upper limb, while higher level cervical injuries and those with brachial plexus injuries present with an extensor pattern coupled with internal rotation. Passive movements, positioning and gentle exercises, along with gentle peripheral mobilisation or scapular movements in side lying, can be beneficial in releasing the pattern (see Chapter 1 for full description of spinal spasticity).

4. *Pressure injuries*: although this is often related to splints, the regular movement of the upper limbs will assist in relieving pressure. The occupational therapist (OT) will remedy the pressure points related to the splints; however, the physiotherapist must know how to apply these splints

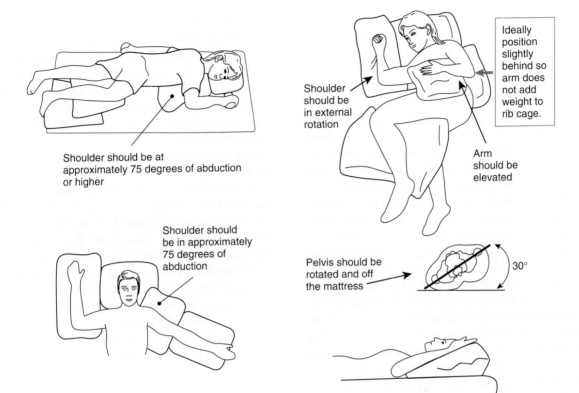

Figure 4.14 Positioning examples.

correctly and what to look for when removing them. Pressure areas from splints occur on the hands and may also be found on the chest and abdomen if the patient habitually adopts a position with hands resting on their chest.

After each treatment check general position, splints and traction. If there is some spasticity present, the patient who is being managed conservatively in traction may 'migrate' up the bed during passive movements and the knot will be resting on the pulley of the traction, thus negating its effect. If this happens, notify the nursing staff and the patient will be moved. (For more information on upper limb range of motion management and splinting, refer to Chapter 17.)

Lower limb

In the acute stage, hip flexion can be restricted depending on the level of the fracture due to possible movement at the fracture site. Patients being managed conservatively may have the following restrictions applied initially depending on the orthopaedic management plan:

- Lumbar fractures are limited to 30°.

- Thoracic fractures are limited to 45°.

- Cervical fractures are limited to 90°.

- SLR is limited to < 45° for the first 6/52 for all levels of injury, although an unstable lumbar fracture will be limited to 30°.

Depending on the healing process and orthopaedic review, this management plan may last for the first 3 weeks following injury, at which point hip flexion can be increased within pain limits to 90°. For those injuries managed surgically, these restrictions are revised postoperatively and direct consultation with the orthopaedic treating team is encouraged.

As spinal shock decreases (see Chapters 1 and 2), muscle tone returns to the leg muscles and careful handling is needed to prevent reinforcement of spasticity. Care should be taken not to elicit either a flexor withdrawal or extensor thrust and the movements should be performed smoothly. Pressure through the heel and long axis of the limb, together with slow rhythmical and smooth movements, tend to elicit a postural response of all deep muscles acting on the knee and ankle. These work in combination to stabilise the joint as they do in normal weight-bearing and total spastic movements are inhibited.

Spasticity can be a challenge to manage if the tone begins to cause pain or discomfort or inhibits the cervical traction when patients are managed conservatively. If this occurs, medications (e.g. Baclofen, Valium) may be given to reduce the spasm.[16] Sometimes more or less elevation or knee flexion may help to break up gross spastic patterns.

For all passive movements, proprioceptive neuromuscular facilitation patterns (PNF)[17] can be used so that combination of all movements is performed. Circumduction of the hip can be started gently and progressed if pain allows. The other leg must be monitored to check that the limb being moved is not being overstretched. Support the knee and ankle and provide gentle smooth passive movements throughout the available range. Never force through spasm or any other restriction.

Hyperextension of the knee should be avoided, particularly with full external rotation of the hip, as this has been thought to be one of the precipitating factors for the development of neurogenic heterotopic ossification (NHO) around the hip and knee (see Chapter 18). The cause of NHO is largely unknown, but the myth persists that it may be due to jerky and rough passive movements causing small haemorrhages and stress to the muscles and connective tissues.

After completing passive movements to both legs, check that the patient is in a good position with the hips extended and in neutral rotation, knees extended but not hyperextended, feet dorsiflexed and in midline with a foam block or pillow to assist with correct alignment. Patients are often managed in slight elevation with single pillows under the legs to prevent swelling. Heels must be kept free to prevent creation of pressure areas. It may be necessary to put pillows under the outside of the transverse pillows to prevent external rotation. Check the catheter position and that any anti-embolitic stockings are pulled up and not wrinkled.

PAIN

Most patients will be in some pain. Possible causes include the fracture site, referred pain, associated injuries, immobility and poor positioning, traction of unopposed muscles. It is important to try to analyse this pain and establish the source in order to relieve it. For more information on pain and pain management following SCI refer to Chapter 18.

TONE AND SPASM

Spinal spasticity is a common presentation following SCI and has been associated with increased pain, functional limitations and can have a significant impact on quality of life and initial rehabilitation if not managed appropriately (see Chapter 1).[18]

Spasticity is multifaceted and therefore requires a combination of measures to adequately assess. Commonly, the Modified Ashworth Scale (MAS) (see Appendix 3) and the Tardieu Scale (see Appendix 4) are used in clinical settings.[1]

As discussed in Chapter 1, in the early stage post initial injury (up to 6 weeks) spinal shock is present, and the limbs involved are usually in a state of flaccidity. Some lesions, especially hyperextension and incomplete injuries, may present with increased tone and spasticity on or soon after admission.

Any sign of increased tone and spasticity may precede neurological recovery, but this is not always the case. Significantly increased tone or spasm may require prescription of muscle relaxants,[16] splinting and specific positioning etc. Tone returns as spinal shock resolves.

CIRCULATION

Immediately post SCI, patients will often present with acute peripheral swelling. In tetraplegics, this involves the hands and lower limbs. For the hands, the OT will fit 'boxing glove' splints and the arms will be elevated on pillows (see Chapter 17).

For the lower limbs of both tetraplegics and paraplegics, graduated elastic anti-embolic stockings are worn that extend from toe to thigh, sequential pneumatic compression devices are applied and the legs are elevated on single pillows. Regular venous thromboembolism (VTE) checks should be performed each time the therapist performs any passive ROM exercises. This involves removing all devices and stockings, feeling for any calf warmth, observing any redness, palpating any isolated areas of pain and assessing for any physiological response to the Homans' sign (i.e. discomfort behind the knee on forced dorsiflexion of the foot).

Nursing staff will perform regular circumferential measurements to detect unilateral swelling, which may indicate a VTE. Any sign of VTE should be reported to the medical staff.

SKIN CONDITION

A thorough skin assessment is an integral component of the initial physiotherapy assessment. It is important to note any areas of redness or skin breakdown, particularly over bony prominences, and determine the cause. Patients are encouraged to keep weight or pressure off these areas until they have disappeared or healed. Below is a diagram of bony prominences vulnerable to breakdown in people with SCI (Fig. 4.15).

Note any areas of scar tissue, particularly on a weight-bearing area. Scar tissue is not as elastic as normal skin and is more vulnerable to breakdown. These areas with reduced skin integrity will affect positioning, length of time sitting, the type of equipment prescribed (cushion, wheelchair, mattress, shower chair, etc.), and may have an impact on the use of orthotics such as ankle foot orthoses (AFOs). Skin breakdown or pressure injuries may delay the rehabilitation process.

Similarly, areas of muscle wasting, particularly over weight-bearing areas, will increase the risk of skin breakdown and need to be considered in the equipment prescription process. This is particularly evident in those patients who suffer a lower motor neuron lesion.

Patients are encouraged to take primary responsibility for the management of their skin as they are the only person who will always be present during an assessment of their skin. Even if they are not able to independently assess the area, they should be taught how to instruct a carer to assess skin changes via palpation and observation. Any anomalies to skin integrity should be reviewed and discussed and where possible a digital image taken to use as reference point or to assist with monitoring the area over time.

The duration and frequency of weight-shift or pressure-relieving strategies should be tailored to the individual. Ideally, an assessment of the individual's daily routine and regular inspection of the skin should guide the frequency and intensity of intentional weight shifts.[19] This will provide an understanding of what unintentional weight-shifting activities are already performed throughout the day while performing functional tasks and when an intentional weight-shift technique should be incorporated (i.e. periods of low functional activity).

Pressure points

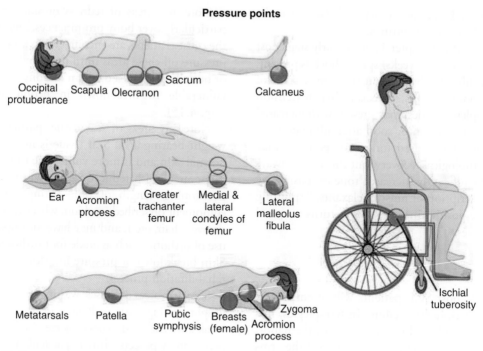

Figure 4.15 **Bony prominences vulnerable to skin breakdown.**

Common pressure-relieving or weight-shift techniques

- Pressure lift via shoulder depression using the wheels or arm rests of the chair, or by placing one arm over the back of the chair then lift the opposite buttock, and repeat on the other side

- Pressure lean via holding onto the hand rim or on a table and lean to the side, or leaning all the way forwards onto their knees, relieving the pressure from the ischial tuberosities

- Patients with high level tetraplegia will require assistance to lean forwards and sideways (Figs 4.16–4.18).

Common pressure-relieving or weight-shift techniques—cont'd

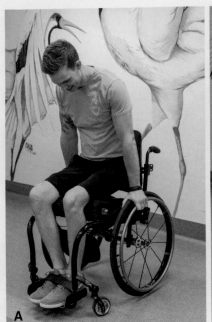
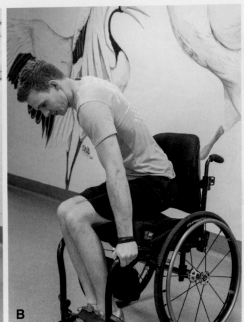

Figure 4.16 A, B Pressure lift.

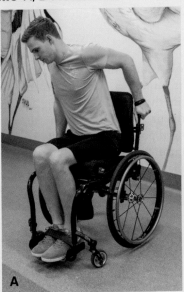
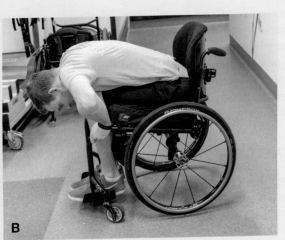

Figure 4.17 A, B Pressure lean.

Continued

Common pressure-relieving or weight-shift techniques—cont'd

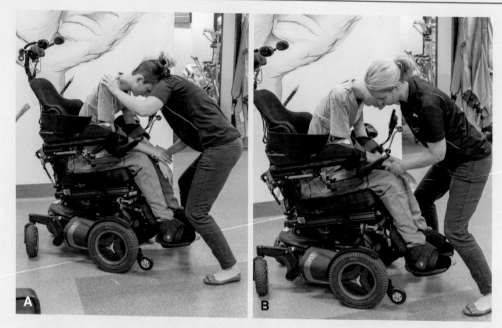

Figure 4.18 A, B High-level tetraplegia pressure-relieving techniques.

The effectiveness of pressure-relieving techniques is best demonstrated to patients by conducting a pressure mapping activity to highlight the significant change in pressure that can be achieved through a simple pressure lean. In fact, the literature suggests that the forward-leaning position is the most effective method of pressure relief.[20]

OSTEOPOROSIS

Immediately following SCI, approximately 75% of patients suffer rapid and severe loss of bone mineral density (BMD) below the lesion level (i.e. sublesional), leading to osteoporosis (OP) in approximately 60% of people 1 year post-injury. The distal femur (DF) and proximal tibia (PT)

are most commonly involved, and 70% of SCI patients sustain a low impact fracture at some point in their lifetime, adding an extra layer of impairment disability to an already physically challenged population.[1] Despite extensive research, mechanisms of this bone impairment are still inadequately understood,[2] although the main reason for SCI-related bone loss in the acute phase is considered to be the loss of mechanical stimuli due to the paralysis. This mechanical unloading results in increased osteocyte expression of sclerostin, suppressed bone formation and indirect stimulation of bone resorption.[4] Risk factors in the SCI population have recently been described as DXA-defined low bone mineral density together with a combination of clinical and demographic factors

Key principles to consider regarding appropriate pressure relief

- Maximise surface area contact to achieve the greatest pressure distribution. Ensure that the equipment is the correct size for the client, especially when including a cushion.

- Bony prominences have peak pressures, so it is important to distribute the pressure over a larger area.

- Flotation/immersion of the patient so that they sit in the cushion/device in order that the whole of the supporting body surface is immersed in the relief medium. Always be mindful to check for bottoming out (i.e. when the bony prominence is no longer supported in the pressure-relieving medium and is touching the firm support surface).

- Shear reduction is hard to measure, therefore ensure the principles of preventing sliding forwards in chair is accommodated through positioning and setup of the chair. For example, tilt in space, squeeze or dump of the chair, use of cushion mediums, as well as covers that have elements of shear reduction. Using slide sheets to reposition people in bed or chairs, even mobile shower commodes, can prevent friction and shear.

- Sitting/lying tolerance should be gradually increased so that the skin integrity is not challenged too much in one session. Often the skin will cope with the stress as a one-off, but will break down if pushed too far too soon or too often.

- Functional independence needs to be incorporated as there is no benefit to ultimate pressure relief if it impacts on the ability to independently achieve functional tasks (balance, transfers, bed mobility, etc). There is a constant assessment between health and function that needs to be undertaken.

- Good positioning/posture is ideal for optimal functioning; however, in some cases it may be an issue if it contributes to a breakdown in skin integrity, whereby the patient's skin should take priority.

- Aim to decrease tone, if possible, by using seating to prevent spasm; this may require a setup that involves the patient sitting in a way that is less upright.

- Moisture control should be managed. Consider managing urinary issues first and don't sit if constantly bypassing, don't use pads or 'blueys' as they can create a hammock effect and may reduce the pressure relieving properties of the cushion/mattress, leading to an increased risk of pressure injury development.

including Caucasian race, female sex, history of prior fractures, medication use (corticosteroids, opioids, anticonvulsants) and SCI-specific characteristics, including duration of injury, paraplegia and completeness of injury.[5]

Non-pharmacological treatment measures on SCI-induced osteoporosis include weight-bearing, electrical stimulation, functional electrical stimulation and vibration therapy, but their effects are inconclusive and the literature describes these methods as being inadequate as sole modalities for osteoporosis prevention.[21–24]

Bisphosphonates are the most common class of drug used to treat SCI-related osteoporosis, but data is mixed on their efficacy for BMD outcomes, and no study has shown a reduction in incident fractures with these medications. Surgical management for lower extremity osteoporotic fractures in SCI may be associated with fewer complications when compared to conservative management.[5,21–24]

INITIAL MOBILISATION

When sitting an acute SCI patient out of bed for the first time it is vital that the initial experience is as pleasant as possible. A negative experience may have a detrimental impact on the therapist–patient relationship and potentially result in a reluctance to engage in the initial stages of rehabilitation. To ensure the experience is positive, limit the initial sit to 1–2 hours. This will minimise fatigue and pain, and provide an opportunity to check that the equipment provided is not causing any inadvertent pressure injuries. The initial mobilisation is an opportunity to provide an orientation to the ward, visit the outdoors and complete a tour of the therapy areas.

Prior to commencing the initial mobilisation:

- review documented mobility instructions from the medical team and be aware of any precautions e.g. bracing, restrictions in flexion, pain

- review documented orthopaedic instructions regarding braces (e.g. +/– cervical collar, thoracic lumbar sacral orthosis (TLSO), etc.)

- discuss with nursing staff/medical team to ensure patient is written up for Sudafed (pseudoephedrine is used to treat orthostatic hypotension by increasing vasoconstriction and peripheral resistance)[25] to be administered 30 minutes prior to the agreed mobilisation time to allow the medication to take effect[26]

- ensure that an abdominal binder has been procured to assist with managing orthostatic hypotension and to assist with breathing

- commence sitting patient up in bed (note: monitor skin, use bed tilt to prevent shearing)

- locate appropriate equipment (recliner wheelchair, ROHO™ pressure-relieving cushion, chest strap, anti-tippers, etc.)

- discuss with patient/family appropriate clothing, which should be loose, comfortable, breathable, seam-free along areas of high risk (e.g. ischial tuberosities, greater trochanter, sacrum, coccyx); and appropriate footwear, which should be enclosed to protect toes and heels, 1–2 times larger than usual to accommodate for any dependent swelling that may develop while sitting and to be wary of areas of pressure in the foot (1st metatarsal phalangeal (MTP), 5th MTP, heel, great toe).

A typical initial mobilisation includes:

- negotiation of appropriate time with nursing staff (e.g. around 11am so the patient can sit up for lunch)

- explanation given regarding mobilisation process

- hoist transfer

- check posture, adjust ROHO eliminate clothing creases

- provide tour of unit and therapy areas

- instruct patient and family on wheelchair use (propulsion, turning, brakes, recline)

- education on pressure relief and skin care, including how to perform pressure lifts and leans in the wheelchair and the importance of a skin check on return to bed

- review skin on return to bed and adjustment equipment, as appropriate, before progressing to sit time.

- emphasise that if a pressure injury is identified, key information needs to be recorded, including the location, a description including colour and size, and how long it takes to fade.

Aim for progression out of the recliner in approximately 2 weeks as able for cervical injuries. Strategies for progressing sitting tolerance include lowering the leg rests, increasing the upright position of the recliner and then removing the head rest. Thoracic injuries should be able to progress more quickly.

STRENGTHENING

Following an SCI, the whole body will be deconditioned due to prolonged bed rest, the initial injury and neurological weakness. A tailored strengthening program should be prescribed based on the clinical presentation and taking into consideration any orthopaedic precautions. Ideally the program will be bilateral and start with light resisted exercise.

To optimise improvements in strength it is advised to follow the simple recipe provided by the progressive resistance training program set out by the American College of Sports Medicine, which involves multiple sets of 8–12 repetition max (RM) with 1–3 minutes rest between sets and a minimum three sessions per week.[27] The reality is that the more training that can be completed the more long-term benefit that is achieved. The literature states that it is unclear whether progressive resistance training improves strength/endurance in muscles with neurologically-induced weakness following tetraplegia.[28] However, the principles described will still achieve the maximum potential of the motor neurons that are still innervated by following the principles of hypertrophy and training.

When developing an exercise program for individuals, it is important to consider whether you are trying to address identified deficits in strength versus endurance. Each type of training has a different physiological effect within the muscle cells. Subsequently, when strength- and endurance-based exercises are performed in the same session or too close together, the body is more likely to respond to the endurance training. As a result, it is important to spend some dedicated time with the patient when first prescribing a program to ensure that they are performing the technique correctly and that the three sets of 8–12 RM is accurate for the patient. Finally, there is now overwhelming evidence that protein supplementation such as whey, casein and milk increases muscle mass and strength gains during prolonged strength training in both younger and older subjects.[29]

While the use of pulleys, springs and weights can be used by all patients to strengthen all muscles, it is important to focus on maximising strength in all active muscles that can assist with functional tasks including rotator cuff (shoulder stability), anterior deltoids (reverse origin insertion to maintain balance in forward lean), latissimus dorsi (shoulder depression during transfers), triceps (maintain elbow extension during shoulder extension) and biceps (wheelchair propulsion).

Strengthening available trunk muscles, including abdominals and long back extensors, assists with improving balance. Prone positioning can be started in the acute setting in preparation for mobilisation if the patient has experienced prolonged bed rest. This can continue in the gym to improve neck strength by the time the soft collar is removed and to strengthen back and neck extensors and scapular stabilisers. This position also allows for propping up on elbows and learning weight transference from shoulder to shoulder while achieving a stretch for the hip flexors. Other techniques include 'sit-ups' on the tilt table, push-ups in prone and Swiss ball activities.

Any identified flickers of lower limb muscle activity should be strengthened. Muscles not strong enough for antigravity work are set up in gravity-eliminated slings and suspension exercises with gradually increasing resistance. Any strength gains may allow the patient to roll and dress more easily, or even manage a standing transfer with assistance.

While concentrating on developing wheelchair skills and independence, the patient is gradually strengthening any other muscles present although a realistic outlook on the functional prognosis is essential (see Online resources for websites with useful strengthening and exercise ideas).

Sitting balance and general balance re-education including mat-based activities, rolling and standing related interventions are all important elements that should be incorporated into the therapy program at this stage. This will be dealt with in more detail in Chapter 6.

EDUCATION

During the patient's time in bed, the physiotherapist is steadily building up rapport with the patient. The physiotherapist teaches them about their injury and setting realistic goals by encouraging them to ask questions and learn about all aspects of their management. At the same time the family is often visiting and asking lots of questions. The patient will be talking to other patients and staff, but most often it will be the therapists to whom they confide their deepest anxieties. This is because of the time the physiotherapist spends with the patient and the fact they are often a more constant face than other staff. The physiotherapist must therefore be well acquainted with every aspect of the patient's case and be ready to answer or refer to the appropriate source any questions which are asked.

Evidence-based practice points

- Maximise ventilation, remove secretions, minimise work of breathing.
- Regularly monitor the efficacy of the management plan by performing regular outcome measures, preferably at the same time each day for consistency.
- An acute SCI patient requires enough breath support to be able to talk, laugh, shout, etc.
- Time interventions to coincide with medications (pain relief, Ventolin etc.) to augment the benefit of both the physiological and the pharmaceutical management.
- Rest and hydration are important components of the healing process and will contribute significantly to any physiological improvements. As such, provide enough rest time between treatments and avoid performing any respiratory intervention after a meal if possible.
- Monitor neurological status.
- Maintain flexibility of all limbs, but particularly pay attention to shoulder and upper limb range of motion.
- Commence a strengthening program that focuses on the key muscles for stability that can assist with functional tasks.
- Pair breathing with movement patterns (active or passive) to facilitate greater respiratory function (flexion with inspiration and extension with expiration), and consider the impact of position changes on respiratory function and passive range.
- Educate at every opportunity at an individual and family level.

SUMMARY

The early hospital physiotherapy management of an acute SCI patient is based on completing a thorough subjective and objective assessment that will allow the development of a patient-centred treatment plan that best meets the needs of the individual and their family or support network, not just the condition. The key principles to follow include setting appropriate levels of expectation without removing hope by explaining what parts work currently, what parts do not and how to adapt. It is imperative to be honest and collaborate on everything and motivate the patient by breaking tasks down into components and making them achievable.

An effective rehabilitation program is one that involves variety, whereby the patient can work on a range of areas but not the same routine every day. Encourage active participation and client focus and set goals so that both the therapist and the patient have an agreed plan of attack with a strong emphasis on functional carryover. Every new skill that is developed in the gym needs to be practised on the ward or in the home environment. The amount of therapy should be directly related to the patient's goals in the context of their rehabilitation plan and take into consideration appropriate rest periods to allow their body to make the most out of every session.

It is impossible for a therapist to prepare their patient for every scenario they may experience, therefore it is important to facilitate the development of problem-solving skills at every opportunity. SCI rehabilitation is a 24/7 experience that does not cease even once the patient leaves the hospital or rehabilitation unit.

Online resources

ASIA. further detailed information on standardised sensory and motor assessments for the ISNCSCI, https://asia-spinalinjury.org/learning

elearnSCI.org, www.elearnsci.org

ISNCSCI impairment scale algorithim, https://www.isncscialgorithm.com/

PhysioTherapy eXercises for people with injuries and disabilities www.physiotherapyexercises.com

Quensland Spinal Cord Injuries Service. Fact Sheet, Management of Autonomic dysreflexia. Information for health professionals and people with spinal cord injury. Queensland Government, 2017, www.health.qld.gov.au/__data/assets/pdf_file/0034/424888/dysreflexia.pdf

References

1. Harvey, L., 2008. Management of spinal cord injuries: a guide for physiotherapists. Churchill Livingstone, Sydney.

2. El Masry, W., 2018. Traumatic spinal injury and spinal cord injury: point for active physiological conservative management as compared to surgical management. Spinal Cord Ser. Cases 4, 14.

3. NSW Agency for Clinical Innovation, 2013. Treatment of autonomic dysreflexia for adults and adolescents with spinal cord injuries, ACI Chatswood, NSW. www.aci.health.nsw.gov.au/__data/assets/pdf_file/0007/155149/Autonomic-Dysreflexia-Treatment.pdf.

4. Berlly, M., Shem, K., 2007. Respiratory management during the first five days after a spinal cord injury. J. Spinal Cord Med. 30, 309–318.

5. Jackson, A.B., Groomers, T.E., 1994. Incidence of respiratory complications following SCI. Arch. Phys. Med. Rehabil. 75, 270–275.

6. Reid, W.D., Brown, J.A., et al., 2010. Physiotherapy secretion removal techniques in people with spinal cord injury: a systematic review. J. Spinal Cord Med. 33 (4), 353–370.

7. Carvalho, C.R., Paisani, D.M., et al., 2011. Incentive spirometry in major surgeries: a systematic review. Rev. Bras. Fisioter. 15 (5), 343–350.

8. Wadsworth, B.M. Abdominal binders – giving breath and voice to people who have suffered a spinal cord injury. MPhil Thesis, School of Health and Rehabilitation Sciences, The University of Queensland.

9. Wadsworth, B., Haines, T., et al., 2008. Abdominal binder use in people with spinal cord injuries: a systematic review and meta-analysis. Spinal Cord 47, 274–285.

10. Hales, M., Biros, E., et al., 2015. Reliability and validity of the sensory component of the International Standards for Neurological Classification of Spinal Cord Injury (ISNCSCI): a systematic review. Top. Spinal Cord Inj. Rehabil. 21 (3), 241–249.

11. Schuld, C., Franz, S., et al., 2015. International standards for neurological classification of spinal cord injury: classification skills of clinicians versus computational algorithms. Spinal Cord 53 (4), 324.

12. Svensson, M., Siösteen, A., et al., 1995. Influence of physiotherapy on leg blood flow in patients with complete spinal cord injury lesions. Physiother. Theory Pract. 11 (2), 97–107.

13. Katalinic, O.M., Harvey, L.A., et al., 2011. Effectiveness of stretch for the treatment and prevention of contractures in people with neurological conditions: a systematic review. Phys. Ther. 91 (1), 11–24.

14. Harvey, L.A., Glinsky, J.A., et al., 2011. Contracture management for people with spinal cord injuries. Neurorehabilitation 28 (1), 17–20.

15. Cratsenberg, K.A., Deitrick, C.E., et al., 2015. Effectiveness of exercise programs for management of shoulder pain in manual wheelchair users with spinal cord injury. J. Neurol. Phys. Ther. 39 (4), 197–203.

16. Reznik, J., Keren, O., et al., 2016. Pharmacology handbook for physiotherapists: Elsevier Health Sciences.

17. Adler, S., Beckers, D., et al., 2014. PNF in Practice, fourth ed. Springer Medizin Verlag, Heidelberg, Germany.

18. Adams, M.M., Hicks, A.L., 2005. Spasticity after spinal cord injury. Spinal Cord 43 (10), 577.

19. National Pressure Ulcer Advisory Panel, European Pressure Ulcer Advisory Panel and Pan Pacific Pressure Injury Alliance. Prevention and treatment of pressure ulcers: clinical practice guideline. Haesler, Emily (Ed.). Osborne Park, Western Australia, Cambridge Media, 2014.

20. Regan, M.A., Teasell, R.W., et al., 2009. A systematic review of therapeutic interventions for pressure ulcers after spinal cord injury. Arch. Phys. Med. Rehabil. 90 (2), 213–231.

21. Trbovich, M., Mack, D., et al., 2019. Osteoporosis in veterans with spinal cord injury: an overview of pathophysiology, diagnosis, and treatments. Clin. Rev. Bone Miner. Metab. 17 (2), 94–108.

22. Dionyssiotis, Y., 2019. Is prophylaxis for osteoporosis indicated after acute spinal cord injury? Spinal Cord Ser. Cases 5, 24.

23. Battaglino, R.A., Lazzari, A.A., et al., 2012. Spinal cord injury-induced osteoporosis: pathogenesis and emerging therapies. Curr. Osteoporosis Rep. 10 (4), 278–285.

24. Zleik, N., Weaver, F., et al., 2018. Prevention and management of osteoporosis and osteoporotic fractures in persons with a spinal cord injury or disorder: a systematic scoping review. J. Spinal Cord Med. 1–25.

25. Blackmer, J., 1997. Orthostatic hypotension in spinal cord injured patients. J. Spinal Cord Med. 20 (2), 212–217.

26. Queensland Spinal Cord Injuries Service. Fact Sheet, Information for general practitioners: Autonomic dysreflexia and blood pressure management after spinal cord injury. Queensland Government. www.health.qld.gov.au/__data/assets/pdf_file/0041/649697/gp-ad-bp-fact-sheet.pdf.

27. Ratamess, N.A., Alvar, B.A., et al., 2009. Progression models in resistance training for healthy adults. Med. Sci. Sports Exerc. 41 (3), 687–708.

28. Glinsky, J., Harvey, L., et al., 2008. Short-term progressive resistance exercise may not be effective at increasing wrist strength in people with tetraplegia: a randomised controlled trial. Aust. J. Physiother. 54 (2), 103–108.

29. Cermak, N.M., de Groot, L.C., et al., 2012. Protein supplementation augments the adaptive response of skeletal muscle to resistance-type exercise training: a meta-analysis. Am. J. Clin. Nutr. 96 (6), 1454–1464.

CHAPTER 5
Biomechanics

Oren Tirosh

INTRODUCTION

Biomechanics is the study of the mechanics of human movement. The field focuses on understanding and implementing mechanical principles to improve human movement performance and reduce injuries.

This chapter will explain the principles of biomechanics that clinicians use to solve the everyday problems they encounter when considering their patients with spinal cord injury (SCI). More specifically, this chapter will focus on rigid body mechanics to explain motion and the forces that are involved in slowing down or speeding up the body and its segments. A segment, for example, can be the trunk, upper arm, pelvis or upper leg. The understanding of how forces can be applied to move or stabilise the body and its segments is important for every clinician. It is essential to understand these forces and how they impact on positioning and transfer tasks, for the wellbeing of both the patient and the clinician.

This chapter will use a series of free-body diagrams, such as the one depicted in Fig. 5.1, to show the relative magnitude and direction of all the forces acting upon an object in a given situation.

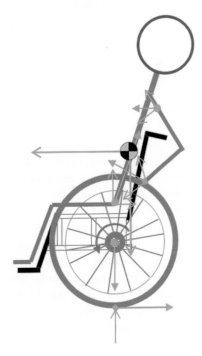

Figure 5.1 Sample of a free-body diagram in wheelchair.

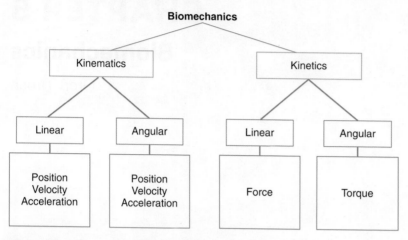

Biomechanics

Kinematics

- Linear
  - Position
    Velocity
    Acceleration
- Angular
  - Position
    Velocity
    Acceleration

Kinetics

- Linear
  - Force
- Angular
  - Torque

Figure 5.2 Flowchart of subdivision in biomechanics.

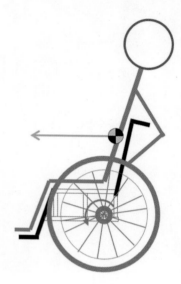

Figure 5.3 Example of kinematics free-body diagram in wheelchair.

DEFINITIONS USED IN BIOMECHANICS

Kinematics and kinetics

Biomechanics is comprised of two subdivisions, kinematics and kinetics (Fig. 5.2).

Kinematics describes the motion of a point, body and systems of bodies without considering the forces that caused the motion. In this case, the wheelchair free-body diagram will be as shown in Fig. 5.3.

Kinetics explains the causes of kinematics, specifically, the relationship between motion and forces and torques that cause the motion. In this case, the wheelchair free-body diagram will be as shown in Fig. 5.4.

When performing a biomechanical analysis, the movement is examined from the perspectives of both linear and angular motion. Linear motion is motion along a line (Fig. 5.5A). Angular motion involves the rotation of an object around its axis. In the human skeleton, for example, the object is a segment and the axis is a joint. Another angular motion can be the rotation of the whole body around an identified axis on the body (Fig. 5.5B).

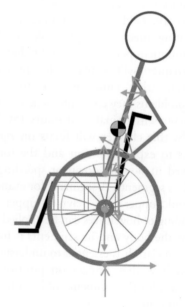

Figure 5.4 Example of kinetics free-body diagram in wheelchair.

The mass

Mass is a measure of the quantity of matter in a physical body. Body mass refers to adding up the molecules of all the materials that makes up a physical body. The mass of a physical body can be measured and reported as a single value without considering each individual molecule within it. This measure is reported in kilograms (kg).

Centre of mass

The centre of mass (COM) is a specific point located within the physical body, which, when a force is applied to that point, will cause linear motion without angular motion (Fig. 5.6A). If the force is not applied directly at the COM, the physical body will rotate (Fig. 5.6B). The COM is the unique point where the weighted relative position of the distributed mass sums to zero. In this chapter, the COM is denoted as ◕.

The location of the total COM of a body comprising multiple segments depends on the distribution of all the masses of its segments. In this case, it is the unique position at which the weighted position of all the segments' COM add up to zero (Fig. 5.7A). The location of the total COM is therefore dependent on its segment's position and orientation relative to each other (Fig. 5.7B). It is possible for the location of the total COM to be outside the physical body (Fig. 5.7C).

Orientation

In biomechanics, movement is described in a two-dimensional (2-D) flat surface plane using the basic spatial reference system known as the *Cartesian coordinate* system, shown in Fig. 5.8. This 2-D coordinate system plane consists of two intersecting lines: one creates a horizontal axis to the ground (often called the *x*-axis), and the other creates a vertical axis to the ground (often called the *y*-axis). Any location on the coordinate system is identified with a pair of coordinates using the format (x, y). The first value, *x*, describes how far the point is along the *x*-axis from origin $(0, 0)$; the second value, *y*, describes how far the point is along the *y*-axis from origin $(0, 0)$. The location of the COM in Fig. 5.8A is therefore described as $(5, 3)$. When the COM moves, its new location can be described in the plane using the coordinate system,

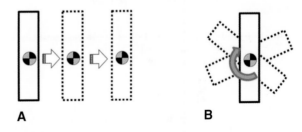

A   **B**

Figure 5.5 A, Linear and B, angular motion.

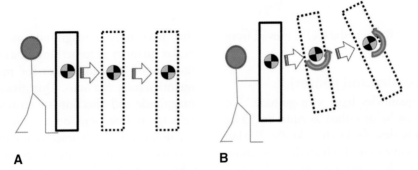

A   **B**

Figure 5.6 Centre of mass (COM) and its relationship to A, linear and B, angular motion

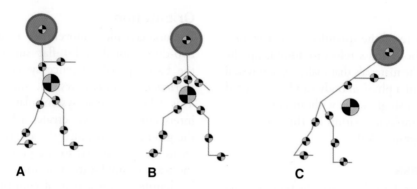

Figure 5.7 A, B, C, Changes in the location of total centre of mass.

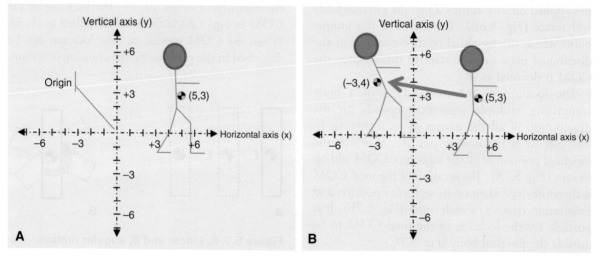

Figure 5.8 A, B Location of the centre of mass in a plane.

as shown in Fig. 5.8B where the COM moved from (5, 3) to (–3, 4).

Illustration (scalar and vector)

In mechanics, quantities have a magnitude. For example, mass can be described as equal to 53 kg and velocity can be described to be 5 km/hr. Within these quantities some may also include a direction. For example, when describing velocity, the direction of the movement is also described, while in the quantity mass there is no direction. Quantities that have only a magnitude are termed *scalars*. Scalar quantity is something described fully by its measure of 'how much', or the magnitude of the quantity, such as a mass. Quantities that have both magnitude and direction are termed *vectors*. Force, velocity and acceleration are the most important vector quantities in biomechanics. In a free diagram, vectors are indicated by an *arrow*, the length of which represents the quantity magnitude, while the direction of the arrow represents the direction of the quantity.

Resolving a vector into components

When performing a biomechanical analysis, vectors are typically broken into two perpendicular horizontal and vertical components. Fig. 5.9 shows that the vertical and horizontal vector components are always smaller than the primary (resultant) vector and the size of these components depends on the direction of the primary vector. For example, Fig. 5.9B shows that the vertical component is larger than the horizontal when the prime vector is primarily in the vertical direction. However, when the prime vector is primarily towards the horizontal direction the horizontal component will be greater than the vertical component.

Composing a vector from components

Vector composition allows for the combination of the horizontal and vertical vectors into a single resultant (prime) vector. The resultant prime vector will always be larger than the two vectors, as can be seen in Fig. 5.9.

STANDARDISING A REFERENCE FRAME

The movement of a body can occur in many directions. In biomechanics the movement is divided into three directions and described as moving in three perpendicular planes, including sagittal, frontal and transverse (Fig. 5.10). When analysing a linear motion, the body is described as moving along a plane. When analysing an angular motion, the body is described as moving about an axis. In the reference frame, an axis of rotation is perpendicular to the plane through which the body or segment moves as it rotates. The same axis will always have the same plane paired with it (Fig. 5.10).

Moving through planes

The whole body and the individual segments of the human body can move in many directions simultaneously. To analyse a multiplane movement pattern the whole body movement and its joint segments are analysed in each plane separately, as shown in Fig. 5.11.

Descriptors of kinematics: displacement, velocity, acceleration

Kinematics is the branch of mechanics concerned with the motion of the mass without reference to the forces that cause the motion. The motion is described as moving in spatial (through space) and temporal (time) characteristics. The motion can be linear, angular, or both. Three vector quantities are used to describe kinematics: displacement, velocity and acceleration.

- Linear *displacement* is measured as a straight-line distance between where the body started and where the body ended up (Fig. 5.12A). Angular displacement is the measured angle between the start and end positions of a rotating body (Fig. 5.12B).

- *Velocity* is the rate of change of displacement, i.e. how fast an object is moving from one location to another. In Fig. 5.12A the linear

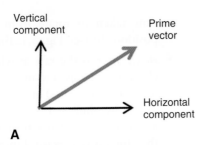

A

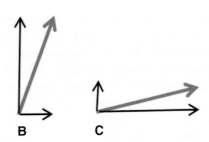

B   **C**

Figure 5.9 A, B, C, A vector and its components.

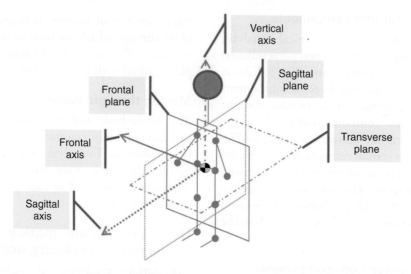

Figure 5.10 The three perpendicular planes and axes – sagittal, frontal and transverse.

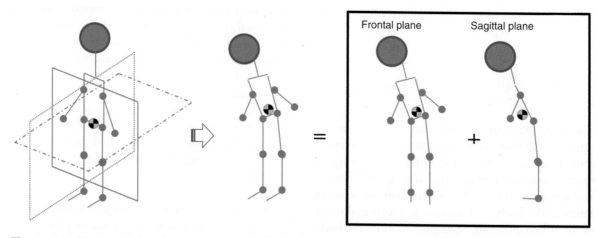

Figure 5.11 Centre of mass movement in multiple planes.

displacement is 9 m, but the performer can translate from point (a) to point (b) in a slow or fast manner. How fast the performer is travelling in a straight line (linear) can be calculated by taking the displacement and dividing it by the time taken to get from point (a) to point (b), i.e. linear velocity. Similar to linear motion, the angular velocity is calculated as the angular displacement divided by the time taken to rotate from position (a) to position (b) (see Fig. 5.12B).

- *Acceleration* is the rate at which the velocity changes with respect to time, how fast an object increases (accelerates) or decreases (decelerates) its velocity. Similar to displacement and velocity, acceleration has a magnitude and direction; therefore, it is a vector. Linear acceleration is the change of linear velocity with time and

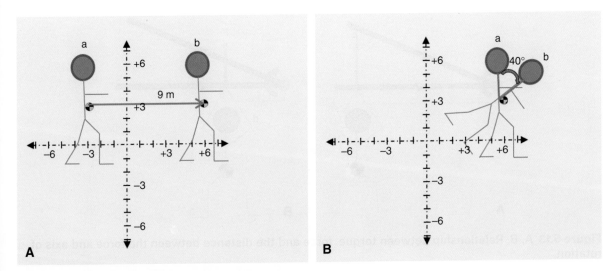

Figure 5.12 A, Linear and B, angular displacement in a plane.

angular acceleration is the change of angular velocity with time. The most commonly used acceleration in biomechanics is the acceleration due to gravity. Gravity is denoted *g*, and its direction is towards the ground. Due to the mechanical relationship between acceleration and force, the gravitational attraction is also known as the *force of gravity* and it acts on the centre of mass.

Descriptors of kinetics: force, torque, impulse

A body's state can be static 'at rest' (zero velocity) or dynamic 'in motion' while moving at a constant velocity. In both states the body velocity does not change. To cause a change to the body's velocity a pushing or pulling action needs to occur, called a *force*. Thus, a body at rest can be made to move when external force is applied to it. Similarly, a body in motion can be slowed down, speeded up, or have the direction of motion altered if external force is acted on it.

Forces can be internal or external. Internal forces are considered to be internal to the system, such as the constriction of a muscle that causes

forces to be exerted on the bones to which it is attached. External forces are considered to be forces coming from other systems, such as the ground, gravity, air resistance, friction and other bodies.

Force has a magnitude and direction; therefore it is a *vector*. The force is generally considered to be linear to cause a linear motion, but when applied away from the centre of mass of an object or from the axis of rotation it creates an angular motion. A force that creates angular motion is called *torque*. The torque magnitude comprises and depends upon two components: 1) the linear force, and 2) the distance between the force and axis of rotation (Fig. 5.13). The torque is the product of the force and the distance between the point of force application and axis of rotation. Fig. 5.13 shows two scenarios while applying the same magnitude of force is applied on the rotating lever but at a greater distance in A as compared to B. The rotating torque in A, therefore, is greater than in B.

The same amount of force can create different torque values. Similar force application can generate more or less torque at the joint. Fig. 5.14 shows an example of the torque at the joint, i.e. less stress can

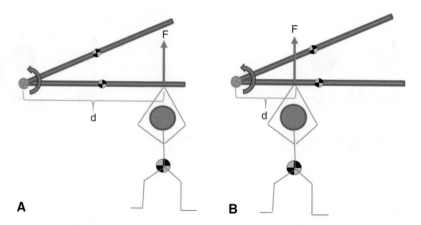

Figure 5.13 A, B, Relationship between torque, force and the distance between the force and axis of rotation.

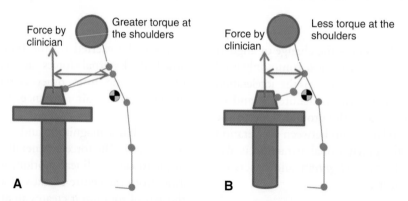

Figure 5.14 A, B, Changes in torque magnitude with changes in segment length.

be minimised by reducing the distance between the force application and the joint.

Time is fundamental when analysing human movement. Displacing an object can be achieved by applying force in short or long duration. The effect of force acting over time on an object is known as *impulse*. An example of impulse is the ground reaction force applied by the foot during walking multiplied by the duration of the force's application, which is equal to the impulse generated by the foot. The magnitude of the impulse linearly relates to body momentum, which describes the body's velocity.

Thus, greater impulse results in greater velocity. It can therefore be seen that to move an object at specific velocity the clinician may choose several options; for example, applying high force in a short time, or applying low force over a long period of time. Both options may result in a similar impulse.

DESCRIBING AND UNDERSTANDING MOVEMENT (THE LAWS OF MOTION)

The prime objective in biomechanics is the ability to describe and understand movement – the cause–effect relationship between bodies and the forces that cause them to move. There are three fundamental laws of motions that guide us in understanding and analysing motion. The three laws were proposed and published by Sir Isaac Newton in the eighteenth century.

- <u>Newton's first law</u> – *inertia:* The body at rest remains at rest and a body in motion continues to move at a constant velocity unless acted upon by an external **force**. In other words, unless an unbalanced force acts on a body, the body does not speed up or slow down.

- <u>Newton's second law</u> – *law of acceleration:* The acceleration of an object is directly proportional to the magnitude of the **net force**, and inversely proportional to the mass of the object. It is important to note here that the sum of all forces acting on the body needs to be estimated and the resultant acceleration will occur if the sum of forces is not equal to zero and the direction of the acceleration will be in the direction of the resultant force.

- <u>Newton's third law</u> – *action–reaction:* for every action (**force**) in nature there is an equal and opposite reaction. It is important to note here that it is not that one force reacts to the other force, but that both forces are acting simultaneously towards each other with similar magnitude but in opposite directions.

BALANCE AND STABILITY

Stability is defined as the resistance to both linear and angular acceleration or resistance to disruption of equilibrium.[1] The level of stability is affected by the relationship between the centre of gravity (COG) and the body's base of support (BOS). The BOS is the area bounded by the outermost points of contact between the feet and the supporting surface. The body is statically stable when the vertical projection of the COG falls inside the area of the supporting base (Fig. 5.15).

One factor that affects stability is the size of the BOS. A larger BOS lowers the likelihood that the

COS will move out of the supporting base. For example, during human walking a longer step with the swing foot will anteriorly increase the BOS and thus will decrease the likelihood of the system to lose balance and fall forwards.

The horizontal location of the COG relative to the BOS is another factor that has an influence over stability. The closer the horizontal location of the COG is to the boundary of the BOS, the smaller is the force required to push it outside the supporting area.

Maintaining stability when walking

A statically stable gait is obtained when the COG is inside the supporting base during the entire cycle. In human walking the gait cycle fluctuates between statically stable and unstable, thus, is 'semi-dynamically' stable (see Fig. 5.16). At heel-contact, for example, the COG is reported to be 7.7 cm behind the BOS, i.e. in an unstable state.[2] However, because the COG has sufficient horizontal velocity, balance is sustained, and the COG progresses forwards and is centred within the BOS during mid-stance. To continue walking, the COG must voluntarily exceed the forward

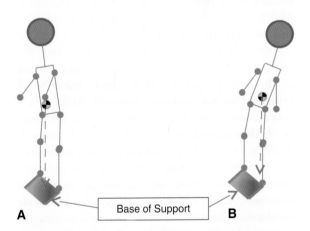

Figure 5.15 A, B, The location and relationship of the base of support (BOS) and the centre of gravity (COG) during double support. The red line illustrates the vertical projection of the COG on to the ground.

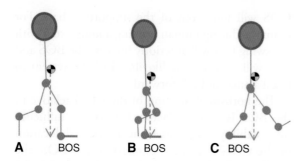

Figure 5.16 The location and relationship of the base of support (BOS) and the centre of gravity (COG) during walking, when A, the COG is behind BOS; B, the COG is inside BOS; C, the COG is ahead of BOS. The blue line illustrates the vertical projection of the COG on the ground.

border of the supporting base, i.e. create a forward fall and accelerate the COG ahead, now statically unstable. This semi-dynamically stable state, therefore, challenges whole-body stability and forces a regulation of the trajectory of the COG so that it remains well within the lateral borders of the BOS.

A further requirement of walking is regulating balance in response to errors of foot placement. McKinnon and Winter[3] suggested a communicative link between the state of the whole body balance system relative to the support surface and the musculature that controls the balance and posture of the large proportion of the body mass. Small errors in foot placement are corrected distally by the subtalar musculature, and large errors are corrected by the hip musculature. Sufficient muscle strength at the hip is, therefore, important to sustain balance and prevent a fall. Other options to assist the distal subtalar musculature are the use of ankle–foot orthoses (AFO) which are suggested to provide mechanical support and alterations in sensorimotor control.[4] Studies provided conflicting results as to whether AFOs reduce the risk of falling, with some reporting no difference in clinical balance scores nor in static or dynamic weight-bearing tasks when wearing an AFO.[5-7] When altering walking speed

and walking direction, fixed AFOs were reported to hinder the generation of propulsion and the regulation of angular momentum; thus, in such cases the prescription of AFOs should be carefully considered.[8]

Transferring

Transferring a patient from one place to another, such as from the bed to wheelchair, is a very stressful task. The lifting and transferring of patients has been perceived by nursing personnel to be the most frequent precipitating factor or trigger of back problems.[9] It is therefore important for the clinician to understand and utilise mechanical principles to reduce the load on their body during patient transfer.

Any transfer requires controlling the movements of the COG away from the centre of the BOS. These movements have the potential of causing a loss of balance and musculoskeletal overloading. Maintaining proper posture during the transfer task is, therefore, crucial to reducing the stress and strain on the musculoskeletal structures. Proper posture and body mechanics are based upon alignment and functioning of the musculoskeletal system. In general, proper mechanics should include the following:

- Maintaining patient stability by having their COG of the body low and close to the centre of BOS.

- Keeping the combined COG of the transferor and patient close and within the BOS.

- Having a BOS that is of the appropriate size and shape.

- Use the principle of torque and levers to minimise the resistance forces, such as reducing the load on the transferor's shoulders by reducing the distance from the shoulders to the patient's COG.

- Use the principle of torque and levers to initiate movement and momentum, such as raising the patient's arm to the side while lying to initiate rotation for rolling.

Applying the above biomechanical principles is important for patients with SCI during sitting, and sitting transfers to upper or lower levels, such as from bed to wheelchair. An example is the use of increased forward trunk flexion during sitting pivot transfers (SPT), which was shown to reduce superior forces compared to a more upright strategy and help preserve upper limb function over time.[10] The increased trunk flexion affects the relationship between the COG and the BOS and the applied forces by bringing the COG further inside the BOS. Although the forward trunk flexion strategy was found to involve significantly greater muscle activity at the anterior deltoid and both heads of the pectoralis major, it was reported to be more dynamically stable, with an increased area of BOS and greater distance travelled.[11] However, the transfer phase when the buttocks lose contact with the initial seat and when they make contact with the target seat was reported to have an impact on dynamic stability (COG and BOS relationship), with the greatest level of instability occurring during this phase.[12]

Sitting balance

The trunk, head and upper extremities comprise more than 50% of body weight that needs to be controlled in order to keep the COG within the BOS and upright sitting position. It is important to recognise that these are separated segments and that their individual movement can dramatically influence the position of the total COG (see earlier discussion at Fig. 5.7). Fig. 5.17 illustrates how the shift of the head can change the overall position of the COG in relation to the BOS. Therefore, a patient who has limited control in their trunk can assist the clinician by shifting their head and/or arms, resulting in shifting the position of the COG in relation to the BOS. The use of neck and head movements can, therefore, be taught by clinicians to assist patients with little or no trunk musculature control for sitting balance tasks. Fig. 5.17 shows an example of shifting the COG forwards towards the edge of the BOS. By doing this, the patient can assist

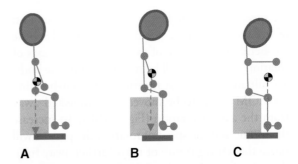

Figure 5.17 A, B, C, The effect of head movement on the overall position of the centre of gravity.

the clinician in moving the head and hands during transfers and reducing the forces and distance from the COG to the edge of the BOS.

BED MOBILITY

Rolling

The ability to roll and turn in bed is one of the most fundamental activities of daily living. Rolling requires intersegmental coordination of the trunk and the upper and lower extremities.[13,14] A wide range of rolling patterns from the supine to side-lying position have been reported, with 32 different combinations of the upper extremities, lower extremities and head and trunk.[15] For example, Sekiya and colleagues[16] observed that the hip adduction angle remained constant throughout the rolling motion when one leg is used to push off the ground, and that the hip rotation angle is in neutral or slightly internally rotated at the beginning of the motion, and externally rotated towards the end of the rolling motion. While the movement in the lower extremities is similar between rolling patterns, it is the variability of the movement of the upper extremities that differentiates between the rolling patterns.[13]

Rolling is initiated by rotational torque when a force is applied on a lever away from the axis of rotation. The further the force is away from the axis of rotation, the greater is the torque and thus the speed of rotation. Fig. 5.18 illustrates a rotation of the body in supine position. In Fig. 5.18A the left-bending leg centre of mass is above the axis of rotation, thus there will be no rotation of the body. To initiate rotation to the right, the left-bending leg COM needs to be moved and projected away from the axis of rotation (Fig. 5.18B). To increase the torque and the speed of rotation the patient will move the left leg centre of mass further away from the axis of rotation (Fig. 5.18C).

Similar to the lower extremity, rolling can be initiated by the upper extremities using comparable mechanical principles. For example, lifting one arm and moving to the side will create a torque that will initiate rolling. In order to maximise the torque, both arms can be moved together accompanied by a coordinated head movement that follows the movement of the arms. Fig. 5.19 illustrates the use of the arms to initiate rolling. The ideal pattern is to move the arms in a diagonal pattern across the trunk from above the ear towards the contralateral hip (like an axe chop or golf swing). This combined movement, using the head to follow the arms, will

ensure that the COG can remain within the BOS throughout the movement. (This describes the proprioceptive neuromuscular facilitation (PNF) pattern, discussed further in Chapter 11.)

Lying to sitting to standing

Fundamental understanding of the principles of balance (BOS and COG), torque and momentum transfer are important to efficiently transfer the body from one position to another. Momentum transfer is the amount of momentum that one segment gives to another segment. As previously mentioned, momentum directly relates to velocity and the term 'momentum transfer', in simple terms, means transferring the velocity of one segment to another with minimal effort or force.

The technique used to raise the body from lying to sitting typically involves a stereotyped sequence in which joints are either stationary or moving in a particular way. The principle of momentum transfer can be used by moving the strong segments to generate velocity that can be transferred to weak segments; for example, moving the strong arm to

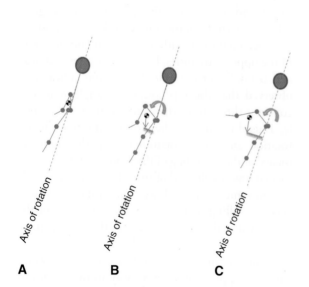

Figure 5.18 A–C, Rotation of the body in supine position.

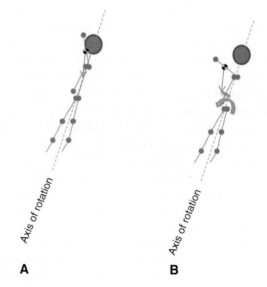

Figure 5.19 A, B, The use of the arms to initiate rolling.

generate velocity that is transferred to the trunk and assisting the weak muscles in moving and lifting the trunk, e.g. sitting to standing (Fig. 5.20).

During lying to sitting transfers it is essential that patients with SCI use their arms to create wide BOS and lift their trunk. To assist with this, initiating a rolling movement will produce COG velocity, which can be transferred to the trunk and assist the arms with lifting it. Bringing the COG forwards outside the BOS will initiate a fall that will promote a forward velocity and shift the body weight forwards until the opposite arm is adjusted to create a new BOS, returning the COG within the new BOS to support the body weight for sitting. See Chapter 6 for an example of this activity in practice (side-lying to sitting).

The same principle can be applied to moving from sitting to standing. Fig. 5.20 shows how the COG is moved forwards towards the end of the BOS to initiate forward movement (A–B), followed by the swing of the arms, which generates momentum (C), which is transferred to the body, assisting with forward velocity (D).

WHEELCHAIR PROPULSION BIOMECHANICS

Wheelchair propulsion is a fundamental movement for lower-limb disabled individuals as it allows for them to be mobile and active; however, this movement is minimally learnt through the rehabilitation process.[17] Wheelchair propulsion is a very complex movement; in order for users to propel themselves in the most efficient way, a desired posture is needed. Boninger and colleagues[18] suggested that the posture of the person should be upright, having the shoulders aligned vertically with the central axle of the wheel (Fig. 5.21). This position allows the user to stretch as far back as possible within their range, grasping onto the rim of the wheelchair and allowing them to propel themselves through a propulsion stoke where flexion and extension occur. For further details on wheelchair prescription refer to Modes of transport, Part 1 in Chapter 8.

Wheelchair propulsion includes two phases: the actual propulsion, which is the push phase, followed by the recovery phase (Fig. 5.22). The push phase is a physical movement performed by the hand while it is in contact with the rim. The push phase is the period beginning with the initial contact of the hand to the top of the rim, and the period ends when the arms are fully extended and the hand leaves the rim. During the period of contact, the hand grasps the rim either at the very top centre of the rim or behind the rim. Push gloves (described in Chapter 21) may be used when when the individual prefers to place their hand on the tyre to propel the wheel. Hand placement is crucial in this period as having it slightly further behind the centre and going through a full movement where the shoulder is rotating and extending can ultimately lead to damage in certain areas within the shoulder joint (discussed in Chapter 15 on ageing with an SCI).[19] This is possibly why wheelchair propulsion has been linked to being a

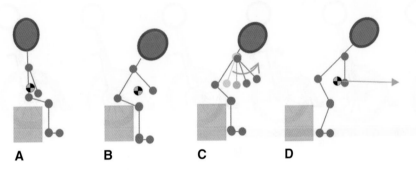

Figure 5.20 A–D, Using arm swing to transfer momentum to the body in sit to stand.

causative factor in shoulder pain and injury.[20] As the propulsion continues, the hand passes the top centre and the arms extend forwards exerting a force onto the rims through the triceps, while the shoulder remains in the optimum position, being vertically aligned to the centre of the rim.

The recovery phase follows after the push phase. The recovery phase, however, differs as the hand is free and not fixed to the rim. The recovery phase is further broken down into four sections: 1) the follow-through, 2) the retrieval, 3) pre-impact, and 4) pre-load. The recovery phase begins at the end of the push phase, when the arms have extended and full force has been applied. The hands continue to follow through further down the rim to complete and maximise the efficiency of the push. Following this, the hands are released from the wheels and the arms are lifted back to counterbalance the inertia; this is the retrieval segment. The retrieval is followed by the recovery phase, then continues with the pre-impact section, where the hands swing back past the centre line of the shoulders, leaving them adjacent to the rim. This is then closely followed by the pre-load phase, where the upper arm returns to a posterior position. Boninger and colleagues[21] suggested that the recovery phase is crucial because individuals were shown to vary in their recovery movement patterns while preparing the hands to hold the rim at the initial pushing phase.

Different types of stroke movement patterns have been discussed in the literature (see Fig. 5.23). Kwarciak and colleagues[22] conducted a study that focused specifically on upper extremity movement patterns in subjects who use wheelchairs as their primary mode of transport. The authors stated that stroke pattern is a prime factor that affects the wheelchair propulsion.

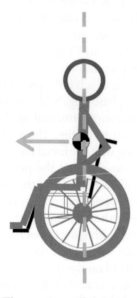

Figure 5.21 The posture of the person should be upright, with the shoulders aligned vertically with the central axle of the wheel.

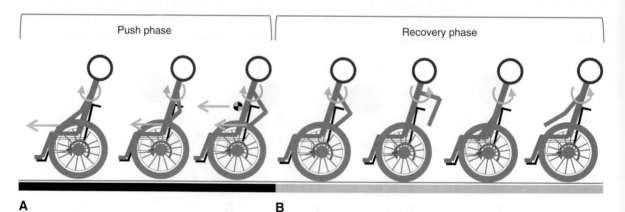

A   Push phase   **B**   Recovery phase

Figure 5.22 The push and recovery phases during wheelchair propulsion.

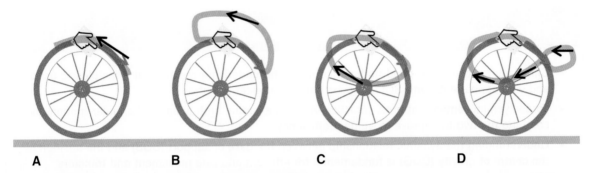

A   **B**   **C**   **D**

Figure 5.23 Different type of stroke patterns identified by Kwarciak et al. (2012): A, Arc. B, Single loop over propulsion (SLOP). C, Semi-circular (SC). D, Double loop over propulsion (DLOP). Red arrow indicates the push phase and the black arrow indicates the recovery phase.

Source: Kwarciak, A.M., Turner, J.T., et al., 2012. The effects of four different stroke patterns on manual wheelchair propulsion and upper limb muscle strain. Disabil Rehabil Assist Technol. 7, 459–463; Sawatzky, B., DiGiovine, T., et al., 2014. The need for updated clinical practice guidelines for preservation of upper extremities in manual wheelchair users: a position paper. American Journal of Physical Medicine and Rehabilitation 94 (4), 313–324.

Kwarciak and colleagues[22] identified four different stroke patterns adopted by wheelchair users: arcing (ARC), single loop over propulsion (SLOP), semi-circular (SC) and double loop over propulsion (DLOP). While they were unable to find any significant differences in forces produced between the four stroke patterns, they did find significant differences in propulsion efficiency.[22] Using propulsion kinematics, Kwarciak and colleagues[22] found more efficient propulsion in the SC and DLOP patterns with longer (by 10–15°) contact angles, lower cadence values (55.9 min^{-1}, 52.2 min^{-1}, 51.3 min^{-1} and 45.2 min^{-1} for ARC, SLOP, SC and DLOP, respectively) and smaller braking moments. Interestingly, the SC and DLOP propulsion patterns were the native patterns chosen by the experienced wheelchair users who participated in the study. Similar results were reported in earlier studies conducted by Shimada and colleagues[23] and Boninger and colleagues[21] showing that Olympian athletes using the SC movement spent 10% less time in recovery and 10% more time in the push phase. This is particularly important for individuals that are seeking to participate in manual wheelchair sport events.

The advantage of the SC pattern was later confirmed by Boninger and colleagues.[21] These authors examined people with paraplegia immediately following their rehabilitation who used manual wheelchairs for mobility. Similarly to Kwarciak and colleagues,[22] this study showed lower cadence values (67.8 min^{-1}, 61.8 min^{-1}, 52.8 min^{-1} and 48.6 min^{-1} for ARC, SLOP, SC and DLOP respectively). Boninger and colleagues[21] also found that manual wheelchair users who utilise both the SC and the DLOP pattern spend less time in the recovery phase and more time in the push phase. Boninger and colleagues[21] indicated that wheelchair users who use both SC and DLOP movement patterns propel less frequently during the push phase while achieving the same speed as others with different movement patterns. Both these patterns of movement had the lowest cadence, as well as the greatest amount of time spent in push phase as opposed to the recovery phase. The findings that SC and the DLOP movement patterns are more efficient suggests that manual wheelchair users with SC and DLOP movement pattern may be less prone to shoulder injury because of their movement and ability to apply less energy into the propulsion over a greater duration of time.

Evidence-based practice points

- Clinicians need to have good understanding of the underlying mechanical principles to assist and educate patients with SCI in movement and transfer activities.
- To analyse movement patterns, clinicians need to examine both linear and angular motion and combine the two to improve movement efficiency.
- Understanding the dynamic relationship between the base of support (BOS) and the position of the centre of gravity (COG) is fundamental for efficient and safe movement and transfers.
- The position of the whole body COG can be translated by repositioning the COG of individual body segments.
- Clinicians need to be familiar with the concept of momentum transfer and identify its use to better initiate whole-body movement using individual body segments such as upper arms, head and neck.
- The movement pattern of manual wheelchair propulsion has a direct relationship to propulsion efficiency and risks to injury.

SUMMARY

Following a description of the basic principles of biomechanics, this chapter has explained the use of biomechanics in solving problems that patients with SCI may encounter while interacting with the environment. Clinicians can, and should, use these mechanical principles to improve patient transfer while reducing their own risk for acute or long-term injury. The basic understanding of the relationship between BOS and COG and how momentum is transferred between body segments may assist clinicians and patients with SCI to use safer and more injury-free movement patterns. Likewise, understanding the mechanical principles behind force and rotary-force (torque) may assist with more efficient manual wheelchair propulsion.

References

1. Hamill, J., Knutzen, K.M., 1995. Biomechanical Basis of Human Movement. Williams & Wilkins, PA, USA.

2. Winter, D.A., 1995. Human balance and posture control during standing and walking. Gait Posture 3, 193–214.

3. McKinnon, C.D., Winter, D.A., 1993. Control of whole body balance in the frontal plane during human walking. J. Biomech. 26, 633–644.

4. Mills, K., Blanch, P., et al., 2010. Foot orthoses and gait: a systematic review and meta-analysis of literature pertaining to potential mechanisms. Br. J. Sports Med. 44, 1035–1046.

5. Park, J.H., Chun, M.H., et al., 2009. Comparison of gait analysis between anterior and posterior ankle foot orthosis in hemiplegic patients. Am. J. Phys. Med. Rehabil. 88, 630–634.

6. Simons, C.D., van Asseldonk, E.H., et al., 2009. Ankle–foot orthoses in stroke: effects on functional balance, weight-bearing asymmetry and the contribution of each lower limb to balance control. Clin. Biomech. (Bristol, UK) 24, 769–775.

7. Wang, R.Y., Yen, L., et al., 2005. Effects of an ankle–foot orthosis on balance performance in patients with hemiparesis of different durations. Clin. Rehabil. 19, 37–44.

8. Vistamehr, A., Kautz, S.A., et al., 2014. The influence of solid ankle–foot-orthoses on forward propulsion and dynamic balance in healthy adults during walking. Clin. Biomech. (Bristol, UK) 29, 583–589.

9. Garg, A., Owen, B., 1992. Reducing back stress to nursing personnel: an ergonomic intervention in a nursing home. Ergonomics 35, 1353–1375.

10. Koontz, A.M., Kankipati, P., et al., 2011. Upper limb kinetic analysis of three sitting pivot wheelchair transfer techniques. Clin. Biomech. (Bristol, UK) 26, 923–929.

11. Desroches, G., Gagnon, D., et al., 2013. Magnitude of forward trunk flexion influences upper limb muscular efforts and dynamic postural stability requirements during sitting pivot transfers in individuals with spinal cord injury. J. Electromyogr. Kinesiol. 23, 1325–1333.

12. Gagnon, D., Duclos, C., et al., 2012. Measuring dynamic stability requirements during sitting pivot transfers using stabilizing and destabilizing forces in individuals with complete motor paraplegia. J. Biomech. 45, 1554–1558.

13. Davies, P.M., 2000. Steps to Follow: The Comprehensive Treatment of Patients With Hemiplegia. Springer Science & Business Media.

14. Hoogenboom, B.J., Voight, M.L., 2015. Rolling revisited: using rolling to assess and treat neuromuscular control and coordination of the core and extremities of athletes. Int. J. Sports Phys. Ther. 10, 787–802.

15. Richter, R.R., VanSant, A.F., et al., 1989. Description of adult rolling movements and hypothesis of developmental sequences. Phys. Ther. 69, 63–71.

16. Sekiya, N., Takahashi, M., 2004. Kinematic and kinetic analysis of rolling motion in normal adults. J. Jpn. Phys. Ther. Assoc. 7, 1–6.

17. De Groot, S., Veeger, D.H., et al., 2002. Wheelchair propulsion technique and mechanical efficiency after 3 wk of practice. Med. Sci. Sports Exerc. 34, 756–766.

18. Boninger, M.L., Baldwin, M., et al., 2000. Manual wheelchair pushrim biomechanics and axle position. Arch. Phys. Med. Rehabil. 81, 608–613.

19. Brubaker, C.E., 1986. Wheelchair prescription: an analysis of factors that affect mobility and performance. J. Rehabil. Res. Dev. 23, 19–26.

20. Koontz, A.M., Cooper, R.A., et al., 2002. Shoulder kinematics and kinetics during two speeds of wheelchair propulsion. J. Rehabil. Res. Dev. 39, 635–649.

21. Boninger, M.L., Souza, A.L., et al., 2002. Propulsion patterns and pushrim biomechanics in manual wheelchair propulsion. Arch. Phys. Med. Rehabil. 83, 718–723.

22. Kwarciak, A.M., Turner, J.T., et al., 2012. The effects of four different stroke patterns on manual wheelchair propulsion and upper limb muscle strain. Disabil. Rehabil. Assist. Technol. 7, 459–463.

23. Shimada, S.D., Robertson, R.N., et al., 1998. Kinematic characterization of wheelchair propulsion. J. Rehabil. Res. Dev. 35, 210–218.

CHAPTER 6

Functional independence

Emilie Gollan and Tiffany Wilson

INTRODUCTION

Following spinal cord injury (SCI), patients must relearn how to perform everyday tasks. The role of the physiotherapist, outlined in Chapter 4, includes a thorough assessment ensuring a good understanding of their patient's injury, including level of injury, type of injury and extent of the neurological impairments associated with that injury. Secondary impairments, such as spasticity and pain, can significantly impede developing new skills aimed at functional independence and have been correlated with poor functional outcomes, limited participation and reduced quality of life for individuals with SCIs (see Chapters 1 and 18).[1] Other secondary impairments, including new or pre-existing orthopaedic injuries and musculoskeletal conditions, must also be considered with respect to their impact on performing activities. Physiotherapists utilise information gained in subjective and objective assessments to assist their clients in establishing individualised goals and tailoring therapy plans for goal attainment (see Chapter 4). This may include optimising normal movement patterns, teaching compensatory strategies and/or utilising equipment, devices or physical assistance from others. The

physiotherapist must frequently review treatment plans in response to progression of strength, task achievement or lack thereof, changing neurological status and refocusing of the individual's goals.

A goal-based, individualised treatment plan aimed at progression of functional skills and management strategies to facilitate hospital discharge should be developed with the patient, their family and the multidisciplinary team. Factors that have been shown to limit functional outcomes include age at time of injury, general health and pre-existing medical conditions, body weight and shoulder pathology.[2] Over the past 15 years the percentage of incomplete and non-traumatic causes of SCI has increased, and individuals are now older at the time of injury,[3] bringing new challenges in relation to predicting outcomes and teaching functional skills.

The International Classification of Functioning, Disability and Health (ICF) assists physiotherapists to establish and monitor rehabilitation programs aimed at teaching functional independence (Fig. 6.1).[4] The patient and the treating physiotherapist work together to set jointly agreed goals to address these limitations and restrictions. Outcomes and successes of therapy programs and goal attainments must be measured.

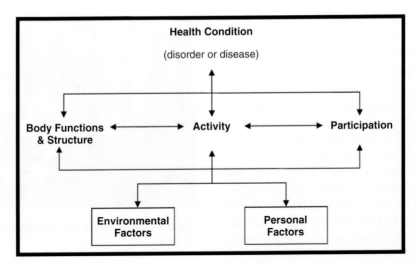

Figure 6.1 The International Classification of Functioning, Disability and Health.
Source: ICF Education CC BY NC SA 4.0

Many challenges are faced with respect to goal setting, particularly in the early stages of rehabilitation. The physiotherapist must educate clients and their families about the implications of objective assessments and their potential impact on goal achievement and functional independence. It is essential to maintain hope and provide motivation by measuring achievable activities for each goal throughout rehabilitation. It can be difficult to find a balance between achievable outcomes and patient-driven goals, while balancing the expectations of the individual, their family and the multidisciplinary team.

TEACHING STRATEGIES AND PROGRESSION OF FUNCTIONAL SKILLS

Teaching strategies for achieving functional skills begins with evaluating the possibility of re-educating normal movement patterns. When normal movement patterns are not possible due to the neurological impairments from the SCI, compensatory strategies should be considered. The outcome is to establish strategies that achieve the highest degree of functional independence. When teaching functional skills, it is imperative to balance the functional independence of an activity with respect to ageing with an SCI and minimising overuse injuries (see Chapter 21). For example, shoulder preservation is key for long-term independence for many individuals with SCI (see Chapter 15, on ageing with an SCI). Consideration is given to the prescription of assistive devices and equipment that may help with energy and joint preservation for activities of daily living (ADLs).

Functional skills retraining commences in therapy areas; however, skills should be integrated into the daily routine as soon as possible. Practising skills outside of therapy areas is essential for evaluating and improving functional independence with respect to everyday life and activities. Wherever possible, rehabilitation programs should include trials away from the hospital setting.

An initial goal of treatment following a newly acquired SCI is to begin sitting out of bed. For many, this involves mobilising in a wheelchair for the first time (see Chapter 4). Once a patient is mobilising in a wheelchair daily and tolerating sitting for at least 1–2 hours, they should progress to early rehabilitation activities. These include basic wheelchair skills training and education, gentle strengthening and stretching exercises and strategies to ensure appropriate pressure redistribution. In the early stages of rehabilitation, activities are often limited by pain, fatigue and endurance. Early rehabilitation activities are also dependent on other individual factors such as emotional and psychological wellbeing (see Chapter 19).

Strength and flexibility are integral to the successful acquisition of performing functional skills for individuals with SCI. Each new functional skill and activity should be broken down into achievable components, allowing assessment of the patient to determine if strength, flexibility or technique are limiting factors preventing successful skill acquisition. Strength impairments can be due to the level of SCI with paralysis or partial paralysis of muscle groups. Weakness can also occur in fully innervated muscle groups due to muscle atrophy and disuse, or to new or pre-existing orthopaedic/musculoskeletal injuries. As discussed in Chapters 3 and 4, it is important to target exercises that increase and maintain strength in fully innervated muscles, but also to target those muscles that have impairments due to denervation from the SCI.[5] Consideration of flexibility is also essential. If flexibility is limiting skill acquisition, interventions can be incorporated to address this. Neural plasticity requires new skills to be taught, practised and learnt, which requires frequent repetition in a variety of ways.[6] The following section will detail key functional skills important for maximising independence with daily activities following an SCI. (See Chapter 5 for the biomechanical principles underlying the teaching of these functional skills.)

UNSUPPORTED SITTING

Sitting balance

a   Teaching the skill

Sitting balance is often the first functional skill that is taught when commencing rehabilitation. Unsupported sitting is inherently important for

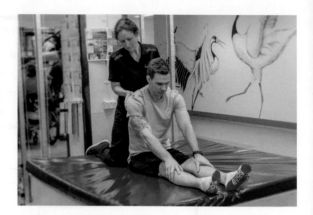

Figure 6.2 Training sitting balance in long sitting.

performing everyday tasks, both in a wheelchair, such as reaching for objects and propelling a wheelchair, and when sitting on a bed, for tasks such as dressing and transferring between surfaces. When training sitting balance, it is important to set up the environment to promote patient confidence and safety. Balance in long sitting (i.e. sitting with legs extended on the bed) will therefore be taught first as this provides the greatest base of support (BOS) (Fig. 6.2).

To commence long-sitting training, the patient should be positioned in the middle of a firm surface, for example, a plinth with a firm foam mattress, with ample space around them. The therapist is positioned behind the patient to support and facilitate movements. The patient needs to lean far enough forwards so that their centre of mass (COM) is in front of their hip joint. Long sitting can be limited by hamstring flexibility and should be modified to avoid excessive neural tension in the early weeks following SCI. For example, knees can be slightly flexed and feet can be off the edge of the bed to compensate for lack of flexibility and to minimise neural tension. Modifying long sitting in this way will also increase stability in sitting (Fig. 6.3).

Depending on the level of injury, the patient may not have voluntary control of the muscles of their trunk and legs. These patients are unable to

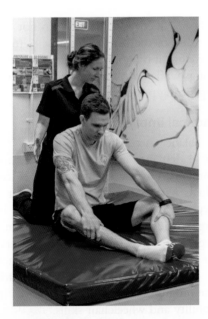

Figure 6.3 Modified long-sitting position.

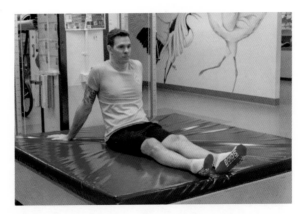

Figure 6.4 Propping with upper limbs in long sitting.

counteract the unstable position of sitting, when displacing their centre of gravity (COG) to perform functional tasks. Therefore, with help from their physiotherapist, the patient must develop strategies to overcome the lack of muscle activation below the level of their injury. Passive tension of hamstring muscles in long sitting can be used to maintain upright posture and prevent falling forwards. Weight shift initiated by head and shoulder movement can be used to compensate for lack of active trunk control. The patient is taught how to use their head and shoulders to initiate weight shift forwards and back, then side to side. This can be done in combination with upper limb movements and facilitated by the therapist. Shifting and exploring their COG is essential for maintaining balance in sitting. Propping, or supporting body position with upper limbs on the bed, can also be used to assist balance and compensate for lack of active trunk control (Fig. 6.4).

Early sitting balance activities include practising maintaining the static position, weight shift and internal perturbations such as head turning, and being able to save themselves from falling. When falling backwards, the patient must learn how to throw their arms backwards, behind their COG, to prop on upper limbs, as shown in Fig. 6.4. This reaction does not come naturally and must be practised before moving onto dynamic activities.

b Progressing the skill

Sitting balance activities progress to include dynamic activities, such as reaching outside their BOS and throwing and catching objects. Patients are taught to reach outside their BOS with one arm, while using the other arm to counteract the loss of stability by reaching behind their body (Fig. 6.5). The focus of all dynamic balance activities is on the individual's ability to return to a position of balance quickly and prevent themselves from falling.

Sitting balance can be challenged further by incorporating more unstable positions, such as high sitting (with feet supported) (Fig. 6.6). Balance in this position is essential for many individuals who will propel a manual wheelchair, utilise this position for showering, toileting or other ADLs, and to transfer between surfaces with feet on the floor. Both static and dynamic activities are practised in high sitting as per long sitting. To replicate the home environment, progression of sitting balance activities should also be performed on softer surfaces, such as inner spring mattresses, when appropriate for the individual's goals.

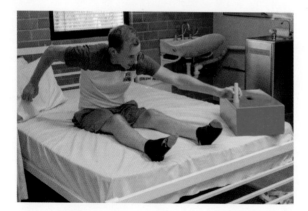

Figure 6.5 Reaching outside base of support in long sitting.

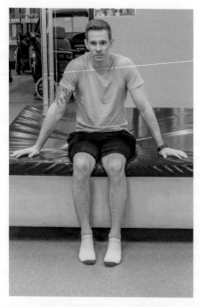

Figure 6.6 High-sitting position on plinth.

c   Modifying the skill

People who lack flexibility in their hamstring muscles may not be able to achieve a long-sitting position and tend to fall backwards when this position is attempted. These individuals may need to modify the long-sitting position and/or focus on improving hamstring flexibility prior to commencing long-sitting training. Those with very flexible hamstring muscles

are likely to fall forwards as they do not have the passive recoil of the hamstring muscles to prevent this. Therefore, it is important not to over-stretch the hamstrings while enabling the patient to maintain the long-sitting position.

d   Practical implications

Sitting balance needs to be trained to replicate functional demands and practised in a variety of environments. High levels of sitting balance allow individuals with SCI to achieve a greater degree of independence. For example, this can include reaching outside the BOS during personal care and hygiene routines and uneven transfers, such as floor or car transfers. Sitting balance activities should be prioritised early in rehabilitation to facilitate progression of other skills, which include bed mobility and wheelchair skills.

BED MOBILITY

Retraining of bed mobility is often demonstrated in smaller achievable components (part-practice). Bed mobility includes rolling from side to side, moving from lying to sitting and moving across the bed. These new skills are then all practised together to achieve the overall goal of bed mobility.

Rolling
a   Teaching the skill

Rolling is an important skill and training should be commenced early. It is important for overnight turns to ensure pressure redistribution, dressing and transitioning from lying to sitting. Without active use of trunk or lower limbs an individual will compensate by using their upper limbs to roll. Rolling practice is commenced on a relatively firm surface, such as a wide treatment plinth or floor mat. The initial focus is on the direction and technique of the arm swing. Starting in a supine position, head and arm movement can be combined and coordinated to create momentum to allow the body to follow. A coil effect is created by swinging arms from up above one ear down towards the opposite hip, in a

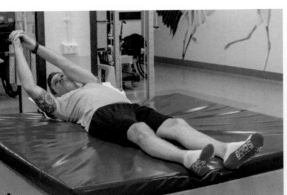
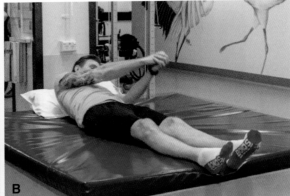
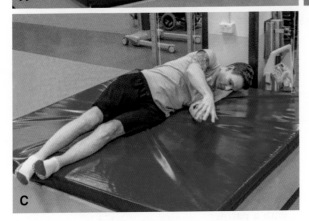

Figure 6.7 A–C Training rolling from supine position.

rapid diagonal movement pattern. These movement patterns replicate the synergic movement patterns used in the proprioceptive neuromuscular facilitation (PNF) techniques (see Chapter 11 for further details on PNF techniques). Arms are repetitively swung rapidly through the arc of movement to create enough momentum to roll. It is vital to ensure that the patient is instructed to tuck their chin to their chest, lift their head off the bed and rotate their neck to follow the position of their arms. Where possible, elbows should remain extended throughout the movement and hands should be clasped together (Fig. 6.7).

b Progressing the skill

The skill of rolling should be progressed to include practice on everyday beds and mattresses, as soon as possible. Over time, each patient will refine the movements required for rolling to incorporate strategies for energy conservation. For example, some individuals will go from sitting to side-lying to avoid the need for rolling.

c Modifying the skill

The supine position can be modified by positioning the patient a quarter turn towards the direction of rolling by propping their hips up with a foam wedge or pillows. Legs can be crossed at the ankles and a weight held in the hands to increase momentum and minimise the effort required to complete the rolling movement. This will allow the patient to focus on the direction of the arm swing (Fig. 6.8).

For patients with impaired upper limb strength or no voluntary control of triceps, shoulder external

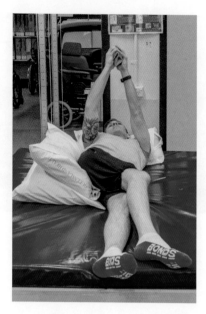

Figure 6.8 Training rolling from modified position.

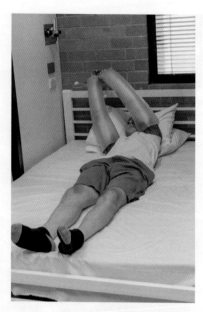

Figure 6.9 Training rolling with air splints for elbow extension.

rotation is used with minimal shoulder flexion to create the required movement pattern. This allows the patient to create the necessary momentum with upper limbs, without their elbows collapsing and hands falling into their face. For teaching purposes, other strategies can be used, such as air splints, to hold elbows extended (Fig. 6.9).

Assistive devices can be used to facilitate rolling, such as bed rails or bed ladders. Devices should be considered when independence would be limited without their addition.

d   Practical implications

Determining how an individual will be able to roll is dependent upon available muscle power and range of movement. As discussed earlier, it is important to consider the type of bed and mattress that will be used, i.e. inner spring mattress versus pressure redistribution mattress, and rolling practice should be progressed to replicate the intended environment where possible. Attention is also given to the amount of space required for rolling and other bed mobility tasks, type of bedding used (sheets, blankets, etc.) and whether the individual will be sharing the bed with a partner.

Moving from lying to sitting
a   Teaching the skill

This activity is essential for tasks such as dressing, moving around the bed and transferring. This task can be completed utilising different strategies. Initial training usually commences with achieving sitting from lying by transitioning through side lying. Other strategies may incorporate the use of electric bed mechanics or moving from lying to sitting without going through side lying.

When transitioning from lying to sitting through side lying, the patient will be taught to use momentum created by the arm swing during rolling to prop up on their elbow in side lying. It is important they keep their head down to ensure their COG remains inside their BOS. The therapist can support the patient from behind, under the axilla, to facilitate weight shift and forward movement. Then

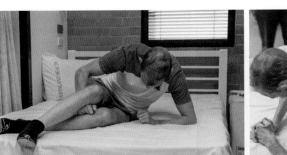
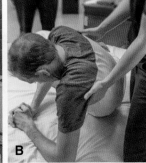

Figure 6.10 A, B Assisting transitioning from lying to sitting through side lying.

the patient shuffles forwards on elbows or hands, in a C-shaped pattern, bringing their head towards their feet until they can push up into long sitting. Pushing up with hands too soon will move their COG backwards and result in the individual, who lacks trunk control, falling backwards (Fig. 6.10).

b   Progressing the skill

With increased skill, moving from lying to sitting can be completed without transitioning through side lying. The more skilled patient may use upper body strength to move from lying directly into a long-sitting position. When performed well, this movement can be quick and efficient. This skill is often taught in reverse to allow the patient to understand the required upper body weight shift and to utilise controlled eccentric activity. For example, starting in long sitting and propping on hands to support body weight, the patient is instructed to shift weight from one hand to the other and slowly walk their hands backwards. They lower themselves towards the bed until they are resting on their elbows. Shoulders are abducted until their trunk is resting on the bed. To move from supine to long sitting, the movement pattern is reversed. Weight is shifted rapidly from side to side, using horizontal momentum, to overcome the force of gravity until the patient is propping up their weight on their elbows. The physiotherapist can facilitate this movement by placing their hands behind the

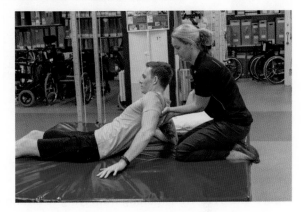

Figure 6.11 Transitioning from lying to sitting with therapist assisting weight shift.

patient's shoulders and assisting them to shift their upper body weight from side to side (Fig. 6.11). The movements must continue to be rapid and utilise momentum until the individual can push up onto their hands. This technique requires a high degree of shoulder flexibility and strength.

c   Modifying the skill

For transitioning from lying to sitting through side lying without active elbow extension or good hand function, the same C-shaped movement pattern is performed as described above. These individuals will need to ensure they keep their COG forward until they can hook a hand behind their knee, i.e. the

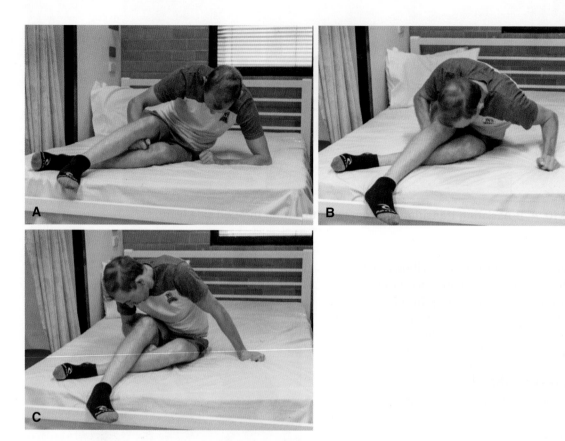

Figure 6.12 A–C Transitioning from lying to sitting with impaired upper limb strength.

right hand will be hooked under the right knee to shift their weight towards the right. They will use active wrist extension, elbow flexion and shoulder adduction to shift their body weight until they can flick the opposite arm out to support their body weight in sitting (Fig. 6.12).

Bed ladders can be used to assist bed mobility tasks such as rolling and moving between lying and sitting. Without active hand function, wrist extension can be used to hook under the loops of the bed ladder. Active wrist extension and elbow flexion are used to pull up on the bed ladder to facilitate weight shift sideways and forwards to assist the movement into sitting (Fig. 6.13). Bed ladders can be useful to increase independence, but must be set up to be available when needed, i.e. attached

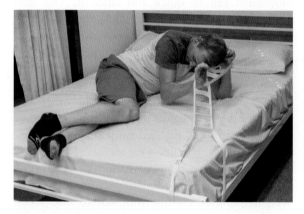

Figure 6.13 Transitioning from lying to sitting using bed ladder.

to side of bed. The use of a bed ladder is one of the most challenging techniques to master for individuals with tetraplegia.

d   Practical implications

Where possible, the home environment should be replicated to progress and practise bed mobility skills. The type of bed and mattress, available space, required devices or assistance needed are all important considerations for discharge planning. Individuals who require physical assistance for bed mobility tasks must ensure that their environment is set up to allow carers to safely assist them. If unable to perform bed mobility tasks independently, a combination of assistive devices and/or electric bed mechanics can be used to complete these tasks.

Moving across the bed
a   Teaching the skill

Moving around the bed is often performed in sitting by performing a series of vertical lifts. Vertical lifts are an important skill to master early in rehabilitation for anyone without active lower limb movement. This is an essential skill for moving to the edge of the bed for transfers and repositioning in bed or in a wheelchair for pressure redistribution. To maintain good skin integrity, it is important to perform an adequate lift when moving around the bed. If unable to lift adequately, shearing forces from skin being dragged across the bed places skin at increased risk of breaking down. An adequate lift is dependent on strong shoulder depression (latissimus dorsi), anterior shoulder stability (anterior deltoid) and sitting balance (Fig. 6.14).

Teaching vertical lifts can be performed in long-sitting or high-sitting positions; however, lift practice is often commenced in the long-sitting position as this is more stable. The technique for the lift is the same. The starting position is dependent on the patient's sitting balance, body dimensions and neurological impairments. In sitting, hands are placed beside and slightly forward of the hips. If hands are positioned too wide it will be challenging to achieve height with the lift. If hands are positioned too close

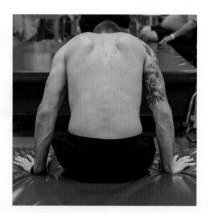

Figure 6.14 Training vertical lifts in high sitting.

to the body, the individual will be more unstable. It is important to consider hand function and provide education to minimise the risk of overuse injuries. For example, some individuals will naturally want to use a fist or fingers to transfer from to provide added height for the lift. Where possible, a neutral wrist position should be achieved, often by having the hand in a stable position over the edge of the bed. For individuals with active wrist extension but no active finger flexion, a tenodesis grasp will be used for independence with hand function. Tenodesis grasp relies on active wrist extension to generate passive finger and thumb flexion. Hand ranging and positioning during practice of functional tasks must pair wrist extension with finger and thumb flexion to ensure the tenodesis grasp is preserved (refer to Chapter 17 for further information on the tenodesis grasp). Hand positioning to maintain a tenodesis grasp is essential for these individuals and should be preserved.

The lift is achieved by using shoulder depression and shoulder flexion/adduction. Elbows should remain extended throughout the movement where possible. Lift height is achieved by leaning forwards and tucking the chin on the chest to keep the head down. This drives the height of the lift. (See Chapter 5 for further information on the biomechanics of lifting.)

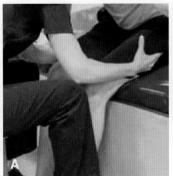
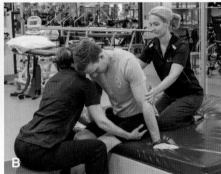

Figure 6.15 A, B Training vertical lifts in high sitting.

In the high-sitting position, vertical lifts can be facilitated by a physiotherapist. The physiotherapist is seated in front of the patient with their hands supporting under the upper thighs. **Do not attempt to lift the patient**. The physiotherapist remains seated with elbows resting on knees to create a closed chain movement and minimise the impact of loading away from the trunk. This position allows the physiotherapist to gently guide the movement as the patient performs the lift. The patient can rest their head on the physiotherapist's shoulder to provide support for their balance and to avoid falling forwards. The focus should be on the correct lift technique, shoulder and hand positioning (Fig. 6.15).

To move across the bed in long sitting, a series of vertical lifts are performed. A lift is performed and the body weight is shifted in the required direction. In order to move across the bed, the hand position is varied. The leading hand (towards the direction of movement) is placed further forward and away from the hip, with the trailing hand behind the hip and in close to the body. This positioning is important to encourage rotation of the trunk. As the lift is performed, body weight is shifted across in the direction of movement. A series of small lifts are performed, then the legs are moved across the bed. Lower limb strength, where possible, may be used to assist the movement, or legs are passively shifted across the bed using upper limb strength (Fig. 6.16).

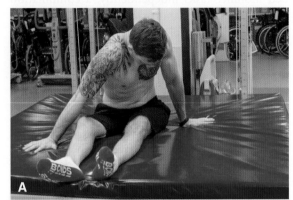
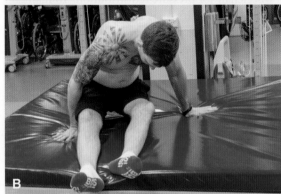

Figure 6.16 A, B Training moving across the bed in long sitting.

b Progressing the skill

Lift practice is commenced on a firm plinth and should be progressed to include a variety of surfaces such as softer mattresses and a variety of hand positions, i.e. hands on different height surfaces as required for high-level transfer practice. For example, lift practice can be completed on an inner spring mattress and incorporate lifting from a variety of stable (e.g. wooden blocks) or unstable (e.g. medicine balls) surfaces (Fig. 6.17). Vertical lifts should be practised from both high- and long-sitting positions, when possible, as this is essential for many everyday functional tasks.

The vertical lift skill is progressed to include moving legs across the bed and on and off the bed, using a variety of strategies. Moving legs without active lower limb muscle activity, can be a difficult task to achieve, particularly for those with impaired

hand function. For example, active wrist extension is used to hook under a knee to shift the leg across the bed (Fig. 6.18).

Lifting legs onto the bed may also be achieved by reaching under both legs from the high-sitting position and rolling back onto the bed (Fig. 6.19). For others, one leg is lifted onto the bed at a time. An individual may need to prop onto one elbow for balance while they reach under the other leg to lift it with their hand or hook under their knee using active wrist extension and elbow flexion (Fig. 6.18) (see Chapter 5 on the biomechanics of lifting). The degree of neurological impairment will influence how these tasks are achieved. Where possible, any preserved muscle power should be used to assist movements, or compensatory strategies can be used, as described above (see Chapter 11 on incomplete lesions).

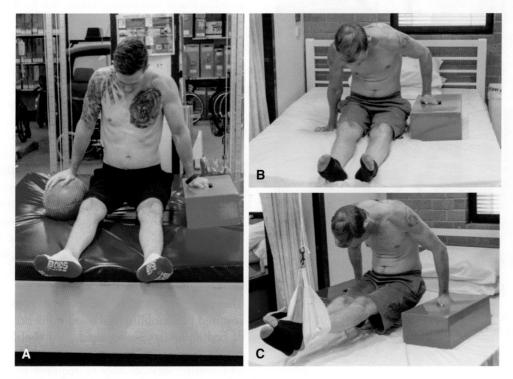

Figure 6.17 A–C Progression of lift practice training.

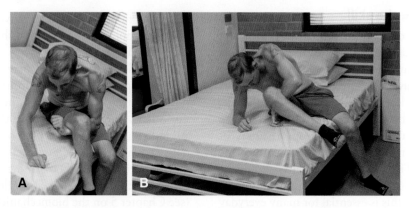

Figure 6.18 A, B Lifting legs onto bed with impaired upper limb strength.

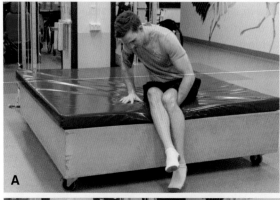

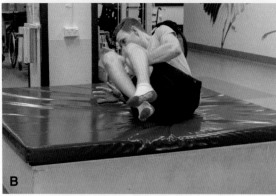

Figure 6.19 A, B Training lifting both legs onto the bed at the same time.

c Modifying the skill

Individuals with impaired tricep muscle function can be taught to maintain an extended elbow for vertical lifts by externally rotating their shoulders and locking out their elbows. With externally rotated shoulders and extended elbows, the COG of the trunk is posterior to the elbow joint thus assisting the elbows to passively extend due to the weight of the body. The physiotherapist can facilitate elbow extension in the early stages of practising this skill. An assistant may be required for safety (Fig. 6.15).

If an adequate lift cannot be achieved, then further strength or balance training may be indicated. Shoulder stability is essential for a good lift technique. Lifting blocks can be considered to assist with achieving an adequate lift, especially when body dimensions or strength are a limiting factor for progression. The ultimate goal is not to rely on assistive devices such as lifting blocks; however, if this allows independence and improves the quality of vertical lifts, it may be considered (Fig. 6.20).

d Practical implications

The ease with which the patient performs all required bed mobility tasks will influence the type of bed and mattress required. Bed mobility tasks can be costly with respect to energy expenditure, and assistive devices may be required to conserve energy for other everyday activities. The need for

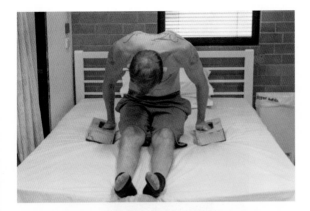

Figure 6.20 Training vertical lifts with lifting blocks.

a pressure redistribution mattress will influence what an individual can achieve as a surface that provides optimal pressure redistribution may prove more challenging in the performance of bed mobility activities. Throughout rehabilitation it is important to consider progression of functional skills in line with equipment prescription. Other factors that need to be taken into account when prescribing beds and mattresses include bladder management, skin integrity, personal circumstances and discharge environment.

TRANSFERS

Transfers are the way in which a person is able to transition between two surfaces. These may include hoist transfers, assisted transfers and independent transfers (with or without devices). Transfers are an important skill and a variety of transfers will be performed daily. (See Chapter 21 for clients' personal reflections on transfers.) Basic transfers can include bed to wheelchair, bed to mobile shower commode chair, wheelchair to toilet or wheelchair to car. Some individuals will also achieve a high level of independence with more advanced skills, such as floor to wheelchair transfers. Transfers are a high-priority goal for individuals with SCI and can often be used as a motivational tool during therapy.

Teaching seated transfers without the use of lifting devices is described in this section. The technique described is modified when trunk and lower limb function can be used to assist transfers. Transfer technique is dependent on body dimensions, skill level and the degree of neurological impairments. Objective assessments of muscle power, range of movement, spasticity and other orthopaedic or musculoskeletal conditions will also influence the type of transfers achieved. Transfer ability is often limited by strength, sitting balance and/or the ability to achieve an adequate vertical lift. The timing to commence transfer practice is dependent on many individual factors. When a reasonable amount of control to lift and shift body weight is achieved, with or without assistance, a transfer may be attempted. A transfer is a high-risk activity and care must be taken to ensure the environment is set up to minimise risk of injury.

Transfer training
a   Teaching the skill
Transfer training is made up of a series of components. Each component may be practised in isolation, then combined to achieve a transfer between two surfaces. Independence with each component is not necessary before progressing to more difficult tasks. Each component should be trialled and practised with or without assistance and/or devices. It is important to review earlier components of the skill to ensure the patient is as independent as possible and only uses assistance or devices if required.

Transfer training should be commenced from a firm, stable surface such as a treatment plinth to the unstable surface of the wheelchair. For most patients, transfer practice is commenced from the high-sitting position. Consideration is given as to when it may be appropriate to teach the transfer from the long-sitting position, with legs up on the bed (Fig. 6.21). This can be useful for patients with limited sitting balance or significant spasticity. Transfers should be slow and controlled. The patient should be able stop at any point during the transfer and return to the starting position to readjust as required. Table 6.1 outlines

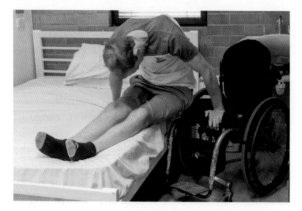

Figure 6.21 Training transfers with legs up.

the steps and considerations for teaching a basic transfer from a treatment plinth to a wheelchair. The therapist is in a seated position in front of the patient throughout the transfer.

b   Progressing the skill

Once the basic transfer from a treatment plinth to the wheelchair is achieved, the transfer from the wheelchair back to the treatment plinth can be attempted. The same basic steps are followed in reverse for this transfer. It is important for the patient to move forwards to the front of the wheelchair seat before attempting to move across to the treatment plinth. This is important to ensure they do not attempt to transfer over the wheel of the wheelchair and risk skin abrasions.

Transfer practice should be progressed to incorporate a variety of surfaces as per individual goals. The same basic transfer technique is used with slight modifications to compensate for uneven and unstable surfaces. The focus of transfer practice is to ensure good technique throughout the transfer and provide the patient with the skills and knowledge to modify the technique as required.

c   Modifying the skill

Depending on upper body strength, some patients may not be able to achieve the forward movement on the wheelchair seat in preparation for the transfer

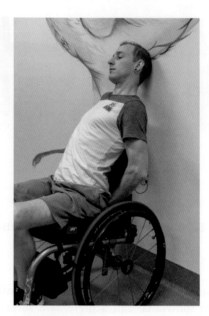

Figure 6.22 Technique to push hips forward in wheelchair.

towards a bed or other surface. They may be required to extend their head and trunk over the back of the wheelchair to move their hips forward on the seat. This is done by positioning the hands behind the hips between their trunk and wheelchair backrest. The hips are pushed forwards by the patient extending their head and trunk over the top of the backrest. By externally rotating the shoulders and extending the wrists, the hips are pushed forwards towards the edge of the wheelchair (Fig. 6.22). (See Chapter 5 for more information on the biomechanics of performing this activity.) The equipment used when completing this task is very important in determining functional outcome. Some cushions make it more difficult to move the hips forward in this manner and might limit functional independence with this technique. The height of the backrest will also influence the ability to perform this task. Consideration of transfer technique to be used is part of trialling and prescribing equipment such as manual wheelchairs, pressure redistribution cushions and back supports. (See Chapter 8, Modes of transport, Part 1, for wheelchair prescription).

Table 6.1 Basic transfer technique training

1. Position wheelchair	• Position the wheelchair as close to the treatment plinth as possible • Front of the wheelchair is angled in towards the treatment plinth • Front corner of the wheelchair cushion and seat should be as close as possible and slightly lower or level with the treatment plinth	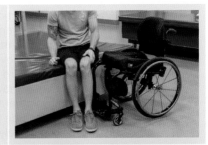
2. Position front castors	• Position the front castors of the wheelchair in the forward position to increase stability of the wheelchair base • If the castors face backwards the wheelchair base is shortened and hence less stable	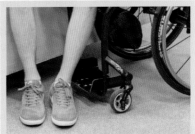
3. Position the patient	• The patient should position themselves on the edge of the treatment plinth, as close as possible to the wheelchair seat • A quarter turn away from the wheelchair is performed so their hips and feet are angled away from the wheelchair • Position hips in front of the wheel so that the greater trochanter is in line with where the wheel and the edge of the bed meet • Position the feet on the floor when possible to provide a stable base • Encourage trunk rotation using hand and foot placement • Leading hand should be placed forwards and away from the body on a stable surface, such as the edge of the cushion or the wheelchair frame • The trailing hand remains on the treatment plinth behind the hip and close to the body	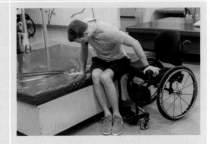

Continued

Table 6.1 Basic transfer technique training—cont'd

| 4. Transfer | • Perform a vertical lift with the focus on the upwards movement before rotating to perform the sideways movement
• During the movement the patient's head must remain forward and angled away from the direction of movement
• The physiotherapist will have their head facing towards the direction of movement so they can closely monitor the patient's body position during the transfer for safety
• The aim is to reach the front of the wheelchair seat, then perform another movement back into the rear of the wheelchair seat | 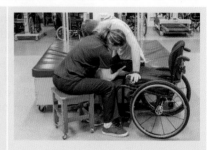 |

The height of the transfer surfaces, equipment used and individual factors will influence foot positioning during the transfer. The options for feet position in a high-sitting position are feet on footplates of the wheelchair, feet on the floor or one foot on the footplate and one on the floor. A variety of both hand and foot positions are trialled when completing transfer training to determine positions that provide the greatest degree of functional independence. For patients with impaired hand function, push mitts may be used for added grip during transfers (see Chapter 21 for a description of the mitts).

Transfer boards can be used to assist transfers. It is important to focus on the required technique of performing a vertical lift then shifting the body weight prior to introducing a transfer board. A transfer board is useful to bridge a gap and decrease the distance to be covered during a transfer, such as car transfers. It will allow a series of small vertical lifts and sideways movements to be performed to achieve the transfer. A transfer board can be used to assist any transfer between level surfaces, such as a wheelchair to bed transfer (Fig. 6.23) or wheelchair to car transfer. Transfer boards are available in a variety of materials and shapes and have various safe working limits. They should be trialled to ensure suitability and safety for the individual. Transfer boards should only be introduced when functional independence is restricted without them.

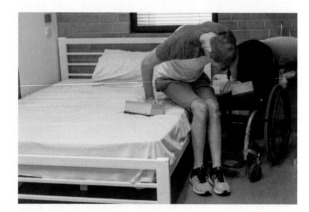

Figure 6.23 Training transfer technique with lifting blocks and transfer board.

As discussed in the previous section, lifting blocks can be used to assist with generating adequate lift height, providing clearance of body weight during vertical lift and assisting the patient to shift their weight across the surface. Lifting blocks can be custom-made to suit the individual's requirements. Lifting blocks are only introduced if functional independence is limited without them and should be trialled to ensure suitability and safety.

Using a variety of lifting blocks of different heights can also be a useful training strategy. For example, lifting from high blocks is beneficial for shoulder stability and strengthening, and lifting from uneven

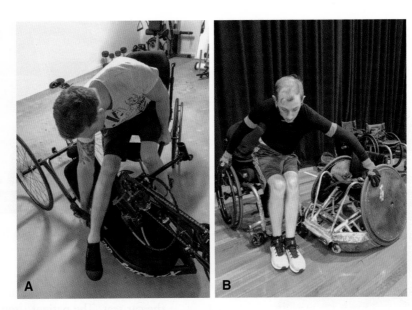

Figure 6.24 A, B Transfer training to sporting equipment.

heights will aid progression of higher-level transfers, such as transferring to or from a low lounge chair or the floor (see Fig. 6.27 on p. 131).

d Practical implications

Once the basic transfer skill has been achieved, transfer practice can be progressed to incorporate a variety of other surfaces. The same basic principles as described above can be applied to a wheelchair to bed transfer, then progressed to bed to mobile shower commode or wheelchair to shower bench and wheelchair to toilet transfer. Initial focus of transfer training will be on achieving transfers to complete personal hygiene care. These transfers should be incorporated into the daily routine on the ward as soon as possible. Transfer practice is then progressed with respect to individual patient goals and may include transfers to other surfaces, such as the lounge chair, car, floor and sporting equipment (Fig. 6.24).

Key considerations for other transfers:

- *Bed to mobile shower commode chair:* Consideration is given to the height and style of the mobile shower commode chair.

This will influence the ability to reach and available space for hand positioning. Since this transfer is performed unclothed, there is a higher risk of damaging skin integrity. It is important that after showering and before attempting the transfer back to bed, the patient should ensure their skin is completely dry. Training for this transfer may initially be practised in a modified (dry) environment. When competent with the basic transfer technique, the skill is then practised as part of the personal hygiene routine. The mobile shower commode is relatively unstable in comparison to the everyday wheelchair. For this reason, it is preferable to teach this transfer to and from the bed, as opposed to a direct mobile shower commode chair to wheelchair transfer.

- *Wheelchair to toilet and wheelchair to shower bench:* These transfers can be challenging due to relatively small surface area of the shower bench and toilet, minimal options for hand placement, the low height of the surface, design of the toilet cistern and circulation

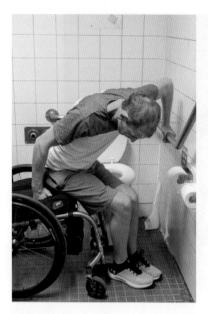

Figure 6.25 Toilet transfer training.

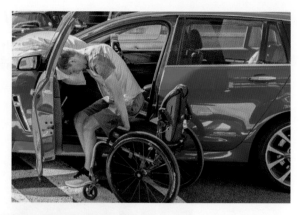

Figure 6.26 Transfer training to front passenger side of car.

space. Where possible, the wheelchair is placed at a 90-degree angle to the shower bench or toilet (Fig. 6.25). The positioning of the wheelchair may be limited by the bathroom design. Since these transfers are also usually completed unclothed extra care must be taken for maintenance of skin integrity. For toilets in an enclosed space without any circulation space for the wheelchair, it is possible to transfer directly to the toilet, i.e. seated backwards on the toilet. A variety of transfers should be practised to ensure strategies are considered for various bathroom and toilet designs to enable clients to manage in all community settings.

- *Wheelchair to car:* Practice is usually commenced towards the passenger side of the vehicle to minimise the complexity of the transfer. Consideration is given to the height of the car seat with respect to the height of the wheelchair. The same transfer technique is to be encouraged. The wheelchair should be positioned on an angle with the front corner of the wheelchair angled towards the car seat. The patient should move to the front corner of the wheelchair seat and reach one hand into the car. A lift is performed to move across and into the car, then legs can be moved into the car (Fig. 6.26). Depending on the distance and height of the transfer and individual body dimensions, it may be necessary to bring legs into the car at various stages of the transfer. The technique can be modified to suit the individual. The driver's side transfer is important for anyone aiming to return to driving. The same technique is used with the added complexity of working around the steering wheel. Another essential skill is being able to dismantle and load the wheelchair into the car or onto a car roof hoist or wheelchair loader for independent driving. (For further details on car transfers and putting wheelchairs into the car, refer to Chapter 8, Modes of transport, Part 2.)

- *Floor to wheelchair:* This transfer is challenging to achieve; however, all wheelchair users need to be taught strategies to complete this transfer in the event of a fall. This may include independently performing the transfer, performing an assisted transfer, utilising an intermediary step, such as a lounge chair, instructing others to be safely lifted from the floor to the wheelchair without injury or contacting emergency services.

A transfer directly from the floor to a wheelchair can be achieved by some patients. The starting position for this transfer is usually sitting on the floor with the wheelchair positioned to the side. Hips and knees are flexed, so feet can be positioned beside the footplate. A strap may be required around the knees to assist holding the legs in position. The leading hand (i.e. the hand closest to the wheelchair) is placed on the far edge of the wheelchair seat with the trailing hand on the floor behind the hip joint. The lift is forwards and up, to pivot around the feet until the individual can return to the wheelchair seat (Fig. 6.27).

This transfer can also be taught from sitting on the floor with the wheelchair positioned behind the individual. Both hands are reached up behind the body on the front edge of the wheelchair frame. The lift is up and back until the wheelchair seat is cleared. Then by leaning forwards and continuing to lift they can return to the wheelchair seat (Fig. 6.28). This technique requires strong and stable shoulder muscles and a high degree of shoulder flexibility. To assist either technique, the individual may choose to sit on their wheelchair cushion on the floor, thereby decreasing the overall height required for the transfer. Both techniques can be reversed for the transfer from the wheelchair to the floor.

Transfer skill practice should focus on establishing a good technique from the beginning. This will provide the patient with the best chance to progress to higher-level transfers. All transfers should be practised in a variety of environments to allow the patient to modify and problem-solve the transfers

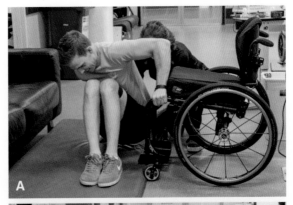
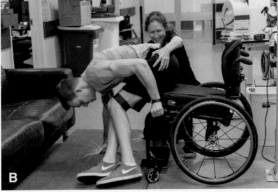

Figure 6.27 A, B Transfer training floor to wheelchair.

required. Small changes in model or style of equipment can have significant implications for the type of transfers achieved and overall independence. Where possible, transfer practice should be completed with the patient's own equipment, such as their manual wheelchair and cushion or own bed. It is imperative that the patient have opportunities to trial the transfers in an environment that replicates the discharge destination, as part of rehabilitation. Small differences in the height of transfer surfaces can have significant implications for functional independence.

At times, a combination of independent transfers, assisted transfers or the use of lifting devices may be required to achieve all transfers throughout the day. This can be due to fatigue at the end of the day, energy conservation strategies, challenges with

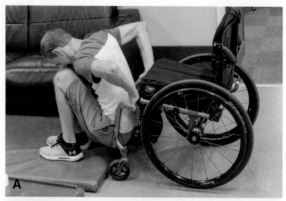

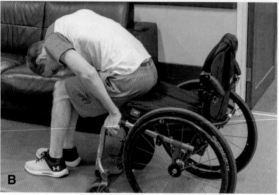

Figure 6.28 A, B Transfer training floor to wheelchair.

achieving higher-level transfers or management of shoulder pathology or other secondary conditions. It is essential to practise as many different transfer techniques as possible to ensure each patient can refine their technique to suit their own individual needs and make informed choices to develop their own unique style (see Chapter 21).

TRAINING OF MANUAL WHEELCHAIR SKILLS

For many individuals with an SCI, a manual wheelchair is their primary means of mobility. (See Chapter 8 for further details on wheelchair prescription.) Numerous studies have described the positive association between manual wheelchair skills,

activity and participation.[7] A high level of manual wheelchair skills is imperative for ADLs, community access and occupational and recreational pursuits. The type of wheelchair skills required are dependent on many individual factors, including the level of SCI, age, weight, shoulder pathology, other injuries and discharge environment. For many individuals with an SCI, a combination of mobility aids may best meet their needs. It is important that all manual wheelchair users have the opportunity to develop skills and are provided with training to ensure they can safely instruct others how to assist obstacle negotiation. Training of the wheelchair user, their family and friends or carers should be incorporated into a wheelchair skills training program as part of rehabilitation.[8,9]

Basic safety education and skill practice are commenced when first mobilising in a wheelchair. Top priority is given to the patient or an assistant being able to safely engage the wheel locks and propel the wheelchair. Education regarding wheelchair propulsion technique is important for preservation of shoulder integrity (see Chapter 5).

Wheelchair skill training will commence with basic skills such as forwards and backwards propulsion over level surfaces, turning and negotiating small lips, kerbs and edges. Advanced skills include back wheel balancing ('wheelies'), negotiating outdoor and uneven terrains, ascending/descending ramps and ascending/descending kerbs. An assistant should be available to act as a spotter during wheelchair skills training to ensure the safety of the wheelchair user at all times. In the early stages of wheelchair skills training a chest strap may be used for safety. Formal wheelchair skills training programs exist, but need to be adapted to the environment and specific goals of the individual.[10]

Lifting the front castors over small obstacles

Once basic wheelchair propulsion has been achieved, wheelchair skills training progresses to lifting the front castors over small obstacles. This is important for negotiating obstacles such as doorways and footpaths. To lift the front castors up momentarily, the wheelchair user will perform a quick, short push forwards on the pushrims. This skill should be practised to ensure efficiency and timing of the movement. If not timed correctly, the castors will hit the obstacle, causing the wheelchair to stop suddenly and shift the bodyweight forwards in the wheelchair. This could cause the wheelchair user to fall forwards out of the wheelchair if the obstacle is hit at speed with enough forward momentum (described in Chapter 21). Small obstacles, such as pieces of dowel approximately 2.5 cm high, can be used to practise this skill in a controlled environment.

Back wheel balancing

Progression of wheelchair skills training should include balancing on back wheels for all active wheelchair users. Back wheel balancing is an essential skill for independent negotiation of uneven terrains, steep declines, kerbs and community access. This skill can be challenging to master and requires practice for the wheelchair user to build confidence. Back wheel balancing, known colloquially as wheelies training, is commenced in controlled environments where the therapist uses a strap attached to the wheelchair to ensure they have control of the wheelchair during skill practice. This is essential for safety as the anti-tippers are removed from the wheelchair when practising this skill.

This skill is performed using the same technique described above to lift the front castors off the ground. In order to find the balance point of the wheelchair, the wheelchair user should keep their body weight back in the wheelchair, so their COG is behind the rear axle of the wheelchair. Small adjustments to maintain the balance point can be completed via the pushrims. With practice, this movement can become quick and efficient.

This skill is first practised in the stationary position, then progressed to propelling forwards and turning the wheelchair while maintaining balance on the back wheels. This movement is useful when manoeuvring a wheelchair in tight spaces. Maintaining balance on back wheels and propelling forwards allows

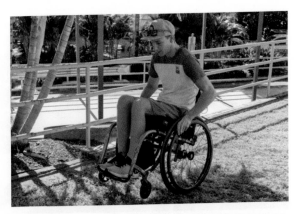

Figure 6.29 Training back wheel balancing over rough terrain outdoors.

the wheelchair user to propel over rough outdoor environments (Fig. 6.29). The small front wheels are lifted off the ground to avoid being caught in the rough terrain and the large rear wheels are used to propel over the surface.

A wheelchair user's ability to back wheel balance is dependent on the type of wheelchair and the wheelchair set-up. Manual wheelchairs, for individuals with SCIs, are custom-made to allow for ease of wheelchair propulsion and provide the greatest opportunity to develop advanced wheelchair skills. It is important that education is provided to ensure the wheelchair user falls safely in the event of the wheelchair overbalancing backwards, to minimise risk of injury.

Ascending a steep incline

To ascend a steep incline, the wheelchair user must modify their propulsion technique to prevent the wheelchair from tipping backwards. Short, sharp pushes are used with the wheelchair user keeping their body weight forwards in the wheelchair. The wheelchair user must have adequate upper body strength, balance and endurance to maintain a suitable propulsion technique for the duration of the incline (see Chapter 5 for further information on wheelchair propulsion). Ascending steep inclines is commonly required in the community and around

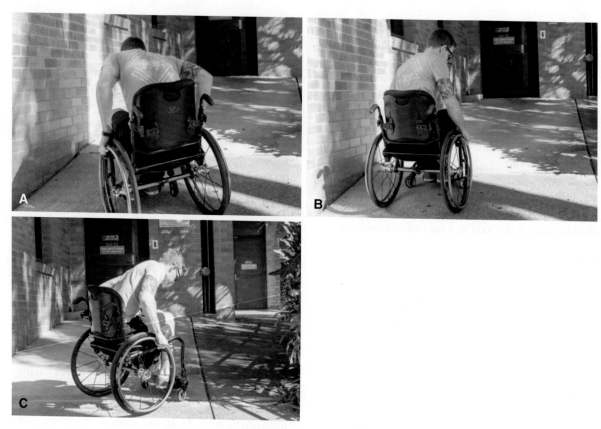

Figure 6.30 A–C Training wheelchair skills to ascend/descend a steep incline.

the home, for example, driveways. If adequate space is allowed, the wheelchair user may ascend the incline by performing a zig-zag pattern to cut the gradient (Fig. 6.30). This skill requires a quick, sharp change of direction in combination with forward propulsion.

Descending ramps and sharp declines

The same technique can be used for descending ramps; however, the wheelchair user must keep their body weight back in the wheelchair and control their speed via the pushrims. For steep declines, back wheel balancing or the zig-zag pattern can be used to descend the ramp and maintain control of the wheelchair. For wheelchair users with impaired hand function, shoulder adduction in combination with elbow flexion can be used to hold palms against

the pushrims, thereby controlling speed. Once at the bottom of the decline, the wheelchair user must monitor the environment as there is often a small change in the gradient to be managed. For example, at the end of the ramp the ground can flatten out sharply, which can cause the footplate to dig into the ground if the front castors are not lifted in a timely manner. If the footplate digs into the ground, the forward momentum of the wheelchair can cause the wheelchair user to fall out forwards.

Negotiating kerbs and gutters

Managing kerbs or gutters is another essential skill for community access. This skill can be completed independently or with assistive devices. To ascend and descend a gutter independently, back wheel balancing

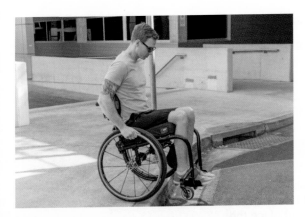

Figure 6.31 Training wheelchair skills to descend an outdoor gutter on back wheels.

is used. The gutter is ascended by approaching the obstacle at speed, the front castors are lifted, and the forward momentum propels the wheelchair up the gutter. This technique is difficult to master and requires practice as the timing of the manoeuvre is essential to successful obstacle completion. Back wheel balancing can be used to descend the gutter by maintaining balance on the back wheels and propelling forwards off the gutter. Active wheelchair users will use this method to quickly and efficiently ascend and descend gutters (Fig. 6.31).

For less active users, a device such as a street pole can be used to assist with ascending and descending gutters (refer to Table 6.2).

This technique can also be used with an assistant to aid the movements. If the wheelchair user can shift their body weight in the wheelchair, less effort is required by the assistant.

Wheelchair skills training is essential for safety and to ensure the wheelchair user can access their community and other environments.[11] It is important that family and carers be taught how to safely assist wheelchair skills to minimise risk of injury to themselves and the wheelchair user. Wheelchair users who progress to the highest level of wheelchair skills training will experience fewer participation restrictions and can be taught how to negotiate stairs in their wheelchair. Wheelchair skill training should

be initiated in controlled environments to ensure safety and build the wheelchair user's confidence before progressing to a variety of environments as guided by their goals. Wheelchair users are taught a range of skills and methods to allow them to problem-solve situations as they arise.

A fair degree of wheelchair skills is required to allow an individual to effectively evaluate wheelchairs during the trialling process. Timing of wheelchair skills training, like other functional skills, will impact on discharge planning and equipment prescription. In addition to wheelchair users being taught how to safely use their wheelchairs, it is also important for them to have an understanding of the implications of wheelchair adjustments and importance of regular wheelchair maintenance.

Efficient transfer and wheelchair skills are based on a good understanding of basic biomechanics, as outlined in Chapter 5.

EARLY STANDING

Early standing can be a motivating rehabilitation tool. The type of standing pattern and posture taught depends on the full results of an objective assessment of the patient's abilities. There are several options for early standing, which include the use of standing devices such as tilt tables, standing frames, orthoses and other devices (Fig. 6.32).

The reported benefits of early standing in SCI rehabilitation include improved bladder and bowel functioning, maintenance of bone health, reduction of spasticity, improved circulation, pressure redistribution, improving fatigue and sleep, maintenance of lower limb range of movement, improved digestion, pain management and psychological wellbeing. The current evidence to support standing is poor and further studies are needed to evaluate efficacy of standing in SCI rehabilitation.[12] However, even though high-quality evidence is poor, there is clinical evidence to justify the incorporation of regular standing into the therapy program. For further details on the importance of standing (and weight bearing) refer to Chapter 3.

Table 6.2 Training wheelchair skills to ascend/descend a gutter using a pole

Ascending	• Propel the wheelchair close to the gutter, leaving space to lift the front castors up	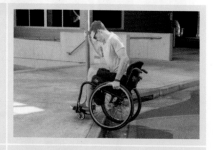
	• The front castors are lifted up, by shifting weight back in the wheelchair, and placed on the gutter • Hold onto the pole with one hand and place the other hand on the pushrim	
	• The hand holding the pole assists to pull the wheelchair user upwards while simultaneously the hand on the pushrim pushes forwards to ascend the gutter	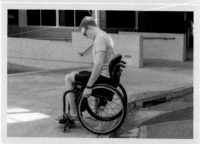
Descending	• The wheelchair is reversed to the edge of the gutter beside the street pole	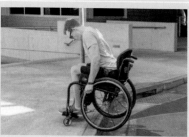
	• One hand is placed on the street pole and the other on the pushrim	
	• The wheelchair user leans forwards in the wheelchair while lowering themselves off the gutter • When the rear wheels are on the lower surface, the wheelchair user can lean back slightly to lift the front castors while propelling backwards to place the castors down	

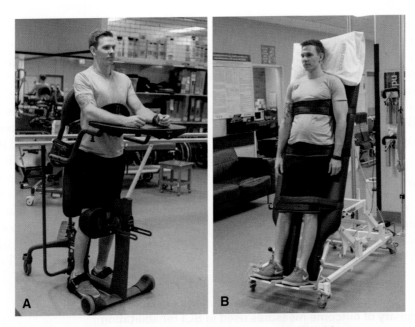

Figure 6.32 A, B Standing devices including standing frame and tilt table.

The tilt table can provide maximal support for individuals with minimal or absent trunk and leg muscle activation to safely commence standing after an SCI. Close assessment is required to ensure safety and to monitor for postural hypotension during standing. For some individuals with incomplete lesions, having neurological function will allow for progression of standing and walking abilities. A variety of orthoses (Fig. 6.33) are available to compensate for lack of active muscle control to progress standing and walking abilities (see Chapter 9). The Toolkit for SCI Standing and Walking Assessment can be used to guide clinical decision-making to determine when it is possible to progress standing and walking activities. This toolkit is a collection of key functional thresholds and outcome measures to assess readiness for walking and to identify deficits to target clinical interventions.[13]

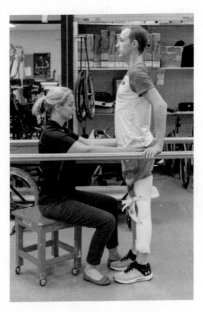

Figure 6.33 Standing with orthoses.

GAIT RE-EDUCATION

Walking is often the ultimate goal for an individual after sustaining an SCI. This goal is often adjusted and modified throughout the rehabilitation continuum of care to be realistic and achievable and is dependent on individual client factors. With the current trend of new spinal cord injuries being classified more often as incomplete injuries with neurological sparing (see Chapter 11), there are more individuals achieving this goal with the use of orthoses, walking aids and compensatory gait patterns (see Chapter 9).

OBJECTIVE MEASURES

A large number of outcome measures are available to assess independence with functional skills, and often a combination of measures is required. The use of consistent, standardised outcome measures is essential for monitoring the efficacy of improvements in rehabilitation, comparison of functional outcomes for research purposes and clinical trials and the prediction of functional recovery.[14] Consistent use of outcome measures also facilitates communication between clinicians and specialised SCI centres nationally and internationally.[15] Experts in the field of SCI data collection have developed the International Spinal Cord Injury Data Sets. The ICF has been used as the framework to develop the data sets in an effort to facilitate comparisons of interventions and outcomes between individuals with SCI and SCI rehabilitation centres internationally.[16] Table 6.3 summarises the usability and limitations of a variety of outcome measures used in SCI rehabilitation.

Table 6.3 Summary of outcome measures used in SCI rehabilitation

Outcome measure	Purpose	Content	Usability	Limitations
Functional Independence Measure (FIM)[17–19]	Developed to assess burden of care	18 items: motor function (13 items) and cognitive function (5 items)	Used broadly in rehabilitation Well correlated when used with SCI	Poor sensitivity in SCI, ceiling and floor effects
Modified Barthel Index (MBI)[20–22]	Developed to assess level of independence with personal care and mobility	10 items (bowels, bladder, grooming, toilet use, feeding, transfer, mobility, dressing, stairs, bathing)	Well correlated when used with SCI	Ceiling and floor effects Less clinically useful when compared to FIM (in SCI)
Quadriplegia Index of Function (QIF)[23,24]	Developed to assess small but clinically significant changes in individuals with tetraplegia	37 items in 10 categories: transfers, grooming, bathing, feeding, dressing, wheelchair mobility, bed activities, bowel program, bladder program, and understanding of personal care. Short form (6 items)	More responsive than FIM or MBI when used with individuals with tetraplegia	Many items are redundant

Table 6.3 **Summary of outcome measures used in SCI rehabilitation—cont'd**

Outcome measure	Purpose	Content	Usability	Limitations
Spinal Cord Independence Measure (SCIM)[20,25-27]	Developed in response to the limitations of the FIM when used in SCI rehabilitation	3 domains: self-care; respiration and sphincter management; and mobility	Reliable, valid, user friendly Sensitive to functional changes in SCI	Ceiling and floor effects for very high or very low lesions
Clinical Outcomes Variable Scale (COVS)[28]	Broader assessment of mobility in rehabilitation settings	General mobility and ambulation subscale	Relevant and comprehensive measure for SCI when compared to FIM, MBI, QIF, SCIM Greater sensitivity to change over time than FIM	Further research is required into the psychometric properties when used in SCI rehabilitation
Wheelchair Skills Test (WST)[29,30]	Designed to measure manual wheelchair skill status, monitor improvements and for research purposes	WST 4.2 contains 33 items Also has versions for power wheelchair users, care givers and a questionnaire	Useful checklist for wheelchair users in general	Not sensitive to manual wheelchair skills for individuals with SCI
Wheelchair Circuit[31,32]	Designed to assess mobility during and after rehabilitation	8 items (3 of which require a wheelchair treadmill)	Valid and responsive to changes in mobility for individuals with SCI	Items are not specific to wheelchair skills only and requires highly specialised equipment
Adapted Wheelchair Circuit[33]	Developed to address limitations of Wheelchair Circuit	6 additional items added to Wheelchair Circuit	Overground pushing replaced wheelchair treadmill	Ceiling and floor effects for individuals with paraplegia and has a complex scoring system

Continued

Table 6.3 Summary of outcome measures used in SCI rehabilitation—cont'd

Outcome measure	Purpose	Content	Usability	Limitations
Obstacle Course Assessment of Wheelchair User Performance[34-36]	Developed for manual and power wheelchair users	10 environmental obstacles replicated	Assesses skills relevant to daily needs of general wheelchair user population	Only used in specially designed, controlled environment High-level skills required by active manual wheelchair users with SCI not well represented
Five Additional Mobility and Locomotor Items Test[37]	Developed specifically for SCI for use with the FIM	5 items (bed mobility, vertical transfer, push on the flat, push on the ramp and negotiate kerbs)	Increases the sensitivity of the FIM and ability to detect functional improvements	Only three items directly relate to wheelchair skills, therefore used as general measure of mobility only
Test of Wheeled Mobility and Short Wheelie Test[38-40]	Developed to assess the wheelchair skills of individuals with SCI during and after rehabilitation	30 items	Able to detect smaller changes in wheeled mobility	Time-consuming to complete and requires extensive equipment
Queensland Evaluation of Wheelchair Skills[41]	Developed specifically to assess manual wheelchair skills for individuals with SCI	5 items: indoor propulsion, ramp, back wheel balancing, gutter and 6 min push test	Shown to be reliable and valid, and sufficiently sensitive to the changes seen as individuals with SCI progress through rehabilitation Quick and easy to use.	Scale for manual wheelchair users only

Table 6.3 **Summary of outcome measures used in SCI rehabilitation—cont'd**

Outcome measure	Purpose	Content	Usability	Limitations
Spinal Cord Injury Functional Ambulation Inventory (SCI-FAI)[42]	Developed to assess walking ability in SCI	3 domains: gait, assistive device and walking mobility Walk maximum of 2 mins with assistive devices and/or walking aid	Reliability, validity and sensitivity established in SCI	Designed specifically for individuals with SCI who possess some ambulatory function
Walking Index for Spinal Cord Injury (WISCI and WISCI-II)[43-45]	Developed for use in clinical trials to evaluate the amount of physical assistance and assistive devices required to walk ten metres	Ranks impairments of walking from 0 (most severe) to 20 (least severe)	Developed specifically for SCI Face validity, concurrent validity and inter-rater reliability have been demonstrated WISCI is more precise and sensitive when compared to the walking items in the FIM and the SCIM, for the measurement of change in walking ability	WISCI/WISCI-II is less sensitive to change when used with chronic SCI (in comparison to the 10MWT, TUG and 6MWT) Additional tests are necessary to assess endurance and walking speed
6-Minute Walk Test (6MWT)[46,47]	Self-paced assessment of walking endurance that was designed for use with patients with respiratory impairments	Measures distance walked over 6 minutes	Good reliability and validity in the SCI population Better reflects ADLs than other walking tests	Normative data available for individuals with coronary artery disease not SCI
10-Metre Walk Test (10MWT)[20,47]	Assesses short duration walking	Measures walking speed over 10 m Used as indication of household or community ambulation ability	High correlation with Walking Index for SCI, FIM locomotor score, 6 min walk test	Threshold values established for stroke not SCI
Timed Up and Go (TUG)[48]	Designed to measure gait speed, balance and functional mobility in elderly individuals	Measures walking ability over 10 m	Excellent correlation between the 6MWT, 10MWT and TUG test	This tool does not consider the quality of gait or assistive devices required

EDUCATION AND TRAINING

It is important for patients/clients to be able to problem-solve with carers, family members and rehabilitation team members, providing them with autonomy, direction and problem-solving and communication skills. Clients, carers and family members should be educated to recognise their limitations and be aware when professional support is required. It is imperative that clients are able to communicate clearly their individual wants and needs to family and carers.

Evidence-based practice points

- Physiotherapists need to have a good understanding of an individual's injury level and extent of neurological impairment to determine whether therapy will focus on attempting to achieve normal movement patterns or compensatory strategies.
- The hierarchy of functional skills acquisition focuses on improving strength and range of movement to allow for new skills to be practised and learnt. Functional skills acquisition is impacted by secondary complications such as spasticity and pain.
- Functional skills retraining must be a top priority in the rehabilitation process. Sitting balance retraining is extremely important as the basis for learning many important skills, such as wheelchair skills, transfers and ADLs. Skin integrity must be considered and closely monitored while learning new functional skills.
- Energy conservation is an essential component to be considered as part of an individual's ADLs after an SCI.
- Preservation of shoulder integrity is vital for individuals after an SCI.
- Wheelchair mobility needs to be taught and practised after an SCI for ADLs, community access, occupational and recreational pursuits.
- Early standing should be commenced in suitable individuals as soon as it is practically possible post-SCI.
- Use of a combination of outcomes measures is required to assess independence with functional skills for individuals with SCI.
- Goal-setting in consultation with the individual, their family and the multidisciplinary team is essential after a SCI.

Please note that these are not necessarily in order of importance, and should be considered in the context of the individual patient.

SUMMARY

Achieving functional independence or strategies to regain independence with ADLs is a key focus of rehabilitation following SCI. For individuals with disability, there is a growing body of research suggesting that life satisfaction is more strongly related to community participation than to impairment and activity limitations.[49] Functional skills training is developed based on impairments and activity limitations and should be progressed with consideration given to the environment and overall participation. A variety of functional skills are important for goal attainment and strategies to achieve ADLs. Regaining a sense of control over daily activities will provide opportunities to further explore participation and community involvement.

Physiotherapists must work collaboratively with their clients and the multidisciplinary team members to develop strategies and goals to facilitate independence, while considering changing function due to ageing with an SCI, changing neurological status and/or the development of secondary complications. Time must be allowed for an individual to build competence in functional skills before final decisions are made on equipment prescription. Strategies are implemented and trialled throughout rehabilitation to allow individuals to make informed decisions regarding future functioning. Problem-solving is a key strategy utilised in functional skills training. This ensures individuals possess the knowledge and skills to achieve optimal levels of independence following an SCI, including the ability to instruct personal support workers to assist functional tasks and to adapt to often new and challenging environments.

References

1. Rivers, C.S., Fallah, N., et al., 2018. Health conditions: effect on function, health-related quality of life, and life satisfaction after traumatic spinal cord injury. A prospective observational registry cohort study. Arch. Phys. Med. Rehabil. 99, 443–451.

2. Chu, J., Harvey, L.A., et al., 2012. Physical therapists' ability to predict future mobility after spinal cord injury. J. Neurol. Phys. Ther. 36, 3–7.

3. Spinal Cord Injury Australia 2015–2016. Canberra Australia: Australian Institute of Health and Welfare. Australian Government.

4. Stucki, G., 2005. International classification of functioning, disability, and health (ICF). Am. J. Phys. Med. Rehabil. 84, 733–740.

5. Martin Ginis, K.A., Jorgensen, S., et al., 2012. Exercise and sport for persons with spinal cord injury. PM R. 4, 894–900.

6. Harvey, L.A., 2016. Physiotherapy rehabilitation for people with spinal cord injuries. J. Physiother. 62, 4–11.

7. Kilkens, O., Post, M., et al., 2005. Relationship between manual wheelchair skill performance and participation of persons with spinal cord injuries 1 year after discharge from inpatient rehabilitation. J. Rehabil. Res. Dev. 42, 65–74.

8. MacPhee, A.H., Kirby, R.L., et al., 2004. Wheelchair skills training program: a randomized clinical trial of wheelchair users undergoing initial rehabilitation. Arch. Phys. Med. Rehabil. 85, 41–50.

9. Kirby, R.L., Mifflen, N.J., et al., 2004. The manual wheelchair-handling skills of caregivers and the effect of training. Arch. Phys. Med. Rehabil. 85, 2011–2019.

10. Keeler, L., Kirby, R.L., et al., 2018. Effectiveness of the Wheelchair Skills Training Program: a systematic review and meta-anaylsis. Disabil. Rehabil. Assist. Technol. 4, 1–19.

11. Hosseini, S., Oyster, M., et al., 2012. Manual wheelchair skills capacity predicts quality of life and community integration in persons with spinal cord injury. Arch. Phys. Med. Rehabil. 93, 2237–2243.

12. Eng, J.J., Levins, S.M., et al., 2001. Use of prolonged standing for individuals with spinal cord injuries. Phys. Ther. 81, 1392–1399.

13. Verrier, M., Gagnon, D., et al., 2016. Toolkit for SCI standing and walking assessment. Rick Hansen Institute, Toronto.

14. Field-Fote, E.C., 2009. Spinal Cord Injury Rehabilitation. F.A. Davis Company, Philadelphia.

15. Alexander, M.S., Anderson, K.D., et al., 2009. Outcome measures in spinal cord injury: recent assessments and recommendations for future directions. Spinal Cord 47, 582–591.

16. Biering-Sorensen, F., Charlifue, S., et al., 2006. International spinal cord injury data sets. Spinal Cord 44, 530–534.

17. Lawton, G., Lundgren-Nilsson, A., et al., 2006. Cross-cultural validity of FIM in spinal cord injury. Spinal Cord 44, 746–752.

18. Cohen, M.E., Marino, R.J., 2000. The tools of disability outcomes research functional status measures. Arch. Phys. Med. Rehabil. 81, S21–S29.

19. Ota, T., Akaboshi, K., et al., 1996. Functional assessment of patients with spinal cord injury: measured by the motor score and the Functional Independence Measure. Spinal Cord 34, 531–535.

20. Wolfe, D., Hsieh, J.T.C., et al. Spinal Cord Injury Rehabilitation Evidence: SCIRE Project / Monkey Hill Health Communications; 2010. Online 19 December 2019. Available: https://scireproject.com/wp-content/uploads/20-Rehab-Practices-v4.pdf.

21. Granger, C., Albrecht, G., et al., 1979. Outcome of comprehensive medical rehabilitation: measurement by PULSES profile and the Barthel Index. Arch. Phys. Med. Rehabil. 60, 145–154.

22. Roth, E., Davidoff, G., et al., 1990. Functional assessment in spinal cord injury: a comparison of the Modified Barthel Index and the 'adapted' Functional Independence Measure. Clin. Rehabil. 4, 277–285.

23. Gresham, G.E., Labi, M.L., et al., 1986. The Quadriplegia Index of Function (QIF): sensitivity and reliability demonstrated in a study of thirty quadriplegic patients. Paraplegia 24, 38–44.

24. Marino, R.J., Huang, M., et al., 1993. Assessing selfcare status in quadriplegia: comparison of the quadriplegia index of function (QIF) and the functional independence measure (FIM). Paraplegia 31, 225–233.

25. Catz, A., Itzkovich, M., 2007. Spinal cord independence measure: comprehensive ability rating scale for the spinal cord lesion patient. J. Rehabil. Res. Dev. 44, 65.

26. Itzkovich, M., Gelernter, I., et al., 2007. The spinal cord independence measure (SCIM) version III: reliability and validity in a multi-center international study. Disabil. Rehabil. 29, 1926–1933.

27. Lam, T., Noonan, V.K., et al., 2008. A systematic review of functional ambulation outcome measures in spinal cord injury. Spinal Cord 46, 246–254.

28. Campbell, J., Kendall, M., 2003. Investigating the suitability of the Clinical Outcome Variables Scale (COVS) as a mobility outcome measure in spinal cord injury rehabilitation. Physiother. Can. 55, 135–141.

29. Kirby, R.L., Swuste, J., et al., 2002. The Wheelchair Skills Test: a pilot study of a new outcome measure. Arch. Phys. Med. Rehabil. 83, 10–18.

30. Kirby, R., Smith, C., et al., 2013. Wheelchair Skills Test (WST) Version 4.2 Manual. Halifax, Nova Scotia. Dalhousie University, Canada. cited 01/01/2015.

31. Kilkens, O.J., Post, M.W., et al., 2002. The wheelchair circuit: reliability of a test to assess mobility in persons with spinal cord injuries. Arch. Phys. Med. Rehabil. 83, 1783–1788.

32. Kilkens, O.J., Dallmeijer, A.J., et al., 2004. The wheelchair circuit: construct validity and responsiveness of a test to assess manual wheelchair mobility in persons with spinal cord injury. Arch. Phys. Med. Rehabil. 85, 424–431.

33. Cowan, R.E., Nash, M.S., et al., 2011. Adapted manual wheelchair circuit: test-retest reliability and discriminative validity in persons with spinal cord injury. Arch. Phys. Med. Rehabil. 92, 1270–1280.

34. Fliess-Douer, O., Vanlandewijck, Y.C., et al., 2010. A systematic review of wheelchair skills tests for manual wheelchair users with a spinal cord injury: towards a standardized outcome measure. Clin. Rehabil. 24, 867–886.

35. Routhier, F., Vincent, C., et al., 2004. Development of an obstacle course assessment of wheelchair user performance (OCAWUP): a content validity study. Technol. Disabil. 16, 19–31.

36. Routhier, F., Desrosiers, J., et al., 2005. Reliability and construct validity studies of an obstacle course assessment of wheelchair user performance. Int. J. Rehabil. Res. 28, 49–56.

37. Middleton, J.W., Harvey, L.A., et al., 2006. Five additional mobility and locomotor items to improve responsiveness of the FIM in wheelchair-dependent individuals with spinal cord injury. Spinal Cord 44, 495–504.

38. Fliess-Douer, O., Vanlandewijck, Y., et al., 2012. Test of Wheeled Mobility (TOWM) and the Wheelie Test. Katholieke University, Leuven.

39. Fliess-Douer, O., Van Der Woude, L.H., 2013. Reliability of the test of wheeled mobility (TOWM) and the short Wheelie test. Arch. Phys. Med. Rehabil. 94, 761–770.

40. Fliess-Douer, O., Van Der Woude, L.H., 2013. Test of Wheeled Mobility (TOWM) and a short wheelie test: a feasibility and validity study. Clin. Rehabil. 27, 527–537.

41. Gollan, E.J., Harvey, L.A., et al., 2015. Development, reliability and validity of the Queensland evaluation of wheelchair skills (QEWS). Spinal Cord 53, 743–749.

42. Field-Fote, E., Fluet, G., et al., 2001. The spinal cord injury functional ambulation inventory (SCI–FAI). J. Rehabil. Med. 33, 177–181.

43. Ditunno, J.F., Ditunno, P.L., et al., 2013. The walking index for spinal cord injury (WISCI/WISCI II): nature, metric properties, use and misuse. Spinal Cord 51, 346–355.

44. Ditunno, J., Ditunno, P., et al., 2000. Walking index for spinal cord injury (WISCI): an international multicenter validity and reliability study. Spinal Cord 38, 234–243.

45. Ditunno, P., Ditunno, J., 2001. Walking index for spinal cord injury (WISCI II): scale revision. Spinal Cord 39, 654–656.

46. ATS Committee on Proficiency Standards for Clinical Pulmonary Function Laboratories, 2002. ATS Statement:

guidelines for the six-minute walk test. Am. J. Respir. Crit. Care Med. 166, 111–117.

47. van Hedel, H.J., Wirz, M., et al., 2005. Assessing walking ability in subjects with spinal cord injury: validity and reliability of 3 walking tests. Arch. Phys. Med. Rehabil. 86, 190–196.

48. Dunaway, S., Montes, J., et al., 2014. Performance of the timed 'up & go' test in spinal muscular atrophy. Muscle Nerve 50, 273–277.

49. Carpenter, C., Forwell, S.J., et al., 2007. Community participation after spinal cord injury. Arch. Phys. Med. Rehabil. 88, 427–433.

CHAPTER 7

Electrotherapeutic techniques

Vanesa Bochkezanian

INTRODUCTION

Neuromuscular electrical stimulation (NMES) is a commonly used intervention in rehabilitation programs for increasing muscle mass and force in individuals with partial loss of motor function, such as following spinal cord injury.[1,2] Functional electrical stimulation (FES) is a type of NMES with the means of producing useful movement and may be used to assist in the performance of a functional task in paralysed muscles. However, both terms NMES and FES are usually utilised interchangeably in the literature, a pattern which will be followed throughout this chapter.

NMES consists of the 'application of intermittent electrical stimuli to superficial skeletal muscles, aiming to trigger visible muscle contractions by activating the intramuscular nerve branches'.[3] The electrical stimuli are delivered by positioning skin-based electrodes at the proximity of motor points and the stimulation is usually delivered by pre-programmed electrical stimulation units.[4] See Fig. 7.1 for an example of positioning electrodes to facilitate movement in the quadriceps muscles.

NMES induces the same action potential as elicited by natural physiological means after reaching the 'stimulus threshold', which is the lowest level of electrical charge required to generate an action potential.[5] To generate muscle contractions through electrical stimulation, the stimulus can be applied from the origin of the nerve to its motor point where it connects with the muscle (Fig. 7.2),[6] thus it is necessary to have an intact lower motor neuron, together with an intact neuromuscular junction.[6]

NMES can be implemented via surface electrodes, percutaneous electrodes or implanted devices. The most common methods used for muscle conditioning within physiotherapy practice are the surface and percutaneous electrodes. Implanted systems, such as intradural electrical stimulation, require surgical intervention and are often used for long-term functional enhancement. These surgical methods can have many side-effects, such as localised infections, extradural haematomas and sepsis.[7]

NMES PARAMETERS, PULSE CURRENT TYPES AND CHARACTERISTICS

NMES parameters are time-dependent attributes for pulse currents and include the waveform or pulse current, pulse duration or pulse width and pulse frequency. These parameters will determine the dose potency of the electrical impulses applied

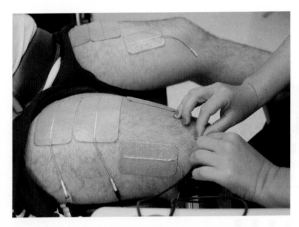

Figure 7.1 Positioning of electrodes at the quadriceps muscles for NMES strength-training.

to the nerves that supply the targeted muscles. These parameters will influence the patient's tolerance and the main results of the NMES application and thus can be manipulated to optimise the response to electrical stimulation.[8] See Fig. 7.3A–C for an illustration of NMES parameters.

The **waveform** or **pulse currents** can be classified into monophasic and biphasic currents (Fig. 7.4).

- *Monophasic currents* consist of a one-directional flow marked by periods of non-current flow; the electrons stay on one side of the baseline or the other and it uses a high-voltage pulse stimulation.

- *Biphasic currents* consist of bidirectional flow of electrons marked by periods of non-current flow, the electrons flow on both sides of the baseline (positive and negative). Biphasic current stimulation is the most common

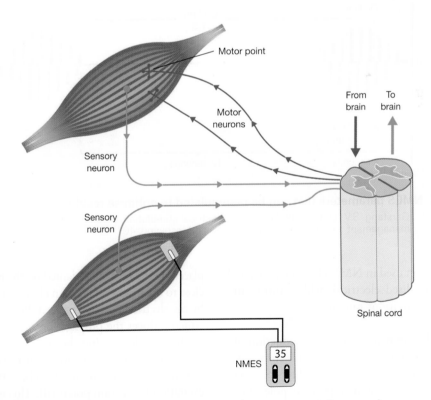

Figure 7.2 NMES uses external stimuli at the motor point to contract the muscle.

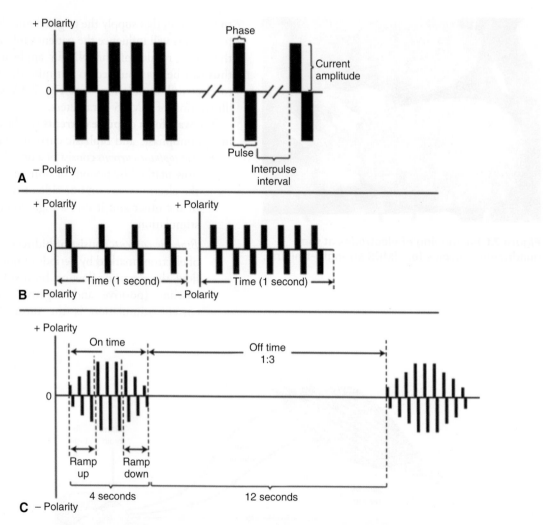

Figure 7.3A–C NMES parameters that can be manipulated to optimise results.

Source: Faghri, P.D., Garstang, S.V., et al, 2009. Functional electrical stimulation. In: S.A. Sisto, E. Druin, et al (eds). Spinal cord injuries: management and rehabilitation. Saint Louis: Mosby; pp. 407–429.

configuration used in NMES because it creates a more localised electrical field resulting in greater selectivity of muscles.[9]

Two electrodes are required for the production of an electrical current flow, which is the force created in the imbalance between a negative pole (high electron concentration, cathode) and a positive pole (low electron concentration, anode). These electrodes can be placed on the skin or implanted on the nerve or muscle close to the motor point.[10] An electric field is generated by the electrical current between the pair of electrodes, which induces the propagation of the nerve impulse to the muscle, causing the muscle contraction.[10] In order for this muscle contraction to occur, the level of stimulation intensity needs to be sufficient to cause excitation (i.e. action potential). This is the threshold of stimulation and follows the all-or-none principle.[10]

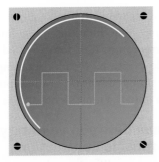

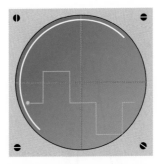

MONOPHASIC CURRENT

Description:
- One-directional flow marked by periods of non-current flow
- Electrons stay on one side of the baseline or the other

Use:
- High voltage pulsed stimulation

BIPHASIC CURRENT

Description:
- Bidirectional flow of electrons marked by periods of non-current flow
- Electrons flow on both sides of the baseline (positive and negative)

Use:
- Neuromuscular electrical stimulation
- Three types of biphasic currents

Figure 7.4 Different waveforms or pulse currents.

The response curve as the intensity increases follows an S-shape, having a steep linear slope over the middle part of the curve, leading to a plateau where the muscle contraction does not increase in response to an increase in intensity (Fig. 7.5).[10]

As previously mentioned, the main characteristics of the electrical pulses are time-dependent attributes and these include the waveform or pulse current amplitude, pulse duration (or pulse width), phase duration, interpulse interval, intrapulse interval, pulse period, pulse frequency and pulse trains (or bursts). The amplitude and pulse width can be considered as the stimulation intensity.

The **pulse duration**, or **pulse width**, is the time (horizontal distance) from when the pulse rises to the baseline to the point where it terminates on the baseline (Fig. 7.6). Changes in pulse width can have a repercussion in the recruitment of motor units. Narrow pulse widths (50–500 microseconds) are often used in FES to recruit motor units, minimising discomfort. The use of wide-pulse width (1000 microseconds) is used in NMES to recruit motor units via direct activation of motor axons that overlie the muscles, and/or via indirect activation through

Ia reflex pathways.[11] Ia reflex pathways refers to the stretch reflex caused by the sensory stimulation of the proprioceptors located in the muscle spindles.

The **pulse frequency** is the number of times a pulse occurs per second (Fig. 7.7). To recruit more motor units, the frequency needs to be enough to produce an optimal muscle force output. However, as the frequency increases, so does the muscle fatigue, thus low-to moderate frequencies are often used to limit the contraction-induced muscle injury, delaying muscle fatigue.

Option 1

The **duty cycle (DC)** is the amount (or percentage) of time that the current is flowing relative to the time it is not flowing. The duty cycle can be expressed as seconds on/off or as a percentage. For example, if the current is on for 20 seconds and off for 40 seconds, it can described as: DC = 20/(20 + 40) × 100 = 33.3%. The duty cycle can be altered based on the specific duration of the desired muscle contraction for a specific functional activity.

A **pulse ramp** can also be used with a duty cycle to gradually increase the current. This will allow for

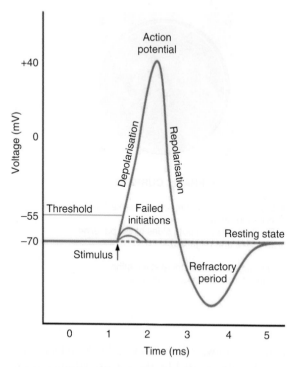

Figure 7.5 Action potential: waves of potential (or voltage) difference that move down and occurs between the inside and outside of a nerve or muscle fibre when it is stimulated. This figure shows the phases of an action potential in relation to the membrane voltage over time.

Source: CC BY-SA 3.0

a more natural and comfortable muscle contraction. For example, long durations at low intensities with a pulse ramp can be used for sustained contractions in a stable position, such as standing, and short durations at high intensities without pulse ramp can be used to initiate a movement, such as 'sit to stand'.

Difference between voluntary and evoked muscle contractions

There are some differences between evoked (i.e. by NMES) versus voluntary muscle contractions that need to be considered to optimise NMES interventions. Table 7.1 describes the main differences between a voluntary muscle contraction and an evoked one (NMES).

Electrical stimulation using standard parameters typically evokes a spatial recruitment pattern of motor units from large to small, which is opposite to that in voluntary contractions, and thus activates fast-fatiguable motor units before fatigue-resistant motor units.[12] For more information about motor unit types, please refer to Fig. 7.8.

NMES also imposes a synchronous temporal recruitment pattern, while motor units are recruited asynchronously during voluntary contractions.[13] In addition, spatial recruitment is limited because NMES imposes a continuous contractile activity to the axonal branches in proximity to the stimulation electrodes. This fixed recruitment diminishes proportionally as distance increases from the electrode.[13]

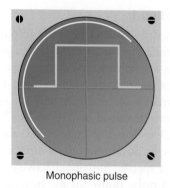

Monophasic pulse

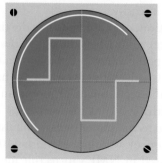

Biphasic pulse

Figure 7.6 Pulse duration or pulse width.

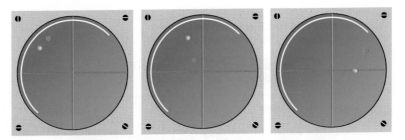

Figure 7.7 Pulse frequency. Pulses moving across the screen.

Table 7.1 Features of a muscle contraction

Voluntary muscle contraction	Evoked muscle contraction
Motor activation orderly	Motor activation non-selective
Near-maximal contraction intensity	Sub-maximal contraction intensity
Synergistic muscle activation	Targeted muscle activation
Internal physiological origin	External physiological origin
Spatial recruitment pattern of motor units from small to large, activating fatigue-resistant fatiguable motor units before fast-fatiguable motor units	Spatial recruitment pattern of motor units from large to small, activating fast-fatiguable motor units before fatigue-resistant motor units
Asynchronous temporal recruitment pattern	Synchronous temporal recruitment pattern

Source: Adapted from Hortobagyi T. Maffiuletti N.A., 2011. Neural adaptations to electrical stimulation strength training. Eur J Appl Physiol 111 (10), 2439–2449.

Precautions associated with using NMES

Using conservative parameters of NMES to evoke isometric muscle contractions in the paralysed quadriceps femoris can elicit higher levels of muscle damage and a greater relative muscle activation than in able-bodied people.[14] In paralysed quadriceps femoris, increases in current intensity would activate more muscle fibres and increase the likelihood of excitability of more nerves closer to the firing threshold and thus more muscle fibres would be activated. Therefore, if NMES produces a tetanic, fused muscle contraction (i.e. a sustained muscle contraction evoked when the motor nerve that innervates a skeletal muscle emits action potentials at a very high rate), muscle fibres will be activated

maximally and thus the only way to increase muscle force would be to increase the current intensity with the consequent effect of muscle damage.[14] Therefore, the use of NMES in paralysed muscles using standard stimulation parameters may elicit early muscle damage and may not be optimum for eliciting broad ranging muscular adaptations, and thus for increasing muscle force production in functionally important muscles.

The force of the muscle contractions and the number of nerve fibres activated during NMES depend on parameters such as the amplitude and duration of the electrical stimulation,[4] and this can affect the effectiveness of the NMES strength training program. However, it is important to note that the muscle force elicited by NMES depends not only

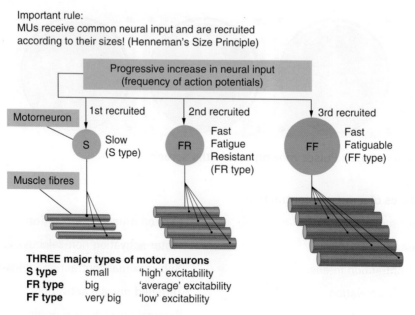

Important rule:
MUs receive common neural input and are recruited according to their sizes! (Henneman's Size Principle)

Progressive increase in neural input (frequency of action potentials)

Motorneuron

1st recruited

S — Slow (S type)

2nd recruited

FR — Fast Fatigue Resistant (FR type)

3rd recruited

FF — Fast Fatiguable (FF type)

Muscle fibres

THREE major types of motor neurons
S type   small   'high' excitability
FR type big   'average' excitability
FF type very big 'low' excitability

Figure 7.8 Motor unit types.

on these external controllable factors, but also on intrinsic anatomical properties of the individual, the inherent length-tension characteristics of the muscle and volume conduction of the current.[5] Nonetheless, the key factor influencing the long-term adaptive response to NMES training is the muscle tension developed during each training session. This muscle tension is the level of evoked force as a proportion of the maximal force capacity of the muscle[15] and can be maximised by appropriately manipulating the frequency and intensity of the NMES pulse burst or trains.[4]

In summary, one of the main problems when using NMES in paralysed muscles is the rapid onset of muscle fatigue due to simultaneous activation of motor axons in repeated muscle contractions and random motor unit recruitment. This requires the use of higher stimulation frequencies and current intensity in NMES to develop a proper muscle contraction. Therefore, in order to obtain optimal muscle contractions during NMES, it is essential to optimise the muscle tension by the manipulation of NMES parameters to delay muscle fatigue.

Some of the strategies to delay muscle fatigue when using NMES/FES protocols include the optimisation of the electrode positioning, using the appropriate electrode size according to length of muscle (e.g. large electrodes for rectus femoris (RF) and medium electrodes for vastus lateralis (VL) and vastus medialis (VM) for the quadriceps muscles); patterns of stimulation and parameters modification; optimisation of the mode and frequency of the NMES/FES training; and the use of biofeedback-controlled NMES/FES devices.[16]

NEUROMODULATION

Electrical stimulation and motor recovery

The use of both central and peripheral electrical stimulation can improve long-term motor and sensory recovery, including standing, walking and hand function. The mechanisms underlying the stimulus-induced recovery are not well-understood, but are thought to be related to training, central pattern generators (CPG) (see Chapter 3) and/or the Hebbian mechanism of synaptic facilitation and stimulation paradigms (for further detail see page 154). These mechanisms aim to facilitate motor function in people with spinal cord injury (SCI) and include the epidural cortical stimulation, epidural spinal stimulation and NMES of peripheral nerves.

Motor cortical stimulation

The motor cortex can be stimulated with epidural electrodes or transcranial electrical currents or magnetic fields. Evidence in healthy and motor incomplete SCI subjects has revealed a modification in lumbar spinal network excitability and a decrease in cervical propriospinal system excitability, facilitating voluntary control and triggered stepping behaviour.[17] However, some of the drawbacks of motor cortical stimulation include the non-specificity effects and the need of a head covering, such as a transcranial direct current stimulator (Fig. 7.9), that may interfere with daily activity.[17]

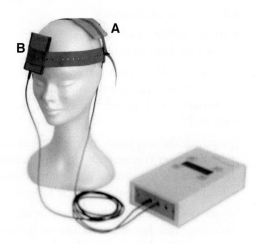

Figure 7.9 Transcranial direct current stimulation procedure. A, Anode electrode displayed in the area of the motor cortex position in the dominant hemisphere, and B, the cathode electrode placed over the contralateral supraorbital region.
Source: Bianchi, M.S., Ferreira, C.F., et al, 2017. Transcranial direct current stimulation effects on menopausal vasomotor symptoms. Menopause 24 (10), 1122–1128.

Epidural spinal cord stimulation

The use of subthreshold epidural spinal cord stimulation is a promising intervention that can activate the lumbar CPG and facilitate voluntary motor control in people with SCI. The underlying hypothesis of the mechanisms for this therapy is the widespread activation of both ascending and descending activity in lumbosacral motor centres.[17] Epidural spinal cord stimulation has many advantages over cortical stimulation. These are related to the nature of the implanted epidural electrodes, which are unobtrusive, can be left on throughout the day and night and do not interfere with daily activities. These electrodes can also be used percutaneously and thus are associated with fewer complications than the surgically placed epidural electrodes.[17]

Peripheral nerve stimulation

Peripheral nerve stimulation can be delivered by stimulator devices, which are available to strengthen muscles for standing and assist gait, activate hand function and relieve seating pressure. It should be noted, however, that NMES/FES requires an intact local nervous system and therefore cannot be used in denervated muscles.[17]

NMES/FES also has central effects, and, as such, can help downregulate spasticity, but can also cause endocrine changes that may induce autonomic dysreflexia (see Chapters 1 and 4). The mechanism on how NMES/FES can promote motor recovery relies on the stimulations of the peripheral motor and sensory axons that return to the spinal cord and activate motor neurons and interneurons, as well as the central nervous system. It can also promote heterosynaptic facilitation of synapses on spinal cord motor neurons and interneurons. In addition, peripheral nerve stimulation can cause antidromic activation of motoneurons and Renshaw neurons, which can induce synapse formation and release neurotransmitters that can consolidate synapses.[17] This is illustrated in the Hebbian facilitation of synapses (Fig. 7.10), which shows that facilitation of synapses can occur at multiple levels in the cortex, brainstem and spinal cord.

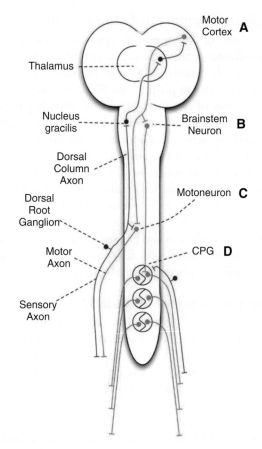

Figure 7.10 Multiple levels of Hebbian learning in the brain and spinal cord: A, Cortical stimulation. B, Brainstem cell stimulation. C, Peripheral nerve stimulation in motoneurons. D, Peripheral nerve stimulation to lumbosacral spinal cord.

Source: Young, W., 2015. Electrical stimulation and motor recovery. Cell Transplant 24 (3), 429–446.

The **Hebbian** theory is a neuroscientific theory claiming that an increase in synaptic efficacy arises from a presynaptic cell's repeated and persistent stimulation of a postsynaptic cell by a presynaptic cell. It is an attempt to explain synaptic plasticity, the adaptation of brain neurons during the learning process. Hebbian facilitation can occur using motor cortical stimulation, epidural spinal cord stimulation and peripheral nerve stimulation. This is produced

by the action potentials activated at different levels: at the peripheral level (i.e. FES) the action potential descends to the muscles, ascends antidromically to activate motoneurons and ascends orthodromically in sensory Ia afferent to enter the spinal cord and activates interneurons and motoneurons; at the central level (i.e. motor cortical stimulation) descending tracts from motor cortex and brainstem activate motoneurons and interneurons.[17]

MANIPULATION OF NMES/FES PARAMETERS IN PEOPLE WITH SCI

The use of NMES parameters in people with SCI has been adapted from evidence-based principles found in healthy people. Current recommendations to maximise muscle tension during NMES in healthy subjects involve:

- biphasic rectangular pulses of 100–400 microseconds delivered at stimulation intensities of 50–100 Hz[13] with the highest tolerated current intensity

- a static loading condition (i.e. isometric) to control the level of evoked force

- altering NMES parameters, which has been documented to influence motor unit recruitment and muscle fatigue in people with SCI[19]

- increasing the amplitude of the current and pulse duration (i.e. pulse width) to increase skeletal muscle recruitment without interfering with the rate or extent of muscle fatigue[18,19]

- longer pulse duration, but not stimulation duration. This has been shown to increase evoked torque when compared to shorter pulse durations. Increasing from 150 microseconds to 500 microseconds resulted in an increase in torque. This was probably due to recruitment of large motor units or high-threshold, usually larger, motor units that added non-linearly to the force. However, increasing the frequency of the pulse stimulation increased torque, but not the activated area[20]

• increasing the pulse width. This increases the number of recruited fibres and thus increases muscle force, whereas increasing the frequency drives the already-active motor units to higher force levels, but therefore also induces more rapid fatigue.[19]

NMES as a high-intensity strength training protocol using wider pulse widths (e.g. ≥ 1000 microseconds) with low-to-moderate frequencies (20–30 Hz) has been shown to improve evoked muscle force, muscle mass and decreasing perceived symptoms of spasticity.[21]

NMES/FES has been found to reduce symptoms of spasticity by 45–60%, evidenced by a decrease in electromyography activity and an increase in range of motion (ROM) in people with SCI.[22] NMES/FES parameters that have been shown to downregulate or reduce spasticity by 40–60% in people with SCI were reported as 20–30 Hz for frequency, 300–350 microseconds for pulse duration/width and >100 mA for amplitude of the current.[22]

The use of NMES has also been investigated for the prevention of pressure sores. The use of NMES targeting the gluteal and hamstring muscles can help decrease the pressure of the ischial tuberosities while sitting.[23] It has been shown that one of the parameters that helped prevent the risk of pressure sores was the duty cycle of 1:4 in comparison to 1:1, which helped reduce the level of muscle fatigue experienced during the electrotherapy.[23]

CLINICAL APPLICATION OF NMES/FES IN PEOPLE WITH SCI

There are two main types of peripheral electrical stimulation: nerve stimulation and muscle stimulation. Nerve stimulation is produced by the delivery of an electrical charge that stimulates the muscle nerve trunk connected to the targeted muscles and muscle stimulation depolarises the terminal axonal branches through surface electrodes placed over the muscles.[24] However, muscle stimulation is the more common method used in the clinical

practice to improve musculoskeletal function in people with SCI.

NMES/FES has been largely used as a muscle stimulation intervention to improve many physical outcomes, such as muscle strength and muscle mass. In individuals with SCI, NMES/FES aims to recruit the paralysed or partially paralysed muscles or to provide sensory stimulation to the nerves enabling voluntary movement. NMES/FES has been shown to improve voluntary strength of muscles directly affected by SCI,[25] improve function and to promote greater independence during activities of daily living[26] in people with incomplete SCI. NMES/FES is also considered a part of the activity-based therapy (ABT) modality and has been widely investigated for this purpose (see Chapter 3 for more detail on ABT).

NMES/FES can be used to improve motor and sensory recovery in the neurological rehabilitation of people with SCI. The therapeutic use of NMES/FES is to minimise muscle atrophy, prevent secondary peripheral nerve deterioration, encourage neural repair and promote healing of pressure sores. NMES has been found to promote cardiovascular and haemodynamic benefits, to reverse muscle atrophy, to improve bone mass, to reduce spasticity and neurogenic pain, to prevent pressure sores and to improve psychosocial outcomes, such as self-image and depression, for people with either complete or incomplete SCI.[27]

NMES/FES DEVICES

Some of the most common NMES/FES devices used in SCI in the clinical setting are the FES bike (RT 300, see Fig. 7.11 for an example) and FES elliptical (RT 600) from Restorative Therapies and the NESS 200 (www.bioness.com). These devices can stimulate up to 16 muscle groups for one or both legs and the trunk and use a smart technology where NMES/FES parameters can be pre-programmed by the user.

Other NMES/FES options to consider are the portable electrical stimulators that patients can use at their homes. These devices have the advantage of being small and allowing therapists to create and

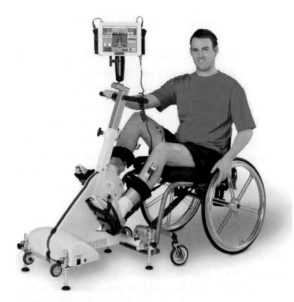

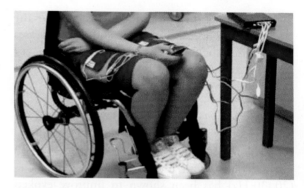

Figure 7.12 Set-up for NMES subtetanic contractions.

Source: Carty, A., McCormack, K, et al, 2012. Increased aerobic fitness after neuromuscular electrical stimulation training in adults with spinal cord injury. Arch Phys Med Rehabil 93 (5), 790–795.

Figure 7.11 FES-assisted cycling. Paraplegia. Device RT 300.

Source: © 2019 Restorative Therapies

save individual-tailored programs based on the patient's goals.[28]

Electrical stimulation to promote aerobic fitness and cardiometabolic health benefits

Maintaining fitness and cardiometabolic health are important priorities for people with SCI. Chronic muscle paralysis can lead to significant reductions in muscle mass, increased intramuscular fat and adipose tissue and metabolic abnormalities that will predispose the person to cardiovascular diseases.[29] Cardiovascular diseases are a major cause of death and thus many cardiovascular risk factors, such as metabolic syndrome, obesity and diabetes, are prevalent among people with SCI.[29] Although the overall physical health in people with SCI has increased in recent years, poor health in the years after injury is still problematic and the mortality rate is still higher than for the general population (see Chapter 15 on ageing with an SCI).[30] Therefore, physical interventions that target a broad decrease

in cardiovascular risk factors are important for the SCI population.

The use of NMES in the legs (i.e. FES leg cycle) has been shown to minimise muscle weakening and even increase muscle strength, reduce the rate of skeletal muscle atrophy and weakness and improve physical health in people with a SCI (see also Chapter 13).[31,32] NMES/FES has been shown to significantly reduce inflammatory markers that are associated with physical health benefits.[31] However, the use of the FES leg cycle to improve aerobic fitness is controversial. This is because FES leg cycling may not have sufficient dose-potency to increase aerobic fitness in people with SCI.

Studies have tried to demonstrate that NMES can improve aerobic fitness. For example, Carty[33] completed a study that used a battery-powered stimulator to deliver subtetanic contractions to quadriceps and hamstrings (Fig. 7.12). This intervention used an overall series of frequencies from 2–4 Hz over phases of 20 minutes and a maximum intensity of 200 mA and found a statistically significant improvement in VO_{2peak} (peak oxygen consumption) and HR_{peak} (peak heart rate) after the intervention.[33] However, this study recruited an untrained cohort and did not have a controlled group, so any other treatment could have similar results. In addition, Bakkum and colleagues (2015) found no significant benefits on metabolic syndrome components from FES-induced leg exercise when compared to handcycling.[34] Finally, a systematic review of the literature about the effects of NMES/FES in aerobic fitness and metabolic health benefits reported low-to-moderate evidence to support improvements in metabolic health and revealed that peak aerobic fitness only improved in those protocols that targeted >50% heart rate reserve ($\approx$ 40% VO_2 reserve).[35]

Use of NMES/FES for aerobic fitness and cardiometabolic health benefits

NMES/FES is usually performed as cycling, which involves the use of electrodes in the major lower limb muscle groups, such as the gluteals, hamstrings and quadriceps in combination with a bike or leg ergometer. FES cycling is usually assisted by a motor until the electrical stimulation of the legs elicits the proper muscle contraction for the pedalling (see Fig. 7.11). Commonly, the leg pedalling power output is modulated by a controlled intensity of the current using fixed values of pulse width (200 and 300 microseconds) and frequency in a range of 10–50 Hz.[12,36] Research studies have used this modality to show the positive effects on muscle strength and endurance adaptations and functional capacity improvements in people with SCI.[2,37] Other studies have documented lower extremity muscle hypertrophy, improved metabolic profiles and decreases in fat mass after FES interventions.[31,38] However, this type of NMES uses low-intensity currents evoking low levels of force during muscle-evoked contractions and cannot optimally stimulate muscular strength and mass improvements, which requires the imposition of a higher load to the muscle to obtain higher force output. Therefore, the use of NMES as a strength training tool may be a more effective physical rehabilitation method than FES cycling if

Important NMES treatment points to improve aerobic fitness and cardiometabolic health benefits

1. Cadence/velocity

- To improve aerobic fitness, the leg exercise (i.e. FES bike) cadence/velocity should be high (i.e. 40–50 rev/min^{-1}).[39]
- If the aim is to improve muscle strength, the cadence/velocity should be low (i.e. 10–20 rev/min^{-1}).[39]
- In both cases, the current intensity should be low to prevent muscle fatigue and allow exercise sessions of longer duration (i.e. 45–60 minutes).[39]

2. Exercise intensity

- To improve aerobic fitness the leg exercise intensity should be between moderate (64–76% HR_{peak}, RPE: 12–13 fairly light to somewhat hard) and vigorous (77–95% HR_{peak}, RPE >18 very hard).[39] This could be challenging as paralysed muscles can fatigue very quickly under higher current intensities, and thus individual characteristics and response to NMES should be taken into account.
- To reduce cardiometabolic risk, the leg exercise intensity should be between light (57–63% HR_{peak}) and the exercise duration should be between 45 and 90 minutes or moderate (64–76% HR_{peak}) and should last between 30 and 60 minutes.[39]

the main aim is to increase muscle force and muscle mass in people with SCI.

Clinicians should use NMES parameters according to 'best practice' guidelines, and carefully plan an appropriate exercise prescription, considering dose-potency to augment outcomes,[16] and consider risk versus benefits based on individual characteristics and treatment goals.

ELECTRICAL STIMULATION TO ELICIT MUSCULOSKELETAL ADAPTATIONS

People with SCI suffer most commonly from muscle atrophy, which is related to the loss of activation and subsequent unloading and alterations in fibre length and composition, impairing the force generating capacity with detrimental consequences.[40] This reduction of muscle force can increase muscle fatigue due to:

- preferential atrophy (or complete loss) of type I (slow) fibres, which are more capable of maintaining an energy balance over repeated contractions
- the requirement for the remaining musculature to work at a higher proportion of its maximum during submaximal activities.[41]

The increased susceptibility to muscle fatigue in people with SCI usually results from a reduced number of fatigue-resistant motor units in the paralysed muscles, which reduces the oxidative capacity of muscle.[41] This ultimately affects the motor output in partially paralysed muscles that are necessary to perform functional activities, such as transfers from the bed to the wheelchair.[42]

The use of NMES/FES as a muscle-strength training intervention can help convert type II into type I muscle fibres.[6] The use of NMES/FES as a muscle-strength modality has been documented to induce many musculoskeletal and physical health benefits in people with SCI. For example, a 12-week NMES twice-weekly strength training intervention using a 450 microseconds pulse width resulted in significant skeletal muscle hypertrophy

and improvements in lipid metabolism and insulin profile.[38]

The use of NMES/FES as a muscle strength training intervention has been utilised in people with incomplete SCI to increase voluntary muscle strength in the lower limbs;[1] however, this NMES modality can also be used in people with complete SCI. A recent study has found that after 12 weeks of NMES as a high-intensity strength-training modality, substantial increases evoked tetanic knee extensor torque (i.e. muscle strength) and quadriceps cross-sectional area (i.e. muscle size).[21] These changes were observed in subjects with complete and incomplete SCI who used other forms of electrical stimulation-based training (e.g. FES bike) regularly before and during the study.[21] Of specific interest in this study was that the mean evoked torque in the last contractions (i.e. at the point of fatigue) in the final week of training was either equal to or higher in all subjects than that during the first contractions (i.e. unfatigued) in the first week of training. This clearly revealed a notable increase in muscle work capacity in paralysed muscles.[21]

Developing a healthier musculoskeletal system through the use of NMES as a strength training modality may also have other long-term advantages in people with chronic SCI. For example, having a strong (and healthy) musculoskeletal system is important if people with SCI wish to utilise new treatments, such as stem cell therapies, epidural stimulation,[43] the use of exoeskeletons and many other promising strategies aiming to repair the injured spinal cord.[44] Having a healthier musculoskeletal system will allow people with SCI to take advantage of these future, innovative therapies and help them improve functional outcomes in the lower limbs, which may allow them to recover greater physical function.

USE OF NMES AS A MUSCLE STRENGTH-TRAINING MODALITY

Similar training programming principles need to be followed when using NMES as a strength training modality as when using voluntary strength training. Muscle force generation varies according to the level of motor unit activation, and the magnitude of strength enhancement with voluntary strength training is known to be highly dependent on muscle action, intensity, volume, exercise selection and order, rest periods and frequency of exercise.[45]

To utilise NMES as a strength training modality, the basic principles of progressive strength training also need to be followed. This involves imposing progressively heavier loads to elicit stronger muscle contractions[46] and a progression of the other parameters during training, such as current intensity, evoked force and training volume.[4] As mentioned previously, the force of the muscle contractions and the number of nerve fibres activated during NMES depend on parameters such as the amplitude and duration of the electrical stimulation[4] and this can affect the effectiveness of the NMES strength training program.

Optimal NMES/FES dosages for muscle strength-training

NMES/FES dosage should be based on evidence:

- 1– 4 times monthly for 2–3 years, 5 days a week, 5 minutes recovery between each interval, total time: 35 minutes.[47]
- 2–3 times per week for 6–18 weeks, total time per session: 30 minutes, 50:50 work to rest ratio; Wide-pulse width/longer pulse duration (500–1000 microseconds).[20,21,48]

Frequency should be enough to obtain an optimal muscle force output:

- Recommendation of low-to-moderate frequencies (20–30 Hz) to prevent contraction-induced muscle injury.[49]

Adequate resting period between sets and between sessions:

- Need to allow 48 to 72 hours after first NMES/FES session for a full muscle fatigue recovery.[50]

Evidence-based practice points

- NMES strength training sessions need to aim for strong muscle contractions (i.e. submaximal or near-maximal) and enough stimuli to elicit musculoskeletal adaptations (i.e. produce hypertrophy and increase muscle force).
- Responses to NMES/FES need to be assessed before prescribing exercise intervention.
- The optimal stimulation parameters for each individual need to be utilised to delay muscle fatigue and obtain the greatest amount of force.
- Muscle strength training principles (progressive overload, specificity, FITT, etc.) need to be followed.
- Isometric contractions may be a good tool for use as a home NMES/FES device and non-isometric contractions are more functional/clinically relevant; however, the latter should be performed in a laboratory or clinic.

SUMMARY

NMES and FES are commonly used interventions in rehabilitation for people with SCI. NMES/FES parameters of stimulation components will influence the patient's tolerance and can be manipulated to improve its effectiveness on different outcomes.

Dosages as described above should be taken into consideration when planning an NMES/FES session in people with SCI; however, clinicians should always apply clinical reasoning skills and consider risk versus benefits based on individual characteristics and treatment goals. Clinicians should also be able to identify in the research literature the population (e.g. consider time since injury, level and completeness of lesion), methodology and dose potency necessary to augment outcomes, in order to make an informed decision on whether that specific intervention would be beneficial for their patients. For example, if a research study found improvements in voluntary muscle strength after applying a certain NMES/FES protocol, this type of intervention would potentially only be applicable for incomplete SCI and may not be adequate for a complete SCI.

Another important aspect to be considered when using any type of NMES/FES interventions are the costs and access to these devices. The optimal and evidence-based NMES/FES protocol for aerobic fitness and muscle strength outcomes in people with SCI can be challenging because the evidence for the use of different NMES protocols is inconsistent.[50] Some of the future directions of NMES/FES would be to perform more clinical trials integrating all strategies to optimise muscle performance and include automated, controlled NMES/FES devices to manage the stimulation parameters in order to suit the fatigue state of the targeted muscles.[16]

The use of electrotherapy as an adjunct to physiotherapy is important to consider when investigating options to integrate evidence into practice and allow patients to have access to the benefits of the electrotherapy. For example, if NMES/FES is routinely prescribed at the same time as standing in a frame, patients may have additional health benefits that could justify the costs of these devices.

Other options to consider are the portable electrical stimulators that patients can use at home. These devices have the advantage of being small and allow therapists to create and save individual-tailored programs based on the patient's goals.[28] However, some of the barriers to using these devices are cost and lack of patient confidence and knowledge relating to how to use them properly. Other considerations when using any type of NMES/FES devices are that the stimulation should be done regularly to obtain the best effects and that in order to observe these benefits, these therapies need to be carried out for weeks and even years.[28]

In terms of the regular implementation of electrotherapy in clinical practice, many limitations have been identified, including expenditure of time, lack of confidence and acceptance from clinicians and patients.[28] Institutions and government agencies can also influence the use of electrotherapy, whereby hospitals and private clinics have available devices, but do not approve any budget for accessories, such as electrodes for each patient, or where, in Australia, for example, the National Disability Insurance Scheme (NDIS) does not support the cost of these devices. These barriers limit the use of NMES/FES in people with SCI, forcing clinicians to consider the cost-effectiveness of these therapies and find alternatives for their implementation.

In conclusion, NMES/FES, when applied judiciously, can be an extremely useful adjunct to therapy for the patient with SCI.

References

1. Harvey, L.A., Fornusek, C., et al., 2010. Electrical stimulation plus progressive resistance training for leg strength in spinal cord injury: a randomized controlled trial. Spinal Cord 48 (7), 570–575.

2. Thrasher, T.A., Ward, J.S., et al., 2013. Strength and endurance adaptations to functional electrical stimulation leg cycle ergometry in spinal cord injury. NeuroRehabilitation 33 (1), 133–138.

3. Hultman, E., Sjöholm, H., et al., 1983. Evaluation of methods for electrical stimulation of human skeletal muscle in situ. Pflügers Arch. 398 (2), 139–141.

4. Maffiuletti, N.A., 2010. Physiological and methodological considerations for the use of neuromuscular electrical stimulation. Eur. J. Appl. Physiol. 110 (2), 223–234.

5. Sheffler, L.R., Chae, J., 2007. Neuromuscular electrical stimulation in neurorehabilitation. Muscle Nerve 35 (5), 562–590.

6. Ragnarsson, K.T., 2008. Functional electrical stimulation after spinal cord injury: current use, therapeutic effects and future directions. Spinal Cord 46 (4), 255–274.

7. Gibson-Corley, K.N., Flouty, O., et al., 2014. Postsurgical pathologies associated with intradural electrical stimulation in the central nervous system: design implications for a new clinical device. Biomed Res. Int. 1, 989175.

8. Faghri, P.D., Garstang, S.V., et al., 2009. Functional electrical stimulation. In: Sisto, S.A., Druin, E., et al. (Eds.), Spinal Cord Injuries: Management and Rehabilitation. Mosby, Saint Louis, pp. 407–429.

9. Grandjean, P.A., Mortimer, J.T., 1986. Recruitment properties of monopolar and bipolar epimysial electrodes. Ann. Biomed. Eng. 14 (1), 53–66.

10. Wood, D., Swain, I., 2014. Functional electrical stimulation. In: Taktak, A., Ganney, P., et al. (Eds.), Clinical Engineering: A Handbook for Clinical and Biomedical Engineers. Academic Press, Oxford., pp. 275–284.

11. Collins, D.F., Burke, D., et al., 2002. Sustained contractions produced by plateau-like behaviour in human motoneurones. J. Physiol. (Lond.) 538 (1), 289–301.

12. Rabischong, E., Ohanna, F., 1992. Effects of functional electrical stimulation (FES) on evoked muscular output in paraplegic quadriceps muscle. Paraplegia 30 (7), 467–473.

13. Vanderthommen, M., Duteil, S., et al., 2003. A comparison of voluntary and electrically induced contractions by interleaved 1H– and 31P–NMRS in humans. J. Appl. Physiol. 94 (3), 1012–1024.

14. Bickel, C.S., Slade, J.M., et al., 2004. Long-term spinal cord injury increases susceptibility to isometric contraction-induced muscle injury. Eur. J. Appl. Physiol. 91 (2–3), 308–313.

15. Lieber, R.L., Kelly, M.J., 1991. Factors influencing quadriceps femoris muscle torque using transcutaneous neuromuscular electrical stimulation. Phys. Ther. 71 (10), 715–721.

16. Ibitoye, M.O., Hamzaid, N.A., et al., 2016. Strategies for rapid muscle fatigue reduction during FES exercise in individuals with spinal cord injury: a systematic review. PLoS ONE 11 (2), e0149024.

17. Young, W., 2015. Electrical stimulation and motor recovery. Cell Transplant. 24 (3), 429–446.

18. Gorgey, A.S., Black, C.D., et al., 2009. Effects of electrical stimulation parameters on fatigue in skeletal muscle. J. Orthop. Sports Phys. Ther. 39 (9), 684–692.

19. Chou, L.W., Lee, S.C., et al., 2008. The effectiveness of progressively increasing stimulation frequency and intensity to maintain paralyzed muscle force during repetitive activation in persons with spinal cord injury. Arch. Phys. Med. Rehabil. 89 (5), 856–864.

20. Gorgey, A.S., Dudley, G.A., 2008. The role of pulse duration and stimulation duration in maximizing the normalized torque during neuromuscular electrical stimulation. J. Orthop. Sports Phys. Ther. 38 (8), 508–516.

21. Bochkezanian, V., Newton, R.U., et al., 2018. Effects of neuromuscular electrical stimulation in people with spinal cord injury. Med. Sci. Sports Exerc. 50 (9), 1733–1739.

22. Bekhet, A.H., Bochkezanian, V., et al., 2019. The effects of electrical stimulation parameters in managing spasticity after spinal cord injury: a systematic review. Am. J. Phys. Med. Rehabil. 98 (6), 484–499.

23. Smit, C.A., Legemate, K.J., et al., 2013. Prolonged electrical stimulation-induced gluteal and hamstring muscle activation and sitting pressure in spinal cord injury: effect of duty cycle. J. Rehabil. Res. Dev. 50 (7), 1035–1046.

24. Neyroud, D., Temesi, J., et al., 2015. Comparison of electrical nerve stimulation, electrical muscle stimulation and magnetic nerve stimulation to assess the neuromuscular function of the plantar flexor muscles. Eur. J. Appl. Physiol. 115 (7), 1429–1439.

25. Aravind, N., Harvey, L.A., et al., 2019. Physiotherapy interventions for increasing muscle strength in people with spinal cord injuries: a systematic review. Spinal Cord 57 (6), 449–460.

26. Popovic, M.R., Kapadia, N., et al., 2011. Functional electrical stimulation therapy of voluntary grasping versus only conventional rehabilitation for patients with

subacute incomplete tetraplegia: a randomized clinical trial. Neurorehabil. Neural Repair 25 (5), 433–442.

27. Beekhuizen, K.S., Field-Fote, E.C., 2008. Sensory stimulation augments the effects of massed practice training in persons with tetraplegia. Arch. Phys. Med. Rehabil. 89 (4), 602–608.

28. Bersch, I., Tesini, S., et al., 2015. Functional electrical stimulation in spinal cord injury: clinical evidence versus daily practice. Artif. Organs 39 (10), 849–854.

29. Bauman, W.A., Spungen, A.M., 2008. Coronary heart disease in individuals with spinal cord injury: assessment of risk factors. Spinal Cord 46 (7), 466–476.

30. Garshick, E., Kelley, A., et al., 2005. A prospective assessment of mortality in chronic spinal cord injury. Spinal Cord 43 (7), 408–416.

31. Griffin, L., Decker, M.J., et al., 2009. Functional electrical stimulation cycling improves body composition, metabolic and neural factors in persons with spinal cord injury. J. Electromyogr. Kinesiol. 19 (4), 614–622.

32. Gregory, C.M., Bickel, C.S., 2005. Recruitment patterns in human skeletal muscle during electrical stimulation. Phys. Ther. 85 (4), 358–364.

33. Carty, A., McCormack, K., et al., 2012. Increased aerobic fitness after neuromuscular electrical stimulation training in adults with spinal cord injury. Arch. Phys. Med. Rehabil. 93 (5), 790–795.

34. Bakkum, A.J., de Groot, S., et al., 2015. Effects of hybrid cycling versus handcycling on wheelchair-specific fitness and physical activity in people with long-term spinal cord injury: a 16-week randomized controlled trial. Spinal Cord 53 (5), 395–401.

35. Hamzaid, N.A., Davis, G., 2009. Health and fitness benefits of functional electrical stimulation-evoked leg exercise for spinal cord–injured individuals. Top. Spinal Cord Inj. Rehabil. 14 (4), 88–121.

36. Peng, C.W., Chen, S.C., et al., 2011. Review: clinical benefits of functional electrical stimulation cycling exercise for subjects with central neurological impairments. J. Med. Biol. Eng. 31 (1), 1–11.

37. Crosbie, J., Tanhoffer, A.I.P., et al., 2014. FES assisted standing in people with incomplete spinal cord injury: a single case design series. Spinal Cord 52 (3), 251–254.

38. Gorgey, A.S., Mather, K.J., et al., 2012. Effects of resistance training on adiposity and metabolism after spinal cord injury. Med. Sci. Sports Exerc. 44 (1), 165–174.

39. Davis, G.M. FES exercise for health, fitness and clinical benefits: the state of the art. Instructional Course: 57th International Spinal Cord Injury (ISCoS) Annual Scientific Meeting, Sydney, Australia, Sept 2018.

40. Castro, M.J., Apple, D.F., Jr., et al., 1999. Influence of complete spinal cord injury on skeletal muscle within 6 mo of injury. J. Appl. Physiol. 86 (1), 350–358.

41. Martin, T.P., Stein, R.B., et al., 1992. Influence of electrical stimulation on the morphological and metabolic properties of paralyzed muscle. J. Appl. Physiol. 72 (4), 1401–1406.

42. Noreau, L., Shephard, R., 1995. Spinal cord injury, exercise and quality of life. Sports Med. 20 (4), 226–250.

43. Harkema, S., Gerasimenko, Y., et al., 2011. Effect of epidural stimulation of the lumbosacral spinal cord on voluntary movement, standing, and assisted stepping after motor complete paraplegia: a case study. Lancet 377 (9781), 1938–1947.

44. Zhang, D., He, X., 2014. A meta-analysis of the motion function through the therapy of spinal cord injury with intravenous transplantation of bone marrow mesenchymal stem cells in rats. PLoS ONE 9 (4), e93487.

45. Kraemer, W.J., Adams, K., et al., 2002. American College of Sports Medicine position stand. Progression models in resistance training for healthy adults. Med. Sci. Sports Exerc. 34 (2), 364–380.

46. Ploutz, L.L., Tesch, P.A., et al., 1994. Effect of resistance training on muscle use during exercise. J. Appl. Physiol. 76 (4), 1675–1681.

47. Shields, R.K., Dudley-Javorski, S., 2006. Musculoskeletal plasticity after acute spinal cord injury: effects of long-term neuromuscular electrical stimulation training. J. Neurophysiol. 95 (4), 2380–2390.

48. Gorgey, A.S., Porach, H.J., et al., 2014. Effect of adjusting pulse durations of functional electrical stimulation cycling on energy expenditure and fatigue after spinal cord injury. J. Rehabil. Res. Dev. 51 (9), 1455–1468.

49. Black, C.D., McCully, K.K., 2008. Force per active area and muscle injury during electrically stimulated contractions. Med. Sci. Sports Exerc. 40 (9), 1596–1604.

50. Ho, C.H., Triolo, R.J., et al., 2014. Functional electrical stimulation and spinal cord injury. Phys. Med. Rehabil. Clin. N. Am. 25 (3), 631.

CHAPTER 8

Modes of transport

Jacqueline Reznik, Joshua Simmons and Kate Walker

Independent mobility, in the form of either a manual wheelchair or a powered wheelchair or scooter, is pivotal to the successful rehabilitation and reintegration of an individual with a spinal cord injury (SCI) back into the community. This is further accentuated and complemented by the method of community access and in particular the ability to return to driving a car. An appropriate assessment of posture and seating forms the basis of any seating solution for a spinal cord injured individual. It is important for the treating therapist to identify and prescribe a solution that meets both the health and the functional needs of the patient. This chapter will explore both the importance of posture and seating and how that applies to the prescription of an appropriate wheelchair or power-assisted device (wheelchair or scooter) and how that may impact on the ability to return to driving a car.

1. WHEELCHAIRS AND POWER-ASSISTED MOBILITY DEVICES

Jacqueline Reznik and Joshua Simmons

INTRODUCTION

Although the introduction of a wheelchair may be seen by the therapist as progression within the rehabilitative status of the patient with an SCI, this might not be the case for the patient themselves, who may view this as a definitive sign that the ultimate goal of walking might never be possible.[1] It is therefore of great importance that the process be undertaken with this is mind and that it might need to be taken relatively slowly, allowing the newly injured patient to gradually accept their new self-image (see Chapter 20 for a personal view on this).

Wheelchair prescription does, however, form an integral part of the rehabilitation of the individual with an SCI.[2,3] Depending upon the setup of the spinal injuries unit (SIU), this process may be facilitated by the physiotherapist or the occupational therapist (OT). Ideally, it should be a multidisciplinary process, allowing the team (including the patient themselves) to decide whether a manual or power-assisted wheelchair or scooter is the mobility aid of choice.

Although it is possibly the most important piece of equipment provided to the patient with an SCI, no formula or 'gold standard' approach exists regarding its prescription. Many wheelchair users and funding organisations confirm that a wheelchair that does not fulfil the needs of the user in relation to potential activities, lifestyle goals and health situation will be discarded.[4,5]

Despite the lack of an agreed gold standard, there are many established processes used by clinicians that have been documented. One of these is guidelines for wheelchair prescription by EnableNSW and Lifetime Care and Support Authority (LTCSA), updated in 2017 (see Online resources).[2] In her more recent update, Lukersmith[2] suggests that although these guidelines inform and guide the therapist, they do not replace the need for clinical supervision or clinical judgement. Many online learning programs are available for wheelchair prescription (see Online resources), however, all have commonalities, which will be outlined here.

This section of the chapter will examine the biomechanics involved in the seating posture, the importance of customised seating systems for this patient group and the various accessories available to complement the manual wheelchair or power-assisted mobility device prescribed. (Pushing and manoeuvring the wheelchair are explained in Chapters 5 and 6)

INITIAL ASSESSMENT

The initial assessment must start with a patient interview, where all personal factors, including age, height, weight goals and preferences, must be taken into account. Since the requirements of the patient will undoubtedly change over time, the components of the wheelchair should be prescribed to accommodate the changes where possible. This is particularly important when prescribing the initial device for a newly injured patient. Even though the additional moving parts associated with an adjustable chair make it slightly heavier than a non-adjustable chair, the health benefits and functional outcomes are far more important than the overall weight of the chair in the earlier years. When a person with an SCI is looking to replace their wheelchair, they

Table 8.1 Seating considerations for SCI

Intrinsic factors	Extrinsic factors
• Neurological level of injury, sitting balance • Age and general health • Body weight • Level of physical function and independence • Pain • Musculoskeletal issues • Abnormal tone and spasticity • Muscle wasting • Skin integrity issues • Continence	• Pressure: vertical force due to gravity • Shear forces: horizontal forces acting between a body and its supporting surface • Personal care requirements • Lifestyle (work, study, recreation) • Financial issues and funding sources • Demographics • Care and maintenance of equipment

are in a better position to understand their postural and functional requirements and, as such, can make a more informed decision about what features and set-up they require.

In order to prescribe an appropriate device, a list of factors should be considered, such as those listed in Table 8.1.

Furthermore, it is very important to conduct a physical examination, both supine *and* sitting, to ensure an accurate understanding of posture, range of motion (ROM), strength, sensation etc. An example of a tool to assist in this type of examination is a MAT evaluation (see Appendix 5), which highlights the need to conduct the assessment using the following process:

Step 1   In current chair
Step 2   Supine on firm surface
Step 3   Sitting unsupported
Step 4   Decision-making/solutions

It is important to observe static and dynamic situations during this assessment, e.g. both sitting and during wheelchair propulsion.

General principles of seating

Using the information obtained from these assessments, the general principles of seating, as outlined by the Queensland Spinal Outreach Team,[6] should be followed:

- Maximise surface area contact
- Maintain or improve postural alignment
- Provide a stable base of support
- Decrease abnormal tone influences
- Promote increased sitting tolerance
- Enhance cosmesis (aesthetically pleasing).

For more detailed information please see Online resources.

These principles will allow the achievement of a background neutral sitting position that allows the patient to not only maintain position or posture (postural stability), but also be able to change it (posture control, movement, balance) for the purposes of function, comfort and pressure relief.

Identifying the correct model for the patient

There are numerous types, makes and models of chairs currently available and it is important when assessing the patient for the most appropriate wheelchair that all available models, irrespective of manufacturer, are considered. For this reason, as mentioned previously, it is important to discuss the purpose of the chair with the patient and ensure that there are clear goals about what the chair or scooter will allow the individual to do. This includes confirming:

- Will this be your primary means of mobility at home, in the community and elsewhere?
- Will you be returning to driving? (This has implications on the types of frame, folding vs rigid, that need to be trialled.)
- What is your home environment like?
- What is your local environment like?
- What is your work environment like?
- What type of transfers do you think you are likely to need/want to do?

Using all this information, it is now possible to identify the type of chairs and set-ups that might be suitable (Fig. 8.1).

Wheelchair specifications

The key measurements to consider when prescribing both manual and powerchair wheelchairs include seat width, seat depth, backrest type (including height and angle), seat to footplate distance, rear seat to floor height, front seat to floor height, and seat angle (Fig. 8.2). (See Appendix 6 for an example of a detailed format to record wheelchair specifications.)

Once a suitable wheelchair has been prescribed and delivered to the patient, it must then be customised to fit that individual. The customisation of seat height includes the correct elbow flexion when the hand is on the highest position of the wheel rim (100–120°) (see Chapter 5 for further details), the wheelchair and arm rests must be designed to fit under a regular table, the position of the footplates must allow the hip and knee to be at an angle of approximately 90°, the height of the footplates should allow clearance of kerbs and the seat height (with cushion) should allow the patient to get his/her feet to the ground during transfers. The position of the seat angle (rake) should allow the patient to sit comfortably and prevent 'jack-knifing' and falling forwards out of the chair when travelling over uneven surfaces.

For propulsive efficiency and preservation of upper limb function there is an optimum position for the client in relation to the rear wheel (Chapter 5 contains more biomechanical detail regarding wheelchair propulsion). If the patient is seated too high above the rear wheel, the length of push stroke is reduced, which requires an increased frequency of pushing, and increased risk of wear in the upper limb joints. If the patient sits too low, there is excessive shoulder abduction, internal rotation and elevation to move through the push phase, and this repetitive movement also increases the risk of shoulder pain (see Chapters 15 and 21 for long-term effects of self-propulsion).

Individuals with SCIs who are long-term wheelchair users advocate the use of aftermarket

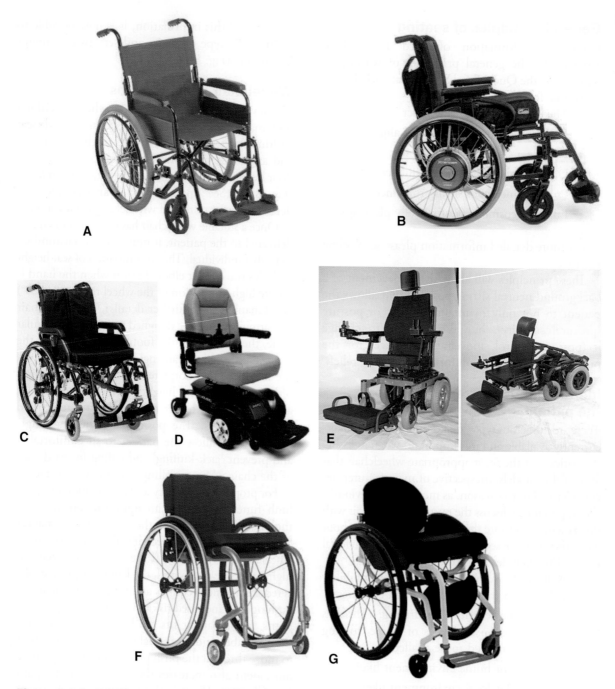

Figure 8.1 **A–G Different manual wheelchair, powerdrive wheelchair and scooter options**
A. Classic manual wheelchair B. Power assist C. Light-weight collapsible D. Power drive E. Power drive collapsible
F. Sports G. Sports with moulded back and wheel guards
Sources: B. © Living Spinal C. © Strive Mobility 2020

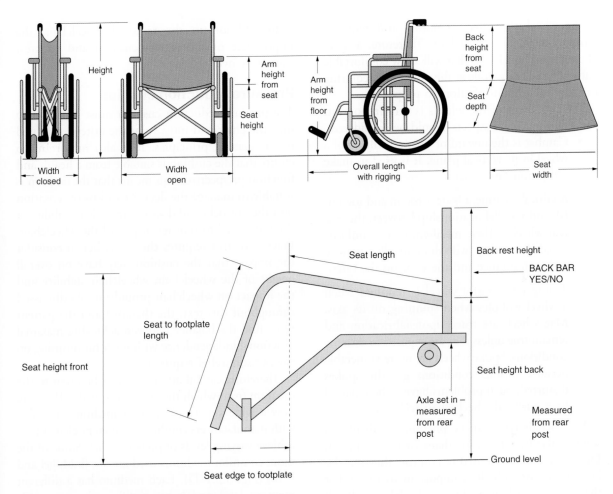

Figure 8.2 Wheelchair specifications

power-assisted devices that can be attached to the chairs in order to prevent persistent overuse injuries of the shoulders. Examples of these devices range from power assist wheels (e.g. Alber, Yamaha), to add-on power assist drives (e.g. Smart Drive, Quickie Xtender), and trike conversion kits (e.g. Firefly, Batec).

When teaching the patient to perform 'wheelies' (see Chapter 6), anti-tippers are recommended; however, they should be removable or at least retractable, as when left in place they make ascent or descent of the kerb impossible.

Other accessories which may add to the usefulness of the wheelchair include a tray-table, push handles, arm rests, clothing protectors or specialised wheel rims.

Wheelchair wheels come in various standardised wheelchair sizes:

- a standard manual adult wheelchair drive wheel size is 24 inches (approx. 61 cm)

- a standard power wheelchair drive wheel size is 18 inches (approx. 46 cm)

- caster wheels start from 3 inches (approx. 8 cm).

The wheel size affects comfort and required effort to move the wheelchair. Therefore, a drive wheel should be selected that will allow comfortable seating in the chair while at the same time requiring a minimum amount of effort to propel it.

The alignment of the wheels is very important. The following three aspects should be considered:

- Camber is the inward or outward tilting of a wheel in its vertical plane. It is used to make self-propulsion easier.

- A critical alignment issue is toe-in and toe-out (the off-parallel relationship between the two rear wheels). These misalignments should be avoided, as they will dramatically increase rolling resistance and the wear on the tyres.

- Truing (aligning) a wheel is required when a wheel wobbles when spinning on its axis. Mag wheels are trued upon fabrication and remain true unless they are exposed to extreme conditions. Spoke wheels are more vulnerable because various conditions get the spokes distorted. Such problems have to be repaired by a qualified wheel-repair technician.

Wheelchair tyres can be pneumatic (air-filled), solid or flat free (foam, urethane or rubber filled). Depending on the desired terrain use, they may be knobbly or smooth. It is important to remember that tyres affect how easily the wheelchair will roll over specific surfaces. The harder the tyre, the easier it will be to propel the wheelchair. The softer the tyre, the harder it will be to propel it.

- Pneumatic tyres will go flat if punctured and will go soft even without any damage but provide soft rides.

- Solid tyres are almost maintenance free and they are unlikely to wear out in the life of the wheelchair, but will be less comfortable on rough terrain.

- Flat free tyres are pneumatic tyres that are filled with a semi-solid material. They are not subject to flat tyres and give a softer ride than a solid tyre.

In addition to the required wheelchair, the importance of the correct cushion and backrest cannot be overlooked.

Pressure reduction cushions

The pressure reduction cushion must fit correctly into the chair and must fulfil the criteria outlined in the general principles. It is also important to ensure that the cushion is suitable from a health and function perspective. This means that the cushion is suitable to manage the decrease or loss of sensation over the buttocks and does not impede the ability of the individual to transfer or propel the wheelchair. Practically, this requires the prescriber to consider the impact that the cushion may have on overall height of the wheelchair, wheelchair stability and the impact on wheelchair propulsion. As discussed throughout this text, the therapist and the patient must find the balance between achieving maximal functional independence without compromising on the pressure relief required.

Therefore, careful attention must be given to the medium from which the cushion is made. There are now a wide variety of cushion mediums available with manufacturers combining different elements to achieve varying levels of pressure relief. Some of the more common mediums used are air, fluid, gel and foam (Fig. 8.3A–D). Each medium has a different memory level and behaves differently to provide pressure redistribution and reduce shearing or friction. (Memory refers to the ability of the medium to return to its original shape once the load is removed. If memory returns quickly, it is likely to lead to higher pressures being generated.) Pressure relief is related to the level of flotation achieved, which is associated with the the degree of immersion of bony prominences in the medium to spread the weight. Shearing is often managed by ensuring that the cushion medium moves with the body and some manufacturers use low friction covers to assist with this principle.

When prescribing a pressure reduction cushion, it is important to ensure that the width of the cushion is based on the patient and not the wheelchair. The way to do this is to measure from greater

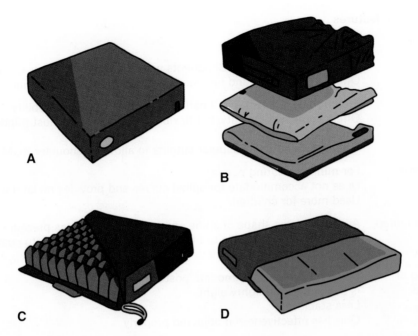

Figure 8.3 Different types of pressure reduction cushions A, Foam B, Fluid C, Air, D Honeycomb

trochanter to greater trochanter, either sitting in the wheelchair, or supine with hips and knees flexed at right angles. This will determine the weight-bearing surfaces of the cushion; however, overall width may also need to consider the soft tissue around the hips.

The depth of the cushion should be measured while the patient is sitting in the prescribed chair with the overall depth designed to maximise the seating surface and spread weight over as large an area as possible. A good rule of thumb is that there should be a gap of 2–3 fingerbreadths between the cushion and the back of the knee.

Lumbar pelvic supports (backrests)

Dynamic seating systems are the preferred choice for long-term wheelchair users, such as the person with an SCI.[7] These systems comprise backrests and seat cushions. As with wheelchairs and cushions, there is also a wide variety of backrests on the market. When prescribing a backrest, it is important to always remember to stabilise the pelvis first before attempting to correct trunk deformity. The key points to consider are, therefore, the overall impact on posture, how the backrest conforms to the patient, how it is fitted to the wheelchair (including the ability to remove it, if lifting it into the car), how heavy it is and the overall effect on function (i.e. balance, propulsion and reach to wheels, transfers, ability to reach the floor) (Table 8.2).

Since back pain is a common complication among wheelchairs users, and particularly problematic in long-term wheelchair users, the importance of suitable supports cannot be overlooked.[6] Wheelchair lateral trunk supports are rectangular- or square-shaped devices which are mounted on the back posts of the wheelchair. They are used to increase stability and balance for the user. Usually they are used in pairs, one on each side of the trunk. Positioning will depend upon the user's problem and in cases of spinal curvature uneven oblique placement may be required. (See Chapter 21 for a personalised

Table 8.2 Backrest features

Backrest feature	Functional implication
Low back	Preferred by low level SCI patients with good strength, active users Offers less stability and less support for thoracic spine, but increased mobility
High back	Preferred by high level SCI patients who use powered mobility Offers increased stability, but flexibility and mobility is lost (hinders use of arms for mobility) Often provided with scapular cutouts to allow for shoulder ROM
Flat/linear/planar back	For minimal seating needs Does not accommodate for spinal curves and provides no lateral stability Used more for children
Generically contoured back	Accommodates shape of spine and back and increases pressure distribution Effectiveness is sensitive to fit to patient (use accessories to customise) Deeper contour provides better lateral support and stability
Soft contouring or upholstery back	Can be used to accommodate postures Is adjustable and lightweight Less stable Only has effectiveness if adjusted properly
Custom-contoured	Labour intensive, takes time and is expensive Tailored to the patient at the time of assessment and construction

view of this complication.) Of the four sitting postures depicted in Fig. 8.4, Li and colleagues[7] demonstrated that the slouched position adopted by many wheelchair users exacerbates metabolite accumulations in intervertebral discs, leading to increased risks of degeneration and pain. They found that the backward thoracic support was the most effective in reducing pain due to the redistribution of interface pressure.

MOBILITY SCOOTERS

A recent survey by Edwards and McCluskey[5] noted that two-thirds of scooter users made their decision without consulting a health professional. The authors of this chapter recommend that the therapist involved with this patient group discuss ALL forms of mobility issues with their clients in order to avoid the possibility of unsuitable modes of transport being sourced. It should, however, be

noted that due to the need for sound postural support and suitable pressure care, parameters which cannot be met by the seating system of a scooter, mobility scooters are not usually recommended for people with SCIs. For many patients with high-level lesions, or some older persons with SCIs, powered wheelchairs with customised seating systems will be the preferred mobility device. However, in some circumstances, such as incomplete SCI lesions with full or partial sensation, a scooter might be appropriate to meet the mobility goals of the individual.

Most of these devices are powered by rechargeable batteries and allow the user to move more freely and independently within the community. A number of both qualitative and quantitative studies have shown that the physical and psychological benefits of these powered devices enable their users greater participation in a wide variety of activities.[7]

Prior to prescription, it is recommended that the therapist trial the scooter with the patient. Factors to

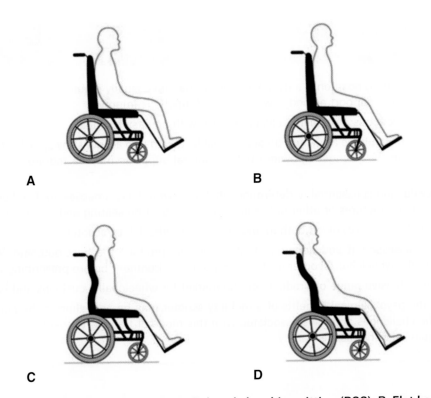

Figure 8.4 **Four different sitting postures. A, Relaxed slouching sitting (RSS). B, Flat back support sitting (FBS). C, Prominent lumbar support sitting (PLS). D, Backward thoracic support sitting (BTS).**
Source: Li, C.-T., Chen, C.-H., et al., 2015. Biomechanical evaluation of a novel wheelchair backrest for elderly people. Biomedical Engineering Online 14 (1), 14.

consider include transport use, seating system, scooter portability, available adjustability, the environment in which the scooter will be used, weight and any limitations in the distances that can be travelled. It is also worth considering the challenges and difficulties associated with learning to drive and manoeuvre the vehicle. It has been suggested that new users of these devices be assessed in a similar way to new car drivers. (Part 2 of this chapter contains a fuller explanation of the driving assessments.) Safety when driving mobility scooters is of great concern not only to the users and their families, but also to the health professionals who prescribe them, members of the public and local councils.

Evidence-based practice points

- When assessing the patient for a wheelchair, whether powered or manual, it is important to involve patient, family and carer(s) in the decision-making process.

Continued

Evidence-based practice points—cont'd

- Adjustment of sitting position is a dynamic process; patients usually require more support in the beginning and less support as body awareness and functions improve.
- Wheelchair selection is a problem-solving exercise with no easy formula.
- Sitting position should be as symmetrical as possible, taking into account any spinal surgery that has occurred. In the younger (growing) patient, lateral supports may be required (see Online resources).
- Physical evaluation is essential to determine whether postural asymmetries are fixed or flexible, the extent of contractures or other deformities which impact on seating and skin condition.
- Each client should be reviewed both in and out of their wheelchair/scooter.
- A thorough assessment and adequate trial period will produce the best outcome. Wherever possible, trial a wheelchair/scooter in the appropriate environment before prescribing one.
- There is an extensive range of products on the market for wheelchairs, cushions and backrests.
- Although the psychological benefits of a mobility scooter may be appealing to the person with an SCI, the challenges and risks associated with this mode of transport must be made clear to the potential user and his/her family.

SUMMARY

An extremely thought-provoking case study by Bates and colleagues[8] describes to therapists that the process of adaptation to wheelchair use may require time on the part of the newly injured patient. What would appear, to the treating therapist, to be a progressive step towards independence may be seen by the patient as an acknowledgement that walking will never be an option. As such, the biomechanical issues of prescribing a wheelchair must be carefully approached.

Although no 'gold standard' for wheelchair prescription exists, there are many useful guidelines that the treating therapist should follow. Wheelchair prescription is an integral part of the rehabilitation process and should remain flexible since the user's needs will change over time.

Dr Rhonda Galbally AO[9]

Wheelchairs and mobility scooters not only remove physical and environmental barriers but can assist with the user's activity and participation in many aspects of life. The appropriate wheelchair, for the person and their environments, can enhance not only their quality of life, but also the lives of families, friends and attendant care worker and carers. In contrast, poor prescription of a wheelchair or mobility scooter can mean the person is more dependent, has fewer opportunities and often will be excluded from participation in their community.

2. RETURN TO DRIVING

Kate Walker

INTRODUCTION

While the provision of equipment to facilitate independent mobility is a step in the SCI rehabilitation process, it is the ability to access the community that has the biggest potential to promote a new level of independence. This section will provide an overview into the best practice procedure for return to, or indeed to begin, driving for people who have had a SCI.

Driving a car is a well-established and important activity,[10] allowing people the freedom to move from place to place and is closely linked to the perceptions of mobility, independence and a sense of wellbeing.[11] Not only is driving an important occupation of itself, it is also the means by which those with SCI can travel to other essential locations and/or their workplaces.[12] People with SCI have long identified mobility issues as being among the most significant factors in their long-term rehabilitation.[13] In their recent study, Lee and colleagues[14] reported that a return to driving independence is an important goal for many individuals following SCI. For persons with SCI the initial driving goal is to be able to travel with family members in the family car as a passenger. Many continue with a further goal of returning to self-driving their own vehicle.[15]

In the majority of developed countries, anyone with a long-term disability that may affect their ability to drive may be required to seek clearance from a licensing jurisdiction to learn or to continue to drive. In these cases, a thorough assessment of the person's off-road and on-road driving skills is required in order to ensure their 'fitness to drive'.[16] Internationally, occupational therapists (OTs), because of their unique skills in the analysis of task performance and the retraining of activities of daily living, are most often the health professionals trained to undertake these assessments.[17,18]

> Driving is my independence. I can get to places under my own steam and don't have to wait for a carer. I've got some of my time back.
>
> SCI Client (age 45)
>
> When I am driving my car, nobody knows I can't walk or there is something wrong with me. I am normal. It is also why I don't want to stow my wheelchair on the roof where people can see it – I would rather throw it in to the backseat. So, nobody knows – just for a little while.
>
> SCI Client (age 23)

While there are variations from country to country and even state to state regarding the process, there are many universal commonalities worth noting. A driver-trained occupational therapist (DTOT) is the leading expert in this field and could use the following format of frequently asked questions and challenges most often faced by clients with SCIs who have a goal of returning to driving.

These questions include:

1. How will I know if and when I am ready to return to driving?
2. What are my alternatives to driving?
3. How do I return to driving?
4. What vehicle modifications are most suitable?
5. What other factors do I need to consider in my return to driving?

HOW WILL I KNOW IF AND WHEN I AM READY TO RETURN TO DRIVING?

You don't need to be Superman to drive a car.

Initially a 'fitness to drive' assessment involves an evaluation by a medical practitioner who ensures that the person meets the appropriate medical standards for driving.[17] For most jurisdictions, clearance from a general practitioner (GP) or rehabilitation specialist is required prior to commencing the return to driving process and the DTOT will also require a doctor's referral to see a new client seeking to return to driving.

The factors outlined in Table 8.3 should be considered by all personnel involved in this decision.

Table 8.3 Factors for consideration of return to driving

Question	Details to consider
Is their condition now stable?	Have medical interventions/surgeries mostly ceased and has the client now plateaued within their rehabilitation and achieved the majority of their functional gains?
What medications are they taking?	Do any of their current medications interfere with their cognitive abilities to a point where safe driving could be compromised?
What is their vision like?	Most jurisdictions have minimum standards for vision for drivers. Visual acuity is the most important and there is a non-negotiable standard for all drivers. In New South Wales (NSW) it is 6/12 on a Snellen chart.[a] Other factors to be considered include complete or near-complete visual fields, as this may impact on peripheral vision, eye movements and eye coordination. Binocular vision is required in order to follow objects, and the ability to change focus quickly from short range objects to long range is also required (e.g. when viewing the road ahead and coming back to check the speedometer).
What is the person's range of motion (ROM) in limbs and trunk?	A DTOT solely assesses functional range – not optimal range. Does the client have the ability to reach and grasp the steering wheel and reach the pedals?
What strength does the person have in their limbs and trunk?	Does the client have the strength to depress the pedals and the proprioception to do so without looking at their feet?
What other medical conditions does the person have?	Does the client have any other medical conditions, aside from their SCI, that could impact their driving – for example have they also had a brain injury which may impact their function for driving?
What is the person's cognitive ability?[b]	Does the client have the ability to process information, maintain attention, use their working memory, problem solve and make decisions quickly and while attending to multiple environmental stimuli?
What level of insight does the person have?[c]	Does the client have a good and consistent knowledge of their capabilities – physically and mentally – and understand how their condition impacts their ability to drive safely?

[a]A Snellen chart is an eye chart that can be used to measure visual acuity. Many ophthalmologists and vision scientists now use an improved chart known as the LogMAR (Log of Minimum Angle of Resolution) chart. Check the standards in your jurisdiction.

[b]Specific assessments tools are discussed later in this section.

[c]See p. 175 for a definition of insight.

How can I return to driving if I do not meet the requirements above and still want to return to driving?

Caveat: Good vision (particularly acuity), sound cognition and a high level of insight are the most important requirements for a return to driving when assessing the capabilities of any future client.

As noted previously, visual acuity is easy to define and measure – as are visual fields. Cognition and insight are, however, often less clear.

Cognition is best defined as a term referring to the mental processes involved in gaining knowledge and comprehension. These processes include thinking, knowing, remembering, judging and problem-solving. These are higher-level functions of the brain and encompass language, imagination, perception and planning.[19] Insight, however, is 'the understanding of a specific cause and effect within a specific context', in this case driving.[20]

Based on these definitions, the following assessments are used by health professionals to assess cognition generally:

- Montreal Cognitive Assessment (MoCA)[21]
- Loewenstein Occupational Therapy Cognitive Assessment (LOTCA)[22]
- Mini-Mental State Examination (MMSE)[23]
- Functional Independence Measure (FIM™)[24]

For driving specifically, however, there are a range of other measures which have proven more relevant and therefore more successful. These include the Occupational Therapy Driver Off-Road Assessment Battery (OT-DORA)[18] and the clinical assessment tool Drive Safe Drive Aware®, computer-based version.[25]

Drive Safe Drive Aware is particularly useful as it assesses both ability and insight. The first component is Drive Safe, which assesses global awareness of the driving environment rather than the visual processing and cognitive skills. Drive Safe is a standardised assessment and is completed on a computer. It has been tested for validity, reliability and predictive accuracy.[26]

Client statements showing insight and awareness such as 'When I am having a bad day I don't drive – I don't want to hurt myself or anyone else' are extremely positive – whereas a statement such as 'I will drive no matter what! If I have things to do I will do them and nobody can stop me – I am going to drive my car when I want' indicate poor insight and possibly a poor candidate for returning to drive.

The person environment occupation model of practice

A useful mode of practice (MOP) for occupational therapy practice and for the occupation of driving in particular, is the person environment occupation (PEO) model (see Fig. 8.5, overleaf).[27]

According to the PEO model, the 'occupational performance' is the task of returning to driving. The factors impacting on a person's returning to driving are represented by:

- person
- occupation
- environment.

These factors are expanded on in Table 8.4 (overleaf).

Personal factors: This represents the function and capabilities of the client and is mostly fixed by the time they come to the DTOT for driving assessment.

Issues with **vision** may arise with clients within the SCI population. This may be due to the fact that during their hospital stay other more obvious problems have been assessed and treated, but vision and/or visual deficits have not been dealt with. Visual acuity should be addressed prior to DTOT assessment by referral to one of the following professionals:

- optometrist for review and perhaps new prescription for glasses or contact lenses

- ophthalmic surgeon for more complex interventions such as cataract surgery

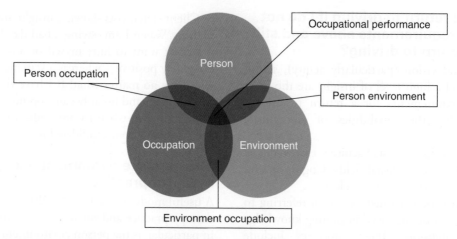

Figure 8.5 Person environment occupation (PEO) model.

Source: Law, M., Cooper, B., et al., 1996. The person-environment-occupation model: A transactive approach to occupational performance. Canadian Journal Of Occupational Therapy 63 (1), 9–23.

Table 8.4 Factors impacting return to driving (PEO model)

Person	Environment	Occupation
Diagnosis/prognosis Level and scale of SCI Cognition ROM Strength Impact of medications Visual abilities – particularly acuity, peripheral vision, eye function Insight into ability to drive safely	Physical – including the car and surrounds Social – supports available Socioeconomic – finances and funding sources available Cultural	Occupational goal – return to driving

- orthoptist – to address disorders of eye movement and assist with diagnoses of eye conditions
- neuro-ophthalmologist – to address visual problems that are related to the nervous system.

Environmental factors: The role of the DTOT is to problem-solve and apply creative solutions, using environmental factors, to enable the person to perform the task of driving despite deficits in the 'person' column. For a person with SCI who wishes to return to driving the environment to be modified is their vehicle.

If a client can wiggle one of their fingers I can get them driving – as long as they have good cognition, vision and insight into their abilities.

WHAT ARE MY ALTERNATIVES TO DRIVING?

As function is regained following SCI, transportation issues become more important. Aids and/or alternatives to walking such as walking sticks, walking frames, manual wheelchairs (MWC), powered wheelchairs (PWCs) and power drive wheelchairs (PDWCs) must be considered (see Part 1 of this chapter and Chapter 6). Similarly, when moving from one position to another, transfers boards, hoists and slings need to be considered. These transport and transfer options of actually accessing a vehicle need to be taken into account prior to the person attempting to return to driving in their private car, either as a passenger or a driver.

Requirements for driving for a person with SCI will depend upon:

- the person's pattern of occupations and their location. Do they travel far from home, and if so, with what frequency? Do they have children who are active in their own occupations, such as school and sport, and who need to be driven?

- their psychosocial situation. This includes factors such as number of people in their household and their ages. Does their spouse drive? Do they have other relatives living nearby who can assist with transport?

- whether they live in an urban or a rural location? Are there many transport options suitable, such as frequent bus services with wheelchair/disabled access? Do they live in a rural area with infrequent transport services such as taxis and accessible buses?

- if there is ongoing funding available to pay for community access such as taxivouchers?

- whether the person has an insurer who will pay for ongoing community transport options, such as wheelchair taxis.

Alternatives to driving
Travelling in a private car as a passenger

This means the vehicle will require access modifications only, which may be as simple as a doorhandle grab bar and transfer board or a full PWC drive-in and dock option. Vans are normally the preferred vehicle for people using PWCs due to the requirement for additional head clearance. PWC users can modify their family car to dock either in the front seat beside the driver or the second or third row. PWC placement depends on personal preference and any requirements to transport other passengers in the vehicle (Fig. 8.6A and B).

MWC users most often transfer into the existing seating of the vehicle and stow their wheelchair on the roof, in the boot space or on the back of the car while they are being driven.

Travelling in wheelchair-accessible public transport

Most states and territories in Australia provide public transport, such as buses, trains and trams, with access for people using both MWCs and PWCs. Some buses are able to lower on their suspension so the person in a wheelchair can access from the footpath on an even surface, with no steps, onto the bus or a retractable ramp may be engaged (Fig. 8.7A). There are wheelchair-safe parking areas at the front of the buses and trains (Fig. 8.7B) for the person to safely park and secure their wheelchair for the journey. Additionally, most train stations have lift access between platforms and available staff to supply accessible ramps; some trams are accessible low-floor trams (Fig. 8.7C), while many tram stops have been raised to allow level access to high-floor trams.

HOW DO I RETURN TO DRIVING FOLLOWING AN SCI?

The steps required to complete successful driving rehabilitation following SCI vary depending upon the individual and where they live, although, as stated earlier, there are many commonalities for all.

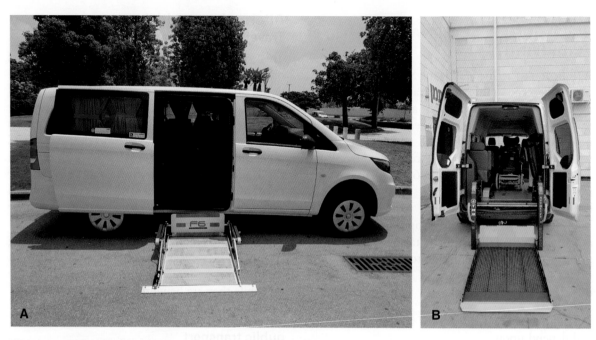

Figure 8.6 Modifications to accommodate PDWC access and travel. A Side entry. B Rear entry.
Source © TMN Driving Systems Industry Ltd

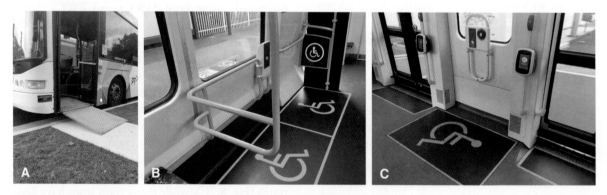

Figure 8.7 Travelling on public transport. A, Bus. B, Train. C, Tram.
Sources: A, courtesy David Reznik B, C, courtesy Marc Wion

These include:

1. **Referral to DTOT** (see prerequisites below).
2. **Full off-road assessment by DTOT** – including cognition, physical function, neurological function and vision.

3. Where it is possible an **on-road assessment in a dual control vehicle** with a range of modifications (mods) in place for the client to trial should also be conducted. If this is not possible due to inability to access a regular car, the DTOT will arrange for the client to have access to a more modified

vehicle (generally a van) that will accommodate their access and driving needs so they can experience driving and start trialling mods.

4. After a series of **trials of mods** the client and DTOT will select those which are most suitable for their driving style and goals.

5. The **DTOT finalises their report** and sends it to the licensing body – listing modifications and licence conditions required for the person to drive safely.

6. **Lessons with a qualified rehabilitation driving instructor (RDI)** will be arranged. The goal of these lessons is for the client to develop their competence and confidence driving with the mods in place. Generally, this will occur in the RDI's vehicle to remove the need for the client to go to the expense of providing modifications to their own car before they are sure the modifications are suitable and they have obtained their licence.

7. **Pass a Disability Driving Test** with the licensing body for their state. For example, in New South Wales it is carried out by the Roads and Maritime Service (RMS). It is similar to a regular licensing test; however, the person is demonstrating that they can drive safely with the mods in place. When they are successful their licence will be endorsed with the conditions relevant for that modification and they can then only drive a vehicle with those modifications in place.

Process for referral to DTOT

As stated earlier, prior to a driving assessment by a DTOT, it is necessary to have:

- a referral from treating doctor (GP or specialist) and
- confirmation from the licensing body that the person has a current licence or if they have never had a licence or had their licence revoked, a provisional licence must be obtained.

It is important to check that a client has a current licence prior to commencing their return to the driving process. The treating rehabilitation physician or GP of the person with a SCI is legally obliged to report their change in medical status, often resulting in licence cancellation or suspension until an assessment is completed. The person may not realise this as they have not been home and received their mail, and may be under the impression that they still possess a current licence.

WHAT VEHICLE IS BEST FOR MODIFICATIONS?

Vehicle choice depends upon whether the person uses a MWC or PDWC and the overall cost of the vehicle compared to the cost of the modification.

- **For a person using a PWC** and with limited ability to transfer independently from their PWC to the driver's seat of the car, they will need to modify a van, rather than a traditional car. This will enable them to drive or winch their PWC into the van and drive from the PWC after docking and securing themselves and the PWC. Some PWC users are able to transfer into the driver's seat of the car and there are modifications to assist with this; however, the PWC still needs to be stowed safely while the person is driving. This requires more space in the vehicle, particularly for head clearance and wider doors.

- **A person using an MWC**, who is able to transfer independently, has a broader range of vehicle options and can drive a regular sedan, hatchback, SUV or station wagon. As all cars have different ergonomics, it is recommended that the driver trial accessing and exiting the vehicle prior to purchase. They will also need to consider how best to stow their wheelchair while they are driving. This is often a very personal choice for the person. Psychologically, many persons with SCIs do not want anyone to see the wheelchair from outside of the car and so choose to transfer to the driver's seat and stow the wheelchair by folding it up and placing it over their shoulder into the back seat. Others prefer to transfer into the driver's seat and have the wheelchair hoisted up to the roof for stowage while driving and others prefer to stow the wheelchair on the back of the car and transfer by walking the short distance to the driver's seat. Clearly choice also depends on physical function of the driver and the weight and type of frame of the wheelchair.

It is not a sound financial decision to install very expensive modifications on a vehicle that is old, has high kilometres on the odometer and is cheap and probably unreliable mechanically. For people with SCI who are covered by insurance there will be guidelines around the value of vehicles and the value of modifications the insurer will fund. It is important to review these prior to commencing the process to return to driving. It is the job of the DTOT to not only prescribe modifications to enable the person with an SCI to return to driving, but also to justify these recommendations, both clinically and financially.

USEFUL EXISTING FEATURES OF UNMODIFIED PRODUCTION CARS

New release cars and motor vehicles are now being sold with many improved options, even on the manufacturer's base models. These features are designed to add to the comfort of drivers and the safety of the vehicle; however, they have the added benefit of assisting people with SCIs, and many other functional challenges, to be able to drive safely and comfortably. These features include:

1. **reverse cameras** – these assist drivers with poor neck and thoracic rotation to safely reverse. They also help people to park closer to their destination as they are more likely to attempt a more difficult parking manoeuvre – such as a reverse park – if they are confident they will be able to do

so safely. From an extremely important safety perspective, these cameras can assist drivers to see children crossing behind the car.

2. **sensor cameras** – used both for parking purposes where the sensors are all around the car and to alert the driver when they are moving out of the lane as they are driving. Sensor cameras assist with safe driving when the driver's range of motion (ROM) is compromised.

3. **lane departure warnings and lane departure assist** – an extension of sensor cameras, which indicate via an alert (can be vibration of steering wheel or audible alarm) if the driver moves out of their lane without using the turn signal.

4. **forward collision warning (FCW) system and automatic braking systems** monitor the car's speed and also the speed of the car in front and the distance between. If the distance lessens, the car sounds an alert to prompt braking. In more advanced systems, the car will also hit the brakes to avoid a collision and can also detect pedestrian hazards.

   Although a useful modality, FCW should be seen as an add-on rather than a prescribed necessity. All drivers must be deemed capable of determining car speed and distance between vehicles, and have the ability to brake independently.

5. **power steering** – vehicles have different levels of power steering and almost all new vehicles have some form of power steering. Steering with a lighter feel is useful for drivers with compromised upper limb strength. Cars can also be modified to have ultralight steering, which is used when drivers require extra assistance with managing steering. When assessing a driver and prescribing this modification, the driver is in the driver's seat and the car is raised on a hoist in order for the

steering to be lightened and to confirm whether the driver can operate the steering wheel.

6. **power brakes** – these can assist the driver with braking if their reaction time is otherwise intact.

7. **air conditioning and climate control** – important in prescribing vehicles for people following an SCI in particular. Climate control is air conditioning where the driver sets the car to a particular temperature, rather than uses a dial to adjust fan force and cooling separately. Some cars also have 'zoned' temperature control, so the driver and passengers can set their own temperature in their 'zone' in the car to their preference.

8. **Bluetooth technology** – in cars allows for voice control of phone function and the vehicle's sound system. This is also an essential safety feature for drivers with SCI as they can call for assistance if required.

9. **keyless entry** – allows the driver to unlock the car remotely without having to insert and turn a key in the door. More advanced versions allow the driver to start the car with the key in the vicinity (such as in a pocket) by pushing a button, or when the person approaches with the key in their pocket or bag.

10. **handbrake switches** – replace handbrake levers and are easier to operate; they are located on the dashboard or the console rather than down the side of the seat or under the dashboard.

11. **automatic wipers** – mean the driver does not have to operate the wiper lever in the car.

12. **cruise control** – very helpful for maintaining speed and avoiding driver fatigue – particularly on longer journeys. Some car manufacturers are also making cars with adaptive cruise control – via radar

signals – which also allows the driver to maintain distance from the car in front, even when they are not using cruise control and are therefore varying their speed.

WHAT VEHICLE MODIFICATIONS ARE AVAILABLE AND WHAT ARE MOST SUITABLE?

As discussed earlier, it is possible for the majority of people with SCI to return to driving, with appropriate vehicle modifications, if their cognition, reaction speed and vision are intact. Deficits in physical function, including ROM, motor control and strength, need to be 'replaced' by modifying their vehicle. There are six types of vehicle modifications needed for people following an SCI:

- accelerator and brake operation
- steering
- operating vehicle controls – indicators, lights, windscreen wipers
- balance
- access and locking in
- wheelchair storage.

The first four of these are required in order to *drive* the vehicle and are known as driving modifications. The last two are known as access modifications and are required to access the vehicle, and are thus also appropriate for a person with an SCI who is travelling as a passenger.

Below is a list and explanation of these types of possible modifications and suggestions for their use.

Accelerator and brake options
Mechanical hand controls

These are a very popular and reliable modification for the brake/accelerator that are installed mechanically (rather than electronically) into the vehicle. They can be installed on either side of the steering wheel and can be push/pull (Fig. 8.8), which means the

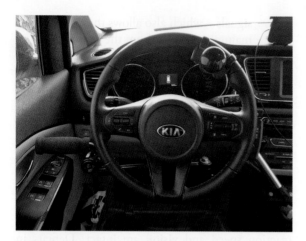

Figure 8.8 Spinner knob and mechanical hand controls (push/pull accelerator/brake and accelerator ring)

Source: Courtesy Arik Vamosh

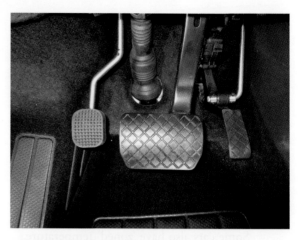

Figure 8.9 Pedal changes and mechanical accelerator-brake mechanism

Source: © TMN Driving Systems Industry Ltd

driver pulls the lever towards themselves to drive and pushes it away to brake, or 'radial' where the driver pushes for the brake and pushes downward for acceleration. These mods need to be used in conjunction with a spinner knob.

Who would use this modification?

Someone with a lower level SCI who has poor or nil motor control of their lower limbs, but has good strength, ROM and fine motor skills in their upper limbs.

Accelerator ring

This is a more recent option for brake/accelerator function, which allows both hands to remain on the steering wheel and facilitates a driving position that allows for easy access to vehicle controls, such as indicators, headlights, gearstick and horn, while maintaining control of the steering wheel and accelerator. This option does not require an additional spinner knob accessory control.

Acceleration is achieved by simply applying pressure at any point of the ring. The accelerator ring can be installed either under or over the steering

wheel. The brakes operate by pushing the handle to the right of the steering wheel.

This conversion is one of the most aesthetically pleasing with the accelerator ring blending in with the vehicle's interior.

Who would use this modification?

Someone with a lower level SCI who has poor or nil motor control of their lower limbs but has good strength, ROM and fine motor skills in their upper limbs.

The left foot accelerator

This is a relatively inexpensive, practical mechanical mod, which enables the driver to accelerate and brake using the left foot only. Fig. 8.9 shows the brake and both accelerators lowered into the operational position; however, when in use, one of the accelerators would be folded well out of the way.

Who would use this modification?

Someone with a lower level, incomplete SCI where the right foot has poor function and motor control, but the left foot has good function.

Steering options

Joystick controls – two-way and four-way

Two-way joysticks are for steering only, the joystick moving to the right and left only. The four-way joystick is for braking/accelerating, as well as steering. This complex modification is also called as 'space drive' and takes many hours of practice with an OT to learn how to use it, prior to licensing. When learning these controls the OT or RBI sits in the front passenger seat and is also able to control all aspects of the vehicle so the driver can practise safely and to ensure they are competent enough to pass their licensing test.

Who would use this modification?

Someone with a high-level SCI with poor control of their limbs, but good fine motor control in their hands. The Joysteer electric driving system has two safety circuits, an active navigation system and an active control system for braking. The electronic steering wheel can be operated in various ways using gripping aids (Fig. 8.10).

Electronic spinner knob

This is attached to the steering wheel at either 10 o'clock or 3 o'clock, depending on handedness, function and/or personal preference. It is easy to remove from the steering wheel for other drivers to use the car and is installed electronically using Bluetooth technology. An electronic spinner knob has

the vehicle controls programmed into the device, so the driver can operate the wipers, horn and blinkers from the device without having to take their hand off the device and therefore remain in control of the steering wheel. These devices are programmable, so individuals can have the buttons set out to suit their preference.

Who would use this modification?

A person with a low level of function in one of their upper limbs but good function in their other upper limb or a person with paraplegia with good bilateral upper limb function who uses hand controls for brake/accelerator and steers using this device with their other hand.

The tri-spinner

This steering device attaches to the steering wheel and is used in conjunction with a hand-operated brake/accelerator device. The three-pronged steering device assists drivers with poor grip strength to grasp and control the steering wheel (Fig. 8.11).

Who would use this modification?

A person with a high, yet incomplete, SCI who has poor fine motor skills but good gross motor skills in their upper limbs.

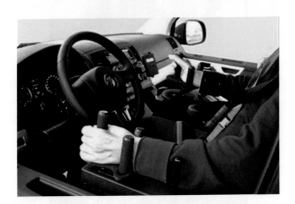

Figure 8.10 Joysteer electronic driving system
Source: © TMN Driving Systems Industry Ltd

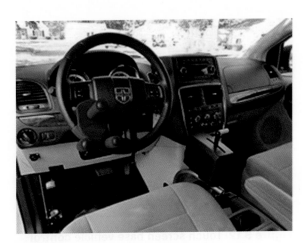

Figure 8.11 Tri-spinner knob
Source: © TMN Driving Systems Industry Ltd

Operating vehicle controls
Indicator extenders

These enable the driver to operate the indicators from the other side of the steering column.

Who would use this modification?

A person who does not have functional hand control on the side where the indicator was originally fitted (Fig. 8.12).

Headrest switches

These enable the driver to operate the indicators and wipers by pressing their head against the switches on the headrest.

Who would use this modification?

A person who is unable to operate the hand controls with their own hands or who is using hand controls for the brake/accelerator but does not have the fine motor skills required to operate a small switch or toggle for indicators.

Voice-controlled vehicle controls

These enable the driver to activate the vehicle controls using their voice. The device is fitted to the car via Bluetooth.

Touch screen control systems

The touch screen control system incorporates the operation functions for driving on a screen in front of the driver. Functions controlled by the touch screen include ignition, gear shift, electric parking brake and wheelchair lock, as well as indicators, horn, lights, windscreen wipers and air-conditioning (Fig. 8.12).

Balance

One issue for people with SCI returning to driving is promoting stability in the vehicle, particularly for people with cervical spinal injuries and poor core control. There is a range of auxiliary seating and seatbelt options for these drivers for use with the car's original driver's seat.

Many postural support harnesses are easily installed with the car's original seat and seatbelt. The straps are adjustable and assist with evenly distributing the person's weight, as well as holding them in the correct driving position. Different options available include a four- or five-point harness (Fig. 8.13). These are often used with side supports/bolsters to provide lateral support to the driver.

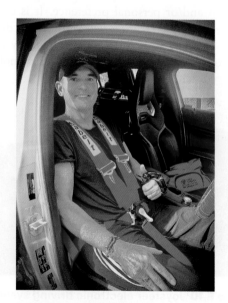

Figure 8.13 Five-point harness

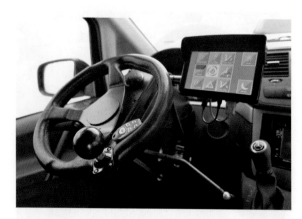

Figure 8.12 Touch screen base vehicle control system, including indicator extensions
Source: © TMN Driving Systems Industry Ltd

Access and locking in

Access modifications are techniques for getting in to the vehicle and include:

- transfer seats
- access ramps and lifts (Fig. 8.17A)
- slings
- transfer boards
- rotating and/or elevating seats (Fig. 8.14)
- wheelchair docks (Figs 8.15 and 8.16B)

Wheelchair storage

Wheelchair storage modifications are required in order to store the wheelchair safely while in transit and include:

- roof mounted loader (Fig. 8.17A)
- boot mounted loader
- boot hoist (Fig. 8.17B and C)

The R11 Robot by TMN (Fig. 8.18B, C) enables wheelchair users to drive by themselves and

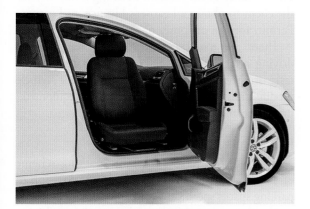

Figure 8.14 Transfer swivel seat
Source: © TMN Driving Systems Industry Ltd

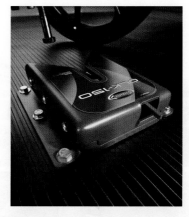

Figure 8.15 Wheelchair dock
Source: © TMN Driving Systems Industry Ltd

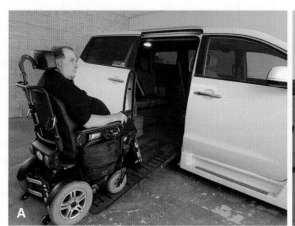

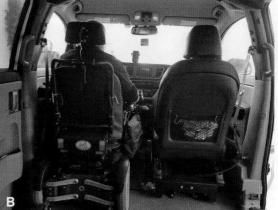

Figure 8.16 A, B Wheelchair transfer ramp and dock in action.
Source: Courtesy Arik Vamosh

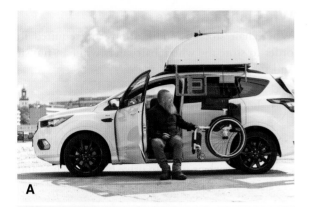

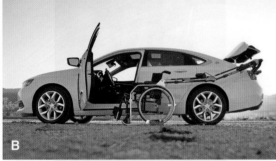

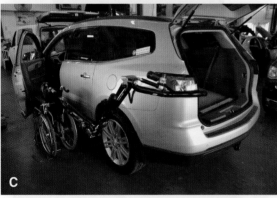

Figure 8.17 Wheelchair storage options. A, Chairtopper™ wheelchair hoist for roof of car with storage. B, C, R11 Robot™, automated wheelchair storage and retrieval system that moves chair to rear of car.

Source: A © BraunAbility B, C © TMN Driving Systems Industry

automatically store their wheelchair in the boot of the vehicle. The robotic retrieval and return of the wheelchair allows the driver complete independence.

WHAT OTHER FACTORS DO I NEED TO CONSIDER IN MY RETURN TO DRIVING AFTER AN SCI?

Caveat: It is illegal for a person to drive on the road without a current licence, even if they are only trying modifications. It is, however, possible, with the assistance of the relevant licensing body, to assist the client to obtain a Learner's Licence, or Learner's Permit, for the purposes of assessment.

There are many complexities in returning to driving after an SCI, including the nature of the task of driving itself, the many types of vehicle modifications; the complex interactions of equipment; insurance and legal issues.

Parking

Many countries have a disability parking scheme or similar. This generally involves the provision of parking spaces specifically for people with a disability and/or their carers. Most people returning to driving after an SCI require more space to access their vehicle. If they are driving their PWC into the vehicle from the rear door they will need additional space behind the car to drop their ramp or hoist and be able to straighten their PWC to access the vehicle. Those using a MWC and transferring independently into the car's existing driver seat will require more room to the side of the vehicle as they need to open the driver's door to its full width to both slide in and then stow their wheelchair (Figs 8.16 and 8.18).

In order to obtain a permit to park in a disabled parking space a letter or form from a GP or specialist is generally needed, which is then taken to the licensing body where a sticker is issued and placed on the vehicle.

Many clients who use wheelchairs are able to use their disabled parking sticker to get parking close to their workplace, including under-building parking

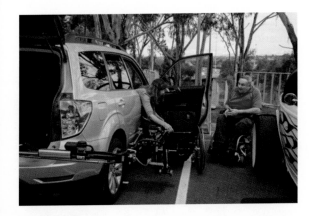

Figure 8.18 Amount of parking space required.
Source: © 2020 Spire Spinal Injury Resource and Support Network

at work. This further assists in the person returning to work and their other occupations.

Insurance

Motor vehicle insurance policies require full disclosure of modifications to ensure full coverage of the vehicle. Most statutory bodies will require all vehicles that have been modified to have an engineering certificate and a certificate of compliance with the licensing authority (e.g. a 'Blue Slip'). The process of returning to driving can be a long, complex and at times frustrating process; however, if the person does not have the correct conditions on their licence or the correct certifications on their car, they may not be covered by their insurer in the event of an accident.

Legal matters

There are different rules for returning to driving after SCI in every jurisdiction, state, territory and country. In Australia, the relevant publication is *Assessing fitness to drive for commercial and private vehicle drivers. Medical Standards for licensing and clinical management guidelines. 2016.*

The guidelines state:[28]

> Driving a motor vehicle is a complex task involving perception, appropriate judgement, adequate response time and appropriate physical capability. A range of medical conditions, disabilities and treatments may influence these driving prerequisites. Such impairment may adversely affect driving ability, possibly resulting in a crash causing death or injury (p. 3).

SCI is classified under 'Musculoskeletal conditions (Part B: 5)' in the guidelines, and the definition of the Austroads/National Transport Commission on the effects of musculoskeletal conditions on driving must be adhered to (S: 5.1.1).

The guidelines further state:[28]

> It is possible to drive safely with quite severe impairment; however, driver insight into functional limitations, stability of the condition and compensatory body movements or vehicle devices to overcome deficits are usually required. Adaptive equipment can be installed in many vehicles (e.g. hand-operated brake and accelerator, automatic transmission and height-adjustable seats) that enable many drivers with impairments to operate vehicles (p. 71).

In practical terms, many people can successfully return to driving following rehabilitation and subsequent assessment and driving instruction by a DTOT.

Refuelling

While refuelling is generally not difficult for MWC users, who can transfer independently into and out of the vehicle and readily access their stowed wheelchair, it can be challenging for PWC users.

If the PWC user has alternative plans for refuelling, such as a family member who can refuel as required, then this is generally not an issue. If, however, the driver wishes to refuel independently the vehicle may require further modifications and/or this needs to be considered when purchasing a vehicle. Generally, the issue with refuelling is the height of the fuel tank opening and the vehicle may have to be lowered, or the position of the fuel tank lowered in order for the driver to safely reach the tank for refuelling.

Safety features

As part of any vehicle modification it is important to obtain the relevant engineering certificates for the vehicle. Of particular interest is that the modifications do not interfere with the inherent safety features of the vehicle, particularly seatbelts and securing systems, and the deployment of the vehicle's airbags.

Reversal of modifications

It is a requirement that modified vehicles are also driveable by able-bodied drivers. This includes both family members and mechanics who service the vehicle. It is recommended that all vehicle modifications are reversible.

For a simple modification such as a left foot accelerator (LFA), this can be achieved by ensuring the LFA can be folded up behind the dashboard structure to the rear of the foot well when not in use – well out of the reach of the driver. When the person requiring an LFA is driving the right foot (or regular) accelerator needs to also be folded up and placed well out of the way of the driver's foot. It is not uncommon for people with an SCI to experience involuntary movements in their legs and it is potentially dangerous if they accidentally depress

the accelerator, particularly if they do not have the sensation to be aware of this or the motor control to remove their foot. If a driver with a complete paraplegia is driving with hand controls (i.e. brake and accelerator operated with their hands), all the foot pedals in the car need to be folded away so they cannot be accidentally depressed. They can then be folded back for an able-bodied person to drive the car.

Vehicle modifications also need to be removed if the vehicle is sold.

THE TECHNOLOGY OF VEHICLE MODIFICATIONS

As the major car companies are rapidly developing their technologies and, in particular, head towards driverless cars, it is useful for anyone who drives a car with modifications to continue to monitor changes in vehicle mods, particularly when upgrading their vehicle. It is possible for people with significant physical disabilities to drive themselves now and this would not have been possible even a few years ago.

Evidence-based practice points

- People with an SCI have long identified mobility issues as being one of the most significant factors in their long-term rehabilitation and a return to driving independence is an important goal for many individuals following SCI.
- Internationally, OTs are most often the health professionals trained to undertake these assessments.
- A thorough assessment of the person's off-road and on-road driving skills is required in order to ensure their 'fitness to drive'.
- For most jurisdictions, clearance from a GP or rehabilitation specialist is required prior to commencing the return to driving process with a DTOT.
- Most jurisdictions have minimum standards for vision for drivers; visual acuity is the most important ability and is a non-negotiable standard for all drivers.
- Other important physical requirements include a functional ROM in upper limbs and lower limbs to allow the client to reach the steering wheel and pedals or hand controls. Suitable strength and proprioception in the upper and/or lower limbs are also required.
- Adequate cognitive ability and insight are also essential.

SUMMARY

Driving as an independent activity and means of transportation is one of the most important rehabilitation issues identified by patients with SCI. Research shows that around 50% of all individuals with SCI return to driving, and it has been suggested that those who are unable to may have additional medical or psychological issues that prevent them from driving. Driving a modified vehicle has been associated with a higher likelihood of employment post-injury, improved re-integration into society and better psychological and general health; all of which lead to better life satisfaction.

It is well recognised that driving rehabilitation together with assistive technologies will positively influence driving outcomes. However, the technology associated with driving modifications is changing so fast that the literature may not always be completely up to date; therefore, it is recommended to always check with vehicle modification companies as to the latest technology available.

Online resources

elearnSCI.org Online learning program for wheelchair prescription, www.elearnsci.org

EnableNSW and Lifetime Care & Support Authority, Guidelines for the prescription of a seated wheelchair or mobility scooter for people with a traumatic brain injury or spinal cord injury. EnableNSW and LTCSA Editor, 2011, Sydney. www.aci.health.nsw.gov.au/__data/assets/pdf_file/0003/167286/Guidelines-on-Wheelchair-Prescription.pdf

Spinal Outreach Team and School of Health and Rehabillitation Sciences University of Queensland. Manual wheelchairs: information resrouce for service providers. 2017. www.health.qld.gov.au/__data/assets/pdf_file/0026/429911/manual-wheelchairs.pdf

United Spinal Association 2016 Wheelchair lateral supports. What do they do? www.unitedspinal.org/wheelchair-lateral-trunk-supports

References

1. Minkel, J.L., 2000. Seating and mobility considerations for people with spinal cord injury. Phys. Ther. 80 (7), 701–709.

2. Lukersmith, S., Radbron, L., et al., 2013. Development of clinical guidelines for the prescription of a seated wheelchair or mobility scooter for people with traumatic brain injury or spinal cord injury. Aust Occup Ther J. 60 (6), 378–386.

3. Lukersmith, S., 2011. Guidelines for the prescription of a seated wheelchair or mobility scooter for people with a traumatic brain injury or spinal cord injury. Sydney.

4. Di Marco, A., Russell, M., et al., 2003. Standards for wheelchair prescription. Aust Occup Ther J. 50 (1), 30–39.

5. Edwards, K., McCluskey, A., 2010. A survey of adult power wheelchair and scooter users. Disabil. Rehabil. Assist. Technol. 5 (6), 411–419.

6. Queensland Spinal Outreach Team, School of Health and Rehabilitation Services University of Queensland. Manual wheelchairs. Information resources for wheelchair providers. 2017. https://www.health.qld.gov.au/__data/assets/pdf_file/0026/429911/manual-wheelchairs.pdf.

7. Li, C.T., Chen, C.H., et al., 2015. Biomechanical evaluation of a novel wheelchair backrest for elderly people. Biomed. Eng. Online 14 (1), 14.

8. Bates, P.S., Spencer, J.C., et al., 1993. Assistive technology and the newly disabled adult: adaptation to wheelchair use. Am. J. Occup. Ther. 47 (11), 1014–1021.

9. EnableNSW and Lifetime Care and Support Authority, Guidelines for the prescription of a seated wheelchair or mobility scooter for people with a traumatic brain injury or spinal cord injury. EnableNSW and LTCSA Editor, 2011, Sydney.

10. Adler, G., Rottunda, S., 2006. Older adults' perspectives on driving cessation. J. Aging Stud. 20 (3), 227–235.

11. Unsworth, C.A., Baker, A., 2014. Driver rehabilitation: a systematic review of the types and effectiveness of interventions used by occupational therapists to improve on-road fitness-to-drive. Accid. Anal. Prev. 71, 106–114.

12. Norweg, A., Jette, A.M., et al., 2011. Patterns, predictors, and associated benefits of driving a modified vehicle after spinal cord injury: findings from the National Spinal Cord

Injury Model Systems. Arch. Phys. Med. Rehabil. 92 (3), 477–483.

13. Whiteneck, G., Tate, D., et al., 1999. Predicting community reintegration after spinal cord injury from demographic and injury characteristics. Arch. Phys. Med. Rehabil. 80 (11), 1485–1491.

14. Lee, R.C.H., Hasnan, N., et al., 2018. Characteristics of persons with spinal cord injury who drive in Malaysia and its barriers: a cross sectional study. Spinal Cord 56 (4), 341.

15. Carpenter, C., Forwell, S.J., et al., 2007. Community participation after spinal cord injury. Arch. Phys. Med. Rehabil. 88 (4), 427–433.

16. Hopewell, C.A., 2002. Driving assessment issues for practicing clinicians. J. Head Trauma Rehabil. 17 (1), 48–61.

17. Unsworth, C.A., 2007. Development and current status of occupational therapy driver assessment and rehabilitation in Victoria, Australia. Aust. Occup. Ther. J. 54 (2).

18. Unsworth, C., Pallant, J., et al., 2011. OT-DORA: occupational therapy driver off-road assessment battery. AOTA Press.

19. Miller, E., Wallis, J., 2009. Executive function and higher-order cognition: definition and neural substrates. Encyclopedia Neurosci. 4, 99–104.

20. Salvi, C., Bricolo, E., et al., 2016. Insight solutions are correct more often than analytic solutions. Think. Reason. 22 (4), 443–460.

21. Nasreddine, Z.S., Phillips, N.A., et al., 2005. The Montreal Cognitive Assessment, MoCA: a brief screening tool for mild cognitive impairment. J. Am. Geriatr. Soc. 53 (4), 695–699.

22. Katz, N., Itzkovich, M., et al., 1989. Loewenstein Occupational Therapy Cognitive Assessment (LOTCA) battery for brain-injured patients: reliability and validity. Am. J. Occup. Ther. 43 (3), 184–192.

23. Folstein, M.F., Folstein, S.E., et al., 1975. 'Mini-mental state'. A practical method for grading the cognitive state of patients for the clinician. J. Psychiatr. Res. 12 (3), 189–198.

24. Hall, K.M., Cohen, M.E., et al., 1999. Characteristics of the Functional Independence Measure in traumatic spinal cord injury. Arch. Phys. Med. Rehabil. 80 (11), 1471–1476.

25. Kay, L.G., Bundy, A.C., et al., 2009. Predicting fitness to drive in people with cognitive impairments by using DriveSafe and DriveAware. Arch. Phys. Med. Rehabil. 90 (9), 1514–1522.

26. Kay, L.G., Bundy, A., et al., 2009. Validity, reliability and predictive accuracy of the Driving Awareness Questionnaire. Disabil. Rehabil. 31 (13), 1074–1082.

27. Law, M., Cooper, B., et al., 1996. The person-environment-occupation model: a transactive approach to occupational performance. Can. J. Occup. Ther. 63 (1), 9–23.

28. Austroads & National Transport Commission. Assessing fitness to drive for commercial and private vehicle drivers. Medical Standards for licensing and clinical management guidelines. 5th edn (rev.) 2017.

Camila Quel De Oliveira and Boaz Shamir

INTRODUCTION

The initial thoughts of the patient with a spinal cord injury (SCI) and their family are most often related to their limitations of mobility and the possibility of a future confined to a wheelchair, without the ability to walk. Walking is possibly one of the most profound and significant issues for these patients and the loss of this elementary function frequently leads to a high level of frustration for this patient group.

The 'fight' starts from the moment of injury and can last forever. Every single manoeuvre that a human being would normally be able to do automatically now requires time and planning.[1] Activities, once performed without any thought, become time-consuming and challenging. The rehabilitation program is a process that aims to lead, as closely as possible, to the normalisation of the life of the patient with SCI. Hence, the task of the physiotherapist in a spinal injury unit (SIU) is to give the patient the necessary tools and education to allow this to take place.

Often as an in-patient at the rehabilitation centre, the individual with an SCI feels comfortable, safe and secure. Some patients feel afraid to return to home and may use excuses, such as *my house is not ready yet; I am waiting for my carer; I do not feel ready yet to leave the centre.* Although the former two reasons may be genuine bureaucratic explanations, the last excuse/reason must also be dealt with thoughtfully and honestly. Due to improved care and better discharge planning, as well as increased costs, the length of stay in an in-patient rehabilitation centre has been dramatically reduced over the years, with the average length of stay in the United States reduced from 106 to 39 days between 1977 and 2004. In Australia, in 2003, the overall median length of stay was 83 days. For individuals with incomplete paraplegia, the median was 43 days, while for people with complete paraplegia it was 96 days, incomplete tetraplegia 64 days and complete tetraplegia 206 days.[2] According to the Australian Institute of Health and Welfare report, in 2015 the median length of stay was 138 days for cervical injuries, 147 days for thoracic and 85 days for lumbosacral injuries.[3]

As discussed earlier in Chapters 2 and 3, incomplete tetraplegia is now the most frequently encountered SCI diagnosis. The frequency of incomplete paraplegia has increased when compared to complete paraplegia over the past 10 years in Australia.[3] However, less than 1% of people experience complete neurological recovery by the time of hospital discharge.[2]

Finally, ambulation is essential to minimise the myriad of complications related to prolonged wheelchair sitting, such as pressure ulcers, shoulder pathologies, loss of bone density in the long bones of the legs, depression and loss of range of motion of the joints of legs and trunk (see Chapters 15, 18 and 21).[4]

AMBULATION/WALKING

The health benefits of standing and walking after SCI include maintenance of bone mineral density (BMD); improved cardiorespiratory function, gastrointestinal function, sitting balance; and decreased pain and spasticity.[5] It is important to note that to improve BMD, loading plus muscle contraction (as provided by functional electrical stimulation [FES]) is required.[6]

Human gait is a complex phenomenon that involves intricate interactions between the trunk, pelvis, hips, knees and ankles. The goal of normal human ambulation is to facilitate travel from one location to another while minimising effort and maintaining adequate stability across a wide variety of environmental conditions. This is possible by complex interactions between central and peripheral neural pathways that coordinate movement of the musculoskeletal system (see Chapter 3 for a detailed explanation of central pattern generators and a more automatic gait).

Gait cycle

Walking is a highly coordinated cyclical series of movements. Several nomenclatures are found in the literature to describe the limb movements and are useful in understanding the functional tasks of the whole limb and in providing a framework for explaining the contributions of the musculoskeletal system at individual joints.[7] The most basic method is to divide the cyclic movement or gait cycle into two parts, a stance phase and a swing phase. Stance phase represents the portion of the gait cycle during which the reference limb is in contact with the ground. During normal walking, this portion accounts for approximately the first 60% of the gait cycle (Fig. 9.1). The second division, swing phase, occurs when the reference limb is not in contact with the ground. During normal walking, this portion accounts for approximately the latter 40% of the gait cycle.

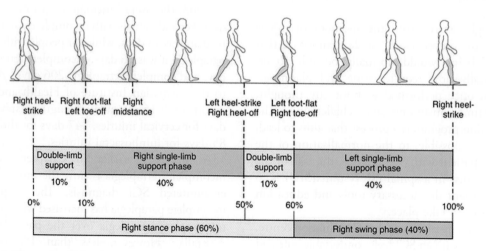

Figure 9.1 The gait cycle.
Source: Muscolino, J.E. 2017 Kinsiology: The skeletal system and muscle function. 3rd edn. Elsevier.

The Rancho Los Amigos (RLA) terminology further subdivides the gait cycle into phases that describe the specific functions.[7] Physiotherapists worldwide frequently use this approach. The RLA nomenclature subdivides stance phase into five parts and swing phase into three parts.

Stance phase

- *Initial contact* is the point at which the foot comes in contact with the ground and serves as the starting point of stance phase and the overall gait cycle. Initial contact is an instant in time rather than a true phase or function of stance.
- *Loading response* starts at initial contact and lasts until the contralateral foot leaves the ground. Loading response is a period of double limb support during which the impact of initial contact is absorbed and weight is transferred rapidly onto the leading limb.
- *Midstance* starts when the contralateral foot leaves the ground and lasts until the ipsilateral heel leaves the ground. During midstance, the body weight moves forward, typically aligned over the foot that is in contact with the ground.
- *Terminal stance* begins when the ipsilateral heel leaves the ground and ends at the time of the contralateral foot's initial contact with the ground. During terminal stance, the body weight continues its forward progression such that normally the heel rises as weight moves over the forefoot.
- *Pre-swing* is the final phase of stance and lasts from the time of contralateral foot initial contact with the ground until the ipsilateral foot leaves the ground (toe-off).

Swing phase

- *Initial swing* is the first phase of swing and encompasses the time from when the foot leaves the ground to ipsilateral foot alignment with the contralateral ankle. During initial swing, the foot lifts off the ground and the limb begins its forward advancement. A critical task of initial swing is positioning the foot such that it clears the ground and any obstacles as it advances.
- *Mid-swing* is the time from ankle and foot alignment until when the swing leg tibia becomes vertical. During mid-swing, the advancement of the limb continues.
- *Terminal swing* is the final portion of swing phase from the time the tibia reaches a vertical position until initial contact of the swing foot with the ground. During terminal swing, the limb completes its forward advancement.[7]

Walking is frequently the ultimate goal of the SCI population and was identified as being in the top five priorities by people with SCI.[8] Furthermore, it has a positive impact on psychological wellbeing, as demonstrated by patient reports:

> 'To see myself walking after so long time it's a dream'; 'It's beautiful'; 'Please, move the computer screen so I can watch myself walking'; 'I don't remember myself walking'.

In general, the overall aim of ambulation for the patient with an SCI is to increase mobility to allow for greater independence and community participation and, ultimately, prevent secondary complications that may result from paralysis. Based on the literature and clinical experience, the success and nature of how people recover ambulation will depend upon many different factors, including the level of lesion, age, sex, height, weight and body mass index (BMI); but most of all, their level of motivation. Normal gait, as defined above, is often unachievable; however, it may be possible to regain a functional gait pattern that is both energy efficient and aesthetically acceptable.

The first decision to be made by the rehabilitation team in conjunction with the patient with an SCI (as the most important member of the team) is whether walking can be a functional activity or a practice activity only.

Although walking is very often the highest goal of the patient, it should not always be the ultimate target. For some, the price of walking may be too high. The high levels of energy consumption, tiredness, sweating or pain may not be compensated for by the experience of walking, nor feasible for daily living and functional activities. In these situations, the practice of walking as a physical activity may be important not only for the joy of the feeling of walking, but also for the benefits of weight bearing in maintaining range of motion achieved by the stretching of the soft tissues.[5]

The primary role of the physiotherapist within an SCI rehabilitation centre is to demonstrate all the possible walking modalities currently available to the patients and help them to decide which would be the most suitable and functional option to meet their goals (Table 9.1). It is vital that the patient is involved in this process and that a third party does not make such decisions for them. To assist the patient to make informed choices, the treating physiotherapist is required to have an extensive knowledge in the area and, as such, the aim of this chapter is to assist the physiotherapist and the patient to come to the most appropriate choice.

WALKING AS A FUNCTIONAL ACTIVITY

Walking as a functional activity is usually dependent upon the level of lesion.

Walking with complete spinal cord injury

Walking for the patient with a complete SCI will require orthotic devices to stabilise the lower limbs and the ability to weight-bear through the upper extremities. Walking aids commonly used are walking frames or forearm-supported (Canadian) crutches.

The amount of stability provided by the orthotic device will vary according to the level of injury and the pre-morbid condition of the patient. The multidisciplinary team, including the orthotist, the physiotherapist and of course the patient, will make the selection of the most suitable type of orthosis.

Walking with incomplete spinal cord injury

Many walking options for the patient with an incomplete SCI are available, since these patients present with a wide range of impairments. Ambulation for the patient with an incomplete SCI can range from requiring only two crutches to walk to functional walking not being a realistic possibility.

Walking with upper motor neuron impairment

As discussed in detail in Chapter 1, the patient with an SCI lesion at the level of T12 or above is described as having an upper motor neuron (UMN) lesion and may demonstrate the signs and symptoms of hyperreflexia and high muscle tone (spinal spasticity). Some patients actually learn how to use their spasticity for functional activities, including standing and walking.

Walking with lower motor neuron impairment

Any patient with a lesion below the level of T12 is described as having a cauda equina lesion that affects the lower motor neurons (described in Chapter 1). The signs and symptoms include areflexia and low muscle tone or flaccidity in the lower limbs. The innervation of the muscles of the trunk and upper limbs remains intact, which allows for ambulatory function with the assistance of fixed long-leg braces.

TRADITIONAL GAIT RE-EDUCATION

A wide variety of orthotic devices is available for the patient with an SCI to assist in functional or non-functional ambulation. Some examples are discussed here.

The decision of which type of brace or orthotic device to use is always a multidisciplinary team decision and many factors, including when and how often the braces will be used, the patient's

Table 9.1 Queensland Spinal Cord Injuries Service physiotherapy standing and walking guidelines

Device	Client physical requirement	Necessary equipment	Physiotherapy intervention	Physiotherapy timeframe	Functional outcome	Approx SCI level
Tilt table (standing only)	Minimal physical ability required 1 or 2 person assist	May need hoist for transfers	Education re: use	2–3 sessions to instruct client/carer on use in the home	Incorporates stretch of trunk/lower limbs Potential to reduce muscle tone	Any level of SCI
Standing frame (standing only)	Ability to transfer onto device or 1 person assist depending on type of frame Good sitting balance Ability to use sit/stand controls	May need hoist for transfer	Education re: use Set-up of device to suit client	2–3 sessions to instruct client/carer on use in the home May also need to learn technique of transfer on/off, depending on device	Self-propel types allow for access on flat, smooth surface	C6 and below
Back slabs (posterior splints usually made of plaster to maintain leg extended during training)	UL function and strength to achieve standing from seated position Assistance to don/doff	Parallel bars	Education re: use Training to achieve sit-stand Standing balance and weight shift	Often done as in-patient 1–2 hour session 3–4 times per week self-practice in parallel bars when safe and sit/stand independently	Stretch (dorsiflexion, hip extension) Standing balance Precursor to other aids (e.g. KAFO if appropriate function)	C8 and below

Continued

Table 9.1 Queensland Spinal Cord Injuries Service physiotherapy standing and walking guidelines—cont'd

Device	Client physical requirement	Necessary equipment	Physiotherapy intervention	Physiotherapy timeframe	Functional outcome	Approx SCI level
• HKAFO (standing and ambulation) e.g. Walkabout, IRGO	• Good sitting balance • Nil upper limb pain/problems • Good shoulder, elbow and hand strength • High level of fitness • Good lower limb range of motion – hip extension, hamstring and calf muscle length • Able to don/doff independently	• Back slabs for initial standing • Parallel bars • Crutches • Full length mirror	• Extensive training to achieve gait outside of parallel bars • Standing balance and weight shift • Home practice with parallel bars set-up (client reliability) • Intensive practice	• 8–12 weeks then review • Continue timeframe if more advanced goals • 3–4 sessions per week, 1–2 hours self-practice in parallel bars, if safe	• Ambulation only achievable on flat smooth surfaces • Issue of safety in crutches • Slow, energy consuming • Wheelchair still primary means of mobility	• Mid-thoracic and below • C8–T1 very difficult – standing only

KAFO (standing and ambulation)	As per HKAFO plus • Good hip extension and lumbar extension range • Normal/near normal trunk function • Quadratus lumborum (T12–L3) allows some hip-hitching for 4-point gait • Hip flexors allow for better 4-point gait • Needs to be able to sit/stand independently	• Back slabs for initial training • Parallel bars • Walking frame • Crutches	• 8–12 weeks then review • Continue timeframe if more advanced goals • 3–4 sessions per week, 1–2 hours • Self-practice in parallel bars, if safe	• As per HKAFO • Training/supervision of technique out of parallel bars, inclines, sit to stand, get off floor • Intensive practice	• Knee locked into extension • Most efficient and safest is 2-point gait (swing-to and swing-through) as compared to 4-point • Highest level may achieve inclines, stairs, on/off floor • Wheelchair still primary means of mobility • Some active lower limb movement may allow for knee flexion during gait as long as able to lock/unlock knee (computerised knee in KAFO)	• T10 and below
AFO	• Able to hold hips/knees into extension without hyperextension	• Parallel bars for training • Various walking aids		• Depending on ambulation goals • Very individual	• May achieve gait without aids • Level of SCI impacts on gait pattern • Gait may become primary mean of mobility	• L2–3 and below

Legend: SCI = spinal cord injury; UL = upper limb; LL = lower limb; ROM = range of motion; IRGO = isocentric reciprocating gait orthosis; AFO = ankle-foot orthosis; HKAFO = hip-knee-ankle-foot orthosis; KAFO = knee-ankle-foot-orthosis

Source: Queensland Spinal Cord Injuries Service with permission

demographic features and the cost of the device must be taken into account. The orthoses that make walking possible for SCI patients are required to give stability to the joints of the lower limbs. The concept behind all orthotics is to keep the range of motion at an angle that will allow standing up with straight legs while not interfering with taking steps.

In general, a patient with an SCI will require upper limb strength to grasp and control the walking aid (walker or crutches) and to stabilise their body while standing or walking. The gait re-education process must be slow and secure; relearning how to walk takes time. Before beginning gait re-education, the patient must be able to balance when standing safely with the orthotic device and walking aid of choice. It is recommended to commence gait re-education sessions between parallel bars with standing only. Standing balance is important and should always be the primary goal; only after the patient has achieved free standing with the preferred orthosis can the first steps be taken. The severity of the injury and other demographic features such as age, height, weight and sex will affect the amount of assistance required. The orthotic device most acceptable to the patient

will be one that is the least restrictive and requires lower levels of energy consumption, allowing for a more functional walking pattern. Moreover, most patients with SCI prefer to use the minimum degree of assistance possible for walking activity.

Hip-knee-ankle-foot orthoses/ reciprocal gait orthosis (HKAFO/RGO)

The hip-knee-ankle-foot orthoses/reciprocal gait orthosis or HKAFO/RGO stabilises the hip and knee joint in extension and the ankle joint in dorsiflexion during the whole gait cycle. Due to a pneumatic mechanism that detects weight-shifting, it facilitates the swing phase by bringing the leg forward when the leg is unloaded. To control this orthosis, the patient must be able to weight-shift through the trunk using the non-affected upper body. It offers maximal support and stability to the lower limbs and may therefore be a good solution for mid or high thoracic injuries. A walking frame or crutches are required when using the HKAFO (Figs 9.2A and B). A reciprocal gait pattern can be achieved, although many patients prefer to use the faster 'swing-to' (jumping up to the line of the crutches)

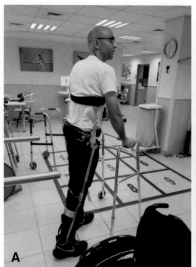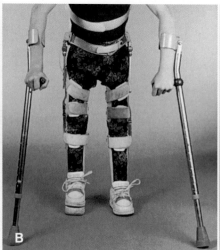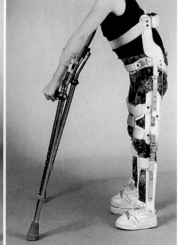

Figure 9.2 A HKAFO/RGO used with A, a walking frame. B, with crutches.
Source: B, Nawoczenski DA, Epler ME 1997 Orthotics in functional rehabilitation of the lower limb. Philadelphia, WB Saunders.

or 'swing-through' (jumping through the crutches) patterns.

The patient with an SCI requires time to adjust to this new situation and the learning process, as the walking pattern will be significantly different from their pre-injury pattern. The author of this chapter recommends that training should begin within the parallel bars, where the patient can learn how to stand and balance with long splints (back slabs) that block the knee joint. Step training begins by walking along the bars in a swing-to, swing-through or reciprocal pattern. A minimum of two training sessions per week for 4–6 weeks for practice of walking is suggested. In addition to gait re-education training sessions, the treating physiotherapist must focus on the strength and flexibility of the muscles of the shoulder girdle as the walking technique relies on the prime muscles of the shoulder girdle and, most importantly, the reversed origin-insertion use of latissimus dorsi. Most often the HKAFO is used only for non-functional gait or with the paediatric SCI population, due to the high-energy cost and the reduced speed achieved, which hinders its use for community ambulation.

Knee-ankle-foot orthosis (KAFO)

A knee-ankle-foot orthosis (KAFO) is a long-leg orthosis that stabilises the knee, the ankle and the foot in an effort to replace the function of the paralysed muscles of the leg (Fig. 9.3). The fixed knee joint maintains the extension of the knee in place of the paralysed quadriceps muscle, the fixed ankle joint maintains the ankle at 90° in place of the paralysed triceps surae and tibialis anterior muscles and the fixed foot joints support the foot in place of the paralysed small muscles of the foot. A person with an SCI classified as T12 complete paraplegia (AIS A) will require a KAFO for each lower limb and will walk with the aid of either two forearm support crutches or a walking frame (see Chapter 4 and Appendix 1 for more details on AIS classifications).

KAFOs may be prefabricated or custom-made in a variety of materials. A variety of locking mechanisms at the knee joint are available. The preferred locking

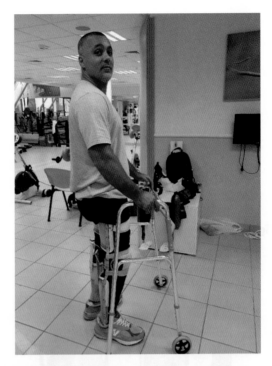

Figure 9.3 Knee-ankle-foot orthosis (KAFO) used with a walking frame.

mechanism for the knee joint is the Swiss lock (Fig. 9.4). This mechanism allows the knee to be firmly locked while standing up and walking, and open or free for sitting down.

As discussed above, all decisions about the type of orthotic prescribed should be a team decision.

Ankle–foot orthosis (AFO)

For lower motor neuron injuries and/or incomplete spinal cord injuries, such as cauda equina syndrome or lower lumbar vertebral column injuries, the residual impairment may be only weakness around the dorsiflexors, resulting in either a unilateral or a bilateral clinical 'foot-drop'. In these cases, an ankle–foot orthosis (AFO) may suffice in achieving the required foot clearance during the swing phase.

A large selection of AFOs are available in a wide variety of materials, either 'off the shelf' or custom-made (Fig. 9.5A–C). It is vital that the least restrictive orthotic device is selected in order

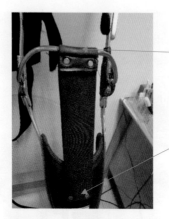

The locking mechanism consists of a centred lock lever and a toothed lock plate. A bolt is placed on the lock plate. The knee angle can be set by adjusting the bolt on the toothed lock

Figure 9.4 **Swiss-locking mechanism.**

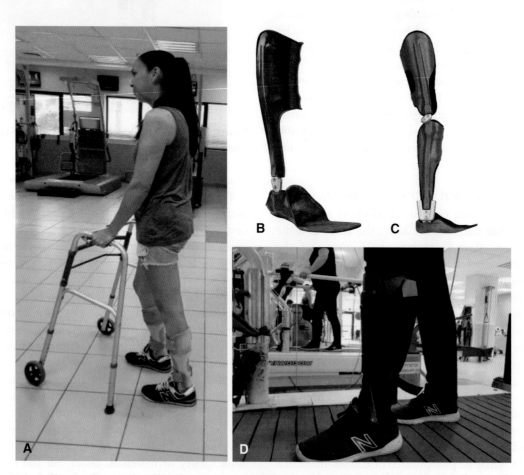

Figure 9.5 **Different types of ankle-foot orthoses (AFO): A, Hinged. B, C, Ventral shell. D, Carbon fibre.**
Source: B, © 2018 FIOR & GENTZ

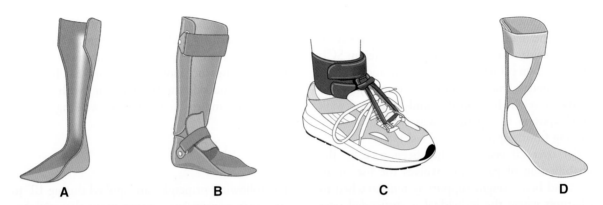

Figure 9.6 Different types of ankle-foot orthoses (AFO): A, Rigid AFO. B, hinged. C, Dictus. D, Posterior leaf spring.

to allow as close to normal gait pattern as possible and facilitate any residual voluntary movement in the joint. The choice of orthotics for this patient group must, therefore, be dynamic and take into consideration neuroplasticity and potential for recovery. Subsequently, the MDT should regularly review all orthoses for this patient group.

When the patient presents with complete paralysis of plantar and dorsiflexor muscles or with spasticity in the plantar flexor muscles that impedes foot clearance during gait, a rigid AFO should be prescribed (Fig. 9.6A). If active dorsiflexion is present, however, and is limited by spastic plantarflexor muscles, a hinged AFO is recommended (Fig. 9.6B). For patients that present with foot-drop due to flaccid paralysis or severe weakness of the dorsiflexor muscles, a Dictus elastic orthosis may be prescribed to assist with foot clearance during the swing phase (Fig. 9.6C). Lastly, the posterior leaf spring AFO (Fig. 9.6D) can assist with propulsion during the push-off phase of the gait as it is made of materials that deform during the terminal stance and recoil during the push-off phase (replacing the action of the gastrocnemius).

NEW PARADIGMS FOR GAIT RE-EDUCATION

There are now a number of possible interventions available for therapists to use in gait re-education programs. These include body weight-supported treadmill training (BWSTT), treadmill training with or without manual assistance and/or functional electrical stimulation (FES), overground walking training with or without body weight support (BWS), manual assistance and/or FES, as well as the growing field of robotic gait training.[9] Collectively these interventions can be classified as activity-based therapy interventions for gait and are an integral component to the shifting paradigm of gait re-education.[10] (See Chapter 3 for further detail on ABT.)

When discussing these interventions, the disadvantages of the BWSTT and treadmill training systems are often highlighted.[11] For example, depending upon how physically capable and cooperative the patient is, between one and three physiotherapists may be needed in order to operate the system. As such, it is not therefore a particularly cost-effective intervention. Furthermore, inconsistent walking parameters make it difficult for the patient to maintain a smooth, coordinated walking pattern. This concept will be discussed further throughout this chapter.

LOCOMOTOR TRAINING FOR GAIT RE-EDUCATION

Locomotor training (LT) is an activity-based therapy (ABT) intervention that aims to improve sensory, motor and autonomic function, health and quality of life. The main focus is to promote recovery of postural control and walking function after an SCI. LT is based on principles derived from studies using animal models that demonstrated recovery of the ability to weight-bear on the hind limbs and walk after exposure to repetitive step training (i.e. by training for the specific motor task).[12]

For over 20 years, LT has been used in the rehabilitation of gait and involves the use of an overhead body weight support system attached to a harness where the individual is suspended over a treadmill (Fig. 9.7).[13] Trained physiotherapists facilitate control of balance and manually assist trunk and leg movement during stepping and standing to generate sensory information that is consistent

with locomotion. In conjunction with BWSTT, LT programs usually include an overground training component, where task-specific training of walking and standing incorporating sensory feedback are performed outside the BWS system, with the aim of contributing to the recovery of walking.[14]

PRINCIPLES OF LOCOMOTOR TRAINING

The following principles are applied during LT to guarantee appropriate sensory input that matches the kinetic and kinematic properties of locomotion:

1 Stepping velocities on the treadmill are set as close as possible to normal walking speeds.
2 The load to the lower limbs is maximised according to the individual's ability to maintain appropriate head, trunk, knee and hip extension during standing and stance phase of gait.
3 Manual guidance is provided to approximate hip, knee and ankle kinematics to normal ranges.
4 Hip extension during the stance phase of gait and the unloading of one limb is synchronised with the simultaneous loading of the contralateral limb.
5 Weight-bearing on the arms is avoided or minimised in order to maximise the load on the lower limbs and facilitate reciprocal arm swing during stepping.
6 Symmetrical interlimb kinematics and kinetics are maintained at all times.[15]

LT was standardised by the Christopher and Dana Reeve Foundation NeuroRecovery Network (NRN) in the United States.[14] Each training session is 90 minutes long and consists of three components: step training, overground assessment and community integration.[16] Each component is as follows:

Step-training

The step training component comprises the initial 55–60 minutes of task-specific training of standing

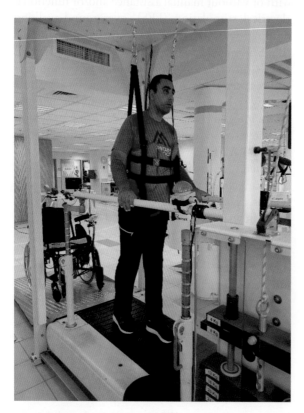

Figure 9.7 Body-weight support treadmill training.

and walking in a controlled environment using a BWS system over a treadmill with verbal and manual facilitation provided by therapists for control of hips and lower limb movements.

The step training is divided into four elements:

1. *Stand retraining:* Consists of retraining posture and balance control in standing by providing manual facilitation at hips, lower limbs and trunk, as necessary. The body weight load is maximised to a point that allows the maintenance of appropriate kinematics of standing with assistance from the therapists. Exercises are performed over a stationary treadmill, involving postural maintenance and weight shifting is facilitated by the therapists (Fig. 9.8).

2. *Stand adaptability:* Consists of retraining posture and balance control in standing with the aim of increasing the patient's independence and reducing external assistance. The percentage of BWS and manual assistance varies according to the patient's ability to control posture and balance in standing. The main goal is to increase the load on the lower limbs as external assistance is reduced. The treadmill is stationary and exercises involving postural control and coordination of the trunk and lower limbs are conducted.

3. *Step retraining:* Consists of step training on the treadmill with manual facilitation of hips and lower limbs to provide sensory cues to optimise the neuromuscular response to the sensorimotor experience (Fig. 9.9). The body weight load is maximised to a point where therapists can maintain the appropriate gait kinematics. The treadmill speed is set at normal walking speed (3.2–4.5 km/h) or greater to promote a stepping pattern as close as possible to pre-injury. The therapists monitor the lower limb joint kinematics and adjust the percentage of body weight and treadmill speed in order to achieve an optimal

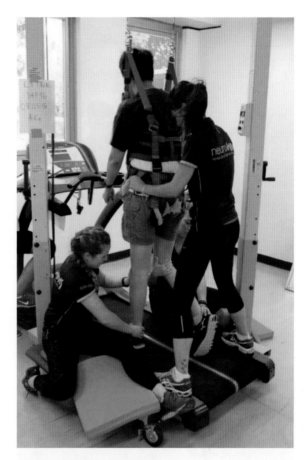

Figure 9.8 Step training.

stepping pattern. An optimal stepping pattern is defined as spatially- and temporally-coordinated stepping pattern that most resembles normal walking.[17]

Therapists provide manual guidance by placing one hand on the patellar tendon to provide proprioceptive input to the quadriceps muscle, facilitating leg extension during the stance phase of gait. During the swing phase, the hand is moved adjacent to the medial hamstring tendon to guide leg flexion. In addition, the other hand is placed over the region of the tibialis anterior tendon to support the

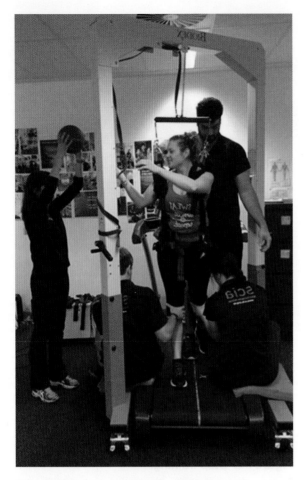

Figure 9.9 An example of a balance task performed during stand adaptability.

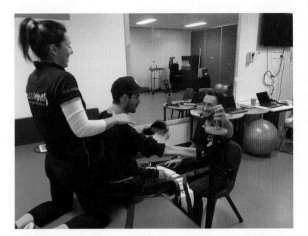

Figure 9.10 Overground training of balance in sitting.

that is achieved, then the focus is to reach normal walking speeds (3.2 to 4.5 km/h).

4. *Step adaptability:* Similarly to stand adaptability, step adaptability aims to increase the participant's independence in trunk control and stepping. Manual facilitation is minimised while maintaining postural control and coordinated stepping. Walking speed is reduced and BWS increased to facilitate voluntary movement.

Overground assessment and training

The second component consists of overground assessment with evaluation of the immediate effects of LT on the patient's abilities when mobilising over ground, allowing the patient and therapist to assess the patient's mobility, and identify critical elements limiting recovery. Each session comprises 30 minutes of training of activities performed out of the BWS system, and targeted at remediating the impairments identified in the initial assessment. Activities involving postural control, muscle strengthening, balance and task-specific training of sitting (Fig. 9.10); moving from supine to sitting; transitioning from sitting to standing; standing with assistance (Fig. 9.11) and walking are performed according

ankle in dorsiflexion for toe clearance during the swing phase and at the calcaneus for appropriate foot placement at heel strike. A third therapist stands behind the participant, with hands on either side of the harness at the approximate level of the anterior superior iliac crests, to assist in weight shifting and maintaining an upright trunk. The participants are instructed to swing their arms reciprocally with the lower limbs. The first aim of the therapists is to provide the optimal stepping pattern by providing sensory cues; once

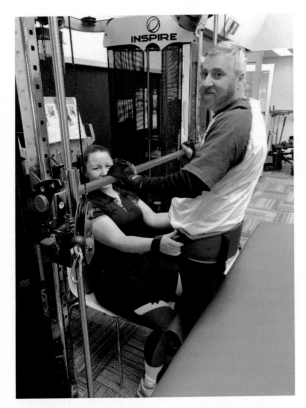

Figure 9.11 Overground training of standing with assistance.

to the participants' abilities and goals. The manual guidance and physical assistance are kept to a minimum during this component.[16]

Community integration

The third component of LT is community integration, where patients are encouraged to use their new neuromuscular capacity outside the clinical environment. The aim is to translate the acquired stepping ability into safe overground mobility for standing and walking in the home and community. If necessary, the therapist will prescribe the least restrictive assistive device to allow for safe ambulation. The patient will then be educated on how to use the device and how to function safely in the home and community.[16]

The Neuromuscular Recovery Scale (NRS) is the outcome measure developed by the NeuroRecovery Network to assess the effects of LT programs and compares the patient's performance during functional tasks to a typical pre-injury movement.[18] It is also a guide to therapists for goal-setting and session planning. It is a measure for classifying lower extremity and trunk recovery after SCI without the use of external devices, physical assistance or compensatory movements.[19,20]

ROBOTIC EXOSKELETAL GAIT RE-EDUCATION

The next challenging global project to offer walking ability for patients with SCI is the exoskeleton.[21,22] Exoskeleton-assisted walking (EAW) refers to a robotic suit that enables a person with paralysis to stand and walk. The device is sensor controlled and responds to the weight shift of the user.

As stated earlier in this chapter, the health benefits of standing and walking after an SCI include maintenance of bone density, improved cardiorespiratory function, gastrointestinal function, sitting balance and decreased pain and spasticity. People with SCI who participated in research-based EAW training programs reported improvements in spasticity, skin health, pain, diabetes, bladder and bowel function and fat loss. Furthermore, small changes in sensation and movement in trunk and legs were reported.[23]

There is a growing interest from consumers with SCI and rehabilitation professionals in EAW. This next section will explore some of the most common devices that are being incorporated into mainstream SCI rehabilitation.

Fixed gait rehabilitation exoskeleton

The best-known fixed rehabilitation exoskeleton currently available is the Lokomat® (Fig. 9.12), a modular, fixed gait rehabilitation exoskeleton that fits around the patient, who is suspended by an overhead harness. The patient carries out gait training over a treadmill. Features of system include:

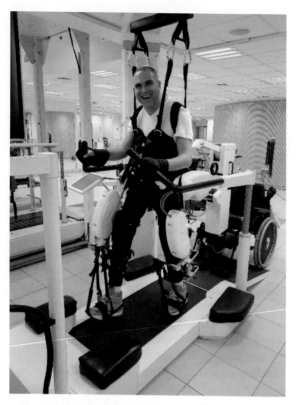

Figure 9.12 The Lokomat®.

Source: © Hocoma

The physiotherapist controls both the kinetic and the kinematic variables at all joints and the amount of unloading at those joints. Depending upon their ability, the client can have between 0% and 100% control of their walking, in conjunction with their physiotherapist.

Following successful treatment, it is often possible to progress the patient to manually-guided BWSTT (but with less assistance provided from the therapists) or other conventional forms of gait re-education.

Training time is approximately 45 minutes per session. Pre-session measurements, including leg length and circumference, are required to ensure appropriate set-up of the device. The system is adjusted to fit each patient individually and silicon sheath protectors are worn on the patient's legs to avoid skin damage. For a patient with tetraplegia, the time taken from sitting in a wheelchair to starting walking has been found on average to be between 7 and 10 minutes (including the more 'complex' patients). For patients with tetraplegia, or those who may suffer from orthostatic hypotension, it is advised that two physiotherapists fit the patient into the device in order to decrease the set-up time (see Chapter 4 for further detail on orthostatic hypotension). The Lokomat® has a safety feature called the 'telestop', which is worn around the physiotherapist's neck and must be pressed every 3 minutes for the system to continue working (Fig. 9.13).

Dynamic overground body weight support

The Andago® is the next generation of robotic-assisted therapy, which utilises mobile robotic technology to sense the patient's movement intention and actively follows them, while providing dynamic body weight support (Fig. 9.14). This device gives the person with an SCI the possibility to achieve a safe, 'near normal' gait pattern in a wide variety of situations, and also allows patients to walk safely on level surfaces. It enables intensive training in a wide range of overground task-specific gait exercises (e.g. starting, turning, stopping, avoiding obstacles) in various daily life environments. However, this

- harness suspension that raises and lowers with each step that accounts for weight shifting
- active hip–knee actuation and passive ankle control
- optional module for pelvis translation and rotation
- visual feedback
- variable assistance
- data collection and interpolation
- a large number of reproducible quality steps provided in each session.

A rigid frame behind the patient supports the exoskeleton, allowing all electrical facilitation to be safely turned off for pre- and post-training evaluation.

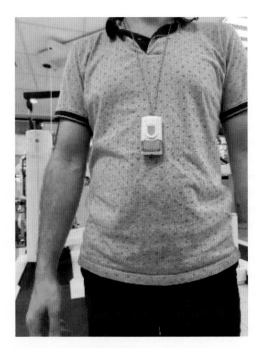

Figure 9.13 The Telestop.
Source: © Hocoma

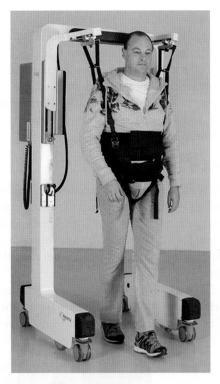

Figure 9.14 The Andago®.
Source: © Hocoma

walking training is only possible indoors, since the apparatus requires special floors.

The Andago's robotic sensor-based system provides the patient with either support or unloading, as required, depending upon the muscle weakness, and allows the user to utilise the reduced body weight in a highly mobile environment. The computerised Andago® follows the patient wherever they choose to walk, offering the required unloading throughout the practice, and giving the patient full confidence and security while they practise walking.

Despite the gait re-education benefits of both the Lokomat® and the Andago® systems, the BWS mechanisms that are involved render them relatively cumbersome and not appropriate for functional walking outside the clinical environment.

Powered robotic exoskeletons

EAW is still in the early stages of its development and, as such, no device is yet available that allows the average person with an SCI to walk with ease and efficiency outside the rehabilitation environment. There are many companies today involved in the development of these devices, but at the time of printing there are no absolute solutions.

More recently, exoskeleton robotic suits that rely solely on sensors to detect the user's shift of body weight have been developed. In this way, patients can use the device to walk quite naturally, using an acceptable amount of energy consumption for a distance of up to a few hundred metres. This is considered to be a much more functional outcome, although there are still limitations to these devices, including weight, size, amount of upper limb function required, battery life, walking speed and the quality of the walking technique of the device.

To date, powered exoskeletons remain primarily exercise devices to prevent secondary complications from paralysis of the large lower extremity muscles.[21] It is, however, a very promising modality and would seem to be the future for ambulation for the SCI population (particularly for those with complete injuries).

Below are some of the common powered robotic exoskeletons that are commercially available on the market and are currently being trialled in spinal units worldwide.

ReWalk™

The ReWalk™ is a unique exoskeletal robotic device that utilises the user's movements to control externally powered gait (Fig. 9.15). It was designed specifically for persons with an SCI, although this technology could potentially be adapted for other neurological conditions.[24]

The ReWalk™ comprises a motorised exoskeleton, a battery unit and a computer-based controller contained in a backpack, a wireless mode selector and an array of sensors that measure upper-body tilt angle, joint angles and ground contact. There is a built-in backup system for both the battery and the main computer. The exoskeleton has bilateral-lateral uprights for the thigh and leg, hinged knee joints and is articulated to foot plates distally and to a sacral band proximally.

It uses a closed-loop algorithm software control. The motors control the movements at the hip and knee joints, but not the ankles which are articulated using a mechanical joint with spring-assisted dorsiflexion.

When in the 'walk' mode, forward flexion of the upper body is detected by the tilt sensor and triggers a step. The resulting gait is a three-point pattern, advancing one step at a time.[24]

Potential benefits include:

- accessibility to confined spaces
- the ability to climb stairs.

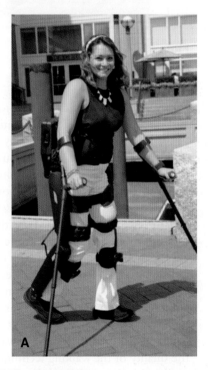
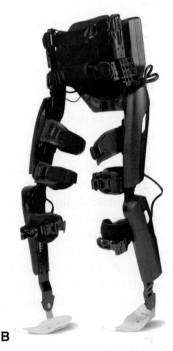

Figure 9.15 A, B The ReWalk™.
Source: © ReWalk Robotics

Limitations include:

- high energy consumption
- difficulty in wearing and adjusting the device
- appears to be more efficient with lower levels of SCI
- requires engagement of upper limbs.

Ekso GT™

The Ekso GT™ is a robotic exoskeleton for comprehensive gait therapy (Fig. 9.16).[22] The use of this exoskeleton allows for a greater number of consistent steps with the appropriate weight shift to be conducted in every rehabilitation session. It is FDA-approved for stroke patients with resultant hemiplegia and SCI at the levels of T4 to L5 and C7 to T3.[25]

Potential benefits include:

- powered hip–knee exoskeleton
- variable assist controls, allowing it to apply power from zero to 100% as needed on a step-by-step basis
- encourages correct body posture.

Limitations include:

- high energy consumption
- difficulty in wearing and adjusting the device
- appears to be more efficient with lower levels of SCI
- requires engagement of upper limbs.

REX™

The REX allows patients with higher lesions to ambulate, as it requires little upper limb function or trunk control (Fig. 9.17). It allows for trunk control and postural training since it can challenge

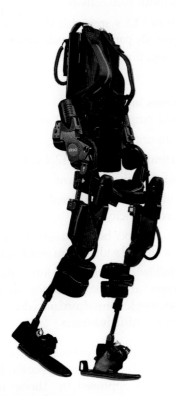

Figure 9.16 EksoNR™.
© EksoNR by Ekso Bionics

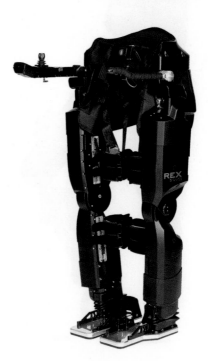

Figure 9.17 REX Bionics.
© REX Bionics Ltd

the trunk in the upright posture and during dynamic tasks, such as lunges, squats and side walking.[25]

Potential benefits include:

- easy to manoeuvre in small spaces
- frees the upper limbs for reaching and manipulation.

Limitations include:

- speed is low, not compatible with community walking
- wearable suit is heavy at 50 kg
- weight and height restrictions (not over 100 kg or 6 ft (182 cm)).

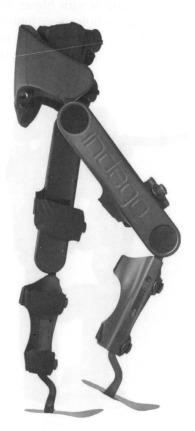

Figure 9.18 Indego®.
© Parker Hannifin Corp

Indego®

According to the manufacturer, the Indego® exoskeleton features a modular design that allows it to be easily stored and transported (Fig. 9.18). It also offers some technology interfaces so the user can collect and export key performance metrics and change the device settings remotely. The Indego® exoskeleton was designed specifically for patients with SCI, in particular those with complete and incomplete SCI at level T4 or below, but is also suitable for individuals with lower limb weakness or paralysis from a variety of neurological disorders.[26]

Potential benefits include:

- powered hip–knee exoskeleton
- lightweight design (12 kgs)
- modular
- ability to export data using an iOS app
- Bluetooth connectivity
- built-in FES system that allows for paralysed or partially paralysed muscles to contract while walking, thus promoting a more physiological gait.

Limitations include:

- height range of 155–191 cm
- maximum weight: 113 kg
- maximum hip width: 42.2 cm
- femur length: 35–47 cm
- should not be considered if the patient has severe spasticity
- enough upper-body strength to balance and move forward with forearm crutches, or a walker.

The following website lists the overall disadvantages of exoskeletons for paraplegics – https://sites.google.com/a/cortland.edu/exoskeletons-for-paraplegics/disadvantages

Caveat: At the time of publication the ReWalk™, Ekso GT™ and Indego® were approved by the US FDA.[22] REX is approved by Therapeutic Good Administration (TGA), Department of Health, Australian Government.

Evidence-based practice points

- The health benefits of standing and walking after SCI include maintenance of BMD, improved cardiorespiratory function, gastrointestinal function and sitting balance; and decreased pain and spasticity.
- Human gait is a complex phenomenon that involves intricate interactions between the trunk, pelvis, hips, knees and ankles.
- Ambulation, whether functional or therapeutic, is an important element of the rehabilitation program for all patients with SCIs.
- A wide range of orthotic devices are available to assist in functional and non-functional ambulation.
- Orthotics are designed to keep the range of motion at an angle that allows standing up with straight legs while not interfering with taking steps.
- The decision of which type of orthotic device to use is always a multidisciplinary team decision. The orthotic device most acceptable to the patient will be one that is least restrictive and requires lower levels of energy consumption, allowing for a more functional walking pattern.
- Advancements in technology have resulted in a variety of new devices that can facilitate gait training for people following a spinal cord injury:
  - BWSTT and BWS (with and without FES)
  - robotic exoskeleton suits – fixed and mobile

SUMMARY

There are many mobility options for people with an SCI; however, the functional outcome varies depending on whether the lesion is complete or incomplete. Considering that injury presentation is multifactorial, it is important to consider these options in principle rather than in practice.

Most walking modalities, apart from the BWSS, the Lokomat™, Andago™ and REX, often require the use of an aid (e.g. crutches or a walking frame). The person with an SCI must therefore possess strong upper limbs and relatively good hand function in order to ambulate. Since their upper limbs are used for weight bearing with the majority of walking modalities, the ambulant person with an SCI is unable to carry anything other than a backpack, which many consider disadvantageous. Table 9.2 lists some of the walking solutions for different SCI levels that have been discussed in the chapter.

Table 9.2 Possible walking solutions for different SCI levels according to severity of injury

Lesion	Cervical	Mid-thorax	Low thorax	Lumbar
Complete SCI	*LOKOMAT	*LOKOMAT, HKAFO, Powered EAW	*LOKOMAT, HKAFO, KAFO, Powered EAW	*LOKOMAT, KAFO, AFO
Incomplete SCI	*LOKOMAT, KAFO, AFO	*LOKOMAT, KAFO, AFO	KAFO, AFO	AFO

All walking solutions except BWSS, LOKOMAT, ANDAGO and REX require crutches or walking frame

Body size, age, sex, motivation and pre-morbid conditions will all influence the outcomes of walking rehabilitation. However, advances in technology are laying a platform that may open new opportunities for functional ambulation for the patient with an SCI.

References

1. Garfin, S.R., Eismont, F.J., et al., 2017. The Spine E-Book. Elsevier Health Sciences.

2. Tooth, L., McKenna, K., et al., 2003. Rehabilitation outcomes in traumatic spinal cord injury in Australia: functional status, length of stay and discharge setting. Spinal Cord 41 (4), 220–230.

3. Australian Institute of Health and Welfare, 2014–15. Spinal cord injury, Australia.

4. Krause, J.S., Clark, J.M.R., et al., 2015. SCI Longitudinal Aging Study: 40 years of research. Top. Spinal Cord Inj. Rehabil. 21 (3), 189–200.

5. Karimi, M.T., 2011. Evidence-based evaluation of physiological effects of standing and walking in individuals with spinal cord injury. Iran. J. Med. Sci. 36 (4), 242.

6. Crameri, R.M., Cooper, P., et al., 2004. Effect of load during electrical stimulation training in spinal cord injury. Muscle Nerve 29 (1), 104–111.

7. Perry, J., Burnfield, J., 2010. Gait analysis: normal and pathological function. J. Sports Sci. Med. 9 (2), 353.

8. Anderson, K.D., 2004. Targeting recovery: priorities of the spinal cord-injured population. J. Neurotrauma 21 (10), 1371–1383.

9. Mehrholz, J., Kugler, J., et al., 2012. Locomotor training for walking after spinal cord injury. Cochrane Database Syst. Rev. (11), CD006676.

10. Jones, M.L., Evans, N., et al., 2014. Activity-based therapy for recovery of walking in individuals with chronic spinal cord injury: results from a randomized clinical trial. Arch. Phys. Med. Rehabil. 95 (12), 2239–2246, e2.

11. Mehrholz, J., Harvey, L.A., et al., 2017. Is body-weight supported treadmill training or robotic assisted gait training superior to overground gait training and other forms of physiotherapy in people with spinal cord injury? A systematic review. Spinal Cord 55, 722–729.

12. Harkema, S.J., 2001. Neural plasticity after human spinal cord injury: application of locomotor training to the rehabilitation of walking. Neuroscientist 7 (5), 455–468.

13. Hesse, S., Bertelt, C., et al., 1995. Treadmill training with partial body weight support compared with physiotherapy in nonambulatory hemiparetic patients. Stroke 26 (6), 976–981.

14. Harkema, S.J., Schmidt-Read, M., et al., 2012. Establishing the NeuroRecovery Network: multisite rehabilitation centers that provide activity-based therapies and assessments for neurologic disorders. Arch. Phys. Med. Rehabil. 93 (9), 1498–1507.

15. Behrman, A.L., Bowden, M.G., et al., 2006. Neuroplasticity after spinal cord injury and training: an emerging paradigm shift in rehabilitation and walking recovery. Phys. Ther. 86 (10), 1406–1425.

16. Harkema, S.J., Behrman, A.L., et al., 2011. Locomotor Training: Principles and Practice. Oxford University Press, USA.

17. Behrman, A.L., Harkema, S.J., 2000. Locomotor training after human spinal cord injury: a series of case studies. Phys. Ther. 80 (7), 688–700.

18. Velozo, C., Moorhouse, M., et al., 2015. Validity of the Neuromuscular Recovery Scale: a measurement model approach. Arch. Phys. Med. Rehabil. 96 (8), 1385–1396.

19. Behrman, A.L., Ardolino, E., et al., 2012. Assessment of functional improvement without compensation reduces variability of outcome measures after human spinal cord injury. Arch. Phys. Med. Rehabil. 93 (9), 1518–1529.

20. Harkema, S.J., Shogren, C., et al., 2016. Assessment of functional improvement without compensation for human spinal cord injury: extending the neuromuscular recovery scale to the upper extremities. J. Neurotrauma 33 (24), 2181–2190.

21. Gorgey, A.S., 2018. Robotic exoskeletons: the current pros and cons. World J. Orthop. 9 (9), 112–119.

22. Gorgey, A.S., Holman, M.E., 2018. The future of SCI rehabilitation: understanding the impact of exoskeletons on gait mechanics. J. Spinal Cord Med. 41 (5), 544–546.

23. Geigle, P.R., Kallins, M., 2017. Exoskeleton-assisted walking for people with spinal cord injury. Arch. Phys. Med. Rehabil. 98 (7), 1493–1495.

24. Zeilig, G., Weingarden, H., et al., 2012. Safety and tolerance of the ReWalk™ exoskeleton suit for ambulation by people with complete spinal cord injury: a pilot study. J. Spinal Cord Med. 35 (2), 96–101.

25. Gorgey, A.S., Sumrell, R., et al., 2019. Exoskeletal Assisted Rehabilitation After Spinal Cord Injury. Atlas of Orthoses and Assistive Devices, fifth ed. Elsevier, pp. 440–447, e2.

26. Indego exoskeleton website. Online 20 December 2019. Available: https://exoskeletonreport.com/product/indego/.

CHAPTER 10
Hydrotherapy

Caroline Barmatz

The surprising science that shows how being near, in, on, or under water can make you happier, healthier, more connected, and better at what you do.

Dr Wallace J. Nichols[1]

INTRODUCTION

'Hydrotherapy', derived from the Greek words '*hydor*' meaning water and '*therapeia*' meaning healing,[2] has been recognised as a treatment modality for many centuries. Originating from a passive modality, it has developed over time to include active patient participation. Physiotherapists are now being encouraged to include hydrotherapy in neuro-rehabilitation treatment principles, making the most of the physical properties of water:[3] mass, weight, density, specific gravity, buoyancy, hydrostatic pressure, surface tension, refraction and viscosity (see Table 10.1). Understanding the correct use of these properties enables the physiotherapist working in a spinal injuries unit (SIU) to prescribe, plan and apply a safe and efficient therapeutic intervention, justifying the benefits of hydrotherapy as compared to land physiotherapy for patients with a spinal cord injury (SCI). Treating patients in water allows those

who need additional support to maintain balance or stability when they move on land the novel experience of being able to move independently in water. They are able to leave walking aids and devices at the poolside and have the opportunity to enjoy the freedom of movement in water.

The pool environment, including water and air temperatures, may affect the treatment. The optimum water temperature for a therapeutic pool is 33–34°C.[4] This temperature enables the patient to perform active exercises without feeling cold or overheated, while allowing the therapist to remain in the pool for up to approximately 2 hours, maintaining thermoregulation.[5] Lower temperatures of 31–33°C are recommended for more active exercise, including aqua-aerobics, swimming, recreation and water sports. Warmer water 34–35°C is prescribed for passive treatment modalities, reducing muscle spasm and pain, thereby promoting relaxation. Higher water temperatures can be disadvantageous to the cardiovascular system and duration of immersion may be limited.

This chapter will discuss the therapeutic effects of hydrotherapy for the patient with an SCI. Included will be a brief overview of techniques that can be applied and taught that utilise the physical

213

Table 10.1 The physical properties of water

Mass	The mass of a substance (human body) is the amount of material it comprises. Mass is measured in kilograms (kg) and cannot be altered.
Clinical significance	*Observe your patient on land before entering the pool; how will the patient's altered body shape and density affect their balance in water?*
Weight	Weight is the effect of gravity upon the mass, and alters according to the position of a body in relation to the earth. Weight is measured in Newtons (N). A mass of 1 kg has a weight of 9.81 N
Clinical significance	*Will the patient be easier to direct by the therapist when in the water?* *Will your patient be able to move with less effort in water?*
Density	The density of a substance is the relationship between its mass and its volume. The average density of the human body is 974 kg/m^3 The density of water is 1000 kg/m^3
Clinical significance	*Observe the differences between the patient's upper and lower extremities, between the right and left sides of the body.* *How will this affect the patient's balance in water?*
Relative density Specific gravity	The relative density or specific gravity of a substance is the ratio of the mass of a given volume of the substance to the mass of the same volume of water.
Clinical significance	*The body is composed of many tissues with varying densities, unique to each individual.* *The trunk, which contains the air-filled lungs, floats better, whereas the lower extremities, which include the denser bone and muscle, have a tendency to sink.*
Buoyancy	**Archimedes' Principle of Buoyancy states:** When a body is fully or partially immersed in a fluid at rest, the body experiences an upward thrust equal to the weight of the fluid displaced. A body with a relative density less than 1 will be able to float. A body with a relative density more than 1 will sink.
Clinical significance	*The relative density of the human body with air in the lungs is 0.97; therefore, supine it floats just below the surface of the water.* *Nose, mouth and chest remain above the water surface allowing the patient to breathe.*
Hydrostatic pressure	**Pascal's Law states:** Fluid pressure is exerted equally on all surface areas of an immersed body at rest at a given depth.
Clinical significance	*A patient standing in shoulder depth water will feel increased resistance to chest expansion in all directions.* *Hydrostatic pressure is directly proportional to the depth of immersion; pressure increases with depth.* *Standing or walking in deep water, together with performing active exercises, decreases peripheral oedema.*

Table 10.1 The physical properties of water—cont'd

Surface tension	The force exerted between the surface molecules of a liquid acts as a resistance to movement.
Clinical significance	*Exercises can be performed while moving a limb in and out of the water. Adapted swimming techniques are a good example. Consider 'streamlined' or 'un-streamlined' objects, body parts or flotation aids.* *As a therapist, this added resistance needs to be taken into consideration when practising passive techniques; implementation of good therapist handling with appropriate therapist footwork reduces water resistance, together with patient/therapist-coordinated breath control.*
Refraction	The bending of a ray as it passes from a less dense medium (air) to a denser medium (water). The pool appears to be shallower than it is, so the range of motion for a limb may be obscured.
Clinical significance	*Is the therapist's vision obscured by being in the water with the patient?* *Is it necessary to observe the patient's position and movements from the poolside or from a different viewpoint?*
Viscocity	Viscosity acts as a resistance to movement, as the molecules of water adhere to the body surface moving through water.
Clinical significance	*As a patient walks through the water turbulence increases, adding resistance to the movement.*

properties of water. References are given at the end of the chapter for fuller descriptions of treatment techniques.

THERAPEUTIC (PHYSIOLOGICAL) EFFECTS OF EXERCISE IN WATER

> A few months after the accident I had an idea for a short film about a [tetraplegic] who lives in a dream. During the day, lying in his hospital bed, he can't move, of course. But at night he dreams that he's whole again, and is able to do anything and go everywhere.
>
> Christopher Reeve (Superman)[6]

Water can provide that medium which allows the paralysed person to move around with greater ease. The aquatic environment can improve body function and performance; pulmonary, cardiac, vascular, renal, musculoskeletal, neuromuscular and psychological systems are all affected by immersion

(see Table 10.2). Therapists should be aware of the physiological changes that occur in patients due to immersion; these same hydrodynamic principles will act on the therapist in water.[2]

Hydrotherapy (HT) can be prescribed as a treatment modality in the multidisciplinary rehabilitation of neurological disorders in general and more specifically following an SCI. A recent systematic review[3] found that hydrotherapy for patients with an SCI improved gait-kinematics, cardiorespiratory and thermoregulatory responses and reduced spasticity. Historically, the therapeutic effects of exercise in water have been well documented by Skinner and Thomson[4] and Harrison.[7] To date, Cole and Becker's comprehensive text on aquatic therapy remains the acknowledged reference text for aquatic therapists.[8]

Therapeutic physiological effects of exercise in water include:

- improved cardiovascular fitness and blood pressure

Table 10.2 Physiological effects of immersion in water by system

Respiratory system

- **Head Out of Water Immersion (HOWI)** results in an inward movement of the rib cage together with an upward movement of the diaphragm due to increased resistance from hydrostatic pressure. Central blood volume increases as blood is returned from peripheral blood vessels to the thorax, resulting in reduced lung volumes.
- High-level lesions involving the cervical and upper thoracic vertebrae will cause respiratory impairment due to the paralysis of the intercostal and abdominal muscles.
- Lesions above C5 will include diaphragmatic involvement and severe respiratory distress may be observed.
- Patients with a vital capacity of less than 1 litre should be treated with extreme care.
- If respiratory distress signals (described later in this chapter in Precautions) occur, these patients may not be suitable for hydrotherapy.
- Respiratory distress is observed more often in patients who were not swimmers prior to their SCI.

Cardiovascular system

- Loss of voluntary movement leads to loss of pumping action of the muscles, with subsequent reduction of circulation.
- Submersion in the warm water dilates the superficial blood vessels, leading to improved blood supply to the skin.
- Deeper circulation can be improved with active movement.
- As described in Chapters 4 and 6, great care must be taken in handling patients with trophic changes.

Lymphatic system

- The pressure of the water on the submerged body part is directly proportional to its depth.
- In a vertical position, standing in water, the pressure exerted distally is greater than proximally, improving circulation and reducing oedema.

Neuromuscular system

Pain	• Full range of motion may be limited due to pain; relaxation is easier to obtain while being floated in warm water. Both the warmth and the support of water help to reduce pain. The causes of pain may be a result of stretching contractures during treatment, active inflammation in the nerve sheaths or meninges, together with the accumulation of metabolites resulting from reduced circulation, due to loss of pumping action of the muscles.
Muscle strength	• In patients with an SCI there may be an alteration in muscle tone; it may be increased (hypertonicity), decreased (hypotonicity) or remain unchanged.
	• The affected muscles offer little protection to the joints; care must be taken when doing passive stretches.

Table 10.2 Physiological effects of immersion in water by system—cont'd

Skeletal system	
Range of motion	• Primary impairment after an SCI can lead to secondary movement problems with significant functional limitations due to pain and limited range of motion. • Warm water 33–34°C helps to relieve spasticity (hypertonicity). • When treating hypertonic muscles, begin the treatment session with slow, rhythmic movements of the trunk from side to side, progress from proximal to distal swaying movements facilitated by the therapist's hands placed laterally on the patient's trunk, continue with rotation of upper trunk on lower trunk, and finally elongate the limbs. • The movements can progress to be given in a greater range and with less discomfort to the patient.
Contractures	• Loss of joint movement can occur as a result of a number of pathologies e.g. fibrosis in joint structures, adaptive shortening due to muscle imbalance or heterotopic ossification. • Stretches are best given slowly in time with the patient's breathing. • Breathing should be deep and calm, increasing relaxation.
Postural system	
Balance and equilibrium	• Buoyancy, together with the turbulence created by movement, make balance in the water difficult. • This may be intensified by the visual effect of refraction, distorting the limbs under water. • Visual input is important for the patient with impaired sensation, since he/she is not able to feel the position of their body in water.
Postural adjustments	• Postural adjustments to changes of gravity are continuous while we move; small changes of equilibrium need to be counterbalanced by changes in muscle tone. • These postural adjustments must be swift, well-timed and in the adequate range of movement. • Adaptive changes in muscle tone as a protection against the forces of gravity can be seen in trunk and limbs. • Reduction of muscle tone in water and increase of muscle strength allows for the improvement of core stability and balance.

- increased respiratory muscle endurance, change of respiratory dynamics
- increased urinary output, together with significant sodium and potassium excretion
- increased ambulation, with significant training
- reduced risk of injury during exercise, fall prevention exercises
- decreased oedema, especially in lower extremities
- decreased pain, generalised and specific
- preservation and protection of health and longevity.

Following the acute phase of an SCI, the dynamic rehabilitation phase is introduced. The activation and strengthening of specific muscle groups and functional movements can be encouraged using the properties of water.

Table 10.3 Comparison of the Oxford Scale of muscle strength (land-based versus water-based)

Land-based		Water-based	
0	No contraction	1	Contraction with buoyancy assisting
1	A flicker of movement	2	Contraction with buoyancy counterbalanced
2	Movement with gravity counterbalanced	2+	Contraction against buoyancy
3	Movement against gravity	3	Contraction against buoyancy at speed
4	Movement against gravity and resistance	4	Contraction against buoyancy + light floating device
5	Normal N.B.: Normal function cannot be tested in water	5	Contraction against buoyancy + heavy floating device

Source: A. Skinner, Duffield's exercises in water, 3rd edn, WB Saunders, 1983.

TREATMENT GOALS

Treatment goals in water are similar to land-based goals, i.e. to increase muscle strength and endurance, to maintain and increase range of motion and to reduce pain, thereby promoting relaxation and improvement of sleep, to improve balance and coordination and finally to increase functional activity and recreation.[9] There are some differences between land-based and water-based muscle strength assessments, as indicated in Table 10.3.

Initially the patient's symptoms, such as pain, spasticity and muscle weakness, are relieved by being supported in warm water (Fig. 10.1); flotation aids should be prepared poolside ahead of time and used as necessary. An exercise program is gradually introduced from buoyancy supported to buoyancy resisted, providing added value to patients whose muscles are weak or paralysed.[10] On land the patient is cumbersome and difficult to move; in water the therapist is able to handle the patient with ease. The buoyancy support allows more freedom, facilitates movement and emphasises the patient's ability in water as opposed to their disability on land. Function, confidence and morale improve daily during the early stages of rehabilitation. In the longer term, 'accelerated ageing', which is an overall decline in both physiological and psychological

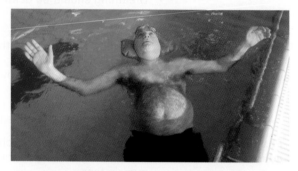

Figure 10.1 Relaxation in a supine float is demonstrated here by a chronic SCI patient. In this position, the support of a neck collar allows the patient to perform active neck movements in all directions without submerging.

mechanisms, leading to a decrease in quality of life, can be prevented or delayed. (For further detail on accelerated ageing see Chapter 15.)

GENERAL PRINCIPLES OF EXERCISES IN WATER

From the author's experience, exercises for upper and lower extremities are usually performed more easily in deeper water. Upper extremity buoyancy-assisted exercises may be performed in shallower water due to

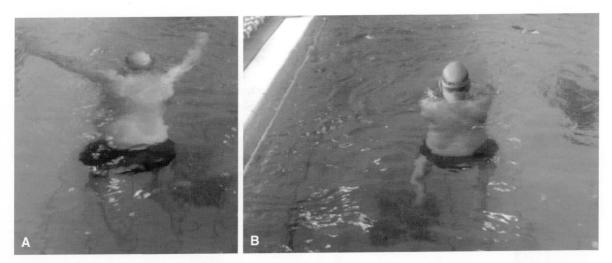

Figure 10.2 A, B The use of buoyancy for upper limb activities. Notice changes in the position of the arms affecting the position of the head.

the resistant drag produced by movement of a limb in water, increasing the effort required by weaker patients. It should also be noted that shape and density of a limb or the torso may alter resistance, making exercises more difficult to perform (Figs 10.2A, 10.2B).

- *Metacentre:* The metacentric principle is concerned with balance in water. In water the Centre of Gravity (COG) interacts with the Centre of Buoyancy (COB) and when equal and opposite the body will float. Any movement of the human body in water will alter the point of reference of these two points causing a rotational effect (Fig. 10.3).[11] In supine position, sitting or standing, any active movements of the patient's arms forwards, backwards, to the sides or raising them above water surface can challenge and improve balance (Fig. 10.4). Turbulence can be added, by movement of the therapist's hands or by walking around the patient.

- *Unilateral or bilateral movements:* One extremity can be used to provide stability e.g. holding onto the handrail, while the other extremity moves. As trunk stability improves,

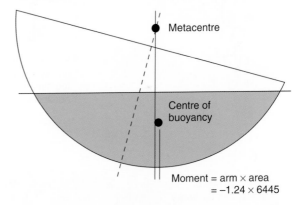

Figure 10.3 The metacentre.

bilateral extremity movement can be initiated, e.g. by standing with their back against the side of the pool, horizontally abducting arms while inhaling (Fig. 10.5A), followed by upper extremity horizontal adduction while exhaling (Fig. 10.5B). The resistance of buoyancy can be increased by lengthening the lever of the weight-arm, adding flotation devices, increasing speed of movement or the number of repetitions (Fig. 10.5C). Closed and open chain exercises can be performed.

- **Buoyancy**

Table 10.4 describes the use of buoyancy principles.

- **Frequency of treatment:** As an in-patient at an SIU patients may receive hydrotherapy two or even three times weekly. Following discharge it is recommended that in order to maintain wellness and prevent physical deterioration, it is recommended that people who have sustained an SCI visit their local swimming pool and perform general exercises in water 30–45 minutes, twice to three times per week. General exercises include walking; strengthening of the core and limbs; active stretches; breathing, including head and chest immersion; together with independent adapted swimming techniques. For safety reasons most people will always need close supervision from a poolside helper or their personal aid. Rehabilitation centres may allow

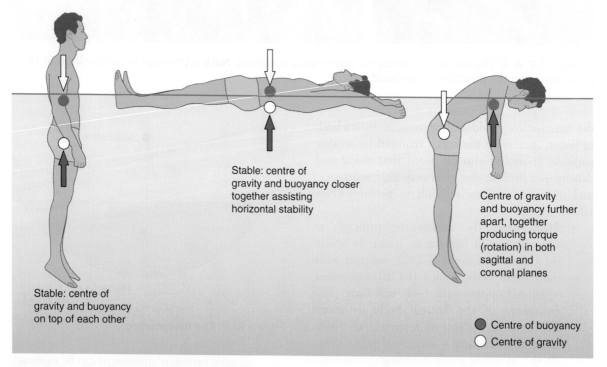

Stable: centre of gravity and buoyancy closer together assisting horizontal stability

Centre of gravity and buoyancy further apart, together producing torque (rotation) in both sagittal and coronal planes

Stable: centre of gravity and buoyancy on top of each other

- Centre of buoyancy
- Centre of gravity

Figure 10.4 Buoyancy: Metacentric effect.

Table 10.4 Use of buoyancy principles

Buoyancy-assisted movement	Buoyancy-supported movement	Buoyancy-resisted movement
Active movement towards the water surface, using buoyancy to assist very weak muscle movement.	As muscle strength increases, active exercises can be performed with the support of water.	Active exercises can be performed by moving against the resistance of water.

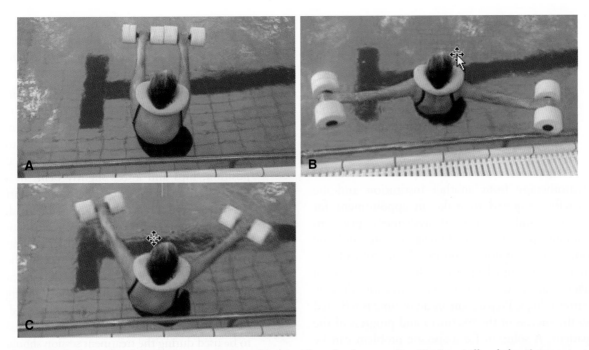

Figure 10.5 A, Active bilateral upper extremity exercises in deep water. Horizontally abducting arms while inhaling. **B** Upper extremity horizontal adduction while exhaling. **C,** Horizontal abduction of upper limbs using flotation devices.

patients to use their facilities after they have been discharged, for a minimal entrance fee. The familiarity with the pool, friendly staff and convenient surroundings have added value.

HYDROTHERAPY ASSESSMENT AND TREATMENT

In most centres, patients are referred to hydrotherapy by their attending physician when they are medically stable, or by the treating physiotherapist on land with the physician's permission.

Inpatients from the SIU require personally-prescribed hydrotherapy sessions. A treatment program is developed based on the digital medical land-based evaluations and treatment goals. It is advantageous for previous swimming competency to be shared with the pool staff, as fear of water may delay mental and physical adaptation to water following an SCI. A water-based assessment should be performed prior to or during the first visit to the pool; considerations that may need to be taken into account include demographics such as height and gender. During aquatic physiotherapy/hydrotherapy/water exercise programs and/or swimming activities, the safety of patients and service providers must be ensured at all times. It is against policy in many hospitals to have a single therapist in the pool.

Prior to commencing the hydrotherapy session, functional goals should be set, taking into consideration precautions and contraindications for aquatic therapy. These include:

- blood pressure must be stable, as on entry to the water a temporary rise in blood pressure occurs due to vasoconstriction; almost immediately vasodilation occurs with a fall in blood pressure due to the warmth of the water.

- the patient must be accompanied by the treating physiotherapist throughout the treatment; the physiotherapist must be aware of respiratory distress signals, e.g. breathlessness and sweating on the face.

- if the patient is too medically unstable to exercise on land, hydrotherapy will be contraindicated.

Outpatients with SCIs may be referred for hydrotherapy from another institution and are therefore required to make an appointment for a land- and water-based assessment prior to commencing treatment. Discharge notes and any other relevant information may be useful to bring along to the initial meeting. This visit to the pool allows patients to familiarise themselves with the new surroundings. Preparation ahead of time is reflected in the success of the treatment and progress of the patient. A solution for a specific problem can be dealt with prior to commencing treatment.

Accessibility of the facility

Most SIUs will have an accessible hydrotherapy facility. If, however, the patient is coming from home or from a different facility, transport to the pool must be planned, and the accessibility of the changing rooms taken into account. Hoists can be used in the changing room and poolside to assist with lifting and transferring patients. Pool rules and regulations should be explained, written information regarding safety should also be accessible to the patient and the person accompanying them, whether family, friend or a professional aide.

Pool entries and exits
Hoist

There are a variety of different strategies available for patients to enter and exit the pool using a hoist, including the following:

- Severely impaired patients can enter and exit on a hydraulic stretcher, if available. The tetraplegic patient with more mobility can make an assisted transfer from the wheelchair

with the help of one or two assistants poolside for safety and is then lowered slowly into the pool on the hoist chair. Fig. 10.6 shows a chair hoist available for pool entry.

- The receiving therapist should be waiting in the water prepared to receive the patient, the ideal water depth being approximately 1.10 m. It is important for the receiving therapist to be stable and to maintain a well-balanced position, hips and knees slightly bent, in a lunge position, arms reaching up to support the patient; eye contact should be maintained, and verbal cues used as necesary. As the patient enters the water, the therapist transfers weight to his/her hind foot in order to receive the patient while maintaining balance. The patient may be received in a saddle position, sitting astride the therapist, supported as needed. Necessary equipment (neck and pelvic floats) to be used during the treatment session should be placed poolside ahead of time.

Ramp

Some hydrotherapy pools are designed with a ramp for easy entry and exit on a shower chair or ease of entry and exit (Figs 10.7A and B).

Independent entry

Given time, and with physical improvement, paraplegics can be taught to enter and exit the pool independently from the poolside; this may also be possible for high-functioning tetraplegics, especially if the lesion is incomplete. Patients with better trunk control can be taught to make a transfer from their wheelchair to a sitting position on to a specially designed metal plate with a handrail (Figs 10.8A, B, C). A forward or combined rotational entry can be made into the water independently (Fig. 10.8D and E) or with support, as needed. An assistant may be needed poolside to provide support or supervise the patient from behind, in order to prevent the patient falling backwards. For the patient with spastic lower extremities, select water depth deep enough to prevent injury from the pool floor.

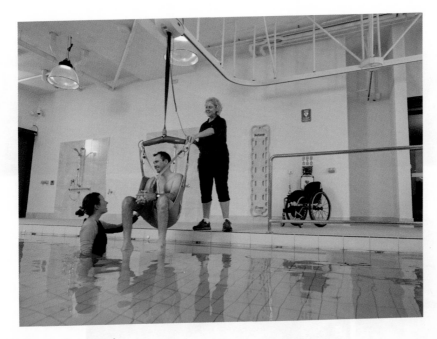

Figure 10.6 Hoist entry into pool
Source: Courtesy Spinal Life Australia

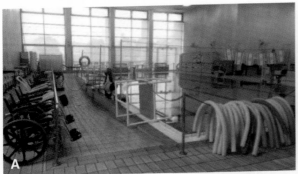

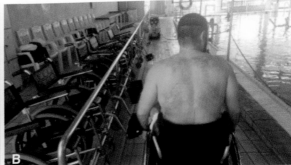

Figure 10.7 A, B, Independent entry via ramp.

Steps

As the patient's land-based functional mobility improves, or for high-functioning patients with incomplete SCI, entry and exit can be via the steps (Fig. 10.9A and B). Handrails should be placed either side with support rails at both 90 cm and 60 cm height, allowing the patient to sit down on the steps while maintaining arm support.

Precautions

Certain precautions must be taken prior to any hydrotherapy session.

These include:

1. **Check open wounds** – open wounds may not necessarily prevent the patient from participating in a hydrotherapy session. Wounds must be small enough to be

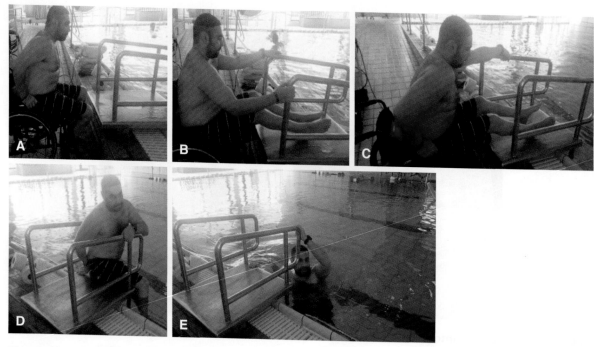

Figure 10.8 A–E, Poolside independent entry.

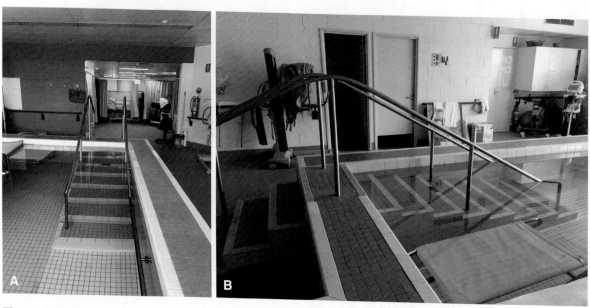

Figure 10.9 Entry steps with handrails for more mobile patients.

covered with waterproof dressings that provide waterproof wound coverage and reduce the risk of infection from airborne bacteria, urine and faeces.

2. **Sensitive skin** – ensure that feet are placed on wheelchair footrests when treating patients with reduced or no sensation. Take special care during transfers in and out of the pool. In the pool, some patients may choose to wear protective socks, shoes or knee pads, to prevent skin damage, when limbs are dragged unintentionally on the rough pool floor in shallow water. Damaged skin/pressure ulcers take time to heal, preventing or delaying further pool therapy (see Chapter 4 on pressure injuries).

3. **Vasomotor** – when moving from one position to another in the water the patient may experience orthostatic or postural hypotension. This is due to the involvement of the autonomic nervous system and may result in a lack of vasoconstriction. The treating therapist must always be prepared to apply

emergency measures, such as pulling the hoist chair into the horizontal position and elevating the patient's lower limbs (see Chapter 4 on orthostatic or postural hypotension).

4. **Cervical instability** – Philadelphia neck collar: If the fracture or dislocation is not stable or has not consolidated the patient must enter the pool wearing a solid neck collar; **extra care must be taken.**

5. **Jewett back brace/halo traction (heads should be kept above water level)** – these patients can be treated with care in water, preferably in a vertical position standing and walking, not swimming.

6. **Tracheotomy** – Ensure adequate flotation equipment is available to keep the tracheostomy site out of water, in the vertical or supine; therapists should be specialised clinical experts (Fig. 10.10A and B).

7. **Uncontrolled bladder and bowel incontinence** – Patients are showered, and bladder and bowel must be emptied before entering the pool. Since most patients are

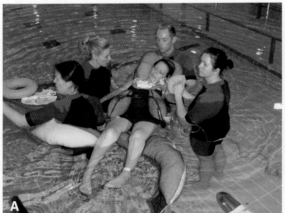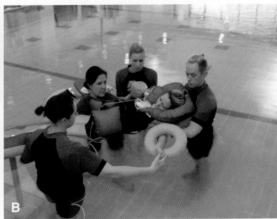

Figure 10.10 A, B, Ensure tracheotomy is kept out of the water by using adequate flotation equipment.

Source: Wegner S, Thomas P, et al., 2017. Hydrotherapy for the long-term ventilated patient: A case study and implications for practice. Australian Critical Care 30 (6), 328–331.

catheterised, catheter bags should be emptied prior to treatment and secured firmly to the patient's leg. Waterproof pants must be worn underneath knee length Lycra tights. Treatment should be delayed if a patient has a urinary infection.

8. **Stomas** – colostomy, ileostomy, urostomy, suprapubic appliances can be allowed in the pool with appropriate handling. The stoma site can be wrapped with plastic wrap, with appropriate clothing worn.

9. **Limited endurance, cardiac involvement, respiratory compromise, orthostatic hypotension** – patients must be closely monitored, starting with shorter treatment sessions.

10. **Autonomic dysreflexia** – a medical emergency that can lead to death. Prior to hydrotherapy, it should be ensured that all the necessary resources are available to carry out a self-management plan in such an emergency, sometimes requiring the assistance of a carer (see Chapter 4).

Screening prior to entering hydrotherapy pool

With the continuing advancement of knowledge in hydrotherapy, infection control and specific benefits of aquatic physiotherapy and water exercise, patients with SCIs where hydrotherapy may previously have been contraindicated can now be safely treated in the water.[12]

GUIDELINES AND STANDARDS

A number of guidelines and standards for aquatic therapy are available worldwide.

A physiotherapy program utilising the properties of water, designed by a suitably qualified Physiotherapist. The program should be specific for an individual to maximise function, which can be physical, physiological or psychological. Treatments should be carried out by appropriately trained personnel, ideally in a

purpose built, and suitably heated Aquatic Physiotherapy Pool.[13]

Guidelines and standards used in this chapter are taken from the Indian Guidelines and Standards booklet.[14] Other guidelines include:

- Australian Guidelines for Aquatic Therapists 2nd edition (2015)
- The Aquatic Therapy Association of Chartered Physiotherapists UK (2015).

(See Online resources at end of chapter for website details.)

Aims of water-based treatment

- Improvement of vital capacity and breath control
- Reduction of hypertonicity/spasticity
- Reduction/prevention of contractures
- Restoration, improvement and maintenance of balance
- Inhibition of abnormal motor patterns, re-education of normal voluntary movement
- Improvement of balance and re-education of postural reflexes
- Encouragement of swimming and independence to improve morale.

CONVENTIONAL HYDROTHERAPY TECHNIQUES

Acute/early rehabilitation phase
Buoyancy assisted, supported and resisted exercises

In the early stages of rehabilitation following an SCI, active exercises can be performed in water while the patient is in supine position or standing with the support of floats. In time, as the patient gains confidence, and their competency and physical adjustment to water improves, exercises can be made more challenging. These can include supine and prone diagonal starting positions, progressing to

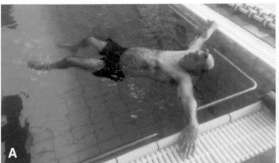
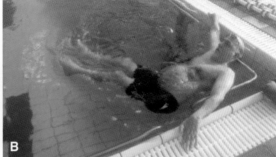

Figure 10.11 A, Supine float active breath control exercises. B, Active trunk side flexion with upper extremity support.

performing assisted active transfers in water, sit to stand, sit to supine or prone lying. Kneeling and half-kneeling can be added, together with more active activities, such as adapted swimming techniques and active transfers initiated by the patient and reaching forward or to the side. Resistance can be increased by lengthening the lever arm, increasing the speed of movement, adding or decreasing flotation devices and increasing the number of repetitions.[8]

Adjustment to the water – supine float position

Treatment should begin slowly, allowing the patient to adjust both mentally and physically to treatment sessions in water. For those patients with SCIs who are unable to stand it is advisable to start in a supine float position. The patient's head is supported by the therapist's shoulder or elbow; a neck float may be useful to free the therapist's hands. Ideally the patient's head can be immersed in a relaxed position, supported by buoyancy without increasing tension of the cervical spine. Try to keep both ears under water; the feeling of having one's ears move in and out of the water may be uncomfortable (earplugs may be recommended). A pelvic float may be necessary as spastic lower extremities have a tendency to sink. The patient gradually adjusts to the water, relaxing and getting used to the feeling of weightlessness, using the rail for guidance as they adapt to body imbalance (Figs 10.11A and B). The patient should be aware

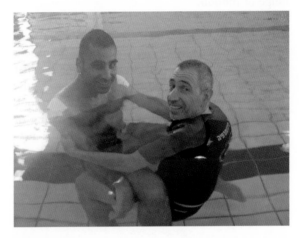

Figure 10.12 Face-to-face saddle position.

that their body will rise and fall as they breathe in and out. Mental and physical adjustment is dependent on acquiring breath control while immersed, together with the control of balance against turbulence.

Seated positions in water

To aid the patient into a seated position, the therapist squats down in the water, with the patient in an upright position facing the therapist, sitting astride the therapist's legs in a saddle position (Fig. 10.12). If lower extremity spasticity does not allow this position, the patient's legs, with knees extended or flexed, can be placed in between the therapist's knees. Allow buoyancy to support the patient, aiming for maximum independence. Keeping the patient's shoulders below water level allows the therapist to give minimum support; the therapist's forearms are supinated, palms up, no gripping. Tension increases density causing the body to sink, preventing flotation. Head out of water immersion (HOWI) is ideal to develop water confidence, while encouraging the inexperienced patient to adapt to the new environment, observing, conversing and adjusting breath and balance control. Treatment sessions can focus on relieving pain, decreasing oedema and improving passive, active and resisted range of motion.

Standing in water

In chest level water, the therapist can assist the patient to stand up (Fig. 10.13A), sometimes for the first time, back against the side of the pool, facing the therapist; this position allows the patient to look around and see what other patients are doing or to generally familiarise themselves with the new surroundings. Being able to see what is going on in the pool reduces anxiety. The acoustics in a swimming pool are sometimes problematic, making it difficult for patients to hear. Standing in the vertical position

with ears out of the water enables the patient to hear the therapist's instructions; having the mouth out of the water allows the patient to communicate verbally. Patients with atrophic lower extremities may need weights to be placed around their ankles to prevent their legs from rising up towards the water surface. The patient can then turn around to face the poolside, and stand reaching for the handrail for support (Fig. 10.13B).

Immersion

Standing by the poolside the patient can begin the treatment session with breathing exercises; initially oral breath control (OBC) is taught by instructing the patient to perform cervical neck flexion, the mouth moving towards the water surface, progressing to exhaling while blowing bubbles (Fig. 10.14A).

Since water exerts pressure on the immersed body, the therapist should be aware of any difficulty in breathing that may occur because of increased pressure on the chest wall (Fig. 10.14B). The venous return is sensitive to external pressure changes, including compression from surrounding muscles and external water pressure. Blood is displaced from the periphery, causing a rise in right atrial pressure, pleural surface pressure rises and the diaphragm is displaced upwards

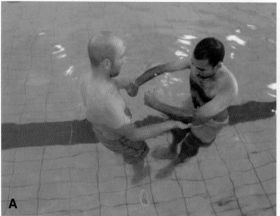
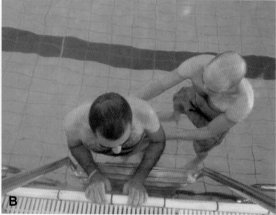

Figure 10.13 A, Standing supported by forearms, focus on improving balance in the vertical position. B, Standing with support of ladder.

into the chest cavity.[2] Central blood volume increases by 0.7 L (60%) during immersion up to the neck. Increasing resistance to inspiration increases cardiac volume by 30% (Fig. 10.15).

To gain nasal breath control (NBC), the patient submerges their nose and mouth while humming, to prevent water from being inhaled up the nose. Progression then continues to total head immersion (THI) while standing, performing a mini-squat and counting the number of seconds the patient is capable of remaining under water. When the patient can confidently remain immersed for 20–30

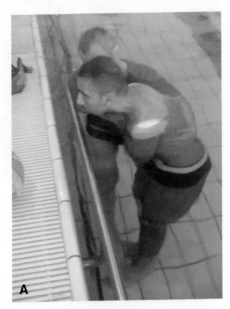
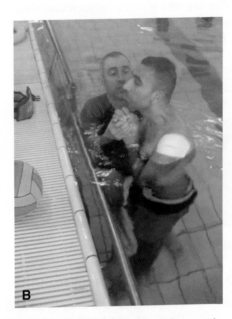

Figure 10.14 A, Early stage supported standing in water. B, Note accessory muscle exertion while patient tries to lift his head.

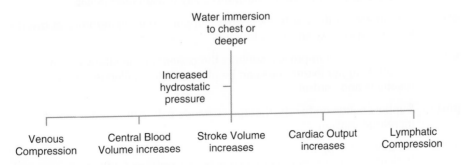

Figure 10.15 HOWI immersion – schematic cardiac changes.

Source: Adapted from Becker, BE, 2009. Aquatic therapy: scientific foundations and clinical rehabilitation applications. PM&R 1 (9), 859–872.

seconds a transfer to a prone float can be introduced. Progressing to prone floating with a snorkel (Fig. 10.16), in this position passive manipulation or myofascial release around the scapula can be included to reduce pain and restore flexibility.

As the patient regains control and balance, the support given by the therapist is gradually reduced. The therapist moves from a hands-on to a hands-off approach, allowing the patient to incresase their confidence and move towards independence in the water (Fig. 10.17, Table 10.5).

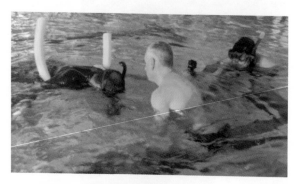

Figure 10.16 Total immersion.

Independence

Patients can be taught to support themselves independently by hooking their elbows over the handrail. In a therapeutic hydrotherapy pool, the rail should be installed 10–15 cm below the

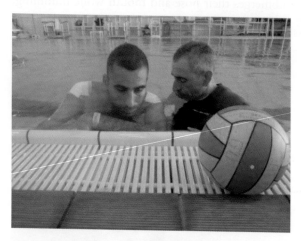

Figure 10.17 Therapist support for SCI patient – support can be given facing the patient while maintaining eye contact, from the side or from behind.

Table 10.5 Supports for patient with an SCI

Full support	For patients with poor head and trunk control, support can be provided by the therapist, one hand supporting the head at the occiput, the other hand on the trunk. A patient with an open tracheostomy should be taken into the pool by an experienced therapist with good handling techniques.
Trunk support	Support can be given on the scapulae; as balance improves support can be provided more distally on the trunk, moving distally towards the pelvis.
Arm support	For patients with poor trunk control, support upper extremities above the elbows, keeping upper extremities adducted.
Elbow support	As trunk control improves, support the patient at the elbows or more distally on the forearms; upper extremities can be abducted to challenge the patient's balance reactions and control.
Hand support	Support hands on hands, therapist's hands palms up, no gripping to prevent increased tension.
Independence	No physical support. Patient progresses from verbal cues to eye contact, finally becoming independent. For safety as a precaution against drowning, a patient with an SCI will almost always need an adult keeping an eye on them from the poolside.

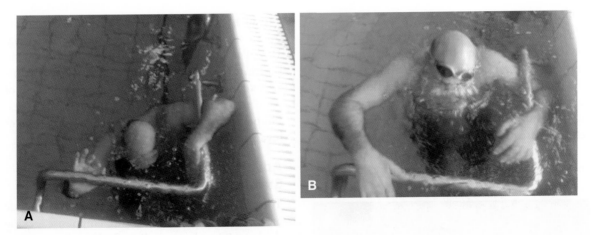

Figure 10.18 A, Oral breath control. B, Nasal breath control.

water surface, approximately 7 cm distance away from the pool wall; in the corners, 14 cm allows elbows to be hooked onto the handrail with the patient's back to the wall. The therapist stands at the patient's side, in order to maintain vision of breath control abilities; the patient can start breathing exercises, immersing chin, mouth, nose, progressing to full head immersion (Figs 10.18A and B); the resistance given from the water is mostly felt during inspiration.

Transfers in water – vertical to supine

To transfer from standing up to supine lying, known as 'transverse rotation control', the therapist moves to shallower water, i.e. water level to the base of sternum. The therapist stands behind the patient, hands palms-up, forearms supinated, hands supporting the patient at the lumbar-sacral level, therapist's fingers flared bilaterally, resting on the patient's iliac crest. The thrapist's hands are then rotated, fingers pointing downwards into a 'backing hold' as the patient bends down into a squat, shoulders in the water. Head movements greatly influence the position of the body in water. The patient looks up towards the ceiling, head slowly extending, while maintaining cervical elongation to avoid neck hyperextension; arms abduct out to the sides as much as possible, depending on the upper

extremity range of motion. The patient lies back while inhaling, slowly relaxing into a 'supine float'. Lower extremities in patients with moderate-to-severe spasticity may need the support of a float under the knees. Recovery from a supine float to the vertical should be practised, commanding the patient to bring their head forwards, chin to chest, looking towards the poolside, reaching forward with the arms, bending the knees, preferably exhaling. Neck collars may be used as necessary. Handling by a specialised therapist is a must, especially after high-level SCIs.

Intermediate rehabilitation phase
Movement in water

Floating supine in the water allows the patient to maintain breath control with greater ease. Balance control must be mastered, and facilitation of active arm movements, known as 'sculling', can be taught to propel the body through the water (Fig. 10.19). Initially the therapist walks slowly backwards, applying pressure to either side of the patient's trunk, facilitating a swaying movement from side to side, a technique call 'seaweeding'. This progresses to the therapist standing at the patient's head and walking backwards while making turbulent movements with the hands, pulling the patient into an area of negative pressure; this movement is known as 'turbulent gliding'.

Rolling over

When the patient is able to maintain a prone float for 10 seconds, transfers from supine lying to prone can be facilitated 'longitudinal rotational control'. The patient is taught to turn the head to one side (e.g. right as in Fig. 10.20A), while protracting the right scapula, if possible reaching forward with the left arm across the midline of the trunk.

The patient is instructed to cross their left leg over the right if possible (lower extremity adduction).

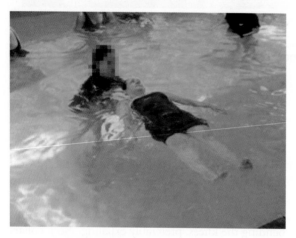

Figure 10.19 Sculling.

Crossing the midline assists the patient while rolling over to a prone float, head immersed, exhaling (Fig. 10.20B). Pressure on the chest is increased and breathing becomes more difficult. Arm movements are encouraged in supine or prone with the use of paddles if necessary to increase palm surface area. Flippers can be used to increase the lever length of lower extremities.

Advanced rehabilitation phase
Standing

The patient can practise standing facing the poolside or between the parallel bars and, emphasise locking the knee joints by extending the hips. Support can be given by holding onto parallel bars or a handrail. The therapist supports manually at the pelvis, knees and feet from in front, at the side or behind. Splints and ankle weights may be used if necessary.

Gait training

Walking forwards, backwards and sideways in water can be introduced before the patient is able to ambulate on land. Support is given by the up-thrust of the water, using the appropriate depth according to the patient's ability. Hip flexion in water is buoyancy-assisted, making it easier to

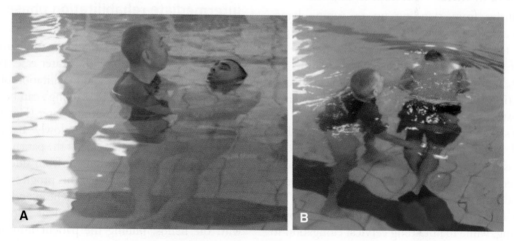

Figure 10.20 A, Teaching the patient to roll – turning the head to one side. B, Teaching the patient to roll – final position.

Table 10.6 Reduction in weight-bearing in water

10%	Shoulders under water	Non-weight bearing, toe touch
30%	Xyphoid	Partial weight bearing
50%	ASIS	Full weight bearing

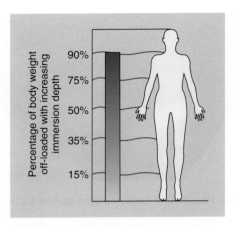

Figure 10.21 Percentage of weight relief according to depth of water.

perform; hip extension is buoyancy resisted, the support of the water allowing the patient more time to react, and assistance can be given by flotation aids or appropriate handling from the therapist. The use of buoyancy and turbulence can be introduced to improve strength, balance and coordination, progressing from deep water ambulation to shallower water and less support. Use the pool floor tiles to walk in a straight line, timing how long it takes to walk across the pool and the number of widths walked.

The degree of proficiency in walking depends on the level of the lesion; with lower level lesions abdominal muscles are retained; in higher levels only the latissimus dorsi muscles are working (for more detail on ambulation see Chapter 9). Buoyancy assists lifting the body in water, an advantage of gait training in the pool.

Re-education of walking can be facilitated in the pool; appropriate depth of water should be chosen, depending on percentage of weight relief (Table 10.6, Fig. 10.21). Weight transference can be practised in stance or stride, altering the base of support.

Underwater treadmills are available in many therapeutic pools and have been shown to be extremely effective in retraining gait after SCI, as well as improving cardiorespiratory and thermoregulatory responses and reducing spasticity.[15]

Balance re-education and falls prevention

Balance re-education and fall prevention exercises can be practised, changing the base of support from wide to narrow, progressing from stance to stride, while gait exercises are performed in water. Falling

is slower in water due to its properties.[12] Energy expenditure has been found to be lower during underwater walking as compared to land-based walking at specific speeds, which allows patients to walk for longer.[15]

Flotation aids

Flotation aids should be used as needed; however, their use delays independence in water, alters balance and can be dangerous. The support given by therapist may be easily altered according to patient ability.

Active exercises for the upper extremities

The strengthening of upper extremity muscle is most important in assisting paraplegics to prepare for wheelchair use or ambulation with crutches and performing push-ups and transfers (strengthens shoulder extensors, adductors and elbow extensors) (Fig. 10.22A and B).

Use of resistance

The water itself can be used as a means of resistance to exercise. In addition, floats, weights, balls and bats can be used to increase resistance, and speed can be increased or lever lengthened (Fig. 10.23).

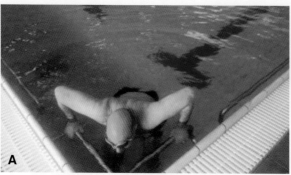 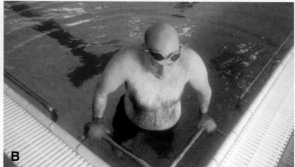

Figure 10.22 A, B, Independent active push-ups.

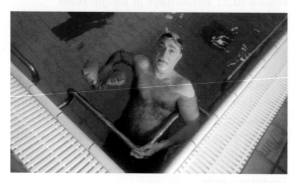

Figure 10.23 Active upper extremity exercises with flotation equipment buoyancy supported, while holding onto handrail independently.

Games (gamification)

Ball games in water help to improve control and speed of reaction, as well as being fun. Water polo can be taught to patients, and participation in group activities can be encouraged.

SWIMMING

Modification of swim strokes

The patient is encouraged to move into a horizontal position by transferring from a sitting position in water to a back float. As balance and breath control improves, sculling bilateral arm movements are introduced, progressing to a basic back stroke, by

lifting the arms slowly up and out of the water, keeping them low, then bringing them down with a propulsive movement. A supine float may be added in order to create movement, improve coordination and progress to adapted swimming.

Paraplegic SCI

A patient with a paraplegic SCI can progress from double arm back crawl to alternate arm back crawl. It should be taken into account that with every stroke of the arm the trunk and pelvis rotate because the paralysed legs cannot counteract the movement. This can be prevented with low sculling movements.

After learning recovery techniques and floating control, patients can advance to learning swim strokes. The neck and upper extremities are used to compensate for the loss of leg mobility. Paraplegics learn to control the roll from prone to supine, supine to prone and prefer to swim adapted front crawl prone (mostly lower motor lesions).

Tetraplegic SCI

The patient with a tetraplegic SCI must learn to exhale when their face is immersed. Swimming prone is more difficult, most patients with tetraplegia preferring to swim supine (Fig. 10.24A and B) or swim an adapted breast stroke. After a few strokes with the head in the water, the neck is hyperextended to bring the head out of the water to breathe (Fig. 10.24C).

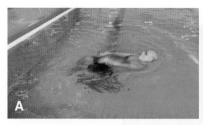 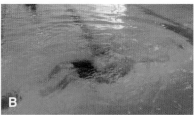 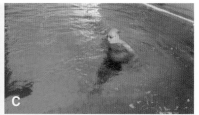

Figure 10.24 A, Transferring from the poolside to supine. **B,** progressing with bilateral arm movements and submersion, requiring good breath control. **C,** performing a forward recovery to the vertical with nose and mouth out of water to breathe.

Swimming training equipment

A flotation belt or noodle can be used to assist the SCI patient who finds it difficult to float independently due to limited motor control. Masks and snorkels can be used in prone swimming to reduce the repetitive strain placed on joints with the breathing technique, or to compensate for poor breath control.

Modified pools
Underwater cameras/virtual reality

The ability of the patient and the clinician to monitor and visually see gait patterns without looking down is essential to regaining normal function. Clinicians can instruct patients on how to correct their movements immediately. For a patient with an SCI to be able to see their legs moving underwater also does wonders for their mental outlook. The virtual reality screen is placed poolside, along with the digital information references (Fig. 10.25A). A camera is placed underwater to record the patient's movements (Fig. 10.25B and C).

Mechanised floor with adjustable depth

Patients recovering from SCIs frequently have mobility issues that make getting in and out of a therapy pool difficult. Moveable floors allow for zero depth entry and can be raised or lowered in just 30 seconds, making them safe and easily accessible for all patients, eliminating the need for ladders or steps.

Resistance jets

Variable speed resistance jets allow clinicians to adjust the level of water pressure and vary the intensity of the workout accordingly.

Family inclusion and education

Where possible, including the patient's family within all aspects of the rehabilitation process and specifically within water-based activities is highly recommended, as this can become a family-based activity.

SPECIFIC HYDROTHERAPY TECHNIQUES

Specific approaches can be introduced together with conventional hydrotherapy techniques.

Caveat: Please refer to the individual websites for further information on all of these specific methods and concepts.

The Halliwick Concept©

The Halliwick Concept was founded by James McMillan in London UK in 1949. The main aims of the program are to teach the swimmers about themselves and their balance control in water and to teach them to swim.

The Association of Swimming Therapy was formed in 1952. Fun is emphasised, including playing games in water, organising races and competitions, open water swims and diving. The Halliwick Concept is

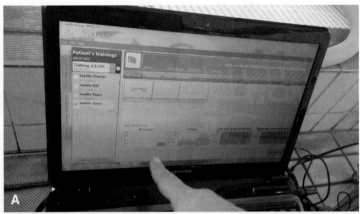

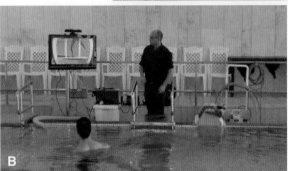
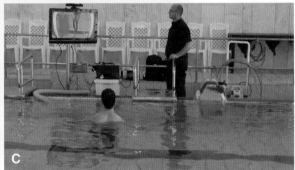

Figure 10.25 A–C, Underwater cameras with monitor.

now practised in many countries throughout the world.[9]

The Bad Ragaz Ring Method©

The Bad Ragaz Ring Method (BRRM) originated in Germany, where it was adapted and developed, before being taken to Bad Ragaz, Switzerland in the 1930s. The primary purpose was to promote stabilisation of trunk and extremities through exercise, while working on resistive exercise patterns of movement with the patient floating, supported at the neck, pelvis and ankles by floats or 'rings'. The BRRM was further developed by physiotherapists Beatrice Eggar and James McMillan,[16] who incorporated the Proprioceptive Neuromuscular Facilitation (PNF) techniques using three-dimensional diagonal movements into the new BRRM.[5]

In the last ten years, the new BRRM has been further developed by physiotherapists Johan Lambeck and Urs Gamper. Treatment is focused on modulation of pain and muscular relaxation. The BRRM is indicated for relatively weak patients.[8]

Aquastretch™ for spinal cord injuries

AquaStretch™, an aquatic form of assisted stretching and myo-fascial release, was created by George Eversaul in the United States. It may benefit both the rehabilitation and wellness maintenance of persons with an SCI.

AquaStretch™ is described as combining the unique properties of water, patient-controlled movement and therapist pressure to break down fascial adhesions.[16]

Clinical adaptation of Watsu©

Watsu began in the early 1980s at Harbin Hot Springs, California, when Harold Dull started floating people, applying the moves and stretches of the Zen shiatsu he had studied in Japan. Watsu has been demonstrated to be effective in the treatment of both old and new injuries. The introduction of Watsu at the beginning of a treatment session to decrease tone and increase soft tissue mobility has been shown to be extremely effective, with its emphasis on trunk elongation and rotation.[17]

Clinical adaptation of Ai Chi©

Created by Jun Kunno, Japan in 1993, Clinical Ai Chi is distinguished as a specialised active form of aquatic therapy. Ai Chi uses breathing techniques and progressive resistance training in water to relax and strengthen the body, based on elements of qigong and Tai Chi Chuan. Attention to posture and breathing with the visualisation and imagery of upright positioning help to place the body in proper alignment. Like Tai Chi, Ai Chi combines slow, fluid, rhythmic movements together with controlled breathing, excellent for fall prevention exercise.[8]

Clinical adaptation of the Jahara® aquatic technique

The Jahara® aquatic technique was developed by Mario Jahara in 1995 and combines body awareness and health body mechanics. It utilises the gentle power of water to perform micro-adjustments to the structural alignment of the body. Aided by a flexible flotation device called the Third Arm, Jahara practitioners provide precise support to the body structure. This support combined with gentle traction elongates the spine and decompresses the neuromuscular system. The head is always leading the movement. The technique is based on The Alexander Technique. The five concepts of Jahara are Expansion, Support, Effortlessness, Invisibility and Adaptability.[8]

Blue mind

Dr Wallace J. Nichols has attempted to link the effects of hydrotherapy with neuroscience, and research including electroencephalogram (EEG) scanning apparatus. The data from the electrodes in a specialised swimming cap were sampled and analysed, allowing neuroscientists to see in real time which areas of the brain were being stimulated during exercises in water.

Evidence-based practice points

- Immersion in water, with all its physical properties, is an exceptional medium in which to treat a person with an SCI, both in the acute, sub-acute and chronic stages of rehabilitation.
- Hydro/aquatherapy has been shown to have positive effects on the respiratory, cardiovascular and musculoskeletal systems of the patient with an SCI.
- In order to qualify to treat patients with an SCI in the water all personnel are required to undergo specialised training.
- Paraplegic patients, tetraplegic patients and high cervical lesions with and without tracheostomy can all be treated in water.
- Specialised hydrotherapy pools with various forms of accessibility are available.
- There are many specialised concepts and methods of treatment in water available, such as Halliwick, Bad Ragaz, AquaStretch, Watsu, Ai Chi.

SUMMARY

Hydro/aquatherapy should begin, where possible, during the acute phase of rehabilitation and be continued through the sub-acute and chronic phases. As discussed in this chapter, the physical and physiological properties of water can be utilised to great effectiveness in the rehabilitation of the person with an SCI. The positive psychological effects of therapy in a medium such as water also cannot be overlooked and often individuals with SCIs will continue to attend a pool long after therapy as such has ceased. As discussed in Chapter 13, watersports is an area that people with SCIs can actively take part in, irrespective of the level of their lesion. It is also a medium where the individual with an SCI can participate with their family.

There is relatively little evidence-based research on hydro/aquatherapy. Further investigation into the benefits of this form of therapy is necessary to prove its effectiveness and to explore the possible carryover of hydrotherapy to functional improvement on land.

CASE STUDIES

Case study 1

A six-year-old girl injured in a motor vehicle accident, with no previous swimming experience, extremely fearful of water. High-level lesion, tetraplegia C4 - ASIA A, very little active motor control, combined with an open tracheostomy. Hydrotherapy was initiated as an addition to land therapy when the patient reached a functional plateau: she was able to steer her wheelchair independently, using an adapted joystick.

The patient had no control of her lower extremities, a hypotonic trunk, with minimal use of her right hand. She was highly intelligent; her fear of the water could be seen in her eyes. Treating her in the water was a challenge for the therapist, who had to be experienced and have excellent handling techniques. Having had little previous experience in water combined with her physical disability it was decided not to continue hydrotherapy for this particular patient.

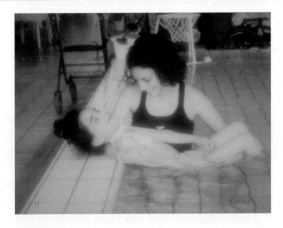

Case study 2

Father of three, aged 42, while riding on his bicycle, he crashed into a parked truck. He suffered from an incomplete SCI together with a fractured pelvis. Highly motivated to recover and return to his daily life, hydrotherapy was introduced into his rehabilitation program early on. He received land physiotherapy on a daily basis, hydrotherapy two to three times a week.

CASE STUDIES—cont'd

On the days when he did not receive hydrotherapy treatment, he came to the pool and practised independently.

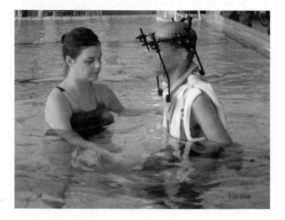

Case study 3
Patient injured in a diving accident, received hydrotherapy twice a week. In order to overcome the mental fear of diving, we organised a diving session with the help of a qualified PADI (Progressional Association of Diving Instructors) diving instructor.

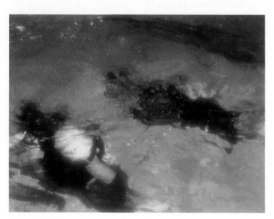

Case study 4
A 33-year-old soldier wounded in battle when a wall collapsed on him, suffered an SCI leaving him totally paralysed in his upper extremities, with partial lower extremity active movement 'walking tetraplegia'. He is wheelchair dependent with an aid 24/7. One of the highlights of his week is his visit to the pool, where he has learnt to swim with a snorkel.

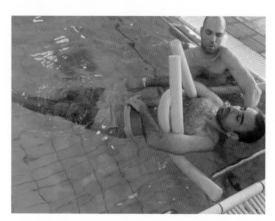

Online resources

The Aquatic Therapy Association of Chartered Physiotherapists UK, 2015. https://atacp.csp.org.uk/content/guidance-good-practice-aquatic-physiotherapy-2015

Australian Guidelines for Aquatic Therapists 2nd Edition, 2015. https://australian.physio/membership/national-groups/aquatic?hkey=625403c5-6db2-430e-99a1-1ab8747bcf64

Guidelines and Standards for Aquatic Therapy India – Aquatic Therapy Network of India 2017

Hydrotherapy techniques

Ai Chi, http://clinicalaichi.org

Aquastretch, https://www.aquastretchcanada.com

Bad Ragaz Ring method hydrotherapy: www.badragazringmethod.org/en/

Blue Mind, https://www.healingwaves.org.je/blue-mind/

Halliwick Concept, halliwick.org

Jahara, https://www.jahara.com

Watsu, https://www.watsu.com

References

1. Nichols Wallace, J., 2015. Blue Mind. Little, Brown and Company, New York.

2. Weston, C.F., O'Hare, J.P., et al., 1987. Haemodynamic changes in man during immersion in water at different temperatures. Clin. Sci. 73 (6), 613–616.

3. Ellapen, T.J., Hammill, H.V., et al., 2018. The benefits of hydrotherapy to patients with spinal cord injuries. Afr. J. Disabil. 7 (0), 450.

4. Skinner Alison, T., Thomson Ann, M. (Eds.), 1989. Duffield's Exercise in Water, third ed. Ballière Tindall, London.

5. Boyle, A., 1981. The Bad Ragaz Ring Method. Physiotherapy 67 (9), 265–268.

6. Reeve Christopher, 1998. Still Me. Cambria Productions, UK.

7. Harrison, R.A., 1980. A quantitative approach to strengthening exercises in the hydrotherapy pool. Physiotherapy 66 (2), 60.

8. Cole, A.J., Becker, B.E., 2011. Comprehensive Aquatic Therapy, thirrd ed. Washington State University Publishing, Pullman WA.

9. Martin, J., 1981. The Halliwick method. Physiotherapy 67 (10), 288–291.

10. Frye, S.K., Ogonowska-Slodownik, A., et al., 2017. Aquatic exercise for people with spinal cord injury. Arch. Phys. Med. Rehabil. 98 (1), 195–197.

11. Campion, M.R., 1997. Hydrotherapy: Principles and Practice. Elsevier.

12. Li, C., Khoo, S., et al., 2017. Effects of aquatic exercise on physical function and fitness among people with spinal cord injury. Medicine (United States) 96 (11).

13. The Aquatic Therapy Association of Chartered Physiotherapists UK, 2015. Online 19 December 2019. Available: https://atacp.csp.org.uk/content/guidance-good-practice-aquatic-physiotherapy-2015.

14. Standards for Aquatic Therapy India – Aquatic Therapy Network of India 2017 Indian Guidelines and Standards booklet 2017. Online 19 December 2019. Available: www.halliwick.net/pdf/2018/Proceedings_4th_ICEBAT_Conference_India.pdf.

15. Dolbow, J.D., Gassler, J., et al., 2016. Underwater treadmill training after neural-paralytic injury. Clin. Kinesiol. 70 (1).

16. Alejo, T., Shilhanek, C., et al., 2018. The effects of an aquatic manual therapy technique, Aquastretch™ on recreational athletes with lower extremity injuries. Int. J. Sports Phys. Ther. 13 (2), 214.

17. Dull, H., 2004. Watsu: Freeing the Body in Water. Trafford Publishing.

CHAPTER 11
Incomplete spinal and peripheral nerve lesions

Julie Vaughan-Graham

INTRODUCTION

Standardised spinal cord injury (SCI) classification is defined by the International Standards for Neurological Classification of Spinal Cord Injury (ISNCSCI), and is able, both from a clinical and a research perspective, to provide an objective neurological distinction between an incomplete and complete SCI based on the presence or not of sacral sparing (see Chapter 4 for more information on the ISNCSCI). Therefore, as per ISNCSCI classification, if a person does not have sacral sparing, even if they have motor and/or sensory function more than three levels below the neurological level of the lesion, the injury is classified as complete. From a physical rehabilitation perspective, this presents challenges as the physical rehabilitation of a person with an incomplete SCI differs significantly from that of a person with a complete SCI injury or a cauda equina injury, irrespective of whether or not they have bladder or bowel control.

INCOMPLETE SPINAL CORD INJURY (ISCI)

The ISNCSI classification defines three different types of incomplete lesions (see Appendix 1):

1. **AIS B Sensory Incomplete**: Sensory but not motor function is preserved below the neurological level and includes the sacral segments S4–5; no motor function is preserved more than three levels below the motor level on either side of the body.

2. **AIS C Motor Incomplete**: Motor function is preserved at the most caudal sacral segments for voluntary anal contraction, or sensory function is preserved at S4–5 and has some sparing of motor function more than three levels below the ipsilateral motor level on either side of the body.

3. **AIS D Motor Incomplete**: Motor function is preserved at the most caudal sacral segments for voluntary anal contraction, with at least half or more of key muscle functions below the single neurological level of injury having a muscle grade greater than or equal to 3.

Incomplete spinal cord injuries are said to account for almost 70% of all traumatic SCIs, the division between paraplegia and tetraplegia being almost equal.[1] The life expectancy for people with incomplete SCI (iSCI) approaches that of the non-injured population.[2] The amount and duration of spinal cord compression negatively relates to neurological improvement,[3] therefore early decompression within 8–24 hours following acute traumatic SCI is advocated and can improve clinical and neurological outcomes, potentially reducing healthcare costs (see Chapter 3 for early treatment paradigms immediately post-injury).[4]

Individuals with an iSCI are an extremely heterogenous group with highly variable residual innervation from a sensory, motor and autonomic perspective; therefore the deficits experienced by this group are highly variable, even with similar levels of injury.[5] Despite the significant differences between iSCI and complete SCI, and their respective recovery patterns, these subgroups of SCI are often not investigated separately.[2] The relatively low overall incidence of SCI, together with the highly heterogenous iSCI population, poses research challenges, as sufficient recruitment of similar clinical presentations is extremely challenging.[6]

A person with an iSCI presenting with any sensory or motor function below the level of the neurological lesion has, from a clinical perspective, an incomplete injury to their central nervous system. Motor control issues, such as the ease, coordination, timing, repeatability, specificity, variability, rhythm, speed and energy cost of movement, are problematic. These motor control issues extend beyond the realm of muscle strengthening and isolated muscle function. The role of the trunk, postural control, balance, atypical muscle tone, including low tone, high tone, clonus and hyper-reflexia, neurogenic pain, age-related issues and comorbidities, are not addressed in the ISNCSCI Classification model (see Chapters 15 and 18 for further information on these issues). However, individually or collectively, these issues will contribute to the complex movement dysfunction experienced by individuals with iSCI and will therefore impact upon functional outcomes.

Spinal cord syndromes

1. **Acute traumatic central cord syndrome (ATCCS):** the most common acute incomplete cervical spinal cord injury (iCSCI), accounting for 70% of all iSCI;

the patient presents with greater weakness in the upper limbs, often resulting in profound functional deficits, varying degrees of sensory loss and sphincter dysfunction.[3,7] Causes of ATCCS include cervical hyperextension, resulting in narrowing of the spinal canal and anterior protrusion of the ligamentum flavum, stenotic spinal canal due to degenerative changes and congenital narrowing.

Hyperextension injuries causing compression of the spinal cord (SC) will result in hypoxia and haemorrhage into the central grey matter of the cord. Since the peripheral rim remains intact, paralysis will typically be more severe in the upper limbs than the lower limbs, the cervical motor tracts being located centrally and lumbar and sacral tracts more peripherally.

The age distribution of ATCCS is bimodal, with the majority of patients being either under 30 years, as a result of high velocity injuries, or elderly patients who have suffered low velocity trauma with associated spinal stenosis.[3]

2. **Brown-Séquard syndrome:** results from a unilateral lesion within the spinal cord, most often due to penetrating lesions, i.e. stab wounds. As a consequence of the layout of the motor and sensory pathways, this lesion results in ipsilateral motor deficits, loss of touch and proprioception ipsilaterally (as the dorsal column medial lemniscal pathway crosses in the medulla), and loss of pain and temperature contralaterally (as the anterior lateral pathways cross in the spinal cord).[6,7] Those who sustain a lateral hemi-section of the spinal cord often demonstrate extensive motor recovery, most likely due to minor ipsilateral components of the affected corticospinal tract or the sprouting of intact contralateral corticospinal axon collaterals.[8]

3. **Anterior cord syndrome:** usually associated with a flexion injury that damages the anterior two-thirds of the spinal cord causing ischaemia in the distribution of the anterior spinal (vertebral) artery. The resultant signs and symptoms include motor paresis below the level of the lesion, due to significant disruption of the corticospinal tract, and loss of pain and temperature due to the interruption of the anterior spinothalamic tracts; light touch and proprioception are preserved.[7]

4. **Dorsal cord syndrome:** results from a posterior injury to the spinal cord with disruption of the dorsal and dorsolateral columns, resulting in loss of fine discrimination, proprioception and vibration.

5. **Syringomyelia:** a disorder in which a cyst or cavity forms within the spinal cord, which may be congenital or acquired. The most common congenital form of syringomyelia is referred to as an Arnold-Chiari malformation (or Chiari malformation). The acquired form of syringomyelia can occur as a complication of trauma, meningitis, haemorrhage, a tumour or arachnoiditis. In this last form, the cyst develops in a segment of the damaged spinal cord. Post-traumatic syringomyelia (PTS) as a diagnosis often proves difficult, as symptoms may appear months or even years after the initial injury. The primary symptom is pain, followed by weakness and sensory impairment, often originating at the site of the lesion, and may extend above and/or below the lesion site. Symptoms may be ipsilateral or bilateral, depending upon the size of the cyst.

(Please refer to Chapter 1 for more information about the anatomical and physiological details related to these syndromes.)

Basic functions of the vertebral column and spinal cord

The human spinal cord contains over 10 million neurons[9] and it is believed that peripheral nerve axons grow at approximately 1 mm per day. Depending upon the level of injury, human axons, therefore, may have to grow substantial distances to reach their former targets (see Chapter 1 for the physiological structure of the spinal cord).[10] Despite considerable research efforts in the field of spinal cord regeneration, successful bridging across the hostile lesion site remains elusive (see Chapter 1).[11–13]

In order to limit injury to the spinal cord and support recovery post-injury, humans have developed a number of other protective mechanisms. The spinal cord has considerable redundancy, with important functions such as walking being possible with approximately only 5–15% of a functional spinal cord.[10] Specific neural networks within the spinal cord, such as the central pattern generator (CPG), serve important functions, such as locomotion, by centralising control (see Chapter 3 for the role of the CPG), with sacral networks controlling bladder, bowel and sexual functions. Lastly, spinal cord plasticity provides a mechanism for uninjured fibres to assume new functions, as well as creating new connections.[8]

Neuroplasticity

Neuroplasticity has been described as: 'the tendency of neural circuits to undergo physiological and/or structural changes in response to changes in patterns of use that are brought about by injury or environmental influences'.[7,14] Neuroplasticity comprises both the adaptive and the maladaptive changes occurring at multiple levels within the nervous system from the peripheral nervous system and muscle to the spinal cord, brain stem and brain (Fig. 11.1), all of which have the potential to influence functional outcomes.[11,14–16]

Functionally successful SCI regeneration requires navigation across the hostile growth-inhibitory injury site, the ability to locate post-synaptic neurons and the creation, reinforcing and strengthening of neural connections that support functionally typical

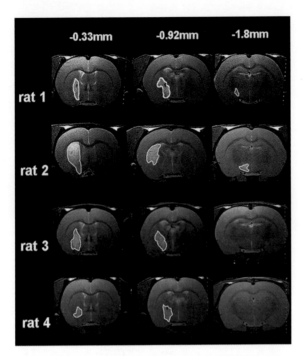

Figure 11.1 Neural reorganisation in rats 7 days after an MCAO.

Source: Mitchell EJ, Dewar D 2016 Is remodelling of corticospinal tract terminations originating in the intact hemispher associated with recovery following tansient ischaemic stroke in the rat? Plos One https://doi.org/10.1371/journal.pone.0152176.

sensory-motor behaviour. Although there have been significant regeneration research efforts, the extent of regeneration has been shown to be modest (see Chapter 1).[11–13]

There is now compelling evidence that the spinal cord is an intelligent structure capable of receiving, integrating and responding independently, as well as being highly plastic.[10]

There has been increasing knowledge and use of the term 'neuroplasticity' over the past three decades, but prior to its usage the concept of being able to make changes within the central nervous system, at both cortical and spinal cord levels, and retrain function was being explored by a number of physiatrists and physiotherapists. Two of the most widely used approaches for patients with neurological deficits, which evolved in the 1950s, were the

Bobath concept[17] and proprioceptive neuromuscular facilitation (PNF).[18] These approaches have been refined over the years and other new ideas added in the form of motor learning, active observation, virtual reality and mirror therapy. All these methods are reliant on the fact that the spinal cord and brain have the ability to rearrange and re-acquire specific functions. An iSCI offers the perfect opportunity for both regeneration and increased plasticity, with neuroscientific evidence supporting both modes. However, recovery profiles are slow and lengthy, with functional recovery continuing for more than two years after the injury.[10]

Neuroplastic change, wherever it occurs in the central nervous system, does not always result in functional recovery and can, in fact, result in maladaptive functions, such as pain, spasticity and atypical motor behaviour.[14,17] Therefore, physical rehabilitation interventions, including technology-based interventions, require careful consideration to ensure optimisation of typical motor behaviour for functional recovery.[14,18]

REHABILITATION POST ISCI

Compensation

As discussed in earlier chapters, SCI rehabilitation has traditionally utilised a focus on learning compensatory strategies. Since the number of iSCIs is increasing, different approaches to the rehabilitation of these individuals must now be considered (see Chapter 2). SCI rehabilitation that focuses solely on strengthening musculature that remains neurologically intact, above the level of the lesion to compensate for the loss of sensory-motor control below the level of the lesion, ignores the potential of the residual intact nervous system.[19]

iSCI – a rehabilitation paradigm shift

The changing demographic of SCI, with increasing numbers of iSCI, specifically incomplete tetraplegia,[20] requires a paradigm shift in SCI rehabilitation (see Chapter 3). iSCI presents significant rehabilitation issues, including: (1) spontaneous discharge from the injured spinal cord tissue; (2) excessive input from particular regions of the CNS; and (3) atypical input from the periphery due to inappropriate proprioceptive and light touch feedback, deprivation of activity-dependent input, excessive feedback due to hypertonia and hyper-reflexia, as well as pain sources.[19] Neuro-rehabilitation is therefore a complex, multifactorial, individualised phenomenon,[21] and outcomes of neuro-rehabilitation post iSCI are dependent upon many factors. Individuals with iSCI should be encouraged to also consider recovery of typical motor behaviour, rather than the exclusive development of compensatory strategies,[13,22] in order to ensure that the optimal level of function is explored.

Recovery following iSCI is believed to be limited to the amount of surviving neural tissue, and level of spinal cord injury that is able to support sensorimotor behaviour.[8,11] Animal studies have shown that the extent of spontaneous recovery is dependent upon the extent of the spinal cord lesion, with only 20% of AIS A (sensory and motor complete) patients exhibiting recovery in comparison to 80% of AIS B or C (sensory/motor incomplete) patients.[8]

Although older patients have similar recovery profiles to younger patients within the iSCI population, the older patients would appear to have more difficulty translating recovery into their daily life.[11] The presence of co-morbidities, which increases with age, but in particular infections such as urinary tract infections (UTIs) and respiratory tract infections, can also negatively affect recovery (see Chapter 15 for more details on ageing with an SCI).[11] Additionally, maladaptive processes post-SCI, such as neurogenic pain (see Chapter 18), autonomic dysreflexia (see Chapter 4) and circulation issues, have the potential to negatively impact on rehabilitation outcomes.[11]

A person with incomplete tetraplegia presents with complex movement problems affecting all four limbs and the trunk. Therefore, when considering rehabilitation of the iSCI person, in order to augment typical movement patterns while minimising compensatory motor behaviour, it is important to consider the sensory consequences of atypical and compensatory movement while simultaneously augmenting appropriate movement-related sensory input to potentiate remaining neural tissue to produce typical movement behaviour.[19,23]

Techniques/concepts that can facilitate neural plasticity

There are many clinical frameworks that can be employed for rehabilitation of the individual with an iSCI, but the challenge is to consider the whole person and the impact of the iSCI on every aspect of that person's life. Outlined below are some of the varied philosophies that employ a neurofacilitation approach to maximise the functional and neurological potential of those who have suffered an iSCI.

- **The Bobath concept** has primarily been utilised and investigated relative to supraspinal lesions such as stroke and acquired brain injury.[24] However, the Bobath concept can provide a useful framework for the rehabilitation of persons with an iSCI.[25] The Bobath concept is based on the principles of experience-dependent neuromuscular plasticity for sensorimotor recovery[26] and provides an overall conceptual framework for the assessment and treatment for persons with movement disorders due to a lesion of the central nervous system, focusing on recovery of typical motor behaviour, not compensation.[25,26] It is based on a systems-based model of motor control and considers the whole person, within their context, with respect to activity limitations, impairments and participation goals.[27] A key aspect of Bobath clinical practice is motor performance, how a task is performed, such that movement analysis considers the role of sensory information in motor control, as well as the relative integration of postural control, selective movement and cognitive/perceptual processes required for a given task.[23] It is currently described as 'an inclusive, individualised, problem-solving, living concept based on a systems approach to motor control, with particular emphasis on movement analysis and motor recovery from the perspective of the integration of postural control, task performance and contribution of sensory inputs'.[26]

- **Proprioceptive neuromuscular facilitation (PNF)** has been one of the most recognised treatment concepts in physiotherapy since the 1940s. It was originally suggested that PNF may promote neuromuscular function through the stimulation of proprioceptive mechanisms using various combinations of movement patterns.[28] The PNF patterns combine motion in the sagittal, coronal and transverse planes, producing a movement that is 'spiral and diagonal'.[29] Resistance is one of the basic procedures used in PNF and when specifically applied the resistance can result in irradiation (overflow) to other muscle groups and, consequently, their reinforcement. In the original PNF concept, resistance was applied manually, allowing the therapist to alter the resistance according to the response of the patient. Patients today are also instructed to self-resist using weight and pulley systems or specialist rubber tubing. The increased muscular activity in the exercised limb and other parts of the body produces an impulse, which is measurable by surface electromyography (sEMG).[30] Axial rotation is the key component to effective resistance and correct resistance will strengthen the entire pattern of movement. The current principles of PNF are described as being 'a combined approach, with each treatment being directed towards the functional rehabilitation of the patient and not towards a specific body segment. Treatment is directed towards attaining the highest level of function for the patient'.[31]

- **Motor relearning:** In 1987, Carr and Shepherd articulated a motor learning model for rehabilitation in which therapy sessions are considered training sessions where patients practise challenging functional tasks in order to 'relearn' their previous skills. Motor learning, motor control, biomechanics and muscle biology form the theoretical framework for this concept. Incorporating context-relevant, task-specific, meaningful activities has been shown to be more effective in the reacquisition of old skills and the learning of new skills as compared to passive activities.[32] Animal studies have shown that cortical changes only occur with learning of new skills and not just with repetitive use. The value in the practice of functional tasks is that it utilises functional synergies specific to the task and including the appropriate postural requirements.

  Motor learning principles provide guidelines for the provision of feedback, and for the structuring of practice. The motor relearning model also takes into account the importance of an enriched rehabilitation environment. Variations on task-specific training are also incorporated into the program and the body parts below the level of the lesion are also incorporated into the regimen. Although historically the term neural plasticity was not used when describing this program, it did adhere to the principles now understood to be required for these changes to occur.[12]

- **Sensorimotor integration** is defined as the ability of the CNS to combine a variety of different stimuli and transform such inputs into motor actions. In 2010 Machado and colleagues[33] reviewed the basic principles of sensorimotor integration, such as its neural bases and its elementary mechanisms involved in specific goal-directed tasks when performed by healthy subjects, and the abnormalities reported in a range of common movement disorders. They concluded that the sensorimotor integration process plays a potential role in elementary mechanisms involved in specific goal-directed tasks performed by healthy subjects and in the occurrence of abnormalities in most common movement disorders. They observed that training strategies, which stimulated the existing neural connections in the sensorimotor regions, played a potential role in the acquisition of functional tasks that depended upon combining different sensory inputs in order to execute the specific tasks.[33]

Other possible adjuncts to therapy that may be employed to facilitate neural plasticity and encourage recovery of typical motor behaviour rather than compensation include neuromuscular electrical stimulation (NMES), functional electrical stimulation (FES), neuromodulation (see Chapters 3 and 7), robotics (see Chapters 3 and 9) and hydro/aqua therapy (see Chapter 10). Furthermore, there are some exercise regimens which may be useful specifically in the longer-term rehabilitation of individuals with iSCI such as Pilates, Feldenkrais and muscle energy techniques.[34] The theoretical concept of all these approaches is based upon retraining typical movement patterns through practice, repetition and task training, and may allow the individual with an iSCI to join in with sessions outside the therapeutic environment, thus acknowledging transfer back into society.

Rehabilitation of the whole person

Movement analysis, and, in turn, intervention, within the neurofacilitatory concepts outlined above, is undertaken from the perspective that movement comprises the whole person and the whole body, not just individual body segments or limbs. From this perspective, intervention is considered within the context of a 24-hour approach.

Movement performance is an essential aspect of any neuro-rehabilitation program.[35] As such, health professionals involved in the treatment of the patient with an iSCI must encourage not only the rehabilitation of the function, but also the quality of the movement used to perform that function. Therefore, while functional outcome measures are important, it is also relevant to consider the qualitative aspect of movement.[27]

The role of the trunk and head in movement recovery post-iSCI

Trunk control in iSCI refers to the function of the trunk in all postures and activities. Depending upon the level of the lesion and the degree of incompleteness, the patient with an iSCI injury will have varying degrees of trunk control. The degree of trunk control will affect all basic activities of daily living (ADLs) and the early stages of the rehabilitation process should include a focus on retraining the postural muscles wherever possible.

This includes consideration of the role and function of the transverse abdominis muscle and the thoracolumbar fascia (Figs 11.2, 11.3), and the implications associated with any upper limb recovery, which is described later in this chapter, as well as recovery of locomotion.

The imbalance of trunk motor control due to an iSCI results in the loss of coordinated activity between both sides of the trunk, as well as the coordination between the upper and lower trunk. Likewise, impaired trunk motor control can result in the development of an extremely rigid and immobile trunk lacking the natural pelvic trunk rotations and flexion extension that usually accompanies typical motor behaviour. The recovery of trunk and head control are integral to regaining postural control and balance, and thus impact upon all ADLs.

Postural control requires multisystem integration and is described in the literature as a complex sensorimotor behaviour.[36] Postural control may be described as: 'the organisation of stability, mobility and orientation of the multi-joint kinetic chain, which is reflective of the individual's body schema in order to maintain, achieve or restore a state of equilibrium during any posture or activity'.[27]

Body schema, also a complex concept, describes the spatial representation of the body including the limbs, which is constantly updated within the brain with respect to the body's configuration in space, the alignment of body segments, as well as the shape of the body surface.[37] Therefore, the relative alignment of body segments to each other, to the base of support, and orientation, will impact on

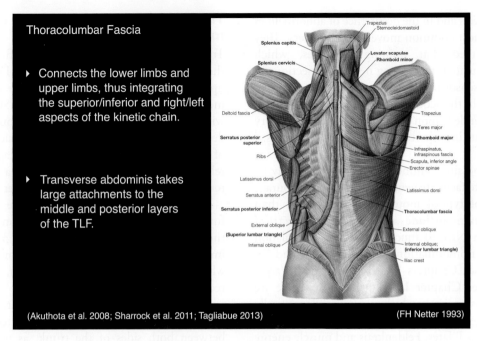

Figure 11.2 Thoracolumbar fascia and transverse abdominis.
Source: Netter, F.H., 2018. Atlas of human anatomy, 7th ed. Saunders Elsevier.

the person's body schema, which in turn influences their postural control and balance.[38]

Thus, attention to active body segment alignment relative to each other, base of support and orientation, as well as careful consideration of the role of the trunk in postural control, balance and ADLs, are required in iSCI rehabilitation, particularly for persons with incomplete tetraplegia.

Postural control/stability and selective movement/mobility

The patient with an iSCI or any of the spinal syndromes described earlier in the chapter may present with a profound loss of postural control through the trunk and proximal limb girdles such that they are unable to posturally stabilise themselves, thereby impacting upon selective distal movement of a limb or limbs. The concept of improving core stability for improved distal motor performance is well documented in the sports science and orthopaedic literature.[39,40] However, there is limited

research into the inter-relationship of sufficient or adequate postural control for selective movement elsewhere, which is the ability to move one body segment in relation to or remote from another body segment.[41,42]

Anticipatory postural control comprises feed-forward mechanisms (postural adjustments that precede the movement by –600 to 0 milliseconds) and seek to minimise the negative consequences of a predicted postural perturbation, such as voluntary movement, breathing or even heart rate.[43] The production of postural responses and their integration in movement is considered to be one of the fundamental roles of the corticoreticulospinal system.[44,45] The magnitude of the anticipatory postural control is influenced by a number of factors, such as direction of the movement, magnitude of the perturbation, body stability, body configuration and characteristics of the movement, including velocity and prediction, as well as training and possibly even fear.[43]

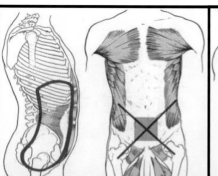
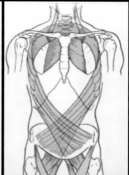
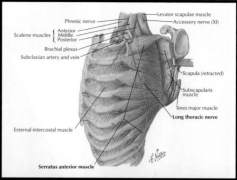

(FH Netter 1993)

▸ Transversus abdominis activation stretches abdominal fascia stabilising centrally on the linea alba.

▸ Through this central anchoring the external oblique can directly influence the ribs.

▸ The stabilisation of the ribs allows serratus anterior to influence the scapula.

▸ The serratus anterior is in anatomic continuation with the rhomboids.

▸ Thus resulting in a belt linking the shoulder girdle with the abdominal mechanism.

(DeRosa & Porterfield 2007)

Figure 11.3 Effect of transverse abdominis.
Source: Netter, F.H., 2018. Atlas of human anatomy, 7th edn. Saunders Elsevier.

Therefore, the consideration of the postural requirements of a task, not only the selective movement components, provides an alternative framework for the potentiation of movement recovery post iSCI. For example, developing the appropriate alignment and postural stability of the trunk may improve upper limb function, standing transfers or locomotion.

The role of the foot in iSCI rehabilitation

Although the foot is the interface between the body and the environment, the role and importance of the foot in the recovery of postural control, balance, standing and locomotion is often overlooked in the rehabilitation of the person with an iSCI. Clinically, one of the most significant problems encountered is cutaneous hyper-reflexia of the foot, such that when the foot touches the floor a flexor withdrawal of the lower limb occurs. Alternatively, or in addition to cutaneous hyper-reflexia, the person with an iSCI may develop increased tone of the posterior tibial musculature, commonly soleus and tibialis posterior as an anti-gravity response, resulting in a plantar-flexed, inverted and supinated posture of the foot (Fig. 11.4), such that appropriate contact of the foot to the floor is not possible. It is therefore important for the clinician to understand the role, function, structure, composition and underlying neurophysiology of the foot in order to appropriately clinically reason through the movement problem.

Tactile somatosensory input from the sole of the foot is important for postural control, balance, perception of standing and boundary-relevant information.[46,47] Weight bearing is an excellent somatosensory input for the foot, hence the emphasis on early standing, as described in Chapter 6. Standing

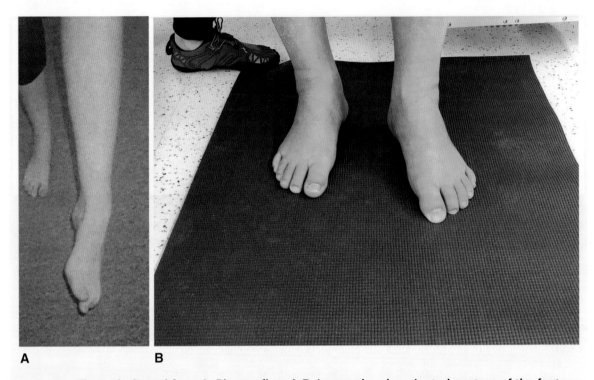

Figure 11.4 The mal-aligned foot. A, Plantar-flexed. B, Inverted and supinated posture of the foot.
Source: A, Umphred, D.A., Lazaro, R.T., 2012. Neurological rehabilitation. Elsevier Health Sciences, Fig. 23-16.

barefoot and on a variety of surfaces, that allow different sensory stimuli is recommended. Where possible, transfers that facilitate weight bearing should also be encouraged.

Recovery of walking

Recovery of walking is often a primary rehabilitation goal following iSCI, not only to restore ambulatory ability, but to reduce physical and psychological complications thereby improving quality of life (see Chapter 9 on ambulation). Due to high-energy cost and low walking speeds, recovery of functional ambulation post iSCI is often very limited.[48,49]

Recovery of upper limb function of the patient with an iSCI

iSCI may present with a profound and devastating loss of arm and hand function, together with a simultaneous loss of postural control, thereby affecting all ADLs and severely compromising independence (see Chapter 17 on the tetraplegic upper limb).[50]

Assessment of upper limb recovery is complicated, as upper limb function requires the coordinated activity of multiple muscles and joints within the limb, truncal stability on which to base limb movement,[51] as well as the environment, motivation and use of atypical/compensatory strategies.[50] Recent evidence suggests that the ability to perform unilateral functional upper extremity tasks after SCI can be predicted from motor testing scores,[50] however, this is affected by confounders such as pain, increased muscle tone and hyper-reflexia, as well as proximal shoulder girdle and trunk control.

The role of the core in upper limb recovery

Functional stability of the upper limb is associated with core control.[39] The thoracolumbar fascia (TLF) is an important structure that connects the lower limbs to the upper limbs integrating the superior/inferior and right/left aspects of the kinetic chain. Stabilisation of the ribs allows serratus anterior to influence the scapula, and as the serratus anterior is in anatomical continuation with the rhomboids, this results in a belt-like mechanism linking the shoulder girdle with the abdominal mechanism.[52] This is very important clinically for the iCSCI patient, as improving core control and abdominal activation can have a positive impact on the alignment and activation of the serratus anterior, which in turn may positively influence selective activation of the upper limb.

The importance of specific joints and muscles in the recovery of function in the upper limb

The scapulothoracic joint is one of the least congruent joints of the body, with no bony attachment, and is solely dependent upon muscle activity for stability and mobility (Fig. 11.5). However, scapula alignment

is critical for providing a stable base for upper limb movement.[53,54]

Scapula movement is complex and includes anterior/posterior tipping, upward/downward rotation, internal/external rotation, elevation/depression, abduction/adduction and the composite movements of protraction and retraction.

The serratus anterior muscle, which receives innervation from C5, C6 and C7, is unique among the scapulothoracic muscles because it contributes to all components of typical 3-D scapular movement during elevation of the upper limb, with its primary function to stabilise the scapula against the thorax and act as the major protractor of the shoulder girdle.[55] The dynamic orientation of the scapula optimises the glenohumeral joint as the prerequisite for shoulder girdle stability and mobility. Along with the serratus anterior, the upper and lower fibres of trapezius are the primary contributors to scapula stability and mobility.[54]

Latissimus dorsi (LD), which receives innervation from C6, C7 and C8, is an extremely important

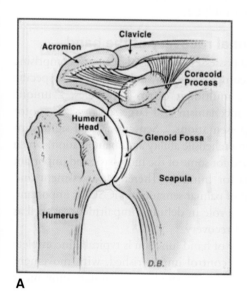

A

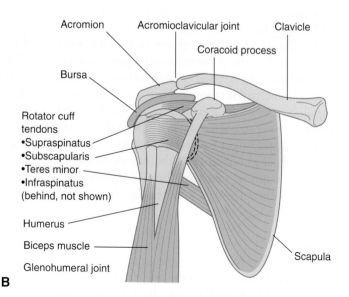

B

Figure 11.5 Scapulothoracic joint. A, Bony configuration. B, With muscles attached.

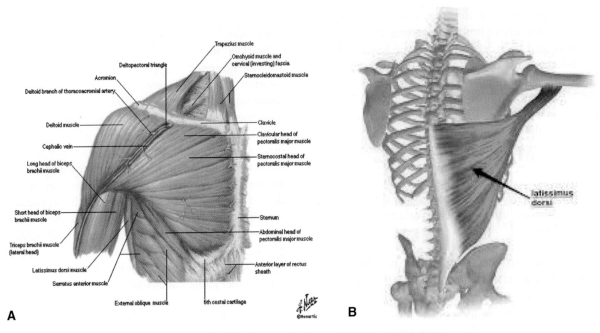

Figure 11.6 A, Muscles of the shoulder (anterior view) and B, latissimus dorsi.

Source: Netter, F.H., 2018. Atlas of human anatomy, 7th edn. Saunders Elsevier.

muscle in the rehabilitation of both complete and incomplete SCIs due to its unique origins and insertions, from the posterior aspect of the iliac crest, to T7–12, TLF, inferior angle of the scapula and ribs 9–12 (Fig. 11.6). LD contributes to compensatory trunk stabilisation in cervical and upper thoracic SCI, although the reversed origin/insertion activation results in internal rotation and inferior subluxation malalignment of the glenohumeral joint. Reduced effectiveness of scapular stabilisers, due to the myriad of neurological signs and symptoms in iSCI, may also result in glenohumeral subluxation. Similarly, reduced scapular mobility directly reduces the acromio-humeral distance increasing the risk for subacromial impingement.[55]

Reach

Reach, the transportation of the hand to an object by the upper limb, requires the integration of object location and body position coordinates, combining both proprioceptive and visual information,[56]

Alignment and activation of the trunk and scapula are critical to redeveloping the reach pattern in a person with iCSCI.

Functional recovery of the hand

The hand possesses unmatched dexterity, comprising a very complex design, including digit-specific intrinsics, multidigit extrinsic muscles, a unique extensor mechanism and large sensory and motor brain representations.[57] Sensation has a significant impact on prehensile ability and manipulation, which are required for some of the most basic and important functions for humans. Therefore, assessment and treatment of palmar sensation in iCSCI is important, as it plays a role in defining impairment, as well as functional recovery.[58]

Recovery of hand function is typically incomplete and motor control impoverished, with movement being poorly fractionated, and voluntary movement being accompanied by unwanted motor activity and increased activation of the wrist and finger flexors.

Tenodesis, a pinch grip achieved through active wrist extension and passive finger-to-palm and thumb-to-fingers flexion, is a different motor skill to typical prehension and requires motor learning of new upper limb coordination.[59] Therefore, careful consideration is required between compensatory tenodesis and remediation of typical hand function. The tetraplegic upper limb (both complete and incomplete lesions) is covered in more detail in Chapter 17.

Evidence-based practice points

- Due to many epidemiological factors, particularly improved pre-admission management, changes in road traffic laws and aetiology of injuries, the majority of SCIs are now incomplete.
- Management/treatment for these iSCI groups should focus on recovery of typical motor behaviour while minimising compensations.
- There are a number of different approaches available to facilitate neuroplastic changes and hence encourage recovery in the individual with an iSCI.
- Many of these approaches emphasise core control; therefore rehabilitation should consider the role of trunk control in the reacquisition of selective limb movement.
- The treating therapist should be familiar with as many of these approaches as possible and use whichever is most appropriate for the individual patient based on a thorough assessment.
- Understanding of the range of typical motor behaviour plays a large role in all treatment approaches for the individual with an iSCI.

SUMMARY

In individuals with incomplete SCI, neuroplasticity can be facilitated and refined by training trunk control simultaneously with upper and lower limb movements, the goal being to improve the functional outcome. Early prognosis of outcome after injury, using clinical and electrophysiological examinations, permits an early selection of appropriate training approaches. These should focus on relearning specific functional tasks contextualised to the individual.

The evidence suggests that maintaining activities that increase muscle activity at regular intervals can minimise the effects of sedentary behaviour in the iSCI population.[5] Therefore, the development of home exercise programs, accessible exercise facilities and equipment to promote increased ADLs are essential for the long-term health of persons with an iSCI.[60]

The ultimate goal of iSCI rehabilitation is to facilitate successful participation in life post injury which is not only influenced by the level of impairment but also by the individual's personality and values, as well as their home/community environment, such that the person can participate in home, work, education and social activities. However, to date there is a paucity of evidence from the perspective of individuals with an SCI on the factors that influence their participation and, in turn, there may be important considerations for rehabilitation programs (see Chapters 13 and 20 on sport and community participation).[61]

References

1. Pickett, G.E., Campos-Benetiz, M., et al., 2006. Epidemiology of traumatic spinal cord injury in Canada. Spine 31 (7), 799–805.

2. Lannem, A.M., Sørensen, M., et al., 2008. Incomplete spinal cord injury, exercise and life satisfaction. Spinal Cord 47, 295.

3. Molliqaj, G., Payer, M., et al., 2014. Acute traumatic central cord syndrome: a comprehensive review. Neurochirurgie 60 (1–2), 5–11.

4. Furlan, J.C., Noonan, V., et al., 2011. Timing of decompressive surgery of spinal cord after traumatic spinal cord injury: an evidence-based examination of pre-clinical and clinical studies. J. Neurotrauma 28 (8), 1371–1399.

5. Dekker, B., Verschuren, O., et al., 2018. Energy expenditure and muscle activity during lying, sitting, standing, and walking in people with motor-incomplete spinal cord injury. Spinal Cord 56 (10), 1008–1016.

6. Harkema, S., Behrman, A., et al., 2012. Evidence-based therapy for recovery of function after spinal cord injury. Handb. Clin. Neurol. 109, 259–274.

7. Kusiak, A.N., Selzer, M.E., 2013. Neuroplasticity in the spinal cord. Handb. Clin. Neurol. 110, 23–42.

8. Serradj, N., Agger, S.F., et al., 2017. Corticospinal circuit plasticity in motor rehabilitation from spinal cord injury. Neurosci. Lett. 652, 94–104.

9. Grau, J.W., 2014. Learning from the spinal cord: how the study of spinal cord plasticity informs our view of learning. Neurobiol. Learn. Mem. 108.

10. Young, W., 2014. Spinal cord regeneration: review. Cell Transplant. 23, 573–611.

11. Dietz, V., Fouad, K., 2013. Restoration of sensorimotor functions after spinal cord injury. Brain 137 (3), 654–667.

12. Silva, N.A., Sousa, N., et al., 2014. From basics to clinical: a comprehensive review on spinal cord injury. Prog. Neurobiol. 114 (Complete), 25–57.

13. Bradbury, E.J., 2012. Re-wiring the spinal cord: introduction to the special issue on plasticity after spinal cord injury. Exp. Neurol. 235 (1), 1–4.

14. Hormigo, K.M., Zholudeva, L.V., et al., 2017. Enhancing neural activity to drive respiratory plasticity following cervical spinal cord injury. Exp. Neurol. 287, 276–287.

15. Isa, T., Nishimura, Y., 2014. Plasticity for recovery after partial spinal cord injury – Hierarchical organization. Neurosci. Res. 78, 3–8.

16. Ding, Y., Kastin, A.J., et al., 2005. Neural plasticity after spinal cord injury. Curr. Pharm. Des. 11, 1441–1450.

17. Zholudeva, L.V., Qiang, L., et al., 2018. The neuroplastic and therapeutic potential of spinal interneurons in the injured spinal cord. Trends Neurosci. 42 (9), 625–639.

18. Jones, T.A., 2017. Motor compensation and its effects on neural reorganization after stroke. Nat. Rev. Neurosci. 18, 267.

19. Brown, J.M., Deriso, D.M., et al., 2012. From contemporary rehabilitation to restorative neurology. Clin. Neurol. Neurosurg. 114 (5), 471–474.

20. Krueger, H., Noonan, V.K., et al., 2013. The economic burden of traumatic spinal cord injury in Canada. Chronic Dis. Inj. Can. 33 (3), 113–122.

21. Vaughan-Graham, J., Cott, C., et al., 2015. The Bobath (NDT) concept in adult neurological rehabilitation: what is the state of the knowledge? A scoping review. Part II: intervention studies perspectives. Disabil. Rehabil. 37 (21), 1909–1928.

22. Darian-Smith, C., 2009. Synaptic plasticity, neurogenesis, and functional recovery after spinal cord injury. Neuroscientist 15 (2), 149–165.

23. Vaughan-Graham, J., Patterson, K., et al., 2017. Conceptualizing movement by expert Bobath instructors in neurological rehabilitation. J. Eval. Clin. Pract. 23 (6), 1153–1163.

24. Winstein, C.J., Stein, J., et al., 2016. Guidelines for adult stroke rehabilitation and recovery: a guideline for healthcare professionals from the American Heart Association/American Stroke Association. Stroke 47 (6), e98–e169.

25. Michielsen, M., Vaughan-Graham, J., et al., 2017. The Bobath concept – a model to illustrate clinical practice. Disabil. Rehabil. 41 (17), 1–13.

26. Vaughan-Graham, J., Cott, C., et al., 2015a. The Bobath (NDT) concept in adult neurological rehabilitation: what is the state of the knowledge? A scoping review Part I: conceptual perspectives. Disabil. Rehabil. 37 (20), 1793–1807.

27. Vaughan-Graham, J., Cott, C., 2016. Defining a Bobath clinical framework – A modified e-Delphi study. Physiother. Theory Pract. 32 (8), 612–627.

28. Voss, D.E., 1967. Proprioceptive neuromuscular facilitation. Am. J. Phys. Med. 46 (1), 838–899.

29. Knott, M., Voss, D.E., 1968. Proprioceptive Neuromuscular Facilitation: Patterns and Techniques, second ed. Hoeber Medical Division, Harper & Row, New York.

30. Sullivan, P.E., Portney, L.G., 1980. Electromyographic activity of shoulder muscles during unilateral upper extremity proprioceptive neuromuscular facilitation patterns. Phys. Ther. 60 (3), 283–288.

31. Adler, S., Beckers, D., et al., 2014. PNF in Practice, fourth ed. Springer Medizin Verlag, Heidelberg, Germany.

32. Galea, M.P., 2012. Spinal cord injury and physical activity: preservation of the body. Spinal Cord 50 (5), 344–351.

33. Machado, L.A., Maher, C.G., et al., 2010. The effectiveness of the McKenzie method in addition to first-line care for acute low back pain: a randomized controlled trial. BMC Med. 8, 10.

34. Janda, V., 1984. Pain in the Locomotor System. A Broad Approach to Aspects of Manipulative Therapy. pp. 148–151.

35. Beyaert, C., Vasa, R., et al., 2015. Gait post-stroke: patho-physiology and rehabilitation strategies. Clin. Neurophysiol. 45 (4–5), 335–355.

36. de Souza, N.S., Martins, A.C., et al., 2015. The influence of fear of falling on orthostatic postural control: a systematic review. Neurol. Int. 7 (3), 62–65.

37. Morasso, P., Casadio, M., et al., 2015. Revisiting the body-schema concept in the context of whole-body postural-focal dynamics. Front. Hum. Neurosci. 9 (83), 1–16.

38. Vaughan-Graham, J., Patterson, K., et al., 2019. Important movement concepts – clinical vs. neuroscience perspectives. Motor Control 23 (3), 273–293.

39. Kibler, W.B., Press, J., et al., 2006. The role of core stability in athletic function. Sports Med. 36 (3), 189–198.

40. Ayhan, C., Unal, E., et al., 2014. Core stabilisation reduces compensatory movement patterns in patients with injury to the arm: a randomized controlled trial. Clin. Rehabil. 28 (1), 36–47.

41. Liao, C.F., Liaw, L.J., et al., 2015. Relationship between trunk stability during voluntary limb and trunk movements and clinical measurements of patients with chronic stroke. J. Phys. Ther. Sci. 27 (7), 2201–2206.

42. Jijimol, G., Fayaz, R., et al., 2013. Correlation of trunk impairment with balance in patients with chronic stroke. Neurorehabilitation 32 (2), 323–325.

43. Santos, M.J., Kanekar, N., et al., 2010. The role of anticipatory postural adjustments in compensatory control of posture: 1. Electromyographic analysis. J. Electromyogr. Kinesiol. 20 (3), 388–397.

44. Sakai, S.T., Davidson, A.G., et al., 2009. Reticulospinal neurons in the pontomedullary reticular formation of the monkey. Neuroscience 163 (4), 1158–1170.

45. Takakusaki, K., 2017. Functional neuroanatomy for posture and gait control. J. Mov. Disord. 10 (1), 1–17.

46. Chiba, R., Takakusaki, K., et al., 2016. Human upright posture control models based on multisensory inputs; in fast and slow dynamics. Neurosci. Res. 104, 96–104.

47. Bourane, S., Grossmann Katja, S., et al., 2015. Identification of a spinal circuit for light touch and fine motor control. Cell 160 (3), 503–515.

48. Louie, D.R., Eng, J.J., et al., 2015. Gait speed using powered robotic exoskeletons after spinal cord injury: a systematic review and correlational study. J. Neuroengineering Rehabil. 12, 82.

49. Benson, I., Hart, K., et al., 2016. Lower-limb exoskeletons for individuals with chronic spinal cord injury: findings from a feasibility study. Clin. Rehabil. 30 (1), 73–84.

50. Zariffa, J., Curt, A., et al., 2016. Predicting task performance from upper extremity impairment measures after cervical spinal cord injury. Spinal Cord. 54 (12), 1145–1151.

51. Gonzalez-Rothi, E.J., Rombola, A.M., et al., 2015. Spinal interneurons and forelimb plasticity after incomplete cervical spinal cord injury in adult rats. J. Neurotrauma 32 (12), 893–907.

52. DeRosa, C., Porterfield, J., 2007. Anatomical linkages and muscle slings of the lumbopelvic region. In: Vleeming, A., Mooney, V., et al. (Eds.), Movement, Stability and Lumbopelvic Pain, second ed. Churchill Livingstone Elsevier, Philadelphia, pp. 46–62.

53. Voight, M., Thomson, B., 2000. The role of the scapula in the rehabilitation of shoulder injuries. J. Athl. Train. 35 (3), 364–372.

54. Kibler, W.B., Sciascia, A., et al., 2012. Scapula dyskinesis and its relation to shoulder injury. J. Am. Acad. Orthop. Surg. 20 (6), 364–372.

55. Struyf, F., Meeus, M., et al., 2014. Interrater and intrarater reliability of the pectoralis minor muscle length measure-ment in subjects with and without shoulder impingement symptoms. Man. Ther. 19 (4), 294–298.

56. Vingerhoets, G., 2014. Contribution of the posterior parietal cortex in reaching, grasping, and using objects and tools. Front. Psychol. 5 (151), 1–17.

57. Perez, M.A., 2015. Neural control of hand movements. Motor Control 19 (2), 135–141.

58. Kalsi-Ryan, S., Beaton, D., et al., 2014. Defining the role of sensation, strength, and prehension for upper limb function in cervical spinal cord injury. Neurorehabil. Neural Repair 28 (1), 66–74.

59. Di Rienzo, F., Guillot, A., et al., 2015. Neuroplasticity of imagined wrist actions after spinal cord injury: a pilot study. Exp. Brain Res. 233 (1), 291–302.

60. Wouda, M.F., Lundgaard, E., et al., 2018. Effects of moderate- and high-intensity aerobic training program in ambulatory subjects with incomplete spinal cord injury–a randomized controlled trial. Spinal Cord 56 (10), 955–963.

61. Amsters, D., Duncan, J., et al., 2018. Determinants of participating in life after spinal cord injury – advice for health professionals arising from an examination of shared narratives. Disabil. Rehabil. 40 (25), 3030–3040.

CHAPTER 12

Overview of sexual function and changes post-SCI

Daniela Mazor and Rafi J. Heruti

INTRODUCTION

Advancement in medical treatment and rehabilitation modalities has prolonged life expectancies following spinal cord injury (SCI) from any cause (traumatic or non-traumatic). Caregivers should be recommended to use a patient-centred model, which has an emphasis on adding life to years, and not years to life, meaning there is a focus on improving quality of life (QoL). Physical limitations caused from SCI affect sexual function and sexuality in broader areas, which in turn has important effects on QoL.[1]

A common misperception is that the disabled person is asexual, with no interest, need or ability to function in this area.[2] Contrary to this myth, extensive clinical scientific evidence shows that interest in sexuality continues to be a major issue in the lives of many people with disabilities.[3] Sexual adaptability of the disabled person is an important and inseparable component of their medical, psychological, social and family rehabilitation process.[4,5] Studies indicate that people with disabilities are very interested in receiving counselling and sexual guidance,[6] but unfortunately this issue is often neglected in people with a disability.

Sexuality changes after SCI are common, complex and confounding.[7] Substantial changes result in altered sexual function and fertility potential, as well as the individual's self-esteem and body image. Alterations with positioning, mobility, incontinence and spasticity introduce unexpected problems, including decreased pleasure and delayed orgasm. Sexual concerns in men can involve erectile function, ejaculation and the ability to reach orgasm,[8] whereas in women they can involve vaginal infections, and the loss of vaginal lubrication and ability to orgasm.[9] People who are able to adapt to their changed bodies and to have satisfying sex lives have better overall QoL.[10] To achieve this goal, sexual issues must be addressed in the acute and chronic phases of rehabilitation after SCI in all age groups, as individuals with an SCI consider sexuality to be a top priority for QoL.[1] This can be best accomplished by a multi-professional interdisciplinary team approach, in which both medical and psychosexual issues are addressed.[11]

This chapter provides an introduction to human sexuality with a clinical overview of the main sexual and reproductive concerns and priorities that men and women face after SCI. It will discuss issues concerning sexuality and disability in general, and the neurophysiological aspects and treatments currently available and specific to the SCI population for sexual rehabilitation. Finally, it will review practical tools for sexual counselling that take into account all consequences of SCI on the individual's sexuality.

BASICS OF HUMAN SEXUALITY

Terminology

Sex: refers to the biological characteristics that define humans as female or male.[12]

Sexuality: a broader term describing everything that expresses our masculinity and/or femininity.[12] Sexuality is experienced and expressed in thoughts, fantasies, desires, beliefs, attitudes, values, behaviours, practices, roles and relationships.[13] It is a multidimensional concept and an integral component of an individual's identity. It is influenced by the interaction of biological, psychological, social, economic, political, cultural, legal, historical, religious and spiritual factors.[14] Happiness is the ability to combine all the elements of our personality, including sexuality.

Sexuality includes the behavioural, biological, psychosocial, clinical and cultural aspects of one's life:

- **Behavioural aspect**: allows us to understand different personal sexual standards, as first described by Alfred Kinsey.[15]

- **Biological aspect**: sexual desire, sexual functioning and satisfaction, conception, birth and the nature of human sexual response, described by William Masters and Virginia Johnson (Fig. 12.1), including the diagnosis and treatment of sexual disorders.[16,17]

- **Psychosocial aspect**: feelings, thoughts, anxieties, personality, which arise in combination with social factors (type of relationship, fatigue, use of drugs or alcohol, etc.). Helen Singer Kaplan, a psychologist and psychiatrist, viewed the human sexual response as a tri-phasic phenomenon, consisting of separate – but interlocking – phases: psychological phase of desire leading

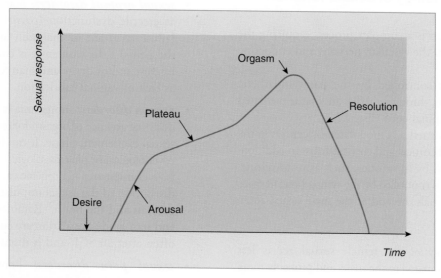

Figure 12.1 Human sexual response.
Source: Masters and Johnson in J.R. Georgiadis, ML Kringelbach, The human sexual response cycle: Brain imaging evidence linking sex to other pleasures. Progress in Neurobiology 98(1):49–81.

to the two organic phases – arousal and orgasm.[18]

- **Clinical aspect**: obstacles that can impair enjoyment, such as diseases, injuries, impairments and disabilities, drugs, emotions, conflicts in the interpersonal relationship and ways of solving the problems created.

- **Cultural aspect**: a wide variety of cultural approaches to sexuality.[19]

Sexual health: a state of physical, emotional, mental and social wellbeing in relation to sexuality; it is not merely the absence of disease, dysfunction or infirmity. Sexual health requires a positive and respectful approach to sexuality and sexual relationships, as well as the possibility of having pleasurable and safe sexual experiences free of coercion, discrimination and violence. For sexual health to be attained and maintained, the sexual rights of all persons must be respected, protected and fulfilled.[20]

Neurophysiology of sexual function
Male
Sexual function is a complex process requiring the involvement of the vascular, nervous and endocrine systems.[21]

Erection is controlled by the parasympathetic nervous system, through a reflex arc that is mediated in the sacral spinal cord (Fig. 12.2).[13]

This complex reflex is modulated by centres in the brain stem, subcortical and cortical areas. In addition, it is influenced by hormones, such as testosterone.

Ejaculation is controlled by the sympathetic nervous system and signals the end of the male sexual act.

Female
The physiology of the female sexual act is less understood compared to the male, and probably more complicated. It depends on a complex interaction between the endocrine and nervous systems, in which psychogenic stimulation plays a major role.[22]

Stimulation of the genital region, including the clitoris, labia majora and the vagina will lead to arousal, which manifests as vaginal lubrication (result of dilation of arteries in the genital area), tightening of the introitus and stimulation of secretion from Bartholin's gland, which aids in vaginal lubrication. The female orgasm is mediated by the sympathetic nervous system and characterised by rhythmic contraction of the pelvic structures. It results in cervical dilation, which may aid sperm transport and fertility.[14]

Sexual dysfunctions
Sexual dysfunction is the difficulty an individual or a couple experiences during sexual activity. According to the DSM-V, sexual dysfunction requires a person to feel extreme distress and interpersonal strain for a minimum of 6 months (excluding substance or medication-induced sexual dysfunction).[23] It has a profound impact on an individual's perceived quality of sexual life. Sexual dysfunction disorders may be classified into four categories:[23]

- *sexual desire disorders:* characterised by a lack or absence of libido for a period of time.[18]

- *sexual arousal disorders:* manifests in men as erectile dysfunction (partial or complete failure to attain or maintain an erection of the penis).[21] In women it is combined with interest and/or desire and manifests physically as lack of vaginal lubrication.[22]

- *orgasm disorders:* anorgasmia is the persistent delays or absence of orgasm following a normal sexual excitement phase. It can have physical, psychological or pharmacological origins.[21] SCI is an example of a neurogenic cause, due to the disruption of the sexual impulse between the genitals and the brain.[9] Retarded ejaculation and retrograde ejaculation are conditions seen often after an SCI, and is discussed below.[24]

- *sexual pain disorders:* known also as dyspareunia (painful intercourse) affect mostly women.[21] Common causes are vaginismus and vulvo-vestibulodynia.[23] Physiotherapists

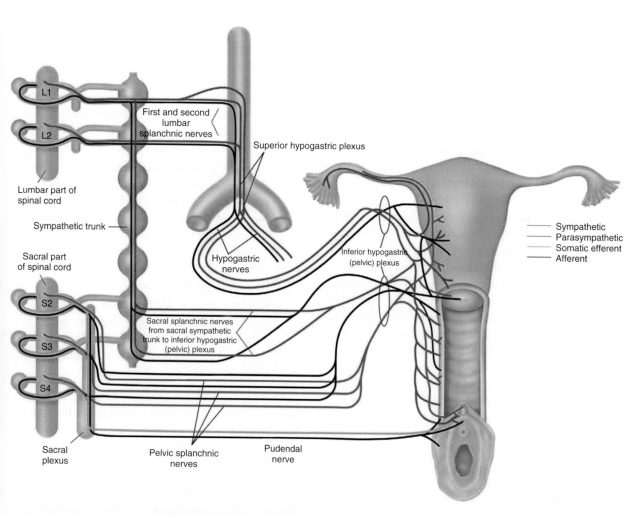

Figure 12.2 Lumbar splanchnic nerves of sexual function in men and women.
Source: © 2020 Elsevier Inc.

specialising in continence and women's health and using treatment interventions such as biofeedback may be critical for a successful treatment.

There are other sexual problems in addition to sexual dysfunction, such as sexual dissatisfaction, lack of social skills, changes due to disability (difficulties in hand function and/or positioning and /or mobility, etc.), sexually transmitted disease, hypersexuality, unhappiness or confusion related to sexual orientation, transsexual and transgender people who may have sexual problems before or after surgery and sexual addiction.[12]

SEXUALITY AND DISABILITY - THE CONSTRUCTION OF SEXUALITY IN PEOPLE WITH DISABILITY

The words 'sexuality' and 'disability' both evoke emotions, values and beliefs that vary in relation to a wide range of contexts.[25] It is possible to speak about sexuality and it is also possible to speak about disability, but if you try to bring together the two subjects as a common reality, suddenly the same old taboos rise up again.[6] The two terms are seen in antithesis to each other, negating each other. Individuals with disabilities are often portrayed as asexual and, as a result, the sexuality of persons with disabilities often becomes a taboo issue.[3]

The social construction of sexuality in people with disabilities

The social constructionist theory of disability, which argues that disability, sexuality and gender are functions of social construction and not biological facts,[2] is rooted in the idea that dominant groups set rules that define normality and deviance. People with disabilities can be marginalised through oppressive societal attitudes and behaviours regarding non-normative appearance and sexuality. Another common perception is that disability renders them sexually unattractive or unqualified to engage in relationships. As a result of such oppressive societal attitudes and behaviours, disabled people of all genders may find that they have fewer opportunities for love, relationships and even parenting.[26]

SEXUALITY AFTER AN SCI

Introduction

An SCI disrupts sexuality and sexual function and it most frequently affects young people who are at a peak of their sexual and reproductive lives.[27] As mentioned above, a common myth from the past regarded people with an SCI as asexual, but research has shown that sexuality is a high priority for them,[9] and certainly an important aspect of QoL.[28] Sexual function was rated as the top priority of all abilities they would like to have return among paraplegics, and second among tetraplegics (after hand and arm function).[29] Sexual function has a profound impact on self-esteem and adjustment to life post-injury.[30]

Sexual dysfunction is common among male and females with an SCI and can be classified into three groups according to their causes:

- ***primary sexual dysfunctions:*** those resulting directly from the impaired neural transmission. Damage to the spinal cord impairs its ability to transmit messages between the brain and parts of the body below the level of the lesion. This damage causes directly impaired vaginal lubrication, erection, ejaculation and orgasm, mostly due to alteration of the sensation.[31]

- ***secondary sexual dysfunction:*** results from factors that follow from the injury, such as physical limitation (e.g. balance, impaired movement, muscle weakness, spasticity), bladder and bowel function, cardiovascular control, temperature regulation, use of medications, hormonal changes, impaired sensation, pain and more.[5]

- ***tertiary sexual dysfunction:*** results from psychological and social factors, such as depression, anxiety, changes in relationships, drug and alcohol abuse, low self-esteem, low confidence and fear of rejection.[32]

Although an SCI causes sexual dysfunction, most individuals are able to have satisfying sex lives[33] by employing a variety of adaptations, and focusing on different areas of the body and types of sexual acts (Table 12.1).[10]

Physical perspective
General considerations regarding women and men with an SCI

In a recent published survey, 75.5% of persons with an SCI reported sexual problems directly due to their injuries.[33] In the population of people with an SCI satisfaction with sexual life was reported to be lower in men compared to women; lower by those who were married compared to being single, and lower by older people compared to younger people.[34] As more time passes since injury, patients attain more sexual satisfaction when compared with recently injured individuals.[30] In general, orgasms were less likely to be normal in males than females. Males had significantly worse psychogenic genital functioning than females and worse reflex genital functioning.[33]

Table 12.1 Potential for sexual response based on SCI

Degree of SCI	Likely to experience, reflexive arousal: erection/vaginal lubrication	Likely to experience, psychogenic arousal: erection/vaginal lubrication	Orgasm	Recommendations
Complete upper motor neuron injury cephalad to T11	Yes	No	Yes	1 Genital stimulation 2 Stimulation of sensate erotic body parts
Complete upper motor neuron injury caudal to T11–L2 with sparing of sacral spinal segments	Yes	Yes	Yes	1 Genital stimulation 2 Stimulation of sensate erotic body parts 3 Audiovisual, tactile gustatory and imaginative stimuli/fantasy
Conus injury/lower motor neuron injury (loss of sensation/voluntary control S4–S5, loss of S4–S5 mediated reflexes)	No	Yes	Yes	1 Assisted lubrication (e.g. KY jelly) 2 Stimulation of sensate erotic body parts 3 Audiovisual stimulation/fantasy
Incomplete injuries	<ul><li>Ability to appreciate pin touch sensation in S2, 3, 4 dermatomes correlates with ability to attain psychogenic arousal and achieve ejaculation</li><li>Ability to perceive T10–L2 dermatomes correlates with the ability to attain psychogenic erection/lubrication, and the better the response to fantasy</li><li>Preservation of sacral sensation or voluntary sacral control of S4–5 correlates with ability to attain reflexogenic erection/vaginal lubrication</li><li>Regardless of level or completeness, approximately 50% of individuals with an SCI experience orgasm</li></ul>			

'Reflexogenic arousal' refers to erection/vaginal lubrication that occurs as a result of genital stimulation. 'Psychogenic arousal' refers to erection/vaginal lubrication that occurs as a result of arousal in the brain (e.g. through hearing, seeing, feeling, or fantasy). 'Orgasm' refers to the perception of a peak feeling of sexual release or climax.

Source: Hess M.J., Hough S., 2012. Impact of spinal cord injury on sexuality: broad-based clinical practice intervention and practical application. J Spinal Cord Med 35, 211–218.

For both genders, problems regarding bladder and bowel management, pressure ulcers, spasticity or pain correlated with lower satisfaction with sexual life. Sexual dissatisfaction increased with increasing age in both genders (see Chapter 15 regarding the effects of ageing).[35]

There are general considerations and factors that affect sexual function in regards to the injury:

- **severity of the injury**: complete versus incomplete neurological classification (see Appendix 1 – INSCSCI for more detail) is an important aspect to determine how much sexual function returns.[36] In an incomplete injury some sensation or motor function is preserved in the rectum, indicating that the brain can send and receive stimuli to the lowest parts of the spinal cord, under the damaged area.[31] In individuals with an incomplete injury, some or all of the spinal tracts involved in sexual responses remain intact, allowing some sexual function, similar to uninjured people. In both injured and uninjured people, the brain is responsible for the way the sensation of climax is perceived. The qualitative experience associated with climax is modulated by the brain, rather than a specific area of the body.[37]

- **level of injury**: upper motor neuron (UMN) versus lower motor neuron (LMN) impairment can influence which sexual function is retained or regained after injury.[38] People with an SCI who have injuries in the sacral region are less likely to achieve orgasm than those with higher level injuries.[39,40] Injuries above the sacral level in men with an SCI are associated with better function in terms of erections and ejaculation, due to reflexes that do not require input from the brain, which sacral injuries might interrupt.[5]

- **psychogenic versus reflexogenic arousal**: arousal (erections in men and vaginal lubrication in women) is usually classified as arising from 'reflexogenic' or 'psychogenic' causes (Fig. 12.3).[41]

In practice, this dichotomy has translated to a distinction between parasympathetic versus sympathetic, pelvic versus hypogastric nerves, or psychological versus somatic. The two separate pathways normally work together in harmony.[31]

Psychogenic arousal is a result of erotic stimuli (fantasies, visual input or other mental stimulation) that results in cortical modulation of the sacral reflex arc (Fig. 12.3).[42] Reflexogenic arousal, on the other hand, is due to physical contact to the genital area, which activates the parasympathetic nervous system. It is mediated by a reflex arc that goes to the spinal cord (not to the brain) and is served by the sacral segments (at levels S2–S4) of the spinal cord (Fig. 12.3). Reflex arousal may increase in frequency after an SCI due to the loss of inhibitory input from the brain, which would normally suppress the response in uninjured individuals.[43]

Desire

Both sexes experience reduced sexual desire in the acute phase after an SCI due to hormonal changes[44] and/or anxiety and/or reactive depression.[4] Almost half of men and three-quarters of women have difficulty becoming psychologically aroused.[29] Depression is the most common cause of problems with arousal in people with an SCI. People frequently experience grief and despair initially after the injury.[32] In the chronic phase desire can be impaired mainly due to secondary causes, such as pain and medications,[45] and tertiary causes, such as depression, anxiety, low self-esteem and fear of rejection.[46]

Sensation

Men and women with an SCI often lack sensation in traditional erogenous areas, such as the genitals and nipples. Stimulating these areas may result in penile erection and vaginal lubrication, but not necessarily in sexual pleasure.[43] However, other areas above the level of the injury may become much more erogenous, such as the ears and the neck, and stimulating them can result in sexual arousal.[39,40] Some individuals with an SCI find the skin around the neurological injury level to have higher tactile sexual response. Neural plasticity probably accounts for the increases in sensitivity in those parts of the body that have not lost sensation.[46]

Neuropathic pain

Neuropathic pain and analgesics may influence life and impair QoL and sexuality (see Chapter 18 for further details).[47]

Urinary and faecal incontinence

Neurogenic bladder is common after an SCI, and the resulting urinary incontinence is a top therapeutic

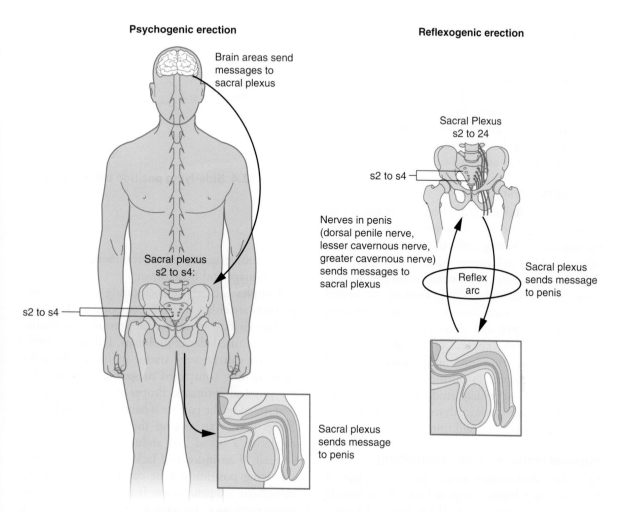

Psychogenic erection

Brain areas send messages to sacral plexus

Sacral plexus s2 to s4:

s2 to s4 —

Sacral plexus sends message to penis

Reflexogenic erection

Sacral Plexus s2 to 24

s2 to s4 —

Nerves in penis (dorsal penile nerve, lesser cavernous nerve, greater cavernous nerve) sends messages to sacral plexus

Reflex arc

Sacral plexus sends message to penis

Figure 12.3 Psychogenic versus reflexogenic erection.

priority of this population. In surveys, it was reported that urinary and/or bowel incontinence at inopportune times were significant concerns and prevented many individuals with an SCI from seeking sexual activity.[46] On the contrary, bladder continence was positively associated with a better satisfaction with sexual life.[34] A bladder or bowel accident may occur at any time – during courtship, sexual activity or social events. The embarrassment, shame and humiliation associated with incontinence creates undue anxiety and is often regarded as a

major reason for social isolation or the termination of a relationship.[48] (See Chapter 18 for further detail on neurogenic bladder and bowel.)

To minimise untimely episodes of incontinence the bladder should be emptied prior to sexual activity.[10] An indwelling catheter, if present, can be taped to the side of the penis with a condom placed over it.[36] In women, taping of the catheter to the abdomen would allow penetration.[5] Despite the best management program, sexual stimulation can cause urinary and/or faecal incontinence. Embarrassing passage of gas from the vagina, bowel or ostomy bag can be avoided by gentle thrusting, coital positioning and a careful diet. Fluids should be limited during the hours preceding sexual activity. Towels should be available at the bedside to manage episodes of incontinence.[30] To better improve sexual satisfaction and QoL for women with an SCI, future research needs to explore the effects of urinary incontinence on various aspects of sexuality.[49]

Autonomic dysreflexia

Autonomic dysreflexia (AD) needs to be taken into account, as some sexual activities, in particular ejaculation (including artificial methods), can be a source of AD (see Chapter 4 for further details on AD). As such, adequate treatments and prophylaxis must be considered in the context of sexual activities. Some medications (such as nifedipine, prazosin, captopril and clonidine) were found to be effective in the context of sexual activities if used in advance, thus limiting spontaneous sexual activities. Nifedipine (a calcium channel blocker) remains the most widely studied and significant treatment of autonomic dysreflexia, whether in acute or prophylactic conditions.[50]

Physical limitations and positioning

Secondary dysfunction results from the physical limitations (e.g. balance, impaired movement, muscle weakness, positioning, manual function).[5] A variety of positions for intercourse should be trialled to determine best comfort and efficacy.[51]

Positioning can be greatly affected by spasticity, contractures and pain.[47] Limitation in hip movement can adversely affect genital stimulation and coital penetration. Thus, the importance of maintaining full range of movement by a skilled physiotherapist should be considered. Positioning may have an effect on the respiratory status and the musculoskeletal and integumentary systems of the individual with an SCI. The weight of the partner can impede chest wall excursion causing respiratory distress and limb fractures in severely osteoporotic limbs. Persistent, unrelieved pressure caused by the combined weight

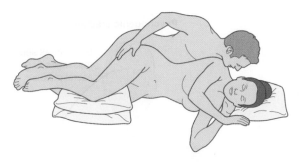

Figure 12.4 Side-lying position using pillows.

of the couple against bony prominences can lead to skin damage and breakdown.[7]

Couples can adjust positioning such that both partners are either side-lying (spooning) (Fig. 12.4) or face to face to maximise pressure distribution and minimise balance problems. Pillows or similar supports can be very useful in lifting the pelvis or sustaining contracted or spastic limbs to allow for physical intimacy. Proper positioning can be performed by the partner if hand function is limited. Slings that wrap around the neck and keep the thighs in a flexed and abducted position can be applied. If an individual lacks pelvic movement, a side-lying position can be conducive to thrusting movement and penetration. If an individual has good upper extremity and truncal strength a gliding seat that glides back and forth can also be considered (Fig. 12.5).[10]

Hand function

Individuals who lack hand function can be evaluated for assistive devices. Limited grasp may be improved by the addition of straps to vibrators, while others with minimal or no grasp can be prescribed custom wrist splints with adaptations to hold vibrators, dildos or other appliances. In the absence of functional arm capability, vibrators can be attached to various body parts, such as the thigh (Fig. 12.6) or pelvis, with the help of straps or a harness, and even the tongue (Fig. 12.7).

If individuals lack strong upper extremities to support their upper bodies, a side-lying or inferior position can be assumed, which also frees up the upper extremities for touching and fondling. Individuals who do not have hand function can guide their partner in trialling various positions as well as stimulation delivery methods.[10]

Spasticity

Spasticity occurs in 65–78% of people with chronic SCI (see Chapters 1 and 4).[48] Sometimes gentle stretching of the affected muscles prior to positioning is sufficient and can easily be incorporated into foreplay. Positioning a pillow or wedge under the individual's pelvis and legs can minimise the stretch on spastic muscle and allow comfortable positioning (see Fig. 12.4). If an individual has severe adductor spasticity in the thighs, pillows should be placed between the knees to prevent rubbing and skin breakdown. The individual and partner may consider carrying out sexual activities in a wheelchair when hip and knee flexion spasms are pronounced. This is a viable option for individuals who have sufficient truncal strength and balance to maintain a seated position without significant external support and for whom sitting does not trigger more spasms or spasticity.[47]

Physiotherapy is the first line of treatment, and also helps to minimise limitations in the range of movement. Often, however, pharmacological treatments need to be considered.[46] Taking a spasmolytic prior to sexual activity may reduce the disruptive effects of spasticity.[1] Intrathecal baclofen pump delivery is an effective method of achieving spasticity control, but may have negative effects on sexual functioning. Reduced libido and difficulty achieving erections and ejaculations have been reported and appear to be dose-related with reversal of symptoms with dose reduction.[52]

Men with an SCI – sexual dysfunction and management

According to a recent study about 75% of younger men with an SCI can achieve erection. About

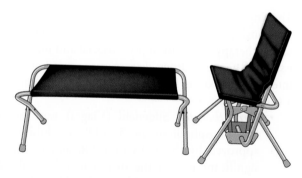

Figure 12.5 Intimate rider.

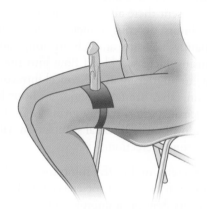

Figure 12.6 Dildo strapped to thigh.

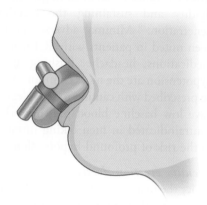

Figure 12.7 Vibrator strapped to the tongue.

44% of this group could also achieve ejaculation. Not surprisingly, significantly more men who had made their partner pregnant were satisfied with their sexual life.[35]

Erectile dysfunction

The ability to achieve an erection depends on the severity (complete versus incomplete) and the level (UMN versus LMN) of the injury.[31] About 80% of men with an SCI recover at least partial erections (psychogenic and reflexogenic) by 2 years after injury, but most of them will have a certain degree of erectile dysfunction.[35] Sometimes the erections do not last long and/or are lost when the stimulus is removed and/or the quality of the erection is insufficient for penetration.[29] Psychogenic erections will occur in men with incomplete injuries (both lower and upper motor neuron), as there is some connection between the brain and the genital region. Reflexogenic erection will occur mainly in UMN motor neuron injuries, as there is a need for the reflex arc.[41]

Men with an incomplete injury, who have some preservation of sensation in the dermatomes at the S4 and S5 levels and display a bulbo-cavernosus reflex, have better chances to achieve erections, usually reflexogenic.[8] Reflex erections may increase in frequency due to the loss of inhibitory input from the brain. These erections may result when the penis is touched or brushed by clothing, even in the absence of psychological arousal.[29] Like other reflexes, reflexive sexual responses may be lost immediately after injury (during the spinal shock period), but return over time as the individual recovers. A man with a complete SCI above T11 may not be able to experience psychogenic erection, but may still have reflex erection if his sacral segments are uninjured.[43] Conversely, an injury below the S1 level impairs reflex erections but not psychogenic erections, if the injury is incomplete.[7]

Erections are not crucial for satisfying sexual activity, but many individuals continue to regard them as necessary,[32] and some reported erectile dysfunction was the main determinant of psychological distress.[53]

Treating erectile dysfunction was seen to improve relationships and QoL, especially if combined with sexual therapy in regard to psychosocial and marital issues.[10] The use of drugs, devices, surgery and other interventions exist to help men achieve and maintain a sufficient erection:[1,29]

- **Oral therapy:** Sildenafil (Viagra) was the first phosphodiesterase 5 (PDE5) inhibitor approved by the FDA in 1998, and had a significant role in the treatment of erectile dysfunction for men with an SCI.[54] Since then treatment of erectile dysfunction through oral pharmacotherapies has been proven to be an effective way to address and treat this concern. At present there about ten variants of PDE5 inhibitors, differing in their pharmacokinetics (mainly half-life and absorption), and all causing increased blood flow into the penis due to interfering in a chemical intracorporal chain. They are taken about an hour before anticipated sexual activity, giving a 12–36-hour window in which sexual stimulation will lead to stronger erection.[7]

- At present, oral PDE5 inhibitors are the first choice in treatment for erectile dysfunction. Patients show great improvement over baseline with the use of these medications. They are less invasive, are well tolerated and are highly effective in men who are capable of achieving reflex erections. It can assist in gaining further rigidity and sustaining the erection for penetration.[10] Minimal adverse effects have been noted in patients with SCI using these medications; headache, flushing and mild hypotension are the most common. It should be prescribed with caution to tetraplegics, who have low baseline blood pressure. They are contraindicated in men taking nitrates, due to the risk of profound hypotension.[36]

- **Vacuum erection device (VED):** With this device the man inserts his penis into a cylinder (Fig. 12.8), then pumps it to create a vacuum around the penis, and as a result blood is

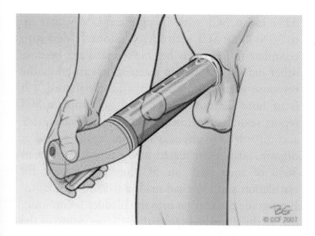

Figure 12.8 Penile vacuum device.

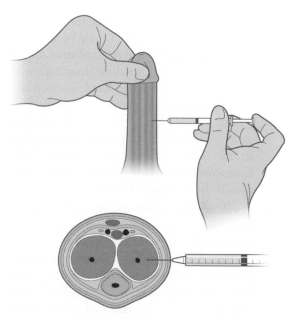

Figure 12.10 Use of intra-cavernosal injection.

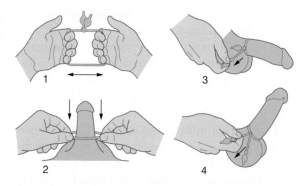

Figure 12.9 Use of constriction ring.

needed with anticoagulant medications. The use of VED requires manual dexterity, so most tetraplegics will need assistance from the partner.[55] VED is more accepted by men in an established relationship. The device is non-invasive, economical and efficacious. Minor side effects includes petechiae, penile skin oedema, colour and temperature change.

- **_Intra-cavernosal injection (ICI):_** If oral medications and mechanical treatments fail, the second choice is the use of local injection to the penis; this alters the blood flow and triggers an erection (Fig. 12.10).[56]
- ICI using papaverin, phentolamine, alprostadil (prostaglandin E_1) or a mixture, is a common practice among patients with erectile dysfunction. The patient is trained in the clinic how to perform the injection correctly, and to find the correct effective dose for a satisfactory erection. ICI resulted in successful erections

drawn into the cavernosal spaces, making it erect.[55]

- A rubber constriction ring is then slipped around the base of the penis, maintaining the erection (Fig. 12.9).

  This ring can be used solely in cases of good reflexogenic erections, which are not maintained long enough. The ring can be placed at the base of the penis, and should be removed within 30 minutes. Caution is

in 88% of patients. No predictive factor for efficacy of a response to ICI could be identified when evaluating type of injected drug, doses, level of injury, age or time since injury. A tetraplegic with impaired hand function will need a cooperative partner to inject. Side effects might include priapism if a higher dose is injected. Local pain at the injection site can occur with incomplete injuries. Penile haematoma and fibrosis (scarring) are potential risks if the technique is wrong.[56]

- *Penile implants:* when conservative treatments have failed, penile implants might be considered.[29] There are a number of different devices, ranging from a simple malleable prosthesis to the more complex hydraulic ones. The procedure is irreversible as the cavernosal bodies are removed and replaced by the implants.[57] Complications occur in about 10% of cases, including the risk of eroding penile tissue (breaking through the skin). It should not be considered in an SCI before emotional adaptation to the injury has occurred.[10] It is also advisable to have sexual therapy first in order to explore less invasive options for sexually satisfying activity.[1]

Other methods, such as topical medications to dilate the blood vessels, inserting a small pellet of medication into the urethra[58] and electrical stimulation of efferent nerves at the S2 level to trigger an erection, may not be as effective, and are not in common use.[29] In total, about 35% of men with an SCI use treatments for erection; of them, 78–94% had a positive effect.[35]

Ejaculatory dysfunction

There is usually a need for more physical stimulation to ejaculate.[59] On the other hand, premature or spontaneous ejaculation provoked only by thinking a sexual thought can be seen in men with injuries at levels T12–L1.[24]

Antegrade ejaculation was reported by 2% of males with an SCI with complete UMN lesions,

32% in an SCI with incomplete UMN and up to 70% in an SCI with LMN lesions.[60] Men with complete injuries may be able to ejaculate, because other nerves involved in ejaculation can affect the response without input from the spinal cord.[59] It is of note that some men with a complete SCI report sexual sensations at the time of ejaculation, accompanied by physical signs normally found at orgasm, such as increased blood pressure.[37] About 56% of men with an SCI used treatment for ejaculation and 19% had made a woman pregnant.[35] Retrograde ejaculation into the bladder is common, due to the disturbed sympathetic innervation of the bladder neck.[59]

Management for ejaculation disorder will be discussed in the fertility section of this chapter.

Orgasm

In a healthy subject ejaculation will follow with an orgasm. Studies show that up to 50% of men with an SCI experience orgasms,[7,33] although it may feel different than it did before the injury.[5] Some with an incomplete injury will describe the same orgasm as prior to the injury. Most report that it feels weaker, and that it needs longer time and stronger stimulation to achieve. Others report of 'para-orgasm' – positive sensation, but not as the burst they felt prior to the injury. Some describe it as an emotional event, and others report orgasm to be non-existent following the injury.[40]

Women with an SCI – sexual dysfunction and management

Women's sexuality after an SCI remains relatively unexamined, though an SCI significantly impairs psychological and physical aspects of female sexual function.[49,61] Studies show that women with an SCI reported that their injury caused many changes in their sex life and affected many aspects of their sexuality in a negative way, but still the majority of subjects reported having experienced intercourse post-injury.[46,61]

Several facets of a woman's sexuality are negatively affected by an SCI, and consequently sexual satisfaction has been shown to decrease, which also negatively affects QoL.[49] Some changes can be of a physical nature (for example, sensation, spasticity, bladder or bowel problems, difficulties to move and position oneself), while other changes are of a psychological nature (for example, feeling unattractive or less attractive, having less self-confidence and difficulties in meeting or finding a partner).[39]

It was found that 94% of women with an SCI had no problems with impaired vaginal lubrication: 22% had given birth after the injury and 69% reported being satisfied with their sexual life. The women who were satisfied with their sexual life were younger than those who were not, and were younger at the time of injury.[35] In another study comparing a group of women who were sexually active with those who were not, the only factors that were found to be related to sexual activity were not having a stable partner and a lack of sensation in the genital area. Variables such as age, neurological level, time since the injury, urinary incontinence, chronic pain and spasticity were found to be unrelated to sexual activity.[62]

As with males who have an SCI, bladder and bowel incontinence, as well as autonomic dysreflexia, negatively impact upon sexual activity and intercourse.[46] Most women report difficulty with positioning during foreplay and intercourse, vaginal lubrication and spasticity during intercourse.[63] Sexual intercourse is much more difficult for females with complete tetraplegia (compared with other women with an SCI), mainly because of autonomic dysreflexia and urinary incontinence.[30]

The age when the SCI was incurred, the importance or surety of one's sexual orientation and the aetiology of the SCI were found to be predictable factors favouring successful sexual rehabilitation.[30] Reasons for not wanting to or not having the courage to be intimate and sexual were physical problems, low sexual desire, low self-esteem and feelings of being unattractive. The motivations for both the women with an SCI and a control group to engage in sexual activity were intimacy-based rather than primarily sexual.[61]

For women who are able to overcome the physical restrictions and mental obstacles due to injury, it is possible to regain an active and positive sexual life together with a partner. Sexual information and counselling should be available, both during initial rehabilitation and later when the woman has returned to her home.[61]

Arousal

Most women with an SCI can achieve some level of vaginal lubrication. Similar to erection, this lubrication can be mediated by reflexogenic or psychogenic factors. Women with complete injuries can achieve sexual arousal and orgasm through stimulation of the clitoris, cervix or vagina, which are each innervated by different nerve pathways.[9] This suggests that even if an SCI interferes with one area, function might be preserved in others.[5] Preservation of sensory function in the T11–L2 dermatomes is associated with psychogenically mediated genital vasocongestion.[9] Individuals with incomplete (both UMN and LMN) injury are more likely to have satisfactory lubrication. If vaginal lubrication is unsatisfactory, then a water soluble lubricant can be used.

PDE5 inhibitors, oral medications for treating erectile dysfunction in men (such as Sildenafil), have been tested for their ability to increase sexual responses, such as arousal, in women. The rationale was that it might increase blood flow to the perineum and increase vaginal lubrication in women with an SCI. Trials with other women of the general population and also women with an SCI yielded only inconclusive results and no clinically meaningful benefit.[39]

An inverse relationship existed between developing new areas of arousal above the level of lesion and not having sensation or movement below the lesion. The most commonly reported sexual stimulation leading to the best arousal involved stimulation of the head/neck and torso areas.[46]

Orgasm

Almost half of the women with an SCI reported experiencing orgasm post-injury and this was positively associated with the presence of genital sensation, usually when their genitals were stimulated.[46,49] Most can experience orgasm with vibration to the cervix, similar to an uninjured woman, regardless of level or completeness of injury.[43,61] Only 17% of women with complete lower motor neuron dysfunction affecting the S2–S5 spinal segments were able to achieve orgasm, compared with 59% of women with other levels and degrees of SCIs. Time to orgasm was significantly increased in women with SCIs compared with able-bodied controls.[9]

Some report the sensation of orgasm is the same as prior to the injury, and others say it is reduced.[63] Those with injuries above the sacral level have a greater likelihood of orgasm in response to stimulation of the clitoris than those with sacral injuries (59% versus 17%).[5] The term 'phantom orgasm' was coined to describe women's perception of orgasmic sensations despite an SCI, but subsequent studies have suggested the experience is not merely psychological.[28] One proposed explanation for orgasm in women, despite complete SCI, is that the vagus nerve bypasses the spinal cord and carries sensory information from the genitals directly to the brain.[64]

Management for birth control, pregnancy and delivery will be discussed in the fertility section of this chapter.

Psychological perspective

Compared with physiological and neurological aspects, less is known about the psychosocial aspects of individuals with an SCI.[34] Recent studies show that psychosocial factors, such as age and partnership status, affect sexual rehabilitation.[65] Sexual identity and body image are important to the overall psychological wellbeing and life satisfaction of all human beings.[66]

Self-esteem, sexual esteem

> 'It is not that before the injury I loved myself, I know I was not the prettiest … but I felt attractive and sexual. Today I need a reminder that I am a woman.'
>
> (Tamara, 32 years old, SCI)

The term 'sexual self-esteem' has been used by several authors to describe the individual's sense of self as a sexual being, ranging from feeling sexually appealing to unappealing, and sexually competent to incompetent. The literature addressing self-esteem among individuals with an SCI strongly suggests that it is not the disability per se, but rather the contextual, social, physical and emotional dimensions that may have an influence on self-esteem and QoL.[67] Negative feedback and stigma attached to physical disability may compromise an individual's self-worth and result in a devalued sense of self. Positive social support and intimate relationships can assist with validating one's worth, particularly for persons with disabilities.[68]

Age at injury has been found to influence reintegration of sexuality after injury. The literature suggests there is a long latency period between time of injury and reintegration of sexuality, although there is little agreement within the literature regarding potential adjustment timeframes.[66]

Body image

> 'Sometimes during the physical treatments, it feels like my body is not mine; I am bringing it to the physical therapy and I am picking it up at the end of the session.'
>
> (Lisa, 23 years old, SCI)
>
> 'You do not understand, a man has to be a man, especially in bed, what can I offer?'
>
> (Eran, 30 years old male, injured at 27)

Body image contributes to sexual self-confidence in both men and women and it impacts on both early experiences and later sexual experience with partners. Men are often troubled by concerns that relate to penis size and women may avoid sex when they feel overweight or physically undesirable.[69] Culturally imposed Western standards stress the importance of characteristics such as being young, thin and beautiful.

Much of the research in SCI and body image has investigated the negative implications, such as changes to sexual self-esteem and overall functionality.

Studies have shown that certain aspects of body image may improve among individuals with an SCI as they adjust to their injury.[45]

Social skills

> 'You do not think it matters that when I turn to people they look down at me? I was 1.83 metres and today I'm barely 1.40.'
>
> (Dan, 40, wounded at age 28)

Social skills, social competence, social intelligence or social performance are terms that are often used interchangeably.[70] Social skills are defined as the ability to interact with other people in a manner that is both appropriate and effective. They are important for people with SCIs, as they help to overcome discomfort and stigmatisation in social situations, to ask for help, to put others at ease in social relationships, to elicit feedback and to develop and foster social relationships.[70] It comprises aspects of verbal and non-verbal communication and includes, for example, styles of social problem-solving, confidence, assertiveness, goal direction or self-monitoring. (Chapter 20 contains a more personal perspective on social skills issues.)

Social difficulties do not always mean that young adults do not wish to pursue social relationships, nor do they indicate a lack of emotion.[71] Social skills do not seem to change after an SCI; however, they are important in the development and maintenance of interpersonal relationships.[32]

Relationships and intimacy

Intimate and sexual relationships have been shown to be the most negatively impacted among the factors that influence QoL in individuals with an SCI.[72] Married men with an SCI reported that relationship factors of partner satisfaction and relationship quality were more predictive of sexual adjustment than erectile function, genital sensation or orgasmic capacity.[73] Married men with an SCI or those with partners who reported low relationship satisfaction or who had a low sexual desire should be referred for sexual counselling and evaluation for marital dysfunction, because sexual satisfaction behaviour is strongly related with quality of the relationship and the partner's sexual satisfaction.[73] (Chapter 20 contains a personal interpretation of relationships and intimacy.)

Dating and relationships among people with an SCI are part of a subject that has far more questions than answers. People with an SCI have the same emotional, psychological and sexual needs as the rest of the population; nevertheless their actual experience of creating or maintaining intimate relationships is often very different and commonly accompanied by difficulties and barriers.[32] Although there is a great deal of literature on the impact of an SCI on the psychological adjustments and social relationships in general, there is a conspicuous lack of research into how it affects the dynamics of adults' intimate relationships. This may be due to the notion that people with an SCI are not perceived as romantic or as sexual partners.[3] Even today, people with an SCI face strong social messages that support the notion they are not worthy of being romantic partners because of their disability. This notion leads to difficulties in their search for a romantic partner. Women with an SCI reported negative changes in their sexuality after the injury, including difficulties in meeting a partner and feelings of lower self-confidence.[61]

Marital status is positively correlated with QoL and wellbeing.[74] Moreover, the greatest predictor of increased wellbeing post-injury for the person with an SCI is partner support.[75] A partner's support is important in the recovery and return to sexual activity after an injury.[76] A phenomenological study that examined the sexuality and relationship in 'lived experiences' followed 15 adult women who sustained complete SCI. Some of the participants reported that they avoided sexual acts with a partner due to their belief in hearsay or other information that sex would not be satisfying. Moreover, most of the participants were not able to talk openly with their sexual partner about what their perceptions of the 'first time' post-injury sexual experience might be like and reported that they did not know what to expect.[34]

Couple relationship and partner support are influenced by the healthcare environment.[65] Several stressors, such as physical, psychological, social and economic factors relating to the living conditions of people with an SCI can greatly affect marital communication, relational stability and sexual intimacy. Other factors contributing to marital and relationship difficulties in people with an SCI can be related to deterioration in health, such as mobility, difficulties in finding employment or maintaining earning capacity and economic situation, such as an increase in the cost of treatments.[77] These factors can contribute to overwhelming feelings by both partners in the relationship. Moreover, it can lead to the partner's decision to become the caretaker; a role that can add an emotional burden and impair the ability to maintain a stable or sexual relationship. Preoccupation with the situation that leads to dependency weakens marital relations. Sometimes couples can be confronted with feelings of frustration, disappointment and a sense of victimisation.

Divorce rates in people with an SCI range between 8% and 48%. Although an SCI represents a major burden to the spouses, partners also report some positive changes, such as more open and honest communication. To strengthen marriage as an important social support system, comprehensive support should be provided to caregivers, for example, in terms of relationship counselling. Traditional social skill techniques use explicit reinforcement to increase appropriate versus inappropriate behaviour. Behavioural techniques such as roleplay, video feedback and cues to assist self-monitoring have increased the number of positive behaviours, such as active listening, and eliminated or significantly reduced the frequency of negative behaviours.[73] Most subjects reported difficulty in becoming psychologically aroused as well as physically aroused, which were both correlated with feeling that their SCI had altered their sexual sense of self.[46] More recent studies have acknowledged that psychosocial factors such as age and partnership status may also affect the successful sexual rehabilitation.[65]

Discussions with women with an SCI in Denmark and Sweden on their reactions to information and counselling offered during rehabilitation revealed an overwhelming need for the exchange of information and experience with other women with an SCI, and a desire for opportunities for counselling after initial rehabilitation.[32]

FERTILITY AFTER AN SCI

Males

An SCI occurs most often in young men at the peak of their reproductive health. Men with an SCI rank the wish to father children among their highest concerns relating to sexuality.[48] Infertility is a common phenomenon following SCI, mostly due to erectile and ejaculatory dysfunction and/or low sperm quality.[78] The reason for these abnormalities is not known, but research points to dysfunction of the seminal vesicles and prostate, which concentrate substances that are toxic to sperm.[59] Leukocytospermia is evident in most patients with an SCI. Additionally, elevated concentrations of pro-inflammatory cytokines and of inflammasome components are found in their semen. Fortunately, the fertility options for these men have notably improved. Neutralisation of these constituents has resulted in improved sperm motility.[7] Without medical intervention, the male fertility rate after an SCI is 5–14%.[79] This ejaculatory failure has prompted the development of various methods for ejaculation procurement.[80]

The first-line method for sperm retrieval in SCI men with an ejaculation is penile vibratory stimulation (PVS).[80] A medical high-speed vibrator is applied to the glans penis to trigger a reflex that causes ejaculation, usually within a few minutes (Fig. 12.11).

The efficacy of PVS ranges from 15–88%, possibly due to differences of level and completeness of the injury, but also due to vibrator settings and experience of clinicians.[7] UMN lesions above T11 are more responsive to PVS, while LMN lesions will not produce a reflex.[59] In addition, the quality of the

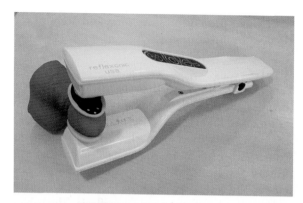

Figure 12.11 Viberect.

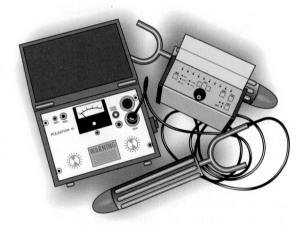

Figure 12.12 Electro-ejaculator.

sperm is better compared to other methods, enabling home insemination.[80] Autonomic stimulation with midodrine enhances orgasm rate, mainly by creating antegrade ejaculation.[81]

Electro-ejaculation (EEJ) is used when PVS has failed or is not suitable.[24,82] With EEJ, a low-current stimulation of the ejaculatory organs via a rectal probe is done, causing induction of seminal emission (Fig. 12.12).[82] Although this would be an unlicensed application of the drug in Australia, the Special Access Scheme (SAS) would allow doctors to obtain

supplies of this medication on a patient-named basis.

In general these electro-ejaculates exhibit high sperm counts, but low motility and poor sperm function.[78,82] Semen collected by EEJ can be used in conjunction with intra uterine insemination (IUI) or in vitro fertilisation (IVF). The use of intra cytoplasmatic sperm injection (ICSI) has raised the pregnancy rate remarkably.[80] The success rate is 80–100%, but the technique requires anaesthesia, and does not have the potential to be done at home.[82]

Both methods carry the risk of autonomic dysreflexia in patients with an injury above T6, so blood pressure monitoring and drugs to prevent the condition may be required.[7]

If these methods fail to cause ejaculation or do not yield sufficient usable sperm, sperm retrieval is also possible via prostate massage or surgical sperm retrieval, such as testicular sperm extraction or percutaneous epididymal sperm aspiration.[59] These procedures yield sperm in 86–100% of cases, but non-surgical treatments are preferred, so couples should be informed of all options, including semen retrieval by PVS or EEJ, before suggesting surgical methods.[79]

Female

Women's fertility is not usually affected, although precautions must be taken for safe pregnancy and delivery. The number of women with an SCI giving birth and having healthy babies is increasing.[83] Half to two-thirds of women with an SCI report they might want to have children, and 14–20% do get pregnant at least once.[84]

In the acute phase after injury 44–58% of women suffer from temporary amenorrhoea due to a stress response that alters levels of fertility-related hormones in the body.[1] Menstruation usually returns to normal 6 months to 1 year post-injury. Neither the level nor the completeness of the injury appears to be associated with interruption of the menstrual cycles. In a small percentage of women with an SCI, there are also changes in cycle length, duration of flow, amount of flow and severity of menstrual pain. After menstruation returns, most women with an SCI become pregnant at a rate close to that of the rest of the population.[85]

Birth control

The issue of birth control can be somewhat problematic for women with an SCI. Condoms provide contraception, as well as diminishing the risk of sexually transmitted infections. A diaphragm may be another option if the individual has adequate hand dexterity or a cooperative partner. Oral contraception is associated with increased incidence of thromboembolism, and must be prescribed with caution in women with an SCI. Oral contraceptives that contain only progesterone may be safer than medications that contain both oestrogen and progesterone. IUDs may be associated with increased incidence of pelvic inflammatory disease, which might lead to autonomic dysreflexia.[83]

Pregnancy

Pregnant women with an SCI are at greater risk of urinary tract infections, leg oedema, thromboembolism, autonomic dysreflexia (if injury above T6), constipation, respiratory infection and premature birth.[86] Since uterine innervation arises from T10 to T12 levels, women with lesions above T10 may not be able to perceive uterine contractions or fetal movements.

In lesions above T6 it may be difficult to detect pregnancy-induced hypertension (pre-eclampsia) in which the blood pressure may increase to dangerously high levels.[41] Autonomic dysreflexia can often be the only clinical manifestation of labour. During the second and third trimesters women may have difficulties in performing functional tasks that were previously completed independently,[84] and urological status is affected and needs closer follow-up.[87] Special considerations during pregnancy should be made to the increased difficulty in moving due to weight gain and changes in centre of balance. Transfers may require the assistance of a caregiver, and a power wheelchair may be necessary for mobility. It is important to maintain proper positioning in a wheelchair, prevent pressure sores and account for changes in medications.[87]

Birth

Labour is recommended to be in a facility that includes a team with accessibility and a supportive attitude and knowledge concerning SCI medicine.[87] The reduced sensation in the pelvic area means women with an SCI usually have a less painful delivery. Sometimes they may experience contractions only as abdominal discomfort, increased spasticity and/or episodes of autonomic dysreflexia. The babies are more likely to be born prematurely small for their gestational time.[86]

TREATMENT ASPECTS – SEXUAL HEALTH ASSESSMENT MODEL

Health professional and client interactions often include issues related to sexuality. Unfortunately, talking about sexuality can be challenging for both clinicians and clients,[10] and broaching the subject is probably the most difficult part for novice providers. By initiating the topic of sexuality as part of the routine SCI assessment, the health professional should create an atmosphere of permission to persons with an SCI and their partners to discuss issues related to sexuality. Communication bridges include the demonstration of respect through providing privacy, asking permission to proceed with more probing questions, being patient and allowing the client time to respond and tailoring the depth of the discussion to the client's readiness. Patients must be informed that sexual healthcare is part of their rehabilitation program and that sexual health services will be offered periodically throughout their rehabilitation process and can also be requested.[10]

Some interactions of health professionals and clients involve intimate contact as part of the therapeutic process. In many other circumstances, sexual issues form part of a required medical history, or are raised as an issue by the client. The availability of oral medication for the management of sexual dysfunctions has raised the important of discussing sexuality with patients on medication or with cardiac problems.[10] It is important to feel comfortable in communicating with the patient about these issues.

Sexuality education should provide basic sexual information and specific suggestions to the client about what changes to expect related to SCI, in order for them to become 'sexually abled' and to feel good about their sexuality.[33] After receiving adequate sexuality education, clients should understand the impact their injury may have on their sexual response and how this can inhibit desire and response. It is important to broaden the client's concept of satisfying sexual experiences. Without help to dispel myths and obtain accurate information, clients may hold onto negative beliefs regarding their sexuality and their sexual potential.[10] They should also be able to identify ways to compensate for the changes in function and to tell a partner what feels good and where, including basic issues such as improving the romantic environment (music, lighting, candles, smells etc). Specifically for people with an SCI, it is important to review issues concerning genital hygiene, bladder and bowel issues (catheterisations and bowel programs prior to sexual activity to avoid accidents, lubricants); mobility and positioning is also important.[36] Patients should be encouraged to explore their own sexuality and what works for them. It is necessary for them to have a specific format in which to address these issues. There are some models for sexual assessment and primary intervention, and elaboration is given on the PLISSIT and Ex-PLISSIT models.

The PLISSIT model, consists of four levels:
1. **P**ermission
2. **L**imited **I**nformation
3. **S**pecific **S**uggestions
4. **I**ntensive **T**herapy

PLISSIT can be used to facilitate the delivery of process-focused counselling by the interdisciplinary rehabilitation team that work with people with an SCI.

This model was designed by Annon[88] as a step-by-step method for gathering sexual health information. The model provides the practitioner with a general framework on how to initiate a dialogue about sexual issues and how to continue the discussion, if warranted. This approach is versatile and can be applied to a wide range of illnesses, situations and settings – both outpatient and inpatient. According to this model, the later levels of treatment build upon the previous ones. However, the health professional can move back and forth between the levels of treatment based on the client's needs.

- **Permission:** *'Sometimes all that people want to know is that they are normal'.* For example, a patient with an SCI asks if it is OK that he has thoughts regarding sex, although he has a disability. In such cases, the clinician can let him know that he is not unusual and the fact that he has a disability does not make him asexual. Permission-giving can be seen as a preventive measure as well as a treatment technique.
- **Limited information:** *Usually given in conjunction with permission-giving.* When giving limited information, it is important for the clinician to do just that – provide 'limited' information that is directly relevant to the client's concern. For example, in response to the above question, after being given the 'permission', the clinician can explain the difference between 'sex' and 'sexuality'.
- **Specific suggestions:** *Before clinicians can give out specific suggestions to a client they must first obtain certain relevant specific information.* This level of intervention involves advanced knowledge of a particular health issue and skills to assess a patient's unique situation in relation to the above-mentioned health issue and to develop a plan.
- **Intensive therapy:** *A minority of patients will require intensive therapy for a particular issue.* This fourth level of intervention may require referral to a specialist. For example, a patient with an SCI who reports several sexual dysfunctions as a result of an injury.

More recently, Taylor and Davis[89] modified Annon's model through the development of the extended PLISSIT model (or Ex-PLISSIT). This model suggests that the 'permission' level should involve requesting permission to discuss sexual issues, as well as providing permission for a person to be a sexual being, and this should be incorporated into each level of the model.[89] Another useful application of the Ex-PLISSIT model is its integration of reflection and review by the clinician after every interaction with the client.

This approach may not adequately emphasise the need for psychotherapeutic interventions or referrals to specialists (e.g. sex therapists, urologists, family and marriage therapists, etc).

This technique helps professionals to learn how to assist with topics that relate to sexuality in people with disabilities. It stresses how important it is to provide information about sexual functioning as well as giving men or women with a disability a safe place where they can go to talk about their fears, hopes and desires and any other topics that relate to psychosexual issues.

It is important to note that the opportunity to receive information and professional advice on the topic of sexuality is limited for people with disabilities, unlike people without. Moreover, it appears that an open discussion in the field of human sexuality allows for clearer sexual communication and thus may improve the ability of people with disabilities to define their sexual needs and the professionals' ability to provide them with a more suitable response. As the caregivers become more comfortable with content related to sexuality and SCIs, they will also be able to legitimise those who ask questions and seek help in the field.

Evidence-based practice points

- Sexuality, including sexual health, sexual functioning, relationships and intimacy are important components of health and wellbeing, thus it is important to relate to those issues in the acute and chronic stages after an SCI in order to achieve better QoL.[10]

- A common myth regards people with an SCI as being asexual, but research shows that sexuality is of high priority for them. It is important to note that sexual function has a profound impact on self-esteem and adjustment to life post-injury.[30]

- Sexual dysfunction is common among male and females with an SCI due to primary causes resulting directly from the impaired neural transmission (such as impaired vaginal lubrication or erection), secondary causes resulting from factors that follow from the injury (such as physical limitation and bladder dysfunction) and tertiary causes resulting from psychological and social factors (such as depression and changes in relationships).[32]

- Initiating the topic of sexuality and informing that sexual healthcare is part of the rehabilitation program creates an atmosphere of permission to persons with an SCI and their partners. The PLISSIT model is a suitable tool to help healthcare givers approach patients in this area.[88]

- Due to the close intensive daily contact with the patients, physiotherapists are often the first healthcare provider the patient will open up to. Furthermore, they have an important role in preventing limitations of range of movement and lower spasticity, thus helping to improve sexual positioning.[47]

SUMMARY

Sexual adaptation following an SCI is a complex and gradual process, involving psychological and physical adjustments. Relationships, self-esteem, sexual function and reproductive ability are all aspects of sexuality, which encompasses a complex array of factors: cultural, social, psychological and emotional influences. The availability of medications, devices and procedures enhance the possibility of having a satisfactory sexual and fertile life after an SCI, and in fact most people with an SCI remain sexually active after the injury, with fulfilling relationships and marriages. Unfortunately, they often experience less sexual satisfaction. Education and counselling about sexuality is an important part of SCI rehabilitation, but is often missing or insufficient.

The rehabilitation process is more efficient when attention is given to the sexual as well as physical aspects of an SCI. Understanding this crucial point makes it clear that successful SCI rehabilitation requires a holistic approach, taking into account the patient's physical, psychological and interpersonal circumstances. The rehabilitation team, including all professional caregivers involved, has the responsibility to provide sexual information, education and counselling during the acute and chronic stages of SCI to all individuals with an SCI, and their partners. To improve sexual rehabilitation services, sexual issues and responses require evaluation during periodical check-ups using validated questionnaires administered by skilled health caregivers.

There are many options and resources to gain more knowledge about sexuality in general and specifically in people with an SCI, including books, the internet and specific courses. There is a need to increase the comfort level of team members in the provision of education during screening, assessment, intervention and discussion of technique.

Online resources

Sexual Health Manual, www.dhrn.ca/files/sexualhealthmanual_lowres_2010_0208.pdf

Sexuality and disability journal, https://link.springer.com/journal/11195

Dr Mitchell Tepper, www.drmitchelltepper.com/media

Sexuality after SCI, www.sexualitysci.org/

References

1. Consortium for Spinal Cord Medicine, 2010. Sexuality and reproductive health in adults with spinal cord injury: a clinical practice guideline for health-care professionals. J. Spinal Cord Med. 33 (3), 281–336.

2. Gergen, K.J., 1999. An Invitation to Social Construction. Sage Publications Ltd, London, England.

3. Tepper, M.S., 2000. Sexuality and disability: the missing discourse of pleasure. Sex. Disabil. 18 (4), 283–290.

4. Committee on Spinal Cord Injury; Board on Neuroscience and Behavioral Health. Institute of Medicine, 2005. Spinal Cord Injury: Progress, Promise, and Priorities. National Academies Press, pp. 56–58.

5. Courtois, F.J., Charvier, K., 2015. Sexual dysfunction in patients with spinal cord lesions. Handb. Clin. Neurol. 130, 225–245.

6. Shakespeare, T., 2000. Disabled sexuality: toward rights and recognition. Sex. Disabil. 18 (3), 159–167.

7. Stoffel, J.T., Van der Aa, F., et al., 2018. Fertility and sexuality in the spinal cord injury patient. World J. Urol. 36 (10), 1577–1585.

8. Dimitriadis, F., Karakitsios, K., et al., 2010. Erectile function and male reproduction in men with spinal cord injury: a review. Andrologia 42 (3), 139–165.

9. Sipski, M.L., Arenas, A., 2006. Female sexual function after spinal cord injury. Prog. Brain Res. 152, 441–447.

10. Alexander, M.S., Courtois, F., et al., 2017. Improving sexual satisfaction in persons with spinal cord injuries: collective wisdom. Top. Spinal Cord Inj. Rehab. 23, 57–70.

11. Heruti, R.J., Ohry, A., 1995. The rehabilitation team. Am. J. Phys. Med. Rehabil. 74 (6), 466–468.

12. Greenberg, S., Bruess, E., et al., 2016. Exploring the Dimensions of Human Sexuality. Jones & Bartlett Publishers.

13. Berry, M.D., 2016. A review of human sexuality: a contemporary introduction. Sex. Marital Ther. 42 (5), 474–475.

14. Whipple, B., 2013. Female sexuality. In: Leyson, J.F.J. (Ed.), Sexual Rehabilitation of the Spinal-Cord-Injured Patient. Springer Science & Business Media.

15. Kinsey, A.C., Clyde, E.M., 1948. Sexual Behavior in the Human Male. Indiana University Press.

16. Masters, W.H., Johnson, V.E., 1970. Human Sexual Inadequacy. Bantam Books, Toronto; New York.

17. Masters, W.H., Johnson, V.E., 1966. Human Sexual Response. Bantam Books, Toronto; New York.

18. Kaplan, H., 1979. Disorders of Sexual Desire. Brunner/Mazel, New York.

19. Graham, C.A., Hall, K., 2012. The Cultural Context of Sexual Pleasure and Problems: Psychotherapy With Diverse Clients. Routledge.

20. WHO, 2006. Defining Sexual Health: Report of a Technical Consultation on Sexual Health, 28–31 2002. World Health Organization, Geneva.

21. Reisman, Y., Porst, H., 2015. The ESSM Manual of Sexual Medicine, second ed. Medix publishers, Amsterdam.

22. Basson, R., Leiblum, S., et al., 2004. Revised definitions of women's sexual dysfunction. J. Sex. Med. 1 (1), 40–48.

23. American Psychiatric Association, 2013. Diagnostic and Statistical Manual of Mental Disorders, fifth ed. rev. APA, Arlington, VA.

24. Soler, J.M., Previnaire, J.G., 2011. Ejaculatory dysfunction in spinal cord injury men is suggestive of dyssynergic ejaculation. Eur. J. Phys. Med. Rehabil. 47 (4), 677–681.

25. Nosek, M.A., Hughes, R., et al., 2004. The meaning of health for women with physical disabilities: a qualitative analysis. Fam. Comm. Health 27, 6–21.

26. Apell, J.M., 2010. Sex rights for the disabled? J. Med. Ethics 36, 152–154.

27. Singh, A., Tetreault, L., et al., 2014. Global prevalence and incidence of traumatic spinal cord injury. Clin. Epidemiol. 6, 309–331.

28. Simpson, L.A., Eng, J.J., et al., 2012. The health and life priorities of individuals with spinal cord injury: a systematic review. J. Neurotrauma 29 (8), 1548–1555.

29. Elliott, S.L., 2013. Sexuality and fertility after spinal cord injury. In: Fehlings, M.G., Vaccaro, A., et al. (Eds.), Essentials of Spinal Cord Injury. Thieme Medical Publishers, New York, pp. 143–157.

30. Lombardi, G., Del Popolo, G., et al., 2010. Sexual rehabilitation in women with spinal cord injury: a critical review of the literature. Spinal Cord 48 (12), 842–849.

31. Wyndaele, J.J., 2010. Neuroanatomy and neurophysiology of sexual function after spinal cord lesion. Spinal Cord 48, 181.

32. Cobo Cuenca, A.I., Sampietro-Crespo, A., et al., 2015. Psychological impact and sexual dysfunction in men with and without spinal cord injury. J. Sex. Med. 12, 436–444.

33. New, P.W., Currie, K.E., 2016. Development of a comprehensive survey of sexuality issues including a self-report version of the International Spinal Cord Injury sexual function basic data sets. Spinal Cord 54 (8), 584–591.

34. Sale, P., Mazzarella, F., et al., 2012. Predictors of changes in sentimental and sexual life after traumatic spinal cord injury. Arch. Phys. Med. Rehabil. 93 (11), 1944–1949.

35. Biering-Sørensen, I., Hansen, R.B., et al., 2012. Sexual function in a traumatic spinal cord injured population 10-45 years after injury. J. Rehabil. Med. 44 (11), 926–931.

36. Hess, M.J., Hough, S., 2012. Impact of spinal cord injury on sexuality: broad-based clinical practice intervention and practical application. J. Spinal Cord Med. 35, 211–218.

37. Courtois, F.J., Charvier, K.F., et al., 2008. Perceived physiological and orgasmic sensations at ejaculation in spinal cord injured men. J. Sex. Med. 5 (10), 2419–2430.

38. Ricciardi, R., Szabo, C.M., 2007. Sexuality and spinal cord injury. Nurs. Clin. North Am. 42, 675–684.

39. Alexander, M.S., Biering-Sorensen, F., et al., 2011a. International spinal cord injury female sexual and reproductive function basic data set. Spinal Cord 49 (7), 787–790.

40. Alexander, M.S., Biering-Sorensen, F., et al., 2011b. International spinal cord injury male sexual function basic data set. Spinal Cord 49 (7), 795–798.

41. Krassioukov, A., Elliott, S., 2017. Neural control and physiology of sexual function: effect of spinal cord injury. Top. Spinal Cord Inj. Rehabil. 23 (1), 1–10.

42. Sipski, M.L., Alexander, C.J., et al., 2007. The effects of spinal cord injury on psychogenic sexual arousal in males. J. Urol. 177 (1), 247–251.

43. Rees, P.M., Fowler, C.J., et al., 2007. Sexual function in men and women with neurological disorders. Lancet 369 (9560), 512–525.

44. Heruti, R.J., Dankner, R., et al., 1997. Gynecomastia following spinal cord disorder. Arch. Phys. Med. Rehabil. 78 (5), 534–537.

45. Burns, S.M., Hough, S., et al., 2009. Sexual desire and depression following spinal cord injury: masculine sexual prowess as a moderator. Assessment of sexual functions after spinal cord injury in Indian patients. Sex Roles 61, 120–129.

46. Anderson, K.D., Borisoff, J.F., et al., 2007. The impact of spinal cord injury on sexual function: concerns of the general population. Spinal Cord 45, 328–337.

47. Andresen, S.R., Biering-Sorensen, F., et al., 2016. Pain, spasticity and quality of life in individuals with traumatic spinal cord injury in Denmark. Spinal Cord 54, 973–979.

48. Abramson, C.E., McBride, K.E., et al., 2008. SCIRE Research Team. Sexual health outcome measures for individuals with a spinal cord injury: a systematic review. Spinal Cord 46 (5), 320–324.

49. Cramp, J.D., Courtois, F.J., et al., 2015. Sexuality for women with spinal cord injury. J. Sex Marital Ther. 41 (3), 238–253.

50. Courtois, F.J., Rodrigue, X., et al., 2012. Sexual function and autonomic dysreflexia in men with spinal cord injuries: how should we treat? Spinal Cord 50 (12), 869–877.

51. Krassioukov, A., MacHattie, E., et al. Pleasureable: sexual device manual for persons with disabilities. Funded Project: Disabilities Health Research Network; 2009.

52. Calabro, R.S., D'Aleo, G., et al., 2014. Sexual dysfunction induced by intrathecal baclofen administration; Is this the price to pay for severe spasticity management? J. Sex. Med. 11 (7), 1807–1815.

53. Barbonetti, A., Cavallo, F., et al., 2012. Erectile dysfunction is the main determinant of psychological distress in men with spinal cord injury. J. Sex. Med. 9, 830–836.

54. Derry, F.A., Dinsmore, W.W., et al., 1998. Efficacy and safety of oral sildenafil (Viagra) in men with erectile dysfunction caused by spinal cord injury. Neurology 51 (6), 1629–1633.

55. Denil, J., Ohl, D.A., et al., 1996. Vacuum erection device in spinal cord injured men: patient and partner satisfaction. Arch. Phys. Med. Rehabil. 77 (8), 750–753.

56. Chochina, L., Naudet, F., et al., 2016. Intracavernous injections in spinal cord injured men with erectile dysfunction, a systematic review and meta-analysis. Sex Med. Rev. 4 (3), 257–269.

57. Linsenmeyer, T.A., 2000. Sexual function and infertility following spinal cord injury. Phys. Med. Rehabil. Clin. N. Am. 11 (1), 141–156.

58. Bodner, D.R., Haas, C.A., et al., 1999. Intraurethral alprostadil for treatment of erectile dysfunction in patients with spinal cord injury. Urology 53 (1), 199–202.

59. Chéhensse, C., Bahrami, S., et al., 2013. The spinal control of ejaculation revisited: a systematic review and meta-analysis of anejaculation in spinal cord injured patients. Hum. Reprod. 19 (5), 507–526.

60. Comarr, A.E., 1970. Sexual function among patients with spinal cord injury. Urol. Int. 25, 134–168.

61. Kreuter, M., Taft, C., et al., 2011. Women's sexual functioning and sex life after spinal cord injury. Spinal Cord 49 (1), 154–160.

62. Otero-Villaverde, S., Ferreiro-Velasco, M.E., et al., 2015. Sexual satisfaction in women with spinal cord injuries. Spinal Cord 53 (7), 557–560.

63. Alexander, M.S., Rosen, R.C., et al., 2011c. Sildenafil in women with sexual arousal disorder following spinal cord injury. Spinal Cord 49 (2), 273–279.

64. Komisaruk, B.R., Whipple, B., 2015. Functional MRI of the brain during orgasm in women. Annu. Rev. Sex Res. 16, 62–86.

65. Freeman, C., Cassidy, B., et al., 2017. Couple's experiences of relationship maintenance and intimacy in acute spinal cord injury rehabilitation: an interpretative phenomenological analysis. Sex. Disabil. 35, 433–444.

66. Ostrander, N., 2012. Sexual pursuits of pleasure among men and women with spinal cord injuries. Sex. Disabil. 27, 11–19.

67. Peter, C., Muller, R., et al., 2012. Psychological resources in spinal cord injury: a systematic literature review. Spinal Cord 50, 188–201.

68. Moin, V., Duvdevany, I., et al., 2009. Sexual identity, body image and life satisfaction among woman with and without physical disability. Sex. Disabil. 27, 83–95.

69. Silvaggi, C., Tripodi, F., 2013. Psychological Barriers to Sexual Functioning. The EFS and ESSM syllabus of clinical sexology. MedixPublishers, Amsterdam, pp. 345–364, (Chapter 15).

70. Muller, R., Peter, C., et al., 2012. The role of social support and social skills in people with spinal cord injury—a systematic review of the literature. Spinal Cord 50, 94–106.

71. Sakellariou, D., 2006. If not the disability, then what? Barriers to reclaiming sexuality following spinal cord injury. Sex. Disabil. 24, 101–111.

72. Anderson, C., Vogel, L., 2003. Domain-specific satisfaction in adults with pediatric-onset spinal cord injuries. Spinal Cord 41, 684–691.

73. Phelps, J., Albo, M., et al., 2001. Spinal cord injury and sexuality in married or partnered men: activities, function, needs, and predictors of sexual adjustment. Arch. Sex. Behav. 30, 591–602.

74. Chang, F.H., Wang, Y.H., et al., 2012. Factors associated with quality of life among people with spinal cord injury:

application of the international classification of functioning, disability and health model. Arch. Physl. Med. Rehab. 93, 2260–2270.

75. Dickson, A., Ward, R., et al., 2011. Difficulties adjusting to post-discharge life following a spinal cord injury: an interpretative phenomenological analysis. Psyc. Health Med. 16 (4), 463–474.

76. Putzke, J., Elliott, T., et al., 2001. Marital status and adjustment 1 year post spinal cord injury. J. Clin. Psychol. Med. Settings 8, 101–107.

77. Angel, S., Buus, N., 2011. The experience of being a partner to a spinal cord injured person: a phenomenological-hermeneutic study. Int. J. Qual. Stud. Health Well-being Internet 6.

78. Ibrahim, E., Lynne, C.M., et al., 2016. Male fertility following spinal cord injury: an update. Andrology 4 (1), 13–26.

79. Bracket, N.L., Ibrahim, E., et al., 2010. Treatment for ejaculatory dysfunction in men with spinal cord injury: an 18-year single center experience. J. Urol. 183, 2304–2308.

80. Fode, M., Ohl, D.A., et al., 2015. A step-wise approach to sperm retrieval in men with neurogenic anejaculation. Nat. Rev. Urol. 12 (11), 607–616.

81. Soler, J.M., Prévinaire, J.G., et al., 2008. Midodrine improves orgasm in spinal cord-injured men: the effects of autonomic stimulation. J. Sex. Med. 5 (12), 2935–2941.

82. Heruti, R.J., Katz, H., et al., 2001. Treatment of male infertility due to spinal cord injury using rectal probe electroejaculation: the Israeli experience. Spinal Cord 39 (3), 168–175.

83. Ghidini, A., Healey, A., et al., 2008. Pregnancy and women with spinal cord injuries. Acta Obstet. Gynecol. Scand. 87 (10), 1006–1010.

84. Lezzoni, L.I., Chen, Y., et al., 2015. Current pregnancy among women with spinal cord injury: findings from the US national spinal cord injury database. Spinal Cord 53 (11), 821–826.

85. Pereira, L., 2003. Obstetric management of the patient with spinal cord injury. Obstet. Gynecol. Surv. 58 (10), 678–687.

86. Bickenbach, J., Officer, A., et al., World Health Organization, 2013. The international spinal cord society. In: International Perspectives on Spinal Cord Injury. World Health Organization, Geneva.

87. Bertschy, S., Geyh, S., et al., 2015. Perceived needs and experiences with healthcare services of women with spinal cord injury during pregnancy and childbirth: a qualitative content analysis of focus groups and individual interviews. BMC Health Ser. Res. 15, 234.

88. Annon, J., 1976. The PLISSIT Model: a proposed conceptual scheme for the behavioral treatment of sexual problems. J. Sex Educ. Ther. 2 (1), 1–15.

89. Taylor, B., Davis, S., 2007. The extended PLISSIT model for addressing the sexual wellbeing of individuals with an acquired disability or chronic illness. Sex. Disabil. 25, 135–139.

CHAPTER 13

Exercise and sport

Greg Ungerer and Jonathan Tang

INTRODUCTION

Spinal cord injury (SCI) and its associated co-morbidities can adversely affect an individual's health, fitness and function. The effects of an SCI can be compounded by a sedentary lifestyle, which is often a result of limited muscle function available, and the challenges encountered by the person with SCI in overcoming the numerous barriers to participation in physical activity or sport. Exercise capacity is reduced in people with an SCI compared to the general population, particularly for those with tetraplegia, due not only to the significant reduction in the muscle mass available for exercise, but also to impaired respiratory function and autonomic dysfunction (e.g. limited maximum heart rate, impaired core temperature regulation).

Physical activity and sport play an important part in the rehabilitation process following SCI. People with an SCI are two to three times more likely to be overweight than the general population.[1,2] Exercise reduces the risk of cardiovascular and metabolic disease, which is the second leading cause of death after respiratory failure in chronic SCI (see Chapter 15).[3,4] Strong evidence supports the premise that regular exercise improves cardiorespiratory fitness, power output, muscle strength and body composition and reduces cardiovascular risk.[5] Emerging evidence suggests that exercise may also reduce the risk of cardiometabolic disease (such as cardiovascular disease, type II diabetes), reduce the incidence of shoulder pain, improve independence in activities of daily living and improve psychosocial wellbeing.[6,7]

ANATOMICAL, PHYSIOLOGICAL AND PSYCHOSOCIAL CONSEQUENCES OF SCI

There are a number of anatomical and physiological changes that occur in the body following SCI (discussed in Chapter 1). Many of these changes can be considered as accelerated ageing, and increase the risk of chronic health conditions that are associated with a sedentary lifestyle.[8] Almost 50% of people with a chronic SCI (> 1 year) have at least one chronic health condition, with hypercholesterolaemia, hypertension and type II diabetes comprising the top three conditions (see Chapter 15). Not surprisingly, cardiovascular disease is the most common cause of death in people with paraplegia, and the second-most common cause of death, after respiratory infections, in people with tetraplegia.[4] Despite potential limitations in cardiorespiratory function and a reduced muscle mass available for exercise, physical activity and exercise have been shown to be effective in reducing the impact and severity of some of these health conditions. People with an SCI can still achieve significant improvements in measures of aerobic fitness and strength, improve respiratory function and reduce risk factors for cardiometabolic disease.

Muscle function

Following SCI, several adaptations occur in muscle physiology. Muscle atrophy occurs below the level of the lesion; there is a change from slow (type I) to fast twitch (type IIb) fibres, a reduction in their oxidative capacity and a reduced number of mitochondria within the cells.[9,10] The result is that these muscles produce less force, have fast contractility and are highly vulnerable to fatigue. Despite these limitations, adaptation to physical activity can still occur. Muscle biopsies taken before and after body weight-supported treadmill training showed reversal of the fibre type change.[11] Endurance training improves muscle oxidative capacity and the ability to utilise fat for energy.[2] There is strong evidence that upper limb aerobic training and circuit training improves cardiorespiratory fitness for people with an SCI. A recent meta-analysis showed there was good evidence that upper-body aerobic exercise could improve cardiorespiratory fitness, power output, muscle strength, body composition and reduce cardiovascular risk in people with a chronic SCI.[5]

Respiratory function

Limitation in respiratory function occurs in individuals with tetraplegia or high paraplegia due to the paralysis of intercostal and abdominal muscles required for forced inspiration or expiration. This can have a significant impact on spirometry measures such as forced expiratory volume (FEV_1) and forced vital capacity (FVC). In addition, dynamic hyperinflation can occur during exercise due to the lack of functioning expiratory muscles. As the respiratory rate increases during exercise, this reduces the time between breaths and thus time available for expiration. In individuals with paralysed expiratory muscles, expiration is mainly reliant on the passive recoil of the lungs and surrounding tissue. In strenuous exercise, this passive recoil is not enough to expel all the air, and results in a cycle of air trapping that can lead to hyperinflation. Despite these complications, individuals with tetraplegia and paraplegia who exercise regularly showed better cardiorespiratory fitness than those who were sedentary. In one study, individuals who exercised for at least 55 minutes twice per week for 6 months had significantly higher FEV_1, FVC and $VO_{2\ peak}$ on cardiopulmonary tests.[12] (For further information on the respiratory impact of tetraplegia or high paraplegia refer to Chapter 16.)

Bone mineral density

Osteoporosis or reduced bone mineral density (BMD) is common following SCI. The lack of mechanical load and weight bearing reduces osteoblast activity, which favours bone resorption over new bone formation. Trabecular bone, particularly in the distal femur and proximal tibia, is most susceptible to demineralisation. SCI-induced osteoporosis may result in low-impact fractures during activities of daily living (ADLs) such as seated transfers. Mimicking mechanical load through electrically stimulated muscle contractions or passive standing does not appear to reverse this loss. A systematic review of exercise, including FES cycling, determined that there was inconclusive evidence regarding whether these modalities could maintain or reverse the loss of BMD after SCI.[5] Similarly, simulated weight-bearing activities, such as body weight-supported treadmill training, have shown limited evidence of success. A 6-week exoskeleton locomotion program (180 min/week) in people with a complete SCI showed improvements in lean muscle mass and reduced body fat, but no significant improvements in BMD.[13] While there is emerging evidence that medications can maintain BMD, to date there is inconclusive evidence that exercise alone can maintain or reverse the loss of BMD in chronic SCI. (For further detail on these issues see Chapters 4 and 18.)

Insulin resistance

Impaired insulin sensitivity or insulin resistance is a growing problem following SCI, and can progress to type II diabetes and metabolic syndrome. Up to 50% of people with an SCI have impaired glucose tolerance, typically associated with insulin resistance.[14] While the mechanisms leading to metabolic syndrome are not completely understood following SCI, a contributing factor is the change in skeletal muscle. Skeletal muscle is responsible for up to 80–95% of daily glucose uptake.[15] Insulin is a key hormone that promotes uptake of glucose into skeletal muscle. Following SCI there is a loss of muscle mass and changes in muscle physiology, reducing the ability of skeletal muscles to uptake glucose. As a result, there is impaired glucose metabolism and a rise in blood insulin levels.[14] However, aerobic exercise and neuromuscular electrical stimulation have been shown to improve glucose metabolism and reduce blood insulin levels. Exercise with FES cycling show short- and long-term effects of improved glucose metabolism, increased glycolytic enzymes and mitochondrial oxidative enzyme activity.[16] Similarly, aerobic exercise has also shown to improve insulin sensitivity. Both a 6-week (180 min/week) and 10-week (90 min/week) arm crank (also known as arm or upper-body ergometers) home exercise program suggested improvements in insulin sensitivity can be achieved in people with an SCI.[6,17]

Lipid profile

People with an SCI have an increased risk of dyslipidaemia; higher levels of triglycerides, LDL cholesterol (LDL – low density lipoprotein cholesterol ('bad' cholesterol)) and lower HDL cholesterol (HDL – high density lipoprotein cholesterol ('good' cholesterol)). This altered lipid profile is a key feature in metabolic syndrome, and associated with increased risk of coronary artery disease and peripheral vascular disease.[14] While there is inconclusive evidence that exercise alone can improve the biomarkers of cardiovascular disease in people with an SCI, there is ample evidence in the able-bodied population. Exercise alone has been shown to reduce triglycerides

and, together with diet, also reduce LDL levels.[18] It is, therefore, not unreasonable to assume these effects might also benefit people with an SCI.

Obesity

Obesity is a major problem following SCI. Recent studies suggest a prevalence between 40% and 83% (BMI ≥ 22 kg/m^2) in people with SCI.[2,19] The BMI cut-off point in people with an SCI is lower because muscle atrophy can give false negative results. Using the World Health Organization guidelines would underestimate the risk of cardiovascular disease in people with SCI.[20]

People with chronic SCI, on average, have a higher percentage of total body fat compared to the general population. Contributing factors include the reduction in lean muscle mass from muscle atrophy, reduced basal metabolic rate, changes in hormones and lifestyle factors (e.g. sedentary behaviour, diet).[21] However, more concerning is that SCI is associated with greater central obesity or visceral adipose tissue. This is fatty tissue deposited around the organs, and is a stronger predictor of obesity-related conditions, such as cardiovascular disease, insulin resistance, dyslipidaemia and may cause mortality.[1]

There is emerging evidence that moderate-to-vigorous leisure-time physical activity is associated with a reduction in visceral adipose tissue.[22] Physical activity plays a vital role in maintaining the homeostatic balance between energy intake and expenditure. In addition to increasing lean muscle mass, physical activity can also increase basal metabolic rate and improve skeletal muscles' oxidative capacity.[2] While physical activity is an important part of a healthy lifestyle following SCI, the need for dietary intervention and behavioural modification is equally important.[21]

Musculoskeletal injuries

Physical inactivity has been linked with increased incidence of shoulder pain.[23] Conversely, participation in physical activity has been associated with reduced musculoskeletal injury, in particular shoulder pain, in people with an SCI. A study of wheelchair athletes showed half the incidence of shoulder pain compared with their non-athletic counterparts.[24] It may appear counterintuitive that sport participation reduces musculoskeletal injury in wheelchair users. It might be expected that physical activity would increase the risk of muscle injuries, particularly in competitive sports. However, a reasonable hypothesis could be that physical activity improves range of motion and muscle strength, in particular in the scapular stabilisers, such as the rotator cuff muscles, which are an important factor in preventing shoulder injuries.[25] A Cochrane review of chronic pain in SCI showed exercise programs had a significant impact on reduction of shoulder pain scores on SF-36 and visual analogue scale (VAS).[26] Health practitioners can therefore be reassured that sporting participation does not significantly increase the risk of musculoskeletal injuries.

Pain

Chronic pain is a common symptom present in 70% of people with an SCI with up to one-third of those having moderate-to-severe symptoms (see Chapter 18).[27] Studies have shown exercise can be an effective non-pharmacological modality in treating chronic neuropathic pain; however, the mechanisms are not well understood. Exercise may have an effect on the endogenous opioid system and endorphins which regulate the perception of pain. The benefits of exercise also include improvement in psychosocial wellbeing and reduction in depression and anxiety, which has a high correlation with pain perception.

Psychosocial wellbeing, community integration and participation

An SCI has a devastating impact on the individual and their family. It is unsurprising that people with an SCI have higher levels of depression and anxiety, and a lower quality of life than the general population. Despite this, exercise and sports literature consistently reports strong associations between physical activity and improvements in psychosocial wellbeing, including reduction in depression and anxiety, improved quality of life and resilience.[7,12]

People with an SCI who exercised regularly had higher self-perceived quality of life and self-reported physical health than their inactive counterparts.[12] Similarly, group exercise programs in the community have been shown to reduce depression and pain scores and improve quality of life and self-esteem.[28]

A more in-depth review of the literature on sport and SCI can be found at the Spinal Cord Injury Research Evidence (SCIRE) project (see Online resources at the end of the chapter).

EXERCISE GUIDELINES FOR PEOPLE WITH AN SCI

Health practitioners have recognised the benefits of physical activity and sport across the domains of health, fitness, wellbeing and participation. Those involved in providing in-patient rehabilitation, which is very physical in its nature, are therefore ideally positioned to promote exercise and its numerous benefits to their patients with an SCI. The challenge many health practitioners face is how to capitalise on the daily routine of exercise that occurs during rehabilitation, and maintain the momentum for regular physical activity beyond the in-patient rehabilitation paradigm, shifting the focus from physical activity and exercise to a greater focus on health maintenance and improvement following discharge into the community.

Community-based health practitioners and exercise and fitness professionals can often be apprehensive about exercise prescription due to the nature of SCI, unfamiliarity with this health condition and the complex co-morbidities that can occur in this population. Difficulties in engaging exercise professionals in prescribing community-based exercise programs was identified as a significant barrier to ongoing regular exercise for people with an SCI.[28] However, this research determined that simple education strategies were effective in reducing this barrier.

The minimum recommended amount of exercise for cardiorespiratory fitness and muscle strength benefits for adults with an SCI are:[29]

- 20 minutes of moderate-to-vigorous intensity aerobic exercise two times per week; and
- three sets of strength exercises for each major functioning muscle group at a moderate-to-vigorous intensity two times per week.

For adults with an SCI the minimum recommended exercise for cardiometabolic health benefits, which reduces the risk for coronary artery disease, stroke, type II diabetes and dyslipidaemia, is at least 30 minutes of moderate-to-vigorous intensity aerobic exercise three times per week.[29]

However, for optimal health, including cardiorespiratory and cardiometabolic benefits, adults with an SCI should aim to complete:[30]

- 30 minutes or more of moderate aerobic exercise on five or more days of the week or
- 20 minutes or more of vigorous aerobic exercise on three or more days a week

and

- strength training on two or more days a week, including scapula stabilisers and the posterior shoulder girdle

and

- flexibility training on two or more days a week, including the shoulder rotators.

High-intensity interval training has been suggested to have superior cardiometabolic benefits when compared to moderate-intensity exercise, and may therefore be better suited to people with an SCI.[31]

When engaging people with an SCI in regular exercise, it may be useful for health practitioners to consider participants as beginners, intermediate and advanced in order to assist in tailoring programs to more individual needs and set realistic exercise goals that are achievable and can progress over time.[30] A long-term view may be required for extremely sedentary individuals.

While there are no tetraplegia-specific guidelines for exercise, it is important for clinicians to be aware of the differences in this subgroup. Firstly, there may be a limitation in physiological response in

motor complete tetraplegia and high paraplegia. As mentioned previously, limitations in maximum heart rate, autonomic dysfunction and respiratory function may alter exercise prescription. For example, heart rate may not be a reliable measure of exercise intensity.

Secondly, this subgroup will have additional barriers to exercise. For example, those with limited hand function will require adaptive equipment. Practical barriers can include transport, organising carers and even the additional time and energy spent physically attending a gym.

Finally, clinicians should understand the difference in energy expenditure between people with paraplegia and tetraplegia. The total energy expenditure in people with an SCI ranges from 900–1500 kcal/day, whereas able-bodied controls average 2200 kcal/day.[14] While both those with paraplegia and those with tetraplegia have lower than predicted resting energy expenditure, in people with tetraplegia his has been shown to be 22% less than able-bodied matched controls.[21] Contributing factors may include reduction of lean muscle mass, which contributes to about a third of cardiac output at rest. More importantly, however, energy expenditure during exercise was significantly reduced in tetraplegia. For the same level of intensity, people with tetraplegia had lower energy output, regardless of exercise modality.[21] This is not surprising considering that people with tetraplegia are exercising with smaller and fewer innervated muscle groups. Therefore, given the reduced energy output in people with tetraplegia, as mentioned above, it is likely that the published guidelines may need to be increased to provide the same cardiometabolic benefits.

This is in line with the WHO Physical Activity Guidelines for Adults, which, while recommending 150 minutes of moderate-intensity physical activity per week, includes a caveat that while these recommendations can be applied to adults with disabilities, they may need to be adjusted for each individual based on their exercise capacity and specific health risks or limitations. Therefore, considering that many people with an SCI are exercising using predominantly smaller upper limb muscle groups, which are not as effective in influencing the biomarkers of metabolic health, it may seem counterintuitive to recommend physical activity levels that are lower than the WHO guidelines.[32]

In this context, it is also necessary to acknowledge the significant barriers to participation in regular physical activity and exercise for adults with an SCI. Therefore, as health practitioners, while it is important to recommend regular exercise for people with an SCI to promote a healthy lifestyle, the barriers needed to be taken into consideration. Some of the most common barriers are summarised in Table 13.1.

Despite the numerous barriers identified, Table 13.2 summarises some simple strategies that may assist in negotiating these barriers. Many of these strategies represent concepts that can be introduced and incorporated into in-patient rehabilitation programs for people with an SCI. Physiotherapists, occupational therapists, leisure/recreational therapists and peer support workers should play a very active role in assisting people with an SCI to achieve their goals of returning to, or embarking on, an active lifestyle.

For example, health practitioners can assist people with an SCI to mitigate the risk of adverse events such as autonomic dysreflexia (AD), pressure injuries due to sensory impairment, thermoregulatory dysfunction, spasticity, orthostatic or exertional hypotension and pain. (For further detail on these issues see Chapters 4 and 18.)

Sport for people with an SCI

Sport is a competitive form of physical activity or exercise that is governed by a set of rules and performed in a social context. For many people with an SCI, particularly those who participated in regular sporting activities prior to their injury, the resumption of sporting activities represents a key goal or milestone in resuming their pre-injury lifestyle.

The term para-sport is collectively used to describe sporting events or activities for athletes who have impairments. Para-sports commonly use adapted rules or equipment to make the sporting activity accessible to the sport's participants. Many para-sports have a 'parallel' equivalent for athletes without impairments, but some, such as wheelchair rugby, have been designed to specifically provide competitive sporting opportunities to a population of athletes with a specific impairment profile. Wheelchair rugby was developed specifically for athletes who have impairments in all four limbs, and was developed to provide competitive opportunities for athletes whose impairment resulted in them being significantly less competitive in other para-sports such as wheelchair basketball.

While sporting events for athletes with impairments can be traced back to the 19th century, para-sport really came to prominence towards the end of World War II. With large numbers of ex-servicemen returning to the United Kingdom with SCIs, the British Government opened a centre for SCI rehabilitation at the Stoke Mandeville Hospital in 1944, under the guidance of neurologist Sir Ludwig Guttman.[33]

Dr Guttman recognised the therapeutic benefits of organised physical activity, and promoted the integration of recreational sporting activities into otherwise conventional rehabilitation programs. Activities such as archery and wheelchair netball (an early form of wheelchair basketball) found a regular place in therapeutic recreation programs, alongside physiotherapy and occupational therapy.

With increasing numbers of athletes participating in these regular sporting activities, competitive sporting competitions were a logical progression, and the Stoke Mandeville Wheelchair Games were born. First held in 1948, 26 athletes competed in a variety of athletic field events and archery. Dutch athletes joined the sporting movement in 1952, giving rise to the first annual international competition.[34] The years that followed would see athletes from other countries and with other impairment types join the movement, with the Stoke Mandeville Games eventually becoming the Paralympic Games in 1960.

The Paralympic Games are the pinnacle of sporting achievement for athletes with impairments and the second largest multi-sport event in the world.

Table 13.1 Barriers to participation in physical activity or sports

Physical factors related to health condition	• Autonomic dysreflexia • Orthostatic/exertional hypotension • Thermoregulation issues • Musculoskeletal injuries • Pressure injuries • Recurrent health issues (e.g. infections) • Pain • Fatigue • Neurological impairment profile (presence of trunk/hand function)
Personal/psychological factors	• Depression • Low motivation • Low energy • Lack of endurance • Lack of confidence • Fear of injury • Fear of exercise environments • Fear of embarrassment or failure • Lack of time • Lack of personal assistance or support • Low value attributed to physical activity
Access/environmental issues	• External access • Internal access • Available and appropriate adaptive equipment • Accessible change rooms and bathrooms • Accessible terrain • Accessible transportation • Impacts of adverse weather
Financial issues	• Cost of transportation • Cost or availability of equipment • Activity or sport program/gym fees
Information/awareness/ education issues: Lack of knowledge/ awareness among people with an SCI	• How to develop an appropriate exercise program • How to execute exercises that need to be modified due to the effects of SCI • How to get involved in organised para-sport or adaptive sport • Understanding classification in para-sport and its implications
Information/awareness/ education issues: Lack of knowledge/ awareness among health practitioners	• How to develop an appropriate exercise/training program • How to prescribe and teach exercises that are modified due to the effects of SCI • How to promote the preservation of upper limb function following SCI • How to minimise the risk of injury or adverse health events • How to access para-sport or adaptive sports • Understanding classification in para-sport

Sources: de Oliveira B.I., Howie E.K., et al., 2016. SCIPA Com: outcomes from the spinal cord injury and physical activity in the community intervention. Spinal Cord 54 (10), 855–860; Martin Ginis K.A., Jorgensen S., et al., 2012. Exercise and sport for persons with spinal cord injury. PM R 4 (11), 894–900; Vissers M., van den Berg-Emons R., et al., 2008. Barriers to and facilitators of everyday physical activity in persons with a spinal cord injury after discharge from the rehabilitation centre. J Rehabil Med. 40 (6), 461–467.

Table 13.2 Facilitators of physical activity/sport participation

Physical Factors	• Action plans for medical issues • Preventative strategies
Personal Factors	• Goal setting • Professional supports • Social supports • Peer supports • Education/information regarding the benefits of physical activity
Access Issues	• Community access training to build confidence and skill • Action plans/strategies for negotiating barriers • Linking with sporting, advocacy and support organisations • Peer supports
Financial Issues	• Information and support to determine subsidies available, low cost options • Support to include provisions for exercise and sport into funded support plans
Information/Awareness/ Education Issues	• Evidence-based resources • Specialist SCI health practitioners and fitness professionals • Peer supports

Sources: de Oliveira B.I., Howie E.K., et al., 2016. SCIPA Com: outcomes from the spinal cord injury and physical activity in the community intervention. Spinal Cord 54 (10), 855–860; Martin Ginis K.A., Jorgensen S., et al., 2012. Exercise and sport for persons with spinal cord injury. PM R 4 (11), 894–900; Vissers M., van den Berg-Emons R., et al., 2008. Barriers to and facilitators of everyday physical activity in persons with a spinal cord injury after discharge from the rehabilitation centre. J Rehabil Med. 40 (6), 461–467.

Elite para-sport

Participation in elite para-sport may be an aspirational goal after SCI. The Paralympic Games now includes athletes with many different impairment types and health conditions. Over the past decade, media coverage and advertising have brought para-sport and many para athletes more into the mainstream, particularly in countries that host the Paralympic Games. In Australia, the Australian Sports Commission provides financial support for established and upcoming athletes in the Paralympic sporting program. Some of the top athletes may be semi-professional. They may train full-time, and supplement their income with prize money, equipment and clothing sponsorship deals. For example, an elite wheelchair tennis athlete may have a racquet sponsor who provides racquets, bags and clothing and a tennis wheelchair sponsor who

will provide a new chair each year. In addition, they may receive government or other funding to subsidise international travel.

Participation at an elite level is challenging, and not dissimilar to able-bodied elite sport. It requires commitment and sacrifice and often involves an arduous competitive and travel schedule. A typical elite athlete would train five to six days per week, and may have multiple sessions per day. In addition, there will be gym sessions, recovery sessions and cross training. The principles of cross training involve the athlete engaging in other forms of physical activity than their usual sport. For example, athletes who compete in track and road wheelchair racing often use swimming and handcycling to improve aerobic fitness.

An international level athlete representing their country may travel overseas up to three to four times per year to participate in training camps, or compete in qualifying events and competitions. However, this can vary dramatically in a world championship or Paralympic year where additional travel to international competitions may be needed to secure qualification for these events. The athlete may spend up to 2 months in a year away from home. Furthermore, sponsored athletes are also required to participate in promotional events, press conferences and interviews.

The athlete commonly works with a team of people, including their coach, physiotherapist, massage therapist, dietitian, sports doctor, sports psychologist and team manager. This team will assist the athlete in managing any injuries that may occur, and help them maintain peak physical performance. The difference between elite para-sport and elite able-bodied sport is that in addition to training and competition, time needs to be set aside to manage living with an SCI. This may include the athlete's personal care routines, the attention to hydration status and prophylactic measures to prevent urinary tract infections, as well as keeping on top of medications and medical appointments. Without maintaining a healthy baseline, a para athlete is unable to excel in their sport.

Participation at an elite level may not be a personal goal, and may not be recommended for every individual with a newly acquired SCI. Elite para-sport may seem glamorous and be an aspirational goal for some people, but the demands on the individual, such as training and competition, will need to be balanced with general health and wellbeing, and other competing demands, such as work and family responsibilities. It may take years of training and dedication to achieve the performance required at elite level. Individuals with an SCI who were previously elite athletes may generally find the transition easier, and may be able to 'get back on the horse' in a shorter space of time.

Some people with a newly acquired SCI may see the Paralympics as their measure of success in 'overcoming' their injury, but the Paralympics should not be seen as the ultimate benchmark for people who want to engage in para-sport. The benefits of exercise and sport can be achieved without the need to progress to this elite level. The framing of sport participation after SCI needs to be carefully considered so as not to promote it as a measure of success above all else. Paralympic participation is a measure of sporting achievement, but is not a requirement for an individual to be successful (Fig. 13.1).

Classification in para-sport

An athlete's success should be determined by a combination of their skill, fitness, power, endurance, tactical ability and mental focus.

However, due to the nature and variety of presentations of SCI, there is a risk that competition will simply be dominated by those athletes with the least impairment, rather than those who are the best at any given moment. This would be a significant barrier to participation for many people with an SCI and, in particular, those people with higher degrees of impairment.

A unique feature of para-sport is the concept of classification. This provides a structure for competition, and ensures that those athletes with the least impairment do not dominate. All athletes who compete in para-sport have an impairment that leads to a competitive disadvantage, and this can vary between sports, being dependent on the sport-specific activities that are the key features of the sport. Measurement of this impairment, and therefore its impact on sports performance, is central to the process of classification. Modern evidence-based classification systems differ significantly by sport, and are developed and managed by each respective sport's international federation.

History of classification systems

Early classification systems were based on the athlete's medical diagnosis, meaning that only athletes with the same (or similar) health conditions could compete against each other.

From the early 1990s, the International Paralympic Committee (IPC) began to promote a

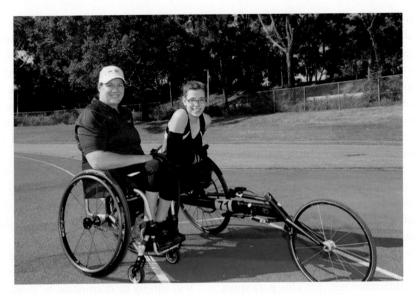

Figure 13.1 Participation in para-sports can foster resilience and independence.
Source: Courtesy Jonathon Tang

more consistent approach to developing classification systems, requiring sporting federations and classifiers to look more closely at how the athlete's impairment may impact upon the performance of activities specific to each sport. This compelled classification systems to move from being impairment-specific to sport-specific. This new approach to classification became known as functional classification.

Due to the time taken to develop the scientific evidence required, early functional classification systems were developed using the expert opinions of classifiers, who were predominantly physiotherapists, occupational therapists, doctors, coaches and athletes.

In the 1990s it was recognised that there was a need for greater consistency and accuracy in classification systems, so in 2007 the IPC Classification Code was released. The Code was revised in 2015, alongside international standards that described technical and operational requirements for classification.[35]

The primary objective of evidence-based sport-specific classification is to ensure that the impact of the athlete's impairment is minimised, thereby ensuring that success is determined by athletic excellence. Classification systems must ensure that athletes who improve their performance through effective training techniques are not penalised for these improvements in performance by moving them into sport classes for athletes with less activity limitation.

Classification for athletes with an SCI

To be eligible to participate in competitive para-sports, athletes must have a permanent and verifiable health condition that falls under one of the IPC's eligible impairment types. For people with health conditions that result in physical impairments, in general terms, this means that athletes must have impaired muscle power, impaired passive range of movement (ROM), limb deficiency, leg length difference, short stature, ataxia, athetosis or hypertonia.

Individual para-sports determine which of the eligible impairment types are eligible to compete in in their respective sport. For example, for athletes who compete in wheelchair rugby, the International Wheelchair Rugby Federation has determined they must have impaired muscle power, impaired passive ROM, limb deficiency, ataxia, athetosis or hypertonia.

Athletes with other impairment types are not eligible to participate in the competitive form of the game, at representative national or international level, but may be permitted to play in social competitions, at the discretion of local sporting clubs.

In addition to having an eligible impairment type, athletes competing in para-sport must meet the minimum impairment criteria prescribed by the international federation for that particular sport. For example, in wheelchair rugby, this means that athletes with an SCI must have a prescribed level of measurable impairment in their upper limbs in order to be eligible. The minimum impairment criteria, in this case, means that athletes who have paraplegia are not eligible to compete in wheelchair rugby. For those athletes who meet the minimum impairment criteria, the degree of the athlete's impairment will determine which of the seven sport classes a wheelchair rugby athlete is allocated, in accordance with the classification rules.

A sport-specific classification process, referred to as athlete evaluation, usually includes two or more of the following components:

- **Measurement of the athlete's impairment:** This component may be referred to as the 'bench test' or 'physical assessment' and includes a physical examination that measures the defining feature of the athlete's impairment. For athletes with an SCI, this will usually include manual muscle testing of the upper and/or lower limbs and assessment of the athlete's trunk function.

- **Activity testing:** This component of the classification process may be referred to as the 'technical assessment', and requires the athlete to perform prescribed activities in a non-competitive environment that would be performed in the sport. For example, for wheelchair rugby, classifiers will evaluate how the athlete propels, turns, accelerates and stops their wheelchair, and how they

pass, receive and dribble the ball. These are considered the key activities performed in the sport, so classifiers are looking at the effect of the athlete's impairment on performance of these activities. The evaluation is also usually conducted both with and without any permitted equipment, such as gloves and strapping, that the athlete uses during play, so that classifiers can observe the extent of assistance the equipment provides.

- **Observation assessment:** also referred to as 'in-competition assessment', this assessment takes place in the competitive environment to ensure that the results of the other components of the athlete evaluation are consistent with the activity limitation that is observed during competition.

Some para-sports require an athlete to be classified only once during their competitive career, while other sports may require classification on more than one occasion.

SCI affects multiple body systems. In addition to impaired muscle power, athletes with an SCI may also present with:

- impaired sensation (including proprioception)
- impaired autonomic function
- impaired respiratory function
- pain.

While it is well recognised that these additional impairments can have a direct impact on sports performance, these are not impairments that can be reliably and consistently measured in the context of classification in the field, and therefore cannot be taken into consideration when determining an athlete's sport class.

When classifying athletes with an SCI, we must also be aware of other factors that can influence the athlete's presentation:

- **Time since injury:** an athlete with a new SCI may not yet have a stable neurological presentation, due to the potential for further recovery. This may not preclude classification, but rather raise a flag for classifiers to review the athlete's sport class at some point in the future.

- **Sport-specific experience:** classifiers need to be able to determine whether the athlete's ability to perform sport-specific activities is due to the impact of the impairment, or rather other factors, such as abilities gained through training and competition, wheelchair set-up or the use of permitted equipment. The risk is that an inexperienced athlete or an athlete with a poor equipment set-up could be placed in a class for athletes who have a higher degree of impairment due to their poorer performance. An athlete's sport class should not change as they develop better strength, endurance and tactical ability, for example, through training.

- **Medical or surgical procedures:** certain medical or surgical procedures can temporarily or permanently change the nature or degree of an athlete's impairment. Nerve or tendon transfer surgeries are not uncommon in athletes with an SCI. Nerve transfer surgeries, in particular, may result in improvements of motor function slowly over time. Botulinum toxin may be used to mitigate the effects of focal spasticity, thereby improving other available motor functions.

Classification systems, by their nature, are complex and evolve over time. Classification research programs, driven by international sporting federations, aim to refine and improve the accuracy of classification systems, based on scientific evidence, sometimes resulting in significant changes to these systems. More information regarding specific classification systems for para-sports can be found on the official website of the Paralympic movement (see Online resources).

Para-sports for athletes with an SCI

Athletes with an SCI are able to compete recreationally or competitively in many para-sports, as outlined in Box 13.1.

Box 13.1 Para-sports

Alpine skiing

Archery

Athletics (track and field)

Badminton

Boccia

Cross country skiing

Cycling (including hand cycling)

Equestrian

Para biathlon

Para ice hockey

Paracanoe

Paratriathlon

Powerlifting

Rowing

Sailing

Shooting

Sitting volleyball

Snowboard

Swimming

Table tennis

Wheelchair basketball

Wheelchair curling

Wheelchair dance sport

Wheelchair fencing

Wheelchair rugby

Wheelchair tennis

Adaptive sports for people with an SCI

Outside of the para-sport programs, a number of other adaptive sporting activities are commonly available, including, but not limited to, those listed in Box 13.2.

State and national disability sports organisations play a pivotal role in linking people who have physical

Box 13.2 Adaptive sports

Bush walking

Cricket

Cue sports

Fishing

Golf

Lawn bowls

Mountain biking

Paddle boarding

Powerchair football

Powerchair hockey

Surfing

Tenpin bowling

Water skiing

Wheelchair Aussie Rules

Yoga

impairments with respective sporting organisations. These organisations provide information and support to new members, offering 'come and try' recreational and sporting opportunities, the loan of sport wheelchairs, linking members with national sporting programs and competitions and linking members with sporting organisations that have an integrated approach to working with athletes who have physical impairments. These organisations may also facilitate classification pathways for new members, where classification is required for sports participation. Peer support also plays a significant role in introducing new athletes to any sport, and these sporting organisations are a rich source of members who have lived experience with their chosen sporting or recreational activity.

In addition to organising the Paralympic Games, the IPC acts as the governing body, or international sporting federation, for 10 sports, including athletics and swimming. For other sports, independent international sporting federations provide governance and, as such, are responsible for all development activities, classification systems, competition structure and management. The IPC and other international sporting federations commonly develop relationships with national sporting organisations, which assume responsibility for managing national competition structures, athlete development and classification. These national organisations may be disability specific, and have responsibility for one or more sports, or may be sport-specific with an integrated model of governance. Integrated models occur in sports where the organisation takes responsibility for the management of the sport for both athletes with and athletes without a disability.

OTHER BENEFITS OF EXERCISE AND SPORT FOR PEOPLE WITH AN SCI

The health benefits of exercise and sport for people with an SCI extend beyond the physiological and psychosocial impacts previously mentioned. Participation in exercise and sport can also foster independence, develop resilience and provide a supportive environment in which individuals can explore and develop new skills. The benefits of exercise and sport participation are therefore much more than muscle hypertrophy, cardiovascular endurance or improved ROM; sport has a positive impact on participation and social inclusion, and can address many of the personal barriers that limit community reintegration. Peer-led learning in areas such as wheelchair skills, equipment maintenance and travel can assist enormously in the development of new skills. (See Chapter 20 for a personal reflection on the importance of participation in sporting activities.)

Fostering independence and developing resilience

Participation in sport can promote independence in daily living. Improvements in muscle strength and cardiovascular endurance can improve ADLs, such as wheeled mobility and transfers. In addition to this, sport can provide a safe environment where individuals are empowered to learn and try new skills. Saltan and colleagues[36] administered a questionnaire to wheelchair basketball players, and found that sports participation was positively associated with improved wheelchair skills.

Another area where sport participation can promote independence is through travel. Travelling after SCI can be a daunting task. There are the logistics of travelling with equipment, the complexities of personal care routines, medications and the uncertainty of accessibility at the destination. If travelling overseas, the added tasks associated with pressure relief and bowel/bladder management on long-haul flights, a foreign health system and foreign language can make the task seem almost impossible. As such, it may take years or even decades after their injury before a person with an SCI attempts to travel. This may have a significant impact on their employment, recreational activities or their ability to see family and friends.

Travelling with a sporting team is one facilitator in overcoming this barrier. While it is not a prerequisite to participation, travelling becomes part of the sporting routine, and most athletes embrace travelling to competitions, training camps or social/recreational reasons, whether overnight, for a few days or even weeks at a time. Travelling fosters independence because it pushes the individual beyond their usual comfort zone by removing their regular supports and challenging their adaptability. For example, staying in a hotel room with limited or no adaptive equipment sounds daunting, but is not necessarily unachievable. Travelling as a team means not everyone will get an accessible room. Usually the accessible room will be allocated to the athletes with the greatest impairment. Peers can teach skills to navigate tight bathroom spaces, including transferring into bathtubs, for example. These skills are transferrable to future travel where 'wheelchair accessible' rooms cannot be guaranteed, and to everyday life, where environmental barriers frequently arise.

Travelling on long-haul flights is difficult for most people, but can be especially daunting for people with

an SCI. For example, there is a fine balance between staying hydrated and minimising the need to use the bathroom. Some people with an SCI choose to travel dehydrated in order to minimise the need to use the bathroom. While it may minimise their use of bathroom facilities, dehydration can lead to adverse events such as increased risk of urinary tract infections, syncope and postural hypotension or acute kidney injury. Regular maintenance of fluids is advised on long-haul flights. On larger aeroplanes there may be larger accessible or double-size bathrooms available, wide enough for individuals with mobility restriction to access with an aisle chair. However, this space can be limited in smaller aeroplanes. One benefit of travelling with a team is learning from peers with experience in how to manage personal care needs, such as bladder management, on a long-haul flight. This may include performing personal care needs without using the bathroom, or advice on using an indwelling catheter for the duration of the flight. Travelling is not only a sport-specific skill, but it is a valuable, transferable life skill.

There is a positive culture in the para-sporting community whereby peers encourage individuals to perform progressively more difficult physical tasks independently without assistance. For example, independently transferring into a rugby or tennis wheelchair is not a skill that is commonly taught in an in-patient rehabilitation environment. Beginners in the sport may find this difficult due to the different positioning required, difficult seat angles and the lack of brakes on these sport-specific chairs. At first, it might seem like an impossible task to perform without assistance. However, the person with an SCI will see their peers overcome these problems, for example, by positioning their chair against the wall to stop it moving. The end result may not be complete independence in all situations, but may see a significant reduction in the amount of assistance required. The benefit of participation such as this is learning from peers, and observing, first-hand, how challenges can be overcome.

In many situations, interaction with peers allows those with similar impairments to share solutions

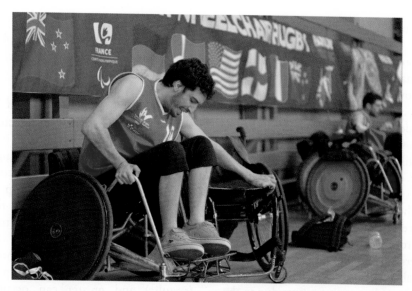

Figure 13.2 Athlete transfers from everyday wheelchair to sports wheelchair.
Source: Luc Percival/IWRF

for common problems. For example, athletes with tetraplegia who have limited hand function may have difficulty holding water bottles. People new to a sporting activity may be used to a friend or carer assisting them with a task such as this. Peers can demonstrate that this problem can be simply resolved with a solution such as adaptive handles or hooks on their drink bottle. Something as simple as this means the person does not have to rely on others to the same extent.

Promoting participation and inclusion

In the sporting environment, people with SCIs are treated not just equally, but are expected to actively participate if they have the ability to perform a task. For example, they may be expected by peers to assist with set-up and packing up of equipment, carrying luggage while travelling or repairing their own equipment. Depending on the individual's degree of impairment, there may be instances where assistance is required, but the expectation exists that the individual will participate to their maximum capacity.

Other seemingly simple interactions in the sporting environment can have a positive impact on the person with an SCI. For example, seeing their peers drive to training in their own car, without relying on family and friends, may prompt the individual to explore this option further for themselves. Hearing about their peer's day at work, the assignments that are due at school or how their housemate keeps leaving dirty dishes in the sink can 'normalise' aspects of life after SCI. Interactions like these can open doors to what is possible after an SCI. It can be extremely empowering for an individual with an SCI to see their peers accomplish a task they are trying to overcome themselves.

CONSIDERATIONS FOR PEOPLE WITH AN SCI PARTICIPATING IN EXERCISE AND SPORT

Autonomic dysreflexia

AD is a health condition that can affect people with an SCI at the level of T6 and above (see also Chapter 4). It is a potentially life-threatening condition, and is an absolute contra-indication to exercise and sport.

The term 'boosting' is used to describe a performance-enhancing practice, whereby athletes with an SCI above T6 try to increase their heart rate and blood pressure, and therefore athletic performance, by deliberately and voluntarily inducing a state of AD. This is achieved by the athlete creating a noxious stimulus below their level of injury, for example, by over-distending their bladder or over-tightening straps on their legs. The practice was banned by the IPC in 2004. It is an extremely dangerous practice that carries the risk of intracranial haemorrhage, stroke and even death. Since 2016, the IPC has determined that athletes with a systolic blood pressure above 160 mmHg should not be permitted to compete in sporting events due to the risk to their health.

Heart rate

The maximum heart rate of an individual with tetraplegia or high paraplegia may be affected due to impaired sympathetic innervation. The body regulates heart rate through the autonomic nervous system. Individuals with injury levels below T5 will have no autonomic dysfunction of their heart, and will be able to elevate their heart rate similarly to an able-bodied individual. Those who have an injury between T1 and T5 or an incomplete tetraplegia may have partial control, and those with a complete injury above T1 will have no sympathetic control. The only method to increase heart rate in these individuals is through withdrawal of vagal tone, and typically results in a maximum heart rate of 100–130 bpm.[37] Reduced heart rate will directly affect cardiac output, limiting cardiorespiratory fitness and exercise performance.[38]

The direct implications for health practitioners is that heart rate may not be a good measure of exercise intensity. For example, conventional measures of maximum heart rate (e.g. 220 minus age) will not be appropriate. Some suggestions to measure exercise intensity may include rated perceived-exertion scales, such as the modified Borg Dyspnoea scale (which measures difficulty in breathing). Understanding the effect of altered cardiac physiology is an important consideration in exercise for people with an SCI.

Orthostatic and exertional hypotension

People with an SCI may be affected by a number of haemodynamic changes that impact on blood pressure, both at rest and during/after exercise. Impaired sympathetic vasoconstriction of peripheral veins and reduced muscle pump during exercise can results in venous pooling in the lower limbs. Reduced venous return, lower stroke volume and impaired blood redistribution during physical activity have been reported as contributing factors. In orthostatic hypotension, drops of 20 mmHg (systolic) and greater can occur with sudden positional changes, such as moving from supine lying to sitting. This may be caused by pooling of blood in the abdominal viscera and lower limbs, where muscle tone is significantly reduced or absent. Exertional hypotension can occur during or after physical activity and similarly may result in drops of 10 mmHg or more (systolic). This is due to the unopposed vasodilation of peripheral blood vessels and increased venous pooling in the abdomen and lower limbs.[38] Symptoms of hypotension include dizziness, light headedness, pallor, vision changes and syncope. Physical activity is contraindicated while symptoms are present. These episodes can usually be managed relatively easily, with leg elevation, recumbency and ingestion of fluids being the first line of management. A range of preventative strategies can be employed to minimise the risk and frequency of hypotensive episodes. These include the use of abdominal binders and gradual introduction to new exercises and increases in exercise intensity.

Impaired sensation

Many people with an SCI have impaired sensation below the level of their spinal cord lesion and it is well recognised that pressure injuries, while often preventable, are one of the most prevalent complications of an SCI.

Therefore, when participating in new physical activities, people with an SCI are often exposed to a range of new risks to their skin. These may include:

- sport-specific wheelchairs, used in wheelchair basketball, rugby and tennis, feature more limited postural and seating options, and are quite different to the seating systems of everyday wheelchairs. Although it is often desirable for people with an SCI to use their regular pressure redistribution cushions in their sports wheelchairs, this may not always be practical or possible due to differences in seat dimensions, or sport-specific rules that limit overall seat height. Additionally, air-filled cushions may result in postural instability, that impacts directly on sport performance. Sport-specific wheelchair upholstery backrests are often quite a different shape to those found on everyday wheelchairs, particularly for those people who regularly use moulded, padded, rigid backrests on their everyday wheelchairs. Due to the repetitive movement that can occur during sporting activities, the spinous processes and ribs can be sites of considerable friction or shearing forces that can lead to skin breakdown.

- strapping and binders to secure legs and stabilise the trunk in sport-specific wheelchairs or other sporting equipment, which can create new locations of potential skin damage.

- for outdoor sporting activities, sporting equipment that is left sitting in the sun for prolonged periods of time can heat considerably, posing a risk of burns to skin with impaired temperature sensation.

- repetitive wheelchair acceleration and braking can result in blisters and friction burns to the hands and forearms.

There are a number of relatively simple preventative strategies that can be employed to mitigate the risks of skin damage while participating in physical activities. These can include:

- regular skin checks, at a minimum both before and after the new physical activity, to assess the condition of the skin in areas at risk due to impaired sensation. Some people with an SCI may require assistance to do this, while others may be able to do this independently. Mobile phone cameras may be useful to document the location and nature of skin damage to assist in identifying the cause and any subsequent remedial action.

- regular pressure relief during exercise. A pressure relief manoeuvre every 15 to 30 minutes is highly desirable.

- appropriate protective equipment to minimise or eliminate the risk of skin damage. This may include padding, gloves, forearm taping or protective sleeves that protect skin from wheel contact.

- where possible, the person with an SCI should use their regular pressure redistribution cushion. However, use of the regular cushion does not preclude the need for regular skin checking, as changes to the person's seating position can result in changes to pressure distribution. If the person's regular cushion is not suitable, an appropriate alternative should be sought. Using a sport-specific wheelchair without a cushion is not recommended in any circumstances for people with impaired sensation, and poses a very high level of risk to skin.

- where possible, new equipment, particularly wheelchairs, should be introduced gradually, for shortened periods at first, in order to assess any adverse impacts on skin.

Impaired pain perception can make it more difficult to detect and diagnose musculoskeletal injuries. In many situations, health practitioners assessing potential injuries in the field will need to look closely for secondary signs of injury, which may include:

- abnormal movement of the injured body part
- AD in those people susceptible to this health condition
- an increase in the degree of spasticity present
- swelling and erythema.

High impact sports such as wheelchair rugby and wheelchair basketball, where falls are common, pose a relatively higher level of risk to the individual, but musculoskeletal injuries can occur in a variety of situations. For example, difficult transfers onto sporting or recreational equipment, particularly manoeuvres that involve twisting of the lower limbs, can pose a risk of fracture in long bones in individuals with reduced BMD. (For further examples of when fractures may occur, see Chapter 21.)

Impaired temperature regulation

Understanding the lack of temperature regulation is an important part of sport and people with an SCI. People with AD, particularly those with tetraplegia, may have impaired body temperature regulation.[39] This is particularly important in hot conditions, as a

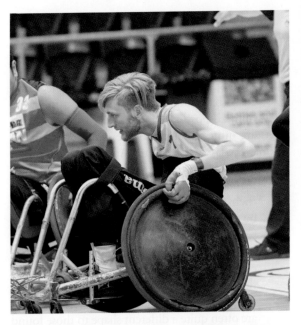

Figure 13.3 Athlete in sports wheelchair. Note sitting position is very different to everyday wheelchair. Strapping for trunk and legs provides stability. Gloves enhance grip on the wheel and protect skin.
Source: Serena Ovens/IWRF

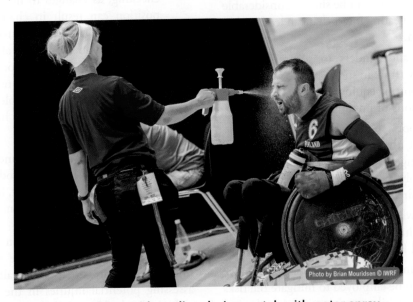

Figure 13.4 Team staff assist athlete with cooling during match with water spray.
Source: Brian Mouridsen/IWRF

lack of peripheral vasodilation to promote heat loss and an inability to sweat in those with high spinal lesions may lead to higher core temperatures and the risk of hyperthermia. In addition, these athletes may have sustained elevated core temperatures after exercise. Practical risk mitigation strategies could include arranging competition and training schedules in the cooler parts of the day, and training indoors instead of outdoors where possible. In situations where heat cannot be avoided (e.g. in competitions), strategies such as pre-cooling with ice vests or cold water immersion therapy, ensuring adequate fluid intake, hand and foot cooling and the use of water spray bottles to mimic the effects of sweating may be of benefit to the athlete.[40,41] While there is evidence that pre-cooling reduces core body temperature in athletes with an SCI, there is inconclusive evidence that pre-cooling improves athletic performance.

Reduced bone mineral density

Following SCI, there is a significant decline in bone mineral density in the hip and knee regions, placing the person with an SCI at risk of low-impact fracture. Some sporting equipment requires the person to perform complex or difficult transfers, or adopt positions that may pose an increased risk of lower limb fracture.

When pursuing new physical activities, particularly those that involve weight-bearing through the lower limbs, medical advice should be sought to assist in quantifying the risk of lower limb fracture.

Acute musculoskeletal injuries of the upper limbs

People with an SCI rely on their upper limbs for all aspects of their mobility and ADLs. While the incidence of musculoskeletal injury is not significantly increased through sport, shoulder and wrist injuries are the most common.[42] Prevention and early treatment of upper limb injury is therefore critical in assisting the person with an SCI to maintain their independence and quality of life. In general terms, the management of upper limb injury in

people with an SCI is the same as the management in the general population. However, relative rest is significantly more difficult to achieve as part of the treatment and recovery process due to the person's reliance on their upper limbs for most of their daily activities. In these instances, the following principles may assist in expediting the recovery process:

- Consider behavioural or environmental modifications to minimise the number of transfers or repetitive activities that need to be performed and limit activities (such as reaching overhead) that could exacerbate the injury.

- Incorporate flexibility exercises, with a particular emphasis on stretching of the shoulder rotators and pectoral muscles within the limits of pain.

- Incorporate strengthening exercises, with a particular emphasis on the muscles of the rotator cuff, scapula and posterior shoulder girdle within the limits of pain.

- Promote a gradual return to the activity that resulted in the injury.

- Try to determine the reason for or contributing factors to the injury and remediate where possible. This may include analysis of seating, propulsion biomechanics and sports-specific techniques.

Spasticity and range of movement

Spasticity and ROM can have an impact on sporting function, just as it can on everyday activities for those with an SCI. However, it is important to consider ROM for sport in the context of functional everyday activities and be wary of compromising existing functional activities when stretching or positioning athletes to participate in their sport; for example, maintaining a tenodesis grip. Conversely, in the context of physical activity, specific positioning and strapping may reduce the incidence and impact of spasticity on sports performance.

Evidence-based practice points

- Strong evidence supports the premise that regular exercise improves cardiorespiratory fitness, power output, muscle strength and body composition, reduces cardiovascular risk and improves psychosocial wellbeing.
- Emerging evidence supports a positive impact of exercise on cardiometabolic risk, incidence of shoulder pain and improved physical independence.
- Participation in physical activity is associated with reduced incidence of musculoskeletal injury and, in particular, shoulder pain.
- Exercise and sports literature consistently reports strong associations between physical activity and improvements in psychosocial wellbeing, including reduction in depression and anxiety and improved quality of life and resilience.
- Published exercise and physical activity guidelines for people with an SCI provide a framework for health practitioners to promote physical activity, but health practitioners may also need to invest time in assisting people with an SCI to overcome significant barriers to participating in these activities.
- Elite competitive (Paralympic) sport may be an aspirational goal for some people with spinal cord injury, but the many benefits of individual or team sporting and physical activities may be realised at all levels of participation.

SUMMARY

Promotion of physical activity and engagement in adaptive sports have long been features of in-patient rehabilitation programs for people with an SCI. Participation in regular exercise or sporting activities has been shown to have numerous physiological and psychosocial benefits for people living with an SCI. However, people with an SCI may experience significant barriers to participation in these activities.

Physical activity and sport provide rich environments to foster the development of physical independence, life skills and psychosocial wellbeing through improved strength and fitness, shared experiences and challenging an individual's perceptions of their physical limitations. Health practitioners have recognised the benefits of physical activity and sport across the domains of health, fitness, wellbeing and participation. However, many people with an SCI do not regularly engage in physical activity or sport due to numerous barriers to participation. Health practitioners and peer-led interventions play a critical role in assisting people with an SCI to overcome barriers to physical activity or sport participation, improving resilience, leading to the many benefits that can positively impact daily life.

Online resources

International Paralympic Committee. https://www.paralympic.org/classification.

Spinal Cord Injury Research Evidence (SCIRE) project. https://scireproject.com.

References

1. Katzmarzyk, P.T., Mire, E., et al., 2012. Abdominal obesity and mortality: the Pennington Center longitudinal study. Nutr. Diabetes 2, e42.

2. Shojaei, M.H., Alavinia, S.M., et al., 2017. Management of obesity after spinal cord injury: a systematic review. J. Spinal Cord Med. 40 (6), 783–794.

3. Saunders, L.L., Clarke, A., et al., 2015. Lifetime prevalence of chronic health conditions among persons with spinal cord injury. Arch. Phys. Med. Rehabil. 96 (4), 673–679.

4. Savic, G., DeVivo, M.J., et al., 2017. Causes of death after traumatic spinal cord injury – a 70-year British study. Spinal Cord 55 (10), 891–897.

5. van der Scheer, J.W., Martin Ginis, K.A., et al., 2017. Effects of exercise on fitness and health of adults with spinal cord injury: a systematic review. Neurology 89 (7), 736–745.

6. Nightingale, T.E., Walhin, J.P., et al., 2017. Impact of exercise on cardiometabolic component risks in spinal cord-injured humans. Med. Sci. Sports Exerc. 49 (12), 2469–2477.

7. Crane, D.A., Hoffman, J.M., et al., 2017. Benefits of an exercise wellness program after spinal cord injury. J. Spinal Cord Med. 40 (2), 154–158.

8. Jorgensen, S., Martin Ginis, K.A., et al., 2017. Leisure time physical activity among older adults with long-term spinal cord injury. Spinal Cord 55 (9), 848–856.

9. Ibitoye, M.O., Hamzaid, N.A., et al., 2016. Strategies for rapid muscle fatigue reduction during FES exercise in individuals with spinal cord injury: a systematic review. PLoS ONE 11 (2), e0149024.

10. Gorgey, A.S., Witt, O., et al., 2019. Mitochondrial health and muscle plasticity after spinal cord injury. Eur. J. Appl. Physiol. 119 (2), 315–331.

11. Stewart, B.G., Tarnopolsky, M.A., et al., 2004. Treadmill training-induced adaptations in muscle phenotype in persons with incomplete spinal cord injury. Muscle Nerve 30 (1), 61–68.

12. Vik, L.C., Lannem, A.M., et al., 2017. Health status of regularly physically active persons with spinal cord injury. Spinal Cord Ser. Cases 3, 17099.

13. Karelis, A.D., Carvalho, L.P., et al., 2017. Effect on body composition and bone mineral density of walking with a robotic exoskeleton in adults with chronic spinal cord injury. J. Rehabil. Med. 49 (1), 84–87.

14. Gorgey, A.S., Dolbow, D.R., et al., 2014. Effects of spinal cord injury on body composition and metabolic profile – part I. J. Spinal Cord Med. 37 (6), 693–702.

15. Tan, B.K.H., Ong, K.W., 2014. Influence of dietary polyphenols on carbohydrate metabolism. In: Watson, R.R., Preedy, V.R., et al. (Eds.), Polyphenols in Human Health and Disease. Academic Press, San Diego, pp. 95–111.

16. Petrie, M.A., Suneja, M., et al., 2014. A minimal dose of electrically induced muscle activity regulates distinct gene signaling pathways in humans with spinal cord injury. PLoS ONE 9 (12), e115791.

17. Bresnahan, J.J., Farkas, G.J., et al., 2019. Arm crank ergometry improves cardiovascular disease risk factors and community mobility independent of body composition in high motor complete spinal cord injury. J. Spinal Cord Med. 42 (3), 272–280.

18. Clifton, P.M., 2019. Diet, exercise and weight loss and dyslipidaemia. Pathology 51 (2), 222–226.

19. Nash, M.S., Tractenberg, R.E., et al., 2016. Cardiometabolic syndrome in people with spinal cord injury/disease: guideline-derived and nonguideline risk components in a pooled sample. Arch. Phys. Med. Rehabil. 97 (10), 1696–1705.

20. Laughton, G.E., Buchholz, A.C., et al., 2009. Lowering body mass index cutoffs better identifies obese persons with spinal cord injury. Spinal Cord 47 (10), 757–762.

21. Shea, J.R., Shay, B.L., et al., 2018. Energy expenditure as a function of activity level after spinal cord injury: the need for tetraplegia-specific energy balance guidelines. Front. Physiol. 9, 1286.

22. Pelletier, C.A., Omidvar, M., et al., 2018. Participation in moderate-to-vigorous leisure time physical activity is related to decreased visceral adipose tissue in adults with spinal cord injury. Appl. Physiol. Nutr. Metab. 43 (2), 139–144.

23. Gutierrez, D.D., Thompson, L., et al., 2007. The relationship of shoulder pain intensity to quality of life, physical activity, and community participation in persons with paraplegia. J. Spinal Cord Med. 30 (3), 251–255.

24. Fullerton, H.D., Borckardt, J.J., et al., 2003. Shoulder pain: a comparison of wheelchair athletes and nonathletic wheelchair users. Med. Sci. Sports Exerc. 35 (12), 1958–1961.

25. Wilroy, J., Hibberd, E., 2018. Evaluation of a shoulder injury prevention program in wheelchair basketball. J. Sport Rehabil. 27 (6), 554–559.

26. Boldt, I., Eriks-Hoogland, I., et al., 2014. Non-pharmacological interventions for chronic pain in people with spinal cord injury. Cochrane Database Syst. Rev. (11), CD009177.

27. Hadjipavlou, G., Cortese, A.M., et al., 2016. Spinal cord injury and chronic pain. BJA Educ. 16 (8), 264–268.

28. de Oliveira, B.I., Howie, E.K., et al., 2016. SCIPA Com: outcomes from the spinal cord injury and physical activity in the community intervention. Spinal Cord 54 (10), 855–860.

29. Martin Ginis, K.A., van der Scheer, J.W., et al., 2018. Evidence-based scientific exercise guidelines for adults with spinal cord injury: an update and a new guideline. Spinal Cord 56 (4), 308–321.

30. Tweedy, S.M., Beckman, E.M., et al., 2017. Exercise and Sports Science Australia (ESSA) position statement on exercise and spinal cord injury. J. Sci. Med. Sport 20 (2), 108–115.

31. Nightingale, T.E., Metcalfe, R.S., et al., 2017. exercise guidelines to promote cardiometabolic health in spinal cord injured humans: time to raise the intensity? Arch. Phys. Med. Rehabil. 98 (8), 1693–1704.

32. World Health Organization, 2011. Global Recommendations on Physical Activity for Health. Online 23 December 2019. Available: https://www.who.int/dietphysicalactivity/physical-activity-recommendations-18-64years.pdf.

33. Buckinghamshire County Council. Sir Ludwig Guttman and his legacy. 2014. Online 23 December 2019. Available: http://www.mandevillelegacy.org.uk/category_id__19_path__0p4p.aspx.

34. International Paralympic Committee. History of the Paralympic movement. Online 23 December 2019. Available: www.paralympic.org/ipc/history.

35. International Paralympic Committee, November 2015. IPC Athlete Classification Code. Online 23 December 2019. Available: www.paralympic.org/sites/default/files/document/170704160235698_2015_12_17%2BClassification%2BCode_FINAL2_0.pdf.

36. Saltan, A., Bakar, Y., et al., 2017. Wheeled mobility skills of wheelchair basketball players: a randomized controlled study. Disabil. Rehabil. Assist. Technol. 12 (4), 390–395.

37. Machac, S., Radvansky, J., et al., 2016. Cardiovascular response to peak voluntary exercise in males with cervical spinal cord injury. J. Spinal Cord Med. 39 (4), 412–420.

38. Hagen, E.M., Rekand, T., et al., 2012. Cardiovascular complications of spinal cord injury. Tidsskr. Nor. Laegeforen. 132 (9), 1115–1120.

39. Price, M.J., Trbovich, M., 2018. Thermoregulation following spinal cord injury. Handb. Clin. Neurol. 157, 799–820.

40. Forsyth, P., Pumpa, K., et al., 2016. Physiological and perceptual effects of precooling in wheelchair basketball athletes. J. Spinal Cord Med. 39 (6), 671–678.

41. Griggs, K.E., Price, M.J., et al., 2015. Cooling athletes with a spinal cord injury. Sports Med. 45 (1), 9–21.

42. Kentar, Y., Zastrow, R., et al., 2018. Prevalence of upper extremity pain in a population of people with paraplegia. Spinal Cord 56 (7), 695–703.

CHAPTER 14

Paediatric spinal cord injury

Shailendra Maharaj and Nicola Thomas

INTRODUCTION

Rehabilitation of children with spinal cord injury (SCI) is a dynamic, long-term journey that focuses not solely on the child but on the whole family. It encompasses the physical, cognitive and psychosocial changes throughout development. It takes a dedicated interdisciplinary team to provide the expert immediate care and long-term anticipatory guidance to see a child and family from the inpatient ward, back to home, school and community; and ultimately into the highest level of independence as an adult. Throughout the developmental journey, SCI rehabilitation in paediatrics seeks to maximise function, adjustment and participation at every age and stage.

INCIDENCE

Paediatric SCI is quite rare (not including spina bifida), but its effects are appropriately described as devastating to both the child and the family. Children represent approximately 3–5% of all those who acquire an SCI.[1] In a recent review of the incidence of paediatric SCI from around the world, New and colleagues[2] found traumatic SCI rates to be 3.3–13.2 per million population per year and non-traumatic rates 2.1–6.5 per million population per year. Variances to incidence rates may be due to age range definitions for children, limited data on non-traumatic causes of SCI and limited data availability in low- and moderate-income countries.[2]

Vogel and colleagues[1] provide a good synopsis on the distribution of children with regards to gender and neurological impairment as a function of age at injury (Tables 14.1, 14.2 and 14.3). The key highlights are:

- gender differences are minimal in the first five years of life; however, they steadily become male-dominated as children approach adolescence and young adulthood

- of children 12 years and younger, approximately two-thirds present with paraplegia

- of children 12 years and younger, approximately two-thirds have complete injuries

- children who have tetraplegia and are 12 years and younger have a higher incidence of upper cervical injuries (C1–3) compared to lower cervical (C4–8), which is attributed to their disproportionate head size and an underdevelopment of muscles around the head and neck.

CAUSES OF SCI IN CHILDREN

Traumatic

Throughout the world, motor vehicle collisions are the leading cause of SCI in children (46–74%), regardless of age.[1,2] Other regularly reported causes include falls (12–35%), sports/recreation (10–25%), medical/surgical procedures and events such as natural disasters.[2,3] The variability in epidemiology around the world may be attributed to environmental, cultural and legislative factors. For example, Galvin and colleagues[3] found a significant difference between paediatric SCI rates resulting from gun-related violence in the United States and Brazil, compared to that in Australia. Traumatic causes of SCI that are particular to paediatrics include child abuse, birth injuries and seatbelt injuries involving a lapsash or lapbelt.[1]

Spinal cord injury without radiographic abnormality (SCIWORA)

Within the traumatic presentations of SCI, SCIWORA is generally considered a paediatric phenomenon,[1] and is considered to be relatively rare in the adult population.[4] The SCIWORA classification arose when children exhibited presentations consistent with an SCI, but without any radiological evidence.[5] This form of injury is

Table 14.1 Gender as a function of age at injury

	Male	Female
0–5 years	51%	49%
6–12 years	58%	42%
13–15 years	69%	31%
16–21 years	83%	17%
22+ years	81%	19%

Source: Vogel L.C., Betz R.R., et al., 2012. Spinal cord injuries in children and adolescents. Handbook of Clinical Neurology, Spinal Cord Injury 109, 131–147.

Table 14.2 Neurological impairment as a function of age at injury

	Paraplegia	Tetraplegia	Complete	Incomplete
0–5 years	66%	33%	68%	30%
6–12 years	64%	34%	62%	36%
13–15 years	44%	54%	55%	43%
16–21 years	47%	52%	56%	42%
22+ years	45%	54%	47%	51%

Source: Vogel L.C., Betz R.R., et al., 2012. Spinal cord injuries in children and adolescents. Handbook of Clinical Neurology, Spinal Cord Injury 109, 131–147.

Table 14.3 Neurological impairment as a function of age at injury

	0–5 years	6–12 years	13–15 years	16–21 years	22+ years
C1-3	8.2%	9.6%	4.3%	4.5%	5.7%
C4-8	26%	24.8%	49.8%	46.8%	48.3%

Source: Vogel L.C., Betz R.R., et al., 2012. Spinal cord injuries in children and adolescents. Handbook of Clinical Neurology, Spinal Cord Injury 109, 131–147.

thought to be related to the added mobility present in the spine of children, where stretch injuries can occur without bony fractures.

The incidence of SCIWORA is reported as ranging from 4.5% to 35% of those with paediatric SCIs.[6] It is highest in children under 9 years, and occurs primarily in the cervical spine (C5–8).[5] Modern forms of imaging such as magnetic resonance imaging (MRI) have enabled better visualisation of soft tissue injuries, which has led to up to two-thirds of cases of previously suspected SCIWORA to be reclassified with a more definitive diagnosis.[6] A high level of suspicion (i.e. spinal precautions to maintain a stable, neutral spine) should be taken for any child, particularly a young child presenting with neurological symptoms that are transient, have central tenderness, particularly in the cervical spine, or have a mechanism of injury where the spinal cord could be stretched (e.g. high-speed accidents or falls).

Non-traumatic

There is less data on non-traumatic causes of paediatric SCI (NTSCI); however, the most common causes are reported to be tumours (30%–63%) and inflammatory/autoimmune disease (28%–35%).[2] (This author does not categorise iatrogenic causes into the non-traumatic category. Medical causes are grouped with traumatic.)

Pruit's[7] categorisation of non-traumatic causes of SCI in children is as follows:

1. Craniovertebral junction abnormalities (e.g. Down Syndrome, Ehlers-Danlos syndrome, skeletal dysplasias)
2. Vertebral anomalies (e.g. spinal stenosis, Klippel-Feil, os odontoideum)
3. Vascular (e.g. arteriovenous malformations)
4. Inflammatory/infectious aetiologies (e.g. spinal cord abscess, transverse myelitis, acute disseminated encephalomyelitis, multiple sclerosis, inflammation post-adenotonsilletomy)
5. Oncological (intramedullary spinal cord tumours, radiation fibrosis syndrome, spinal cord compression).

Although the causes of NTSCI differ from traumatic presentations, the rehabilitation goals remain the same. It is important to note that with some non-traumatic presentations there is the potential for progressive disease, in which case the use of validated traumatic SCI classification and standardised examination can be used for neurological surveillance.[7]

CLASSIFICATION

The International Standards for Neurological Classification of Spinal Cord Injury (ISNCSCI), developed by the American Spinal Injury Association (ASIA) (see Appendices 1 and 2), is a routinely used examination of neurological function for any person who has suffered an SCI. The assessment consists of a motor, sensory and anorectal examination (see Chapter 4). The measure was developed for an adult population and hence assumes a certain level of cognition and maturity to be able to follow the instructions and give subjective responses to the sensory stimuli assessment. Not all children have the requisite ability to give accurate responses, such as the very young child or the child with SCI and traumatic brain injury. In cases where reliable assessment is compromised, it may be best to use observational motor assessment to determine the level of neurological function.

The motor and sensory components of the ISNCSCI have been reported by Mulcahey and colleagues[8] to have moderate-to-strong reliability in children as young as 6. Similarly, the ASIA Impairment Scale (AIS),[1] which determines the completeness of the injury, is only recommended in children aged 6 and over. Consideration must also be given regarding the anorectal component of the examination, as young children may not have developed continence before sustaining their injury, or may be too young to understand the test instructions.

For children under 6 years of age, it is recommended that observational muscle assessment be used to determine motor function.[9] For the very young age group, it is acknowledged that more accurate and valid methods of assessment of neurological function need to be developed. Novel methods of assessment for the younger age group (0–5 years), such as diffusion tensor imaging, are being investigated as alternatives to observational assessment.[10]

PROGNOSIS

In the majority of cases, an SCI leads to lifelong impairments, making discussions on prognosis a difficult task to conduct with families. The use of standardised assessments, such as the ISNCSCI, enables the treating team to more objectively and accurately discuss the current level of neurological impairment and prospects of future recovery. Even though much of the information shared with families regarding recovery and prognosis is extrapolated from adult-based studies, it is still of value because it gives both the family and the treating team a place from which to monitor recovery. The ISNCSCI examination can be administered daily after the initial injury; however, its highest prognostic value is shown to be at 72 hours post-injury.[11]

Neurological recovery is most likely to be seen in the initial months following injury, as healing occurs and swelling subsides (for further details see Chapter 1). Functional recovery continues beyond this timeframe, particularly in paediatrics, and hence rehabilitation goals need to adapt and change in line with the child's development.

Life expectancy for children with an SCI is reported as being slightly shorter than that of adults with an SCI.[12] Although no specific reasons for these changes have been clearly identified, the literature does postulate that scoliosis development and related pulmonary complications; incipient respiratory failure and sleep disordered breathing; hip dislocation causing increased risk of pressure injuries; and metabolic effects, are possible contributing factors for this difference. Shavelle and colleagues[12] report that life expectancy can range from 83% of normal for those with incomplete lesions with minimal deficit (AIS D/E) to 50% of normal for

children with high cervical injuries who are not ventilator dependent. Life expectancy for children with ventilator dependency has not been reported.

PREVENTION

As an SCI is a devastating, life-changing event at any age, government and non-government organisations go to significant efforts to reduce incidence through prevention.

Motor vehicle collisions remain the highest cause of traumatic SCI in children, which has led to legislative changes and the development of standards for child restraints and seatbelts in many countries. Personal responsibility has been promoted through education programs such as 'Don't Drink and Drive', 'Buckle Up for Safety', and 'ThinkFirst'. In the modern era of social media and advancing technologies, more targeted initiatives continue to emerge to reduce risk-taking behaviour seen in adolescence and young adulthood.

In the sporting arena, changes are regularly being debated, particularly in popular high-impact sports such as rugby, ice hockey and American football. Administrators of sport, referees, coaches and players continue to work together to maintain player safety; however, SCI remains a risk wherever speed, force and contact are present.

ACUTE SETTING – PREPARATION FOR REHABILITATION

As it is in adult acute SCI management, early stabilisation of the spine is important to limit further injury and allow early commencement of rehabilitation (see Chapter 4).[13] Current literature does not support neuroprotective approaches such as early steroid use or hypothermia in traumatic presentations.[13,14]

Prior to the commencement of formal rehabilitation, the focus of acute management is to maintain respiratory function, manage urinary and bowel function, ensure adequate fluid and nutrition and prevent secondary complications (e.g. pressure injuries, contractures). Though the child may not be ready to commence rehabilitation, it is prudent, where possible, that the rehabilitation team work closely with the acute team. Early engagement not only enables optimal care and preparation for rehabilitation, but also aids the family in the transition from acute to rehabilitation services.

EARLY REHABILITATION AND PSYCHOSOCIAL SUPPORT

Rehabilitation commences once the child is considered medically stable, but does not conclude once their inpatient stay is over. As indicated previously, rehabilitation in paediatrics spans from the time the child first meets the rehabilitation team until their transition to adult-based services. A further point of differentiation in the rehabilitation of children with SCI is that children will always have some level of dependency on their parent/caregiver. For this reason, rehabilitation goals need to focus on both child and family.

Goal setting in the early phases is difficult for both the child and the family, due to the disorientation and grief they experience from such a catastrophic event. It is at this time that the expertise of a paediatric rehabilitation team is most necessary. The multidisciplinary team (MDT) is essential in orienting the child and family to their new situation. This is primarily achieved by educating both the child and the family and addressing their immediate psychosocial needs. Depending on the age of the child, education and adjustment may take the form of play-based therapy, social stories or modifying medical information to an age-appropriate level. Hospital procedures, therapy sessions, disruptions to routine, as well as their physical limitations, can provoke anxiety in infants as well as young adults. For the school-aged child, where independence in some tasks (e.g. feeding, bathing, dressing, toileting) would have occurred prior to the SCI, frustration is often seen. Some children at this age may grasp the permanence of their injury but can still speak about wanting to get better.[1] School-aged children

can also be acutely aware of the impact of their injury on social interaction with peers.

For the adolescent age group, independence from parents is a primary driver. Becoming dependent on parents again for basic cares and having to spend significant time with them can lead to acting out. Other considerations of this age group are the importance of appearance, self-esteem and social standing. Consequently, re-establishing contact with peers is important within the initial rehabilitation phase.

Education and adjustment for the parents, siblings and wider family are also primary goals of rehabilitation. Early conversations will focus on gaining an understanding of the injury and prognosis. As families shift their focus to new roles and expectations, which involve maximising function and independence and preventing secondary complications, hope can still be maintained for neurological improvement. (Chapter 20 provides a personal interpretation of this sociological issue. Also see Samuel's case study at the end of this chapter to gain a perspective from parents and the child.)

Rehabilitation approach

Paediatric SCI rehabilitation has steadily progressed from a purely compensatory approach to including restorative or activity-based (i.e. below level of injury) therapy (ABT) (see Chapter 2).

In a review of current work within the field of activity-based therapy (ABT), Behrman and colleagues[15] found that there was preliminary evidence that locomotor training can improve trunk control, as well as foster participation in children with an SCI. Their clinical practice recommendations acknowledge the challenges in the developing and growing child, but still advocate rehabilitation approaches that activate the central nervous system at all levels with intense task-specific practice.

Factors that impede the integration of ABT into current models of care are the fact that it is labour intensive (locomotor training can require 60 or more sessions involving multiple persons; see Chapter 9), has limited accessibility in terms of specialised equipment required and location (rehabilitation setting), and it is difficult to sustain when children return home (as there are costs involved).

OUTCOME MEASURES

In many forms of clinical practice and research, adult-based measures are either used or modified to accommodate children. An example of this is the adult functional independence measure (FIM), which has been adapted for children as the WeeFIM. The FIM is also the basis of the Spinal Cord Independence Measure III (SCIM-III) (see Appendix 3), which has been adapted specifically to the adult SCI population. The SCIM-III has been shown to have moderate-to-strong reliability and validity and is responsive to change in adults, but to date no large-scale studies have been reported in paediatric populations.[16]

The International Classification of Function (ICF) provides a good framework in which to consider body structure and function, activity and participation, and quality-of-life domains, in paediatric SCI. As outlined in Table 14.4, there are a number of tools which can be used to measure the ICF. These may be expanded as follows:

- Body structure and function – ISNCSCI, manual muscle testing, range of motion, respiratory function tests.

- Activity measures – WeeFIM or SCIM-III. Specific tools for paediatric SCI are being developed, such as the Child Needs Assessment Checklist (ChNAC),[17] but as yet are not widely used.

- Participation measures – The Children's Assessment of Participation and Enjoyment (CAPE), and the Preferences for Activities by Children (PAC) are paediatric measures, but not SCI-specific. Other suggestions include: The Lifestyle Assessment Questionnaire, Activities Scale for Kids and the paediatric version of the Assessment of Life Habits.[16]

- Quality of life measures – Paediatric Quality of Life Inventory.

Table 14.4 Examples of tools that may be used to measure the ICF

Body structure and function	Activity measures	Participation measures	Quality of life measures
ISNCSCI	WeeFIM	CAPE	PQLI
MMT	SCIM-III	PAC	
RoM	ChNAC	LAQ	
Respiratory function tests		ASK	
		ALH (paediatric version)	

KEY: ASK – Activities Scale for Kids; ALH – Assessment of Life Habits; CAPE – Children's Assessment of Participation and Enjoyment; ChNAC – Child Needs Assessment Checklist; FIM – Functional Independence Measure; ICF – International Classification of Function; ISNSCI – International Standards for Neurological Classification Of Spinal Cord Injury; LAQ – Lifestyle Assessment Questionnaire; MMT – Manual Muscle Testing; PAC – Preferences for Activities by Children; RoM – Range of Movement; PQLI – Paediatric Quality of Life Inventory; SCIM – Spinal Cord Independence Measure.

Sources: Mulcahey M.J., 2014. Assessment of children with spinal cord injury. In Vogel L.C., Zebracki K., et al. (eds). Spinal cord injury in the child and young adult. Mac Keith Press, pp. 41–66; Webster G., Kennedy P., 2007. Addressing children's needs and evaluating rehabilitation outcome after spinal cord injury: the child needs assessment checklist and goal-planning program. J Spinal Cord Med. 30 (Suppl 1), S140–S145.

Using tools that can capture the individual needs of children and their families across so many domains and ages is difficult. Tools such as the Canadian Occupational Performance Measure (COPM) and the Goal Attainment Scale (GAS) (see Chapter 17) have benefit because goals can be individualised and change quantified; however, their utility may be most useful in the later stages of rehabilitation.[18,19]

As paediatric SCI is rare, pooling data from consistently used outcome measures is imperative in deriving meaningful information. Work in developing common data elements and international data sets for paediatric SCI is well underway.[20] By developing consistency and accuracy with data collection globally, paediatric SCI standards of practice may emerge to better guide practice, as seen in adult SCI.

MEDICAL ISSUES WITHIN PAEDIATRIC SCI

The impairments to various systems within the body, seen in children with an SCI, although similar to those in adults, may have to be managed differently because of the age, size and cognition of the child. Key areas that require early development of a management plan include: autonomic dysreflexia (AD) (see Chapter 4), bladder management and bowel management. Respiratory function is influenced primarily by the level of injury and requires immediate attention and regular surveillance, as it remains the leading cause of death for children with an SCI.[21] (See Chapter 16 for further details on respiratory management and ventilator supported patients.) Assessment of spasticity and skin care are issues that also require early observation and will require lifelong monitoring. Other medical issues that require awareness, education and monitoring are summarised in Table 14.5.

Respiratory function

Complications related to respiratory function remain the highest cause of morbidity and mortality for children.[21]

A child without diaphragmatic innervation will require ventilator support.[13] For those children, the need for ventilator support often leads to longer inpatient stays and families potentially having to relocate home to be within close proximity of a specialised paediatric medical facility that can manage their ventilatory needs. These children will require monitoring and adjustment to ventilator settings throughout their childhood, in step with physical changes that take place within the thorax.

Children who do not require ventilator support but have impaired respiratory function will require age-appropriate education on how best to reduce pulmonary-related risks. These include teaching physical techniques such as assisted airway clearance, as well as promoting engagement in active pursuits and exercise to maintain good respiratory health.

Sleep studies and chest X-rays may be required throughout the growing years to monitor and ascertain both the physical impacts (e.g. scoliosis) and ventilator requirements of the child with an SCI. (For further detail on sleep apnoea see Chapter 18.)

Autonomic dysreflexia (AD)

AD can be life-threatening at any age. It requires all caregivers (family, school staff, sports coaches, etc.) to be acutely aware of not only the observable physical manifestations of AD, but also how the child may communicate these symptoms. Although it may be difficult for a very young child to understand AD, age-appropriate education is still essential. Role-play may be used to help a child become familiar with the procedures they would undergo if AD was suspected. Family and health professionals need to be mindful that baseline blood pressures for a child with an SCI will change as the child grows.[22,23] (See Chapter 4 for further details on AD.)

Bladder management

Intermittent catheterisation remains the standard of practice for children presenting with a neurogenic bladder.[1]

Intermittent catheterisation by the family can commence around 3 years of age, or earlier if urinary

Table 14.5 Medical issues in SCI with paediatric considerations

Medical issue	Age-related considerations	Age-related management
Deep venous thrombosis	Rare in children under 12 years of age (0–1.9%). Uncommon in adolescents (7.9–9.1%).	Similar to adult management – use of appropriate anticoagulation medication; use of graduated stockings (avoiding latex).
Temperature regulation	As with adults, issues with regulation will be related to level of neurological impairment. Younger children with limited communication and cognitive abilities may be more vulnerable to changes in ambient temperature. Adolescents may be more at risk because of their judgement and unpredictable behaviour.	Children at levels T6 and above require specific focus on understanding, planning and management strategies for AD. Education of family and caregivers about minimising the risks of hyper- or hypothermia. Early education about AD and risks associated with extremes in environmental temperature. Empowering child to develop strategies to minimise risk and self-monitor.
Hypercalcaemia	Most commonly seen in adolescent and young adult population. Noted to be mainly in males. Occurs within first 3 months after injury.	Similar to adult management – using hydration and medications to facilitate renal excretion of calcium. Some studies indicate the use of bisphosphonates.
Hyperhidrosis	Related more to level of injury than age (i.e. seen primarily in those with tetraplegia or high paraplegia).	Management considered if child/family report impaired function, increased risk of pressure injuries or embarrassment as a result of increased sweating.
Latex allergy	6–18% of children with an SCI reported as having allergy to latex. Having an increased exposure to latex, such as in a hospital environment, can lead to the development of an allergy.	Latex allergy to be suspected if child has had unexplained intraoperative allergic reactions; allergy to foods such as bananas, kiwi fruit, avocadoes or chestnuts. Some paediatric hospitals have moved to eliminate, where possible, the use of latex in gloves and other medical supplies.

Source: Adapted from Vogel L.C., Betz R.R., et al., 2012. Spinal cord injuries in children and adolescents. Handbook of Clinical Neurology, Spinal Cord Injury 109, 131–147.

tract infections are prevalent. Self-catheterisation can commence as early as 5–7 years if the child is developmentally ready and has adequate hand function.[1] For those with limited hand function or issues of access, alternatives to adult options (e.g. suprapubic catheter) include the Mitrofanoff procedure.[24] This procedure gives access to the bladder through the abdominal wall by creating a non-refluxing conduit made from either the appendix or the small bowel. As procedures like this are not common in the adult SCI population, families need to be aware that the current bladder management plan may be altered as they transition to adult services.

Bowel management

Bowel routines for typically developing children commence between the ages of 2 and 4 years. For a child with an SCI, bowel routines will require ongoing adult involvement, which may gradually reduce as the child enters school age. For those with the physical capacity for carrying out bowel care, 10–12 years of age is around the time that children may develop independence. For those children where physical independence may not be achieved, autonomy by directing care should be pursued.

As with adult bowel programs, routine is key. Developing a routine may prove challenging for some families with younger children. In adolescence, complying with any routine can be a challenge. With physical growth, optimising bowel care may require surgical intervention (e.g. antegrade continence enema procedure).

Spasticity

Approximately half of the children with an SCI will exhibit spasticity (see Chapter 4 for more information on managing spasticity).[25] Spasticity management in the growing child requires careful initial assessment and ongoing monitoring to determine its impact on function. As children are skeletally immature, spasticity may have an even greater impact on contracture development than in the adult population, and can negatively affect function. Pain and spasticity can also occur together to influence posture, comfort and function. Where spasticity aids function (e.g. for standing or transfers), care should be taken when considering management options. In the paediatric population, because of the growth issue, the use of splinting and casting is more prevalent in the paediatric population compared to the adult population.

The main forms of surgery that are considered are related to scoliosis and hip instability. Other forms of lower limb surgery are only pursued if pain or deterioration of function is noted – so in the lower limb it will be higher for the incomplete ambulant/ semi-ambulant; more than for those who are not walking/standing or transferring through standing.

In the upper limb, surgery is more related to muscle function and if surgery does occur, it is around the time of skeletal maturity (see Chapter 17). Surgeons are often more cautious of surgery in the upper limb as there is a greater risk of functional loss.

Skin care

Pressure injuries can have a significant impact on a young person's independence, function, access to schooling, social engagement, community and sporting participation and, as such, can have a considerable health, economic and personal burden.[26] Prevention needs to be an important component of any rehabilitation program, beginning early in the acute phase and continuing throughout the child's life.

In the acute setting, appropriate pressure redistribution devices (e.g. mattresses, cushions) should be incorporated into treatment immediately, combined with frequent and thorough skin assessment. As children transition into a rehabilitation setting, education regarding skin care needs to remain a high priority. What were once innocuous activities (e.g. moving on the floor, getting into the car, outdoor play) may now pose a significant risk to skin integrity.

Infants and young children cannot accurately participate in sensation assessments, therefore it is often safest to assume that the child has impaired sensation and take appropriate precautions to prevent the development of a pressure injury. They are also reliant on caregivers for pressure injury management and inspection of skin integrity. Children should be encouraged to wear long pants and socks when crawling or using other forms of floor mobility to minimise the impact of friction and abrasions (e.g. carpet burn). Other common causes of skin injury in children with an SCI are burns and scalds from hot showers or baths, hot food being placed in the child's lap or sitting on hot surfaces such as slides or hot concrete in playgrounds. Significant skin breakdown can result in skin grafting and prolonged hospitalisation (see Chapter 21).

As the child develops, it is imperative that education of pressure injury prevention and self-skin checks are taught in an age-appropriate way to promote a gradual transition to independence. Adolescence can prove to be a difficult time for prevention of pressure injuries as poor compliance, together with an increasing expectation of independence and self-responsibility, have the potential to increase pressure injury risk.

ANTICIPATORY GUIDANCE

As the child and family acclimatise to the rehabilitative phase following injury, the MDT's role includes providing necessary information and direction about challenges and opportunities that will arise during growth and development. This advice, given throughout the child's development, is known as anticipatory guidance.

Guidance around discharge and return to school are covered early, but topics of ongoing discussion include shared mobility, skin care, upper limb functioning, sport, recreation and leisure and, at a later stage, musculoskeletal issues. The guidance given is personalised to the level and completeness of injury, age of the child and the family's unique circumstances. Having some idea of what the future holds helps to give hope, but also mitigates against feelings of failure or loss. Anticipatory guidance also enables children and their families to better plan timing of interventions to maximise function and/or reduce disruption; for example, developing mobility skills prior to starting schooling or timing surgical procedures to limit time spent out of school.

DISCHARGE PLANNING

Discharge planning for the child with an SCI has both similarities to and differences from adult management. Issues around modification of the home (i.e. safety and access) may be similar, but participation and level of independence for everyday tasks is age-specific. Parents provide significant care for the child and will need to develop competency in a range of areas (e.g. respiratory, bladder and bowel, AD, orthoses, skin care, etc.). The level of care will diminish over the course of the child's cognitive and motor development. Parenting and psychosocial considerations are also important components of discharge planning.

SCHOOLING

A key aspect of discharge planning within the paediatric population is on return to school.

Schooling is one of the primary contexts of development for a child, and it is therefore important to incorporate schooling within inpatient rehabilitation. Ideally, it is helpful for school staff and students to visit the child during rehabilitation.

Hospital schooling provides the environment where a child can learn how to adjust, problem solve and experience graded success, in preparation for returning to school out of hospital. It is preferable to have the child return to their own school where possible, in order to benefit from a familiar environment and established social networks. Unfortunately, not all schools are accessible and significant changes to classroom allocations and travel paths need to be assessed and accommodated. Access to appropriate toilet/change facilities is often available, but in locations not readily accessible to students (e.g. staff rooms). Therefore, transitioning back into school will often require appropriate investigation of safety, access and participation by the healthcare team with the family, as well as psychosocial preparation of all involved. School staff will need specific education on caring for the child, for example where AD is a concern, and will require access to the healthcare team as appropriate. Having a graded return to school is recommended (i.e. incremental increase of time spent at school to foster success).

As the child transitions from one level of schooling to another (e.g. junior to middle to high), similar levels of preparation are required to enable a safe and successful transition. Children may require a review of their mobility to ensure they are able to be independent in new schooling environments (e.g. travel distances and paths).

MOBILITY

Understanding the importance of early mobility, as well as the concept of 'shared mobility', is key when providing therapy and anticipatory guidance for the child with an SCI. Families and funding bodies need to be aware that throughout development the child with an SCI will use a variety of means to negotiate their environments. Sharing their mobility may mean using upright mobility (i.e. walking or moving in a standing frame) and wheeled mobility (e.g. buggies, castor carts, wheelchairs) in certain circumstances, such as walking short distances indoors, and using wheeled mobility, such as a powerchair, within the community (see mobility case study at the end of this chapter). Families also need to be prepared for the time when wheeled mobility may take precedence over upright mobility because of growth, energy efficiency or environment. Through appropriate anticipatory guidance, transitioning from upright to wheeled mobility should not always be seen as a failure of the child or family, but rather a natural progression.[27]

Early development

The presence of an SCI will affect a child's development, depending on the level of the injury and the age at which the injury occurred. For children with an SCI, a limitation in independent mobility may restrict their ability to actively explore their environment and consequently have an impact on their acquisition of important skills. These children can become overly reliant on others for the provision of activities, leading to a learned helplessness and lack of motivation to move and explore. Self-initiated mobility allows the child to experience opportunities for success, leading to improved motivation and engagement in play activities, which in turn provides stimulus for the development of fine motor, language, social and cognitive skills.[27] It is therefore important that children, particularly very young children with spinal cord impairments, are provided with opportunities to develop self-initiated movement.

Encouraging the development of floor mobility, such as rolling, creeping and crawling, is an important goal of therapy in the first year. For some children, this will not be achievable due to their level of impairment and in such cases the use of early wheeled mobility should be promoted. Current recommendations encourage the clinician to consider providing independent mobility opportunities around the age that typically developing children would begin to crawl.[28]

Wheeled mobility

Providing wheeled mobility at an early age will require appropriate levels of supervision and training. Teaching good propulsion techniques will promote good habits and will help mitigate against shoulder dysfunction and pain in the future. Where self-propulsion does not enable a meaningful experience of mobility, powered mobility should be considered. Developing simple skills, such as stopping, starting and turning, form the foundation from which more advanced skills can follow. It is important to provide age-appropriate wheelchair skills training to maximise the child's level of independence, while ensuring safety. Chapter 5 contains more detail on wheelchair propulsion.

For the self-propeller, skills such as back-wheel balancing and negotiating slopes and gutters safely are important skills to learn, as children seek independence in community settings.[29] Individual training for children can be enhanced through wheelchair skills programs, which have been shown to improve skills for young people with spinal cord impairment.[30]

When deciding between manual and powered mobility, neurological level does guide decision-making; however, other considerations, such as age, body shape, finance, transportation and the ability to participate fully in the environment, also need to be considered. In motor complete (AIS A) or sensory incomplete (AIS B) injuries, Calhoun and colleagues[27] recommend the following: C1–4 level injuries require powered mobility; C5–C8 utilise either power bases, power add-ons to manual chairs or simply an ultra-light chair; T1–S5 utilise ultra-lightweight manual chairs. The appropriate wheelchair set-up for the C5–C8 group will evolve throughout their development and relate to their specific environment. For example, a child may be able to self-propel on flat ground around school, but may be too exhausted to concentrate in class, in which case considering a power add-on or power base may be the better option in that environment.

With wheeled mobility, monitoring and guidance is required because of growth. As the child grows, their fit within their chair will alter and it is necessary to modify equipment to reduce risk of injury, as well as ensuring efficiency and function. Families also need to be advised about keeping schoolbags off wheelchairs and checking tyre pressures as these can make self-propulsion difficult and lead to future shoulder injury.

Upright mobility

Pursuing upright mobility starts with developing regular standing (Fig. 14.1). Children at all levels of injury, particularly younger children, will benefit from standing. For the child who has a high cervical injury, standing will require the use of a tilt-table with postural supports. Some standers will allow a child to self-propel short distances, from which they can experience upright mobility. For these children, mobility may be limited to experience and therapy rather than function as there is a high energy cost involved.[31]

Standing, which may be either passive or active on a tilt-table or stander, swivel walking with a parapodium, and/or ambulating in more conventional

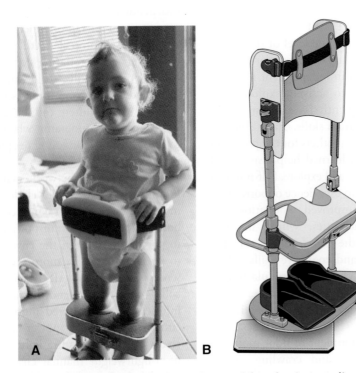

Figure 14.1 A, Child in a standing frame, which can be used for play in standing and swivel walking. B, Parapodium, which allows swivel walking.

ways in the home or community with the assistance of orthoses and mobility aids are all beneficial. It is well documented that standing has the potential to reduce the risk of pressure injury, maintain lower limb range of motion, improve bladder and bowel function and improve bone density, which may result in a reduction in the incidence of lower limb fractures, improve cardiovascular fitness and as such increase independence (see Chapter 9 on ambulation).[32,33] Even if a child is unlikely to achieve functional ambulation upon discharge, it is worth attempting upright mobility during rehabilitation for the psychosocial and physiological benefits it gives to the child and family. The sense of achievement that the child and family have when the child first learns to 'walk' should not be underestimated.

To assist with realistic goal-setting, it is important to be able to predict ambulatory potential in children with an SCI and be aware of the aids and orthoses that will promote meaningful mobility. Key factors that influence what form of ambulation a child may be capable of include neurological level, completeness of injury and age at injury. Factors such as level of cognition and motivation, access to therapy with a focus on ambulation, appropriate and well-fitting orthoses, lower limb deformities, presence of spasticity, obesity and skin breakdown should also be considered.[32]

In determining whether the child with an SCI will be a therapeutic, household or community ambulator, a summary of studies by Calhoun and colleagues[27] reflects current clinical practice. If the child has an injury at a younger age, particularly before the age of 5, they have a greater likelihood of achieving functional mobility, compared to when injuries occur later in childhood. The following recommendations were made regarding neurological level for those with AIS A (motor complete) or AIS B (sensory incomplete) injuries: C1–C8 ambulation not indicated; T1–T9 therapeutic walking; T10–L1 therapeutic or household mobility; and L2–S5 functional household and community ambulation.[27]

For those with motor incomplete injuries (AIS C and D), the ISNCSCI assessment or manual muscle testing can be used to assist in determining mobility capacity. From adult data, Waters and colleagues[34] showed that motor scoring less than or equal to 20 in total for the lower limbs indicated limited or household mobility, while scores greater than or equal to 30 indicated community ambulators.

Chaftez and colleagues[35] reported that strength of quadriceps muscles can predict community ambulation in children with spinal cord impairment. These children will often require ankle–foot orthoses to compensate for weakness in the foot and ankle muscles. Upper limb strength is also important to consider for children with an SCI as they will often need to utilise walking aids that rely on upper limb strength.

Children with upper lumbar and thoracic level lesions who do not have antigravity quadriceps strength will require significant bracing above the knee to achieve ambulation. Devices such as a reciprocating gait orthoses (RGO) or hip–knee–ankle–foot orthoses (HKAFOs) may be considered for children with hip, knee and ankle weakness, or even complete lower limb paralysis. Some children may be able to achieve a reciprocal stepping or swing-through pattern to achieve functional ambulation with the use of these devices,[36] but they will often be slow and have a high energy expenditure, which may make functional community ambulation difficult.[37] The prescription of these complex and expensive devices should be done on an individual basis and in conjunction with an experienced orthotist, particularly for those with incomplete injuries. Care must be taken when looking at orthotic prescription as poor orthoses can lead to poor mobility outcomes.

It must be remembered that these are only recommendations and functional mobility for the child must remain an ongoing personalised assessment by their treating allied health professional. Whatever the goal may be at each age and stage of development, supporting upright mobility in rehabilitation is essential. Realistic goal-setting combined with an understanding of natural progression (e.g. upright mobility may progress to wheeled mobility later on) will help ensure the best outcomes for child, family and team.

UPPER LIMB FUNCTION

Maximising upper limb function will enhance independence in a variety of areas, such as ADLs (including bladder and bowel care), socialisation (e.g. technology, phone use) and mobility (e.g. power chair control) (see Chapter 17 for more information on upper limb function in patients with tetraplegia).

Management of upper limb function in children is similar to adults; however, there are several notable considerations. The main risks of contracture of young children who have injuries before the age of five are around the shoulders and within metacarpophalangeal extension.[38] Children's trunk and upper limb proportions are such that they have better reach and access when young and hence their shoulder range may not require great excursions of movement. As they grow, trunk and upper limb proportions change, and children may use deformity within their trunk (e.g. neuromuscular scoliosis) to maintain function, such as self-feeding. Careful consideration of function is required when assessing options and timing of interventions throughout development.

Children will often utilise a variety of adaptive devices and splints that are similar to those used by adults, but smaller; however, their purpose of use may be different. Above self-care needs, the child's occupation is play and their context includes schooling. Enabling meaningful play and maximising participation at school are key goals. Trialling various options in the context of improving play or functional skill development will help tailor devices to each individual and increase acceptance for future use.

Surgical options, such as nerve and tendon transfers, may be required for the child with tetraplegia. Surgical principles that apply to adults also apply to children; that is, to enable elbow extension, grasp and release. Once recovery is considered to have plateaued, early surgery has been shown to produce high gains, low risks and sustained function through growth and development.[38] For further detail on surgical options for the tetraplegic hand please refer to Chapter 17.

ASSISTIVE TECHNOLOGY

Assistive technology covers a wide variety of items. Equipment prescription and review is one of the more obvious areas of differentiation between paediatric and adult care. The rapid growth seen in childhood requires assistive technology prescribers to factor in expected physical and cognitive changes and its potential impact on function.

For items such as upper or lower limb orthoses, where maintaining posture may be the key goal, growth may lead to ill fit, which may in turn lead to pressure injuries and skin breakdown. The child, family and other carergivers need to be vigilant to monitor skin integrity. Poor fit, discomfort or pain may be the first indicators of growth and hence the need for review and/or replacement of orthoses. For splints and aids that are used to promote function, growth and ill fit may cause the child to perform activities less efficiently and/or predispose them to injury.

When considering more substantial and costly pieces of assistive technology, such as wheelchairs and shower chairs, it is vital to factor growth into the prescription. Many pieces of paediatric equipment will have some level of adjustment for size, such as seat depth and width, axle position and foot plate height. Care must be taken to identify which features may be most beneficial to achieve longevity, without adding unwanted weight to the chair.

Reviewing equipment regularly will enable early planning for replacement, as well as alllowing for appropriate set-up throughout its time of intended use. For example, an initial manual wheelchair set-up must take into account a variety of considerations, including safety, function and efficiency. As the child grows, their posture and position within the chair frame will alter, leading to inefficiency in propulsion, increased risk of pressure areas and overuse injuries.

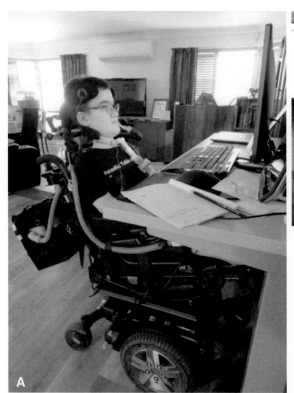

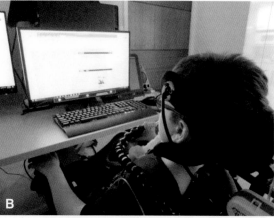

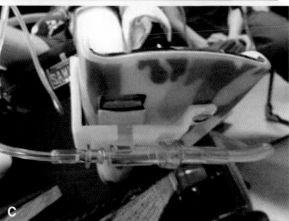

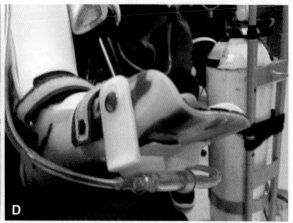

Figure 14.2 **A, B,** Assistive technology – Samuel using eye-gaze technology to do his homework.
C, D, Ankle foot orthosis with in-built switch to activate portex valve and enable vocalisation through tracheostomy.

Continued

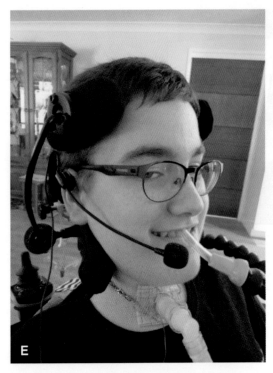

Figure 14.2, cont'd **E,** Voice amplification head set and suction unit that is foot-controlled to enable independent removal of saliva, as Samuel is unable to swallow.

Other forms of assistive technology, such as environmental controls, switches and software all need to take into consideration the age of the child at the time of prescription, as well as anticipating their future needs as they transition towards adulthood.

MUSCULOSKELETAL ISSUES

Neuromuscular scoliosis

Families need to be aware that scoliosis is practically a certainty (98%) for children who have an SCI prior to skeletal maturity, and that two-thirds go on to have surgery.[39] For children who have an SCI after skeletal maturity, scoliosis risk drops to 20%, with around 5% going on to have surgery.[40]

Vogel and colleagues[1] recommend monitoring the spine through regular (3–6 monthly) X-rays up to puberty, then 6–12-monthly until skeletal maturity and then every 2 years. The conundrum with neuromuscular scoliosis, following SCI, is not in the monitoring, but in the management. Adopting a watch-and-see approach is not recommended. Competing goals within the team mean that careful consideration must be given to each individual presentation and intervention option. For example, the orthopaedic surgeon might be aiming to achieve maximal correction to obtain maximal height, but the physiotherapy preference is not always to achieve maximal height, as this can lead to less function. Similarly, the patient may not want fusion as this can lead to less flexibility and reduced function.

The key biomechanical principle governing surgical intervention is to delay surgery to attain maximal truncal height (and associated lung development), but not delay it so long that spinal deformity leads to neurological complications from any corrective surgery.

The three main methods of slowing or correcting scoliosis have been through the use of external devices such as a thoracolumbar sacral orthosis (TLSO), internal implantation of growing rods to provide correction yet enable growth, and internal spinal fusion, which arrests growth and immobilises the spine. Each approach has its advantageous and disadvantages, which must be clearly communicated to the family (see Table 14.6). Flexible cabling is a developing approach that seeks to partially correct scoliosis in a way that enables both flexibility in the spine and bony correction during growth.

Treatment note

Children will be accustomed to the biomechanics of their posture and may use deformity to facilitate function. By changing alignment through surgery, independence with activities such as self-feeding, perianal care and transfer ability may be compromised. Whenever spinal surgery is being considered, a neurological and functional assessment prior to and following the surgery is recommended.

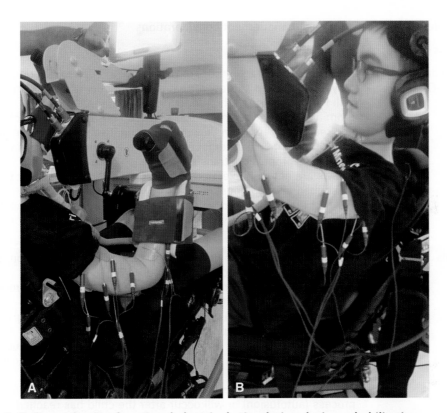

Figure 14.3 **A, B, Samuel using functional electrical stimulation during rehabilitation.**

Hip instability

Hip instability (subluxation/dislocation) is often associated with neuromuscular scoliosis in children with an SCI. As with scoliosis, children whose injury occurs at a young age are at higher risk of hip deformities.[43] As hip development occurs in the early years, hip instability is a near certainty for children having an SCI early in life (100% for injury before 5 years of age; 93% risk for injury before 10 years of age).[44,45] Unlike scoliosis management, surgical intervention may be less related to degree of subluxation or dislocation, and more related to factors such as potential functional gain, pain in the incomplete presentation or postural issues such as seating. Common surgical procedures include muscle balancing, tendon releases and reconstructive bony surgery.

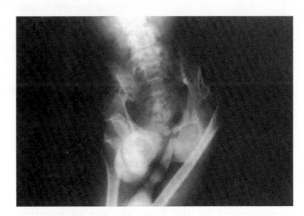

Figure 14.4 **Spinal deformity, dislocation of hip and pelvic tilt revealed at the age of 14.**

Source: Yashimura O., Murakami T., et al., 1995. Spinal cord injury in a child: A long term follow-up study. Case report. Paraplegia 33 (6), 362–363.

Table 14.6 Neuromuscular scoliosis management considerations

Management option	Considerations
Thoracolumbar sacral orthosis (TLSO)	• May prevent surgery in 50% of patients with curves < 20 degrees • May delay time to surgery for patients with curves < 20 degrees • Will have little or no effect for curves > 40 degrees[41] • From a functional perspective, TLSOs can assist in areas such as posture and respiratory function; however, the negative features often far outweigh the potential gains. External bracing to the spine often interferes with ADLs, self-propulsion, transfers and reach.[42] • TLSOs are not well tolerated and children often do not meet the regimens prescribed (e.g. 23 hours per day or 'whenever upright'). • Risks of pressure area development and intolerance due to heat mean that TLSOs are usually not well tolerated or worn for the amount of time prescribed.
Growing rods	• The child undergoes spinal surgery for the initial implantation, and then subsequent surgeries to grow the rods (every 6–12 months). • The benefit of this approach is that it enables the spine to grow, while trying to correct or limit the development of the scoliosis. • Surgical risks, as well as interruption to the child's schooling, are key detractors from this approach. • Magnetised systems of growing have been developed to reduce surgical risks; however, children will still need to return to medical facilities to have the rods grown. • Whatever the method of growth, spinal fusion either will result during the process (autofusion) or will occur after the child has reached skeletal maturity.
Spinal fusion	• This is considered when the progression of scoliosis is significant and respiratory function is declining. • Spinal growth is arrested, and functional ability is reduced due to loss of movement.
Flexible cabling	• New approach that seeks to address scoliosis without spinal fusion. • Flexible anterior scoliosis correction uses pedicle screws with a flexible cable to tether the spine. The technique seeks to correct the scoliosis utilising growth and allowing the child mobility for functional tasks.

Understanding early childhood development is important in order to address present or future hip instability. This may include assessment of patterns of movement on the floor; the use of standing frames to assist hip joint development and bone density; positioning in prone positions (e.g. for sleep) to counteract time spent in hip flexion when in the chair; use of abduction wedges; as well as strengthening programs for those with incomplete presentations.

Fragility fractures

As children can be high-spirited in the early years and engage in risk-taking behaviours in adolescence and young adulthood, it is necessary to help children and families understand the risks of osteopenia and fragility fractures. Everyday activities, such as transfers, can lead to the pathological fractures in bones with severe osteopenia.

Degradation of bone mineral density commences from the time of injury, plateauing at around 6–12 months after injury.[1] Engaging in weight-bearing and/or muscle-stimulating activities is encouraged throughout rehabilitation, in conjunction with good nutrition and exposure to sunlight. In the early years, this may involve the use of standing frames or parapodiums for those with higher level lesions, and assisted mobility through orthoses and walking aids for lower and incomplete lesions. Combining weight-bearing activities (e.g. cycling, standing, stepping) with FES (e.g. cycling or locomotor training) can achieve up to 25% increase in bone mineral density.[1]

Pathological fracture rates in children are reported to be approximately 14%.[40,43] The most common areas of fracture tend to be the distal femur or proximal tibia. Children, families and carers need to be on the lookout for swelling in the extremities accompanied by a fever.

Should fractures occur, casts should be applied with caution, due to the risk of causing pressure areas. Removable casts can achieve the immobilisation required for bone healing while still allowing carers to monitor skin condition.

Heterotopic ossification

Vogel and colleagues[1] indicate that heterotopic ossification (HO) does occur in children, but incidence is 3% compared to the 20% often documented for the adult population (see Chapter 18). The other major difference is when onset occurs – in children onset appears to be on average at around 14 months, while in the adult population it is much earlier, at 1–4 months.

SPORTS, RECREATION AND LEISURE

A key area of guidance for children with an SCI and their families is engagement in age-appropriate, sports, recreation and leisure pursuits (see Chapter 13 for more information). From a medical perspective, engaging in sports and leisure will limit the risk of cardiovascular disease and have positive health benefits throughout development.[1] From a psychosocial perspective, engaging in activities that expose children to new people, especially those with similar presentations, can be of great benefit.

When it comes to choosing appropriate pursuits, it must be noted that typically-developing children will have exposure to a wide variety of activities throughout their childhood. Children with an SCI, like their typical peers, are more likely to pursue an activity if afforded the choice and allowed to develop their own preferences.

Within the education setting, a key goal is to maximise participation in peer activities, which may involve modification of tasks or rules. Children tend to participate more fully when they perceive that their engagement is meaningful, hence where possible avoid relegating them to tasks such as time-keeping and scoring in school physical education sessions. The TREE model is a practical tool that can be used in schools to improve inclusion by considering modification of:

- teaching style
- rules
- equipment
- environment.

Many community-based organisations run programs that specifically cater to both children and adults with disability; for example, Sporting Wheelies and Disabled Association. Children are encouraged to participate and explore activities that maximise their function and participation e.g. boccia, wheelchair rugby, wheelchair basketball, etc. Many mainstream sports (e.g. athletics, swimming) also embrace children and adults with disability by having events in specific sports classifications.

Classification for specific sports enables children with an SCI to be matched against those with similar levels of impairment. Children can then pursue sporting prowess at state, national and international levels, in a similar way to their peers (see Chapter 13).

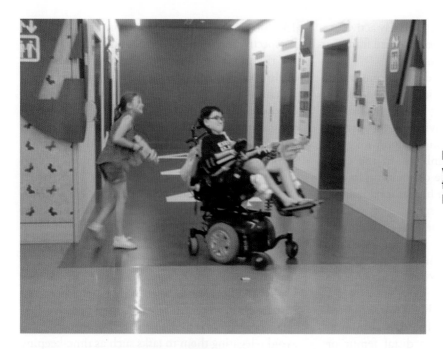

Figure 14.5 Samuel playing with friends – shooting foot-switch-enabled Nerf Blaster.

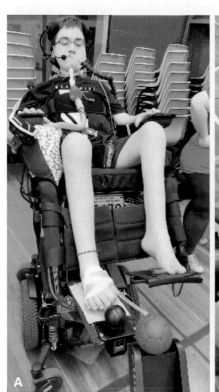

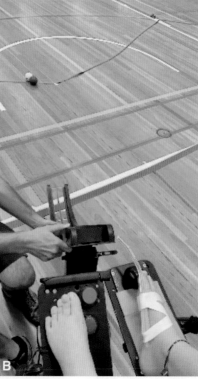

Figure 14.6 A, B, Sports and recreation – Samuel playing boccia (Paralympic sport).

For children who are not keen on sporting pursuits, exploration of leisure and recreation options is recommended for their psychosocial benefit and development of specific skill sets. These might include musicianship, craft and painting.

Screen-based play has a place as a leisure option for children with very high lesions. Gaming with peers may enable similar psychosocial benefits as those who meet face to face. Mainstream gaming for those with minimal movement capacity is now

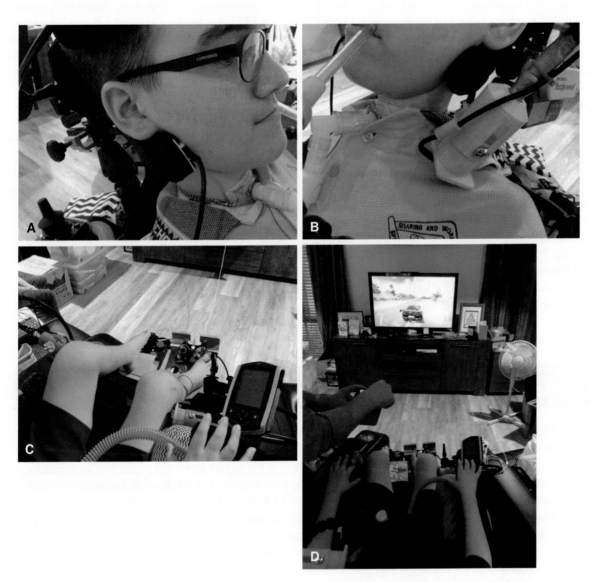

Figure 14.7 **A–D, Assistive technology – Samuel playing Xbox with switch set-up and adaptor.**

possible through technological advances in switches, buttons and interfaces.

TRANSITION TO THE ADULT SETTING

Transition is a process that commences from the moment the MDT meets the child and family. Key goals, such as bladder and bowel care, and medical literacy, are introduced early, and are specifically addressed at relevant stages of development. Having a planned approach to transition, from parental dependency towards young adult independence and autonomy, will help to lessen feelings of being overwhelmed as child and family transition from paediatric to adult setting.

Developmentally, specific matters such as driving will arise (see Chapter 8). Depending on the level of injury, most young adults with an SCI will need a driving assessment to determine what modifications may be needed to make their vehicle suitable for them to learn to drive. Like their peers, young adults with an SCI have to undergo the necessary training and examination required to acquire a driver's licence.

Other topics that may have been initiated earlier in development that need specific focus in this transition phase include sexuality and vocation.

Sexuality

Sexuality is an example of an issue that is generally discussed in the initial episode of care, particularly with parents of the younger child, but which requires further input as the child approaches puberty and subsequently engages in sexual activity (see Chapter 12 for further information). The adolescent or young adult will need to be afforded greater independence from the family as they transition to be able to freely discuss such matters.

Within a schooling context, discussions about sexuality are to be given in an age-appropriate context and followed up with opportunities for the child to ask questions of health professionals or informed adults, about the way the SCI will affect them.

Vocation

Employment is considered a crucial predictor for life satisfaction for adults with an SCI.[1] Guidance in vocational pathways is a component of most scholastic institutions. Adolescents and young adults with an SCI will need exposure to a range of possibilities and should be encouraged to pursue what they believe will give them greatest satisfaction in the employed world. Guidance relating to specific factors (e.g. safety, access) around their SCI should be discussed early on, with an attitude of inclusion and productivity (for more detail see Chapter 20).

Evidence-based practice points

- The management of children with an SCI is significantly different to that of the adult population due to growth and development.
- It takes a dedicated interdisciplinary team to provide the expert immediate care and anticipatory guidance required to see a child and family from the inpatient ward, back to home, school and community; and ultimately into the highest level of independence as an adult.
- The motor and sensory components of ISNCSCI are only recommended in children aged 6 and over. Consideration must also be given regarding the anorectal component of the examination as young children may not have developed continence before sustaining their injury, or may be too young to understand the test instructions.

Evidence-based practice points—cont'd

- Although it may be difficult for a very young child to understand AD, age-appropriate education is essential for the child and all caregivers.
- It is preferable to have the child return to their own school to benefit from a familiar environment and established social networks.
- Understanding the importance of early mobility, as well the concept of 'shared mobility', are key when providing therapy and anticipatory guidance for the child with an SCI.
- The prescription of these complex and expensive devices should be done on an individual basis and in conjunction with an experienced orthotist, particularly for those with incomplete injuries.
- Scoliosis is practically a certainty (98%) for children who have an SCI prior to skeletal maturity, of which two-thirds go on to have surgery. For children who have an SCI after skeletal maturity, scoliosis risk drops to 20%, with around 5% requiring surgery.

SUMMARY

The management of children with an SCI is significantly different from that of the adult population due to growth and development. Despite being a small population group, they require an expert MDT to address the challenges that arise from physical, cognitive and psychosocial perspectives as they transition from infancy to early schooling and go through growth spurts, puberty and adolescence into young adulthood.

Anticipatory guidance is a key concept in the management of children with an SCI. Being aware of the challenges and opportunities that present themselves throughout development helps children and families overcome hurdles and enrich their lives as they transition to adulthood.

The goal throughout development is to maximise quality of life and participation at each and every stage. Through careful and intentional planning, the intended result is to have a young adult who is emotionally and physically healthy; is literate and confident in the management of their own healthcare needs; has developed autonomy in decision-making, daily living and mobility; and ultimately has a strong sense of self.

CASE STUDY 1   MOBILITY FOR MOLLY

Molly presented with a flaccid paralysis of her lower limbs at birth. She was subsequently diagnosed with an intraspinal mass and underwent surgery at 3 days of age to remove the mass. As the lesion was benign, no further treatment was required. On early physical assessments, Molly had complete paralysis of her lower limbs, but with time she began to

Continued

CASE STUDY 1 MOBILITY FOR MOLLY—cont'd

demonstrate some activity in her quadriceps, hip adductors, tibialis posterior and, to a lesser extent, hamstring muscles. She had weak but present abdominal muscles. Molly developed progressive hip flexion contractures and equinovarus deformities of her feet due to the presence of muscle imbalance.

Early therapy interventions focused on maintenance of joint range and facilitation of age-appropriate motor skill acquisition. Compensations and adaptations were required to achieve some motor skills that required lower limb strength. Throughout her first year, Molly demonstrated an inherent desire to move and explore her surroundings. She was able to roll by 6 months using her upper limbs to initiate, and commando crawl by 12 months. She commenced upright mobility in a dynamic custom-made standing frame by 12 months of age and thoroughly enjoyed the new movement experiences that this provided for her. She was taught to initiate movement in the standing frame, initially through rocking in parallel bars before progressing to a swivel walk and jumping

action with the use of a posterior-wheeled walker. Because of the desire of Molly and her parents to explore upright mobility, she was fitted with a HKAFO before 3 years of age. Early manual-wheeled mobility was introduced at around 15 months of age and the use of a custom-fitted manual wheelchair was introduced by 2 years of age.

Throughout her preschool years, Molly used a combination of mobility options to explore her environment and to use as functional community mobility. A combination of floor mobility, upright mobility and wheelchair were used in the home and kindergarten setting, while the manual wheelchair was the preferred mobility option for the community setting. As Molly continues to progress through her primary education, she uses her AFO/HKAFO and walker for periods within the classroom, and her MWC within the playground and community. She is a keen and motivated young wheelchair athlete and continues to inspire many with her determination and independence with all forms of mobility.

CASE STUDY 2 SAMUEL

Parents' perspective (Craig and Jane)

At 9 years of age, Samuel acquired transverse myelitis which extended the length of his spinal cord and into his brain stem.

While our experience may be summarised as a non-traumatic C1/C2 SCI, we have given some consideration to different levels of injury and outcome because we remained ever-hopeful of

a better result for our son, Samuel, who remains PEG-fed (incapable of swallowing) and on ventilator life support.

It must be acknowledged that we were under no misapprehension that major implications would result, impacting on Samuel's physical wellbeing because of his age. Our rehabilitation team had on many occasions discussed with us

CASE STUDY **2**   SAMUEL—cont'd

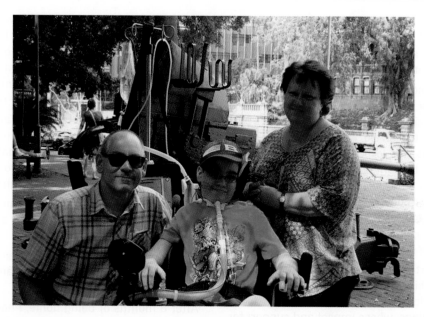

Figure 14.8 Samuel with his parents on his first drive out of the hospital in his foot-controlled power wheelchair.

how normal growth and development would physically alter over time and no doubt be affected also by what could be considered large steroid therapies early in his treatment. It would not be a single care strategy but one which would need to evolve over time, remaining responsive to Samuel's maturing needs.

Throughout explanation of diagnosis and resultant treatments, it was always important to us that the treating team direct conversations with nine-year-old Samuel. Clearly this approach should be determined with the family prior to any given conversation and also bearing in mind the age and comprehension potential of the child.

We also thought it important to not underestimate Samuel's capacity to understand the diagnosis and other information with an ongoing preparedness (for therapists/medical staff) to explain and elaborate multiple times as required. One would expect that adults, with their filter of life experience, would have a better initial understanding of the totality or finality of the SCI and resultant understanding of adult-world losses that could become a reality. But Samuel's knowledge and experience could only be filtered with a child's life experience.

As a mature ten-year-old at the time, Samuel's discharge planning had considered elements of future-proofing to account for his expected growth spurts and cognitive functioning. This included arm splints and AFOs (with at least two updates because of growth), multiple rehabilitation engineering team updates to his wheelchair to account for worsening scoliosis because of growth patterns demanding chair adjustments/corrections and also the advancing

Continued

CASE STUDY 2   SAMUEL—cont'd

psychological support. Samuel, as time progressed, became ever more capable to articulate and express psycho-emotional developments and needs.

Family life now needs constant, often complex, planning for what would otherwise have been simple family activities. Despite our best intentions to shield Samuel from these complexities, his exposure to this necessity elevates his thought processes to a level higher than should be expected of a child of his age. He is also in a constant state of 'risk assessment' – Will I be too far from my support workers if my life-support ventilator tubing suddenly disconnects? Is the ground/pathway level enough?

Our support considerations extended beyond Samuel to his sister. It should not be forgotten the dynamic of a paediatric case will likely include siblings, whose impact and support for the patient may well be integral to their rehabilitation journey.

Samuel's prognosis was never put forward as a 'status' without a plan for an evolving and supported journey. Together.

Child's perspective – Samuel (at 12 years)

In the first month after transverse myelitis left me with an SCI, I was more concerned about watching 'Shark Week' on Discovery Channel than what was happening to my body. About three months in I knew I wasn't going to get much better because of my right foot moving such a little amount, my left toe moving even less and I had some facial muscle movement.

For 480 days in hospital, I used arm and leg splints every day and I regularly used the tilt table, FES arm and leg cycling that made my limbs hurt a bit, but was important as it heightened the chance of fuller rehabilitation.

'Bloody amazing' are the rehab team, orthotists and engineers who made my AFOs and adapted my power chair.

I was over so many trials of equipment in hospital and was pleased to discharge and use the equipment at home.

After 8 months of being home, I had a growth spurt of about 12 cm. This caused scoliosis to worsen and my chair to not correctly support my body so my physio and the rehab engineers helped modify my back rest to support my scoliosis.

Next, I'm off to the Scoliosis clinic – another team to help care for me. For now though ... back to the Xbox.

References

1. Vogel, L.C., Betz, R.R., et al., 2012. Spinal cord injuries in children and adolescents. Handb. Clin. Neurol. 109, 131–147.

2. New, P.W., Lee, B.B., et al., 2019. Global mapping for the epidemiology of paediatric spinal cord damage: towards a living data repository. Spinal Cord 57 (3), 183–197.

3. Galvin, J., Scheinberg, A., et al., 2013. A retrospective case series of pediatric spinal cord injury and disease in Victoria, Australia. Spine 38 (14), E878–E882.

4. Boese, C.K., Lechler, P., 2013. Spinal cord injury without radiologic abnormalities in adults: a systematic review. J. Trauma Acute Care Surg. 75 (2), 320–330.

5. Pang, D., 2004. Spinal cord injury without radiographic abnormality in children, 2 decades later. Neurosurgery 55 (6), 1325–1343.

6. Leonard, J.C., Bachur, R.G., et al. Spinal cord injury without radiographic abnormality (SCIWORA) in children. UpToDate. Online 10 December 2019. Available:

www.uptodate.com/contents/spinal-cord-injury-without-radiographic-abnormality-sciwora-in-children.

7. Pruit, D., 2014. Non-traumatic pediatric spinal cord injury. In: Vogel, L.C., Zebracki, K., et al. (Eds.), Spinal Cord Injury in the Child and Young Adult. Mac Keith Press, pp. 111–123.

8. Mulcahey, M.J., Betz, R., et al., 2011. The international standards for neurological classification of spinal cord injury: psychometric evaluation and guidelines for use with children and youth. Phys. Med. Rehabil. 92, 1264–1269.

9. Calhoun, C., Chafetz, R., et al., 2009. A pilot study of observational motor assessment in infants and toddlers with spinal cord injury. Pediatr. Phys. Ther. 21, 62–70.

10. Mulcahey, M.J., Samdani, A.F., et al., 2012. Diffusion tensor imaging in pediatric spinal cord injury: preliminary examination of reliability and clinical correlation. Spine 37, 1–7.

11. Brown, P.J., Marino, R.J., et al., 1991. The 72-hour examination as a predictor of recovery in motor complete quadriplegia. Arch. Phys. Med. Rehabil. 72 (8), 546–548.

12. Shavelle, R.M., Devivo, M.J., et al., 2007. Long-term survival after childhood spinal cord injury. J. Spinal Cord Med. 30 (Sup 1), S48–S54.

13. Consortium for Spinal Cord Medicine, 2008. Early acute management in adults with spinal cord injury: a clinical practice guideline for health-care professionals. J. Spinal Cord Med. 31 (4), 404–479.

14. Parent, S., Mac-Thiong, J.M., et al., 2011. Spinal cord injury in the pediatric population: a systematic review of the literature. J. Neurotrauma 28, 1515–1524.

15. Behrman, A.L., Ardolino, E.M., et al., 2017. Activity-based therapy: from basic science to clinical application for recovery after spinal cord injury. J. Neurol. Phys. Ther. 41 (Suppl. 3 IV STEP Spec Iss), S39–S45.

16. Mulcahey, M.J., 2014. Assessment of children with spinal cord injury. In: Vogel, L.C., Zebracki, K., et al. (Eds.), Spinal Cord Injury in the Child and Young Adult. Mac Keith Press, pp. 41–66.

17. Webster, G., Kennedy, P., 2007. Addressing children's needs and evaluating rehabilitation outcome after spinal cord injury: the child needs assessment checklist and goal-planning program. J. Spinal Cord Med. 30 (Suppl. 1), S140–S145.

18. Gustafsson, L., Mitchell, G., et al., 2012. Clinical utility of the Canadian Occupational Performance Measure in spinal cord injury rehabilitation. Br. J. Occup. Ther. 75 (7), 337–342.

19. Doig, E., Fleming, J., et al., 2010. Clinical utility of the combined use of the Canadian occupational performance measure and goal attainment scale. Am. J. Occup. Ther. 64 (6), 904–914.

20. Mulcahey, M.J., Vogel, L.C., et al., 2017. Recommendations for the National Institute for Neurologic Disorders and Stroke spinal cord injury common data elements for children and youth with SCI. Spinal Cord 55, 331–340.

21. Devivo, M.J., Krause, J.S., et al., 1999. Recent trends in mortality and causes of death among persons with spinal cord injury. Arch. Phys. Med. Rehabil. 80, 1411–1419.

22. Hickey, K.J., Vogel, L.C., et al., 2004. Prevalence and etiology of autonomic dysreflexia in children with spinal cord injuries. Top. Spinal Cord Inj. Rehabil. 6 (Suppl.), 85–90.

23. McGinnis, K.B., Vogel, L.C., et al., 2004. Recognition and management of autonomic dysreflexia in paediatric spinal cord injury. J. Spinal Cord Med. 27, S61–S74.

24. Mitrofanoff, P., 1980. Trans-appendicular continent cystostomy in the management of the neurogenic bladder. Chir. Pediatr. 21, 297–305, (in French).

25. Vogel, L.C., 1996. Spasticity: diagnostic workup and medical management. In: Betz, R.R., Mulcahey, M.J. (Eds.), The Child With Spinal Cord Injury. American Academy of Orthopaedic Surgeon, Rosemount IL, pp. 189–212.

26. Kinsman, S.L., Doehring, M.C., 1996. The cost of preventable conditions in adults with spina bifida. Eur. J. Pediatr. Surg. 6 (Suppl. 1), 17–20.

27. Calhoun, C., Schottler, J., et al., 2013. Recommendations for mobility in children with spinal cord injury. Top. Spinal Cord Inj. Rehabil. 19 (2), 142–151.

28. Livingstone, R., Paleg, G., 2014. Practice considerations for the introduction and use of power mobility for children. Dev. Med. Child Neurol. 56 (3), 210–221.

29. Sol, M.E., Verschuren, O., et al., 2017. Development of a wheelchair mobility skills test for children and adolescents: combining evidence with clinical expertise. BMC Pediatr. 17, 1–18.

30. Sawatzky, B., Rushton, P.W., et al., 2012. Wheelchair skills training programme for children: a pilot study. Aust. Occup. Ther. J. 59 (1), 2–9.

31. Calhoun, C., Harvey, L.A., 2014. Mobility for children with spinal cord injury. In: Vogel, L.C., Zebracki, K., et al. (Eds.), Spinal Cord Injury in the Child and Young Adult. Mac Keith Press, pp. 307–328.

32. Mazur, J.M., Shurtleff, D., et al., 1989. Orthopaedic management of high-level spina bifida. Early walking compared with early use of a wheelchair. J. Bone Joint Surg. Am. 71 (1), 56–61.

33. Liptak, G.S., Shurtleff, D.B., et al., 1992. Mobility aids for children with high-level myelomeningocele: parapodium versus wheelchair. Dev. Med. Child Neurol. 34 (9), 787–796.

34. Waters, R.L., Adkins, R., et al., 1994. Prediction of ambulatory performance based on motor scores derived from standards of the American Spinal Injury Association. Arch. Phys. Med. Rehabil. 75 (7), 756–760.

35. Chafetz, R.S., Gaughan, J.P., et al., 2013. Relationship between neurological injury and patterns of upright mobility in children with spinal cord injury. Top. Spinal Cord Inj. Rehabil. 19 (1), 31–41.

36. Gerritsma-Bleeker, C.L., Heeg, M., et al., 1997. Ambulation with the reciprocating-gait orthosis. Experience in 15 children with myelomeningocele or paraplegia. Acta Orthop. Scand. 68 (5), 470–473.

37. Cuddeford, T.J., Freeling, R.P., et al., 1997. Energy consumption in children with myelomeningocele: a comparison between reciprocating gait orthosis and hip-knee-ankle-foot orthosis ambulators. Dev. Med. Child Neurol. 39 (4), 239–242.

38. Mulcahey, M.J., Zlotolow, D.A., et al., 2014. Upper extremity function. In: Vogel, L.C., Zebracki, K., et al. (Eds.), Spinal Cord Injury in the Child and Young Adult. Mac Keith Press, pp. 282–294.

39. Dearolf, W.W., 3rd, Betz, R.R., et al., 1990. Scoliosis in pediatric spinal cord injured patients. J. Pediatr. Orthop. 10, 214–218.

40. Betz, R.R., 1997. Orthopaedic problems in the child with spinal cord injury. Top. Spinal Cord Inj. Rehabil. 3 (2), 9–19.

41. Mehta, S., Betz, R.R., et al., 2004. Effect of bracing on paralytic scoliosis secondary to spinal cord injury. J. Spinal Cord Med. 27 (Suppl. 1), S88–S92.

42. Sison-Williamson, M., Bagley, A., et al., 2007. Effects of thoracolumbosacral orthoses on reachable workspace volumes in children with spinal cord injury. J. Spinal Cord Med. 30 (Suppl. 1), S184–S191.

43. Schottler, J., Vogel, L.C., et al., 2012. Spinal cord injuries in young children: a review of children injured at 5 years of age and younger. Dev. Med. Child Neurol. 54 (12), 1138–1143.

44. Betz, R.R., Mulcahey, M.J., 1994. Spinal cord injury rehabilitation. In: Weinstein, S.L. (Ed.), The Pediatric Spine: Principles and Practice. Raven, New York, pp. 781–810.

45. Miller, F., Betz, R.R., 1996. Hip joint instability. In: Betz, R.R., Mulcahey, M.J. (Eds.), The Child With a Spinal Cord Injury. American Academy of Orthopaedic Surgeons, Rosemount IL, pp. 353–361.

CHAPTER 15
Ageing with a spinal cord injury
Jacqueline Reznik

INTRODUCTION

More people than ever are now living for much longer (possibly decades) with spinal cord injury (SCI).[1,2] It is therefore increasingly important that all medical and allied health professionals working with this patient group understand the ageing process following SCIs and its ramifications.

Ageing, broadly defined as a time-dependent process leading to functional decline, is characterised by a progressive loss of physiological integrity of all body systems, ultimately leading to increased vulnerability of death.[3] Clinical observations have led to the conclusion that due to the slow decrease of many of their biological mechanisms, chronic SCI patients may be prone to premature ageing,[4] a term now described in the literature as 'accelerated ageing'.[5] The results of many longitudinal studies, however, undertaken over the past four decades do not confirm these assumptions. The majority of these studies have shown that the hypothesis that ageing in this population will inevitably be accompanied by overall decline in both physiological and psychological mechanisms, leading to a decrease in quality of life (QOL), may in fact be misleading.[1,6]

TRENDS RELATING TO THE NATURAL COURSE OF AN SCI

Four important trends related to the natural course of an SCI have been identified: (1) the survivor effect; (2) changing trends in activities, satisfaction and health over time; (3) the multifaceted nature of subjective wellbeing (SWB); and (4) outcomes reflecting successful employment.[1]

Survivor effect

In his longitudinal study on ageing, Krause and colleagues[1] suggested that those individuals who were gainfully employed, and more active, had a better psychosocial adjustment and were therefore more likely to complete the study; they termed this the 'survivor effect'. Self-reported physical and psychological health problems, reliance on caregivers and financial difficulties represented significant risk factors to life expectancy. By definition, this 'survival bias' can lead to false conclusions due to self-selection bias, questioning the validity of these results. The authors themselves imply that survivors are not representative of the total SCI population, but rather indicate the importance of the need for

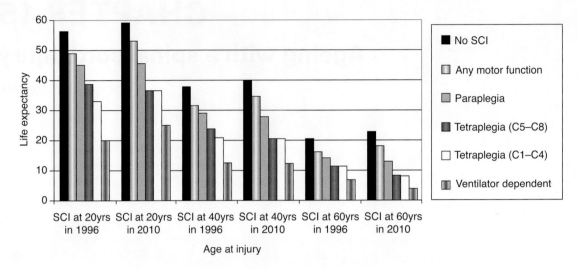

Figure 15.1 Trends in life expectancy for those surviving the first year after SCI.

Source: Groah S.L., Charlifue S., et al., 2012. Spinal cord injury and aging challenges and recommendations for future research. American Journal of Physical Medicine and Rehabilitation 91 (1), 80–93.

intervention at the levels described above in order to promote longevity.[1]

As shown in both United States (US) and European studies[2,7] survival-time post-injury is on the increase. Older age at the time of injury is still associated with higher mortality rates in the acute and chronic stages, following traumatic SCI.[8] The higher mortality rates in this population may be linked to pre-existing medical conditions or general deconditioning due to age. As indicated in Fig. 15.1, a 20-year-old who sustained a high-level SCI in 2010 had a longer post-injury lifespan compared to if they had sustained the same injury in 1996. Conversely, and perhaps of more concern, the life expectancy of the tetraplegic or ventilator-dependent SCI person at 60 years was lower in 2010 than it was in 1996. This trend is secondary to a multiplicity of causes, among them the changes in the delivery of health services during the first year post-injury.[2]

Changing trends in activities, satisfaction and health over time

In this same study, Krause and colleagues further demonstrated that activities and general lifestyle satisfaction improved significantly over the first 11 years post-injury, remaining at a similar level at the 20-year follow-up.[1,9] Interestingly, the 25-year follow-up revealed an important reversal; in particular, a decrease in the areas of social participation, satisfaction with social activities and overall health.[10] Krause and colleagues speculated that the effects of ageing and the passage of time appeared to have the greatest impact on social and medical outcomes, whereas employment outcomes were more likely to be maintained. Three chronic health conditions – diabetes, hypertension and high cholesterol – are significantly linked to people with long-term traumatic SCI and regular screening and, where necessary, regular maintenance strategies for these conditions is recommended.[11] This demonstrates the importance of local GPs being up-to-date with the most recent studies in these areas and lends weight to the value of targeting diet and exercise regimens soon after injury. It has also been reported that additional 'subsequent' injuries (in the form of musculoskeletal damage and/or syringomyelia) are frequent among persons with an existing SCI, possibly leading to further significant complications and added disability.[12] (See the end of this chapter and chapter 21 for lived experience examples.)

Subjective wellbeing

Subjective wellbeing (SWB) is a multidimensional concept, which, within the SCI community, has been shown to change over time.[1] The impact of ageing on SWB would appear to be directly related to the age at which the SCI occurred; chronologically older patients reported lower levels of SWB than the general population.[1] Molton and Yorkston, in their recent study,[13] highlighted four key areas for successful ageing with a disability; 1) resilience/adaptation; 2) autonomy; 3) social connectedness; and 4) physical health. Studies have also shown that the more assistance required for daily activities such as bathing, dressing and meal preparation etc, the greater the negative impact on SWB.[14] In a longitudinal study conducted on over 800 traumatic SCI individuals, more than 22% were found to have symptoms of probable major depression (PMD). (See Chapter 19 for further information on psychological issues.)[15]

Trends in employment

In his most recent paper on the natural course of ageing in SCI, Kraus and colleagues[16] restated what they had found in earlier studies, i.e. that the proportion of SCI individuals working full-time increased significantly over the first 20 years post-injury, but then began to decline at the 30-year follow-up. This trend continued at the 40-year follow-up.[16] Strategies designed to enhance employment possibilities within the SCI community have been found to be useful in increasing the number of SCI individuals in paid employment.[17] The strategies outlined in this study include the integration of vocational staff with individual placement and support expertise into the clinical rehabilitation teams. Similar strategies might also prove useful in supporting SCI individuals to remain in paid employment longer. Unfortunately, barriers to implementation include lack of self-confidence, lack of motivation on the part of the potential employee and lack of understanding of the condition on the part of the employer (see Chapter 20 for a personal account of these issues).[17]

ACCELERATED AGEING

The term 'accelerated ageing' was first used in a study describing 301 middle-aged men and women living with the effects of three disabling conditions: polio ($n = 124$), rheumatoid arthritis (RA) ($n = 103$) and stroke ($n = 75$).[5] This study presented reliable evidence that middle-aged individuals with chronic physical disabilities demonstrated significant signs of accelerated ageing. In the SCI population, Groah and colleagues[2] suggest that both the rate and the characteristics of ageing are affected, leading to significant disparities in life expectancy with and between this and the general population.

Within the SCI population, 'accelerated ageing' describes the unusually rapid physiological processes of maturation by many of the body systems following the initial damage to the spinal cord.[18] In a systematic review addressing the issues of ageing of the body systems following SCI, Hitzig and colleagues[19] refer to all relevant literature published from 1980 through to December 2009. From the 74 articles included in this review, the authors were able to demonstrate that the hypothesis that SCI represents a model for premature ageing is supported by a large proportion of low-level evidence for the cardiovascular and endocrine systems, stronger evidence for premature ageing in the musculoskeletal system, but only limited low-level evidence for the immune system. Only a few studies of low-level evidence were found for the respiratory system. The evidence on the genitourinary system, gastrointestinal system and for skin and subcutaneous tissues demonstrated that in these systems premature ageing might not be occurring. However, in a recent review analysing data from a number of clinical trials there is a suggestion that higher intake of animal–protein foods, either alone or in combination with a physical active lifestyle, is associated with a slowing down of the ageing process, with preservation of muscle mass and functional performance in the general population of older adults.[20]

With respect to the nervous system, only studies related to chronic pain were identified and the clearest finding from these was that the presence of pain at an earlier point in time after SCI appeared to be the best predictor of future pain. Overall, it would appear that there continues to be a lack of knowledge regarding any different physiological ageing process within the nervous system of the person with an SCI compared to the general population.[19]

Mortality and causes of death

Although both acute and long-term survival rates of people with an SCI have improved considerably since World War II, life expectancy for most people with an SCI remains below that of the general population.[2] Cardiovascular disease (CVD) is now considered to be the primary cause of morbidity and mortality within the ageing SCI community, exceeding renal and respiratory complications, which were previously regarded as the leading cause of death in this population.[21] The main risk factors for CVD include sedentary lifestyle, obesity, lipid disorders, metabolic syndromes with insulin resistance and diabetes. The incidence of death in the patient with an SCI from sepsis (a life-threatening infection in which large amounts of bacteria are present in the blood, potentially leading to organ failure, shock and death), pneumonia and influenza, diseases of the urinary system and suicide have been shown to be significantly higher within this group.[22] Interestingly, fatal complications associated with autonomic dysreflexia (AD), a relatively common complication of SCI, are more prominent in the earlier years post-injury, but incidence does not appear to be related to ageing (discussed in more detail in Chapter 4).[23]

A recent systematic review and meta-analysis[24] of patients with thoracolumbar spinal cord injuries (TLSCI) demonstrated an overall range between 0 and 37.7% as compared to an in-hospital (i.e. acute) range between 0 and 10.4%.

In the tetraplegic subgroups, patients with complete lesions were found to be more likely to die of septicaemia, pneumonia, influenza and urinary system-related diseases than those with incomplete lesions, whereas in the paraplegic subgroup this was true only for septicaemia.[22] A systematic review of crude standard mortality rates revealed that the overall mortality rate in people with an SCI is up to three times higher than that of the general population.[25] For understandable reasons relating to the disease process, survival rates were statistically lower in the non-traumatic SCI population than in the traumatic SCI population, with respiratory system failure being the leading cause of death in both groups.[25] Predictors of survival for people with an SCI include younger age at the time of injury, lower neurological level, incompleteness of lesion and more recent year of injury.[25,26] Table 15.1 (overleaf) provides a summary of some of the more notable key findings and recommendations from a variety of retrospective studies of SCI populations around the world. It would appear from these studies and recommendations that recognition and early preventative measures for CVD may reduce mortality in this 'at-risk' population.

CHANGES IN FUNCTIONAL ABILITY ASSOCIATED WITH AGEING

Within the general population, advancing age may bring with it resultant loss or decrease of independence.[18] There is a close correlation between changes in functional ability and ageing, leading to an increased need for physical assistance.[1] Age-related atrophy of the motor cortical regions and corpus callosum may precipitate or coincide with declining motor abilities such as balance and gait deficits, coordination deficits and movement slowing.[27]

Problems in functional abilities associated with ageing are strongly related to factors including pressure injury, long-term bladder and bowel concerns, postural and musculoskeletal changes, other joint changes and pain.

Tissue viability – pressure injury

The natural ageing process may induce changes in structure and function of the cardiovascular system.[28] These changes cause attenuated microvascular

Table 15.1 Summary of key findings and recommendations to improve survival rates for the person with an SCI

Year/author/title	Type of study	Country and population	Key findings	Recommendations
2013 Rabadi, Mayanna, Vincent Predictors of mortality in veterans with traumatic SCI.	Retrospective	United States 147 veterans with TSCI over 12-year period	• Survival at the end of 12 years was 60%. • Three main causes of death were infection (46%), cardiovascular disease (25%) and cancer (16%). • Older age at the time of injury was the main predictor of mortality. • There was a trend towards an increase in cardiovascular deaths and a decrease in infection deaths. • The standardised mortality ratio (SMR) was 3.1 times greater than the control population.	Preventative strategies, such as cardiovascular risk factor management, in order to decrease long-term mortality.
2012 Middleton, Dayton, Walsh et al. Life expectancy after SCI: a 50-year study	Retrospective	Australia 2014 patients with TSCI over 50-year period	• Overall 40-year survival rates among first-year survivors were 47% for persons with tetraplegia and 62% for those with paraplegia. • Three main causes of death were cancer (14.5%), ischaemic heart disease (13.2%) and pneumonia and influenza (12.7%).	Survival related strongly to the extent of neurological impairment – need to explore causative background circumstances.
2010 Hagen, Lie, Rekand, et al. Mortality after traumatic SCI: 50 years of follow-up	Retrospective	Norway 401 patients with TSCI over 50-year period	• Survival at the end of 50 years was 56.8%. • The SMR was 1.85 compared to the control population. • There was a high cause specific SMR for suicide including accidental poisoning, particularly for women (SMR of 37.59).	Greater attention required for psychological issues – identification of patients at risk for suicide.

Continued

Table 15.1 Summary of key findings and recommendations to improve survival rates for the person with an SCI—cont'd

Year/author/title	Type of study	Country and population	Key findings	Recommendations
2004 Imai, Kadowaki, Aizawa Standardised indices of mortality among persons with spinal cord injury: accelerated ageing process	Retrospective	Japan 960 males with SCI over 30-year period	• Mortality elevated compared to population norms (SMR of 2.8). • Among the leading causes of death were malignant neoplasms, cardiovascular disease and suicide.	Malignancies and age-related diseases appear to be the major causes of death.
2005 Garshick, Kelley, Cohen et al. A prospective assessment of mortality in chronic SCI	Prospective	US 361 males with chronic SCI over a period of 6 years	• Mortality elevated compared to US rates (SMR of 1.47). • Most common underlying and contributing causes of death were diseases of the circulatory and respiratory system.	Recognition and treatment of risks such as cardiovascular disease may reduce mortality in chronic SCI.

TSCI traumatic spinal cord injury; SMR standardised mortality rate

reactivity and poor soft tissue viability, increasing the risk of pressure injuries (terminology changed by the National Pressure Ulcer Advisory Panel from pressure ulcers in 2016 as it more accurately describes pressure injuries to both intact and ulcerated skin).[29] Tissue breakdown is a direct result of compromise to the integrity of the regional capillary blood supply and lymphatic drainage. Although many factors may adversely affect tissue viability, the primary cause of pressure injuries is generally considered to be externally applied pressure leading to local capillary occlusion and consequently to prolonged tissue ischaemia.

Due to impaired mobility and loss of sensation, together with repetitive exposure to pressure, friction and ischaemia/reperfusion cycles, people with an SCI of any age have an increased potential risk for the development of pressure injuries.[30,31] As longevity in people with an SCI advances, pressure injury incidence is expected to rise in parallel with other functional impairments.[31] Identifying the exact cause of pressure injury formation in people with an SCI may be difficult due to sensory loss, with no specific injury being noted by the sufferer. For those individuals with very limited mobility, there may be problems in actually identifying the position of the pressure injury; those on the sacrum or lower back are often overlooked. People with an SCI may lack awareness of the early signs and symptoms signalling pressure injury formation or fail to recognise the severity of what initially presents as a minor problem (e.g. redness over area, abrasion). Finally, there are many disincentives for early reporting of pressure injury onset, including the prospect of a long stay in hospital. In addition, it has been suggested that pressure injuries that remain resistant to treatment for more than 24 weeks might have unidentified factors hindering wound healing.[32] For strategies regarding the management of pressure injuries in the acute and sub-acute lesions please refer to Chapters 4 and 6. These strategies should become part of the daily routine for the person with an SCI and remain a top priority for all persons with an SCIs. (For a personal account see Chapter 21.)

Long-term bladder and bowel concerns

Although strong evidence on the effects of accelerated ageing on the genitourinary system and gastrointestinal system has not been well established, urological dysfunction will undoubtedly increase the risk of long-term complications and decrease the psychological and subjective wellbeing in the person with an SCI. It is important that regular monitoring and suitable management be put in place in order to prevent any long-term complications such as infections, vesicourethral reflux, renal failure, renal calculi or bladder cancer.[33]

Neurogenic bowel dysfunction is discussed in detail in Chapter 18 and has been reported as a major cause of constraints to social activities and QoL in a large proportion of people with an SCI. Non-surgical interventions for the management of bowel dysfunction include special dietary regimens, abdominal massage, manual evacuation, oral laxatives, transanal irrigation, rectal suppository and other pharmacological agents. Functional electrical and magnetic stimulation of perineal muscles has been shown to be beneficial. Surgical intervention is an option if all other methods prove to be unsuccessful; these include the implantation of electrodes, colostomy and Malone antegrade continence enema (MACE), a surgical procedure used to create a continent pathway proximal to the anus that facilitates faecal evacuation using enemas.[34]

Postural changes

Postural deviations in people with an SCI have been associated with pain,[35] skin breakdown,[32] respiratory insufficiencies[36] and functional disabilities.[37] Abnormal curvature of the spine may occur in the sagittal plane (kyphosis, lordosis) or in the coronal plane (scoliosis).[37]

Kyphosis: In the ageing population of people with an SCI it has been shown that there is increased thoracic kyphosis compared to a similar able-bodied cohort.[38] No significant difference was found of an increased kyphosis for older and longer duration participants versus younger, shorter duration participants with an SCI.[38]

Lordosis: Prolonged sitting with increased posterior pelvic tilt in the ageing population with an SCI can lead to a loss of lumbar lordosis or 'flat-back syndrome'. This, in turn, may lead to chronic low back pain and sacral pressure injuries in this population.

Scoliosis: Lateral curvature of the spine with rotation of the vertebrae and deformity in the sagittal plane, described as scoliosis,[37] may be observed in persons with an SCI who have poor trunk control when using a wheelchair seating system. As the person with an SCI ages the scoliosis may become progressively more severe due to loss/imbalance of muscular support to maintain good sitting posture.[39] Increased spinal curvature may also be a result of sagging upholstery or old poorly fitting wheelchairs. A clinical trial conducted on 17 persons with an SCI with scoliosis demonstrated that lateral trunk supports in a special seating system improved scoliotic spinal alignment in the frontal plane and reduced lumbar angles in the sagittal plane.[39]

These postural problems highlight the need for ongoing wheelchair review. Unsuitable wheelchairs may be an outcome of poor financial resources/disability funding. The importance of good seating systems for this population cannot be underestimated (see Chapter 8).

Spasticity of the trunk may also be responsible for adverse postural alignment (Fig. 15.2) (further discussed in Chapters 1, 4, 6 and 11).

Musculoskeletal changes

Within the general ageing population, the musculoskeletal ageing phenotype comprises four, often interwoven key elements – osteoporosis,

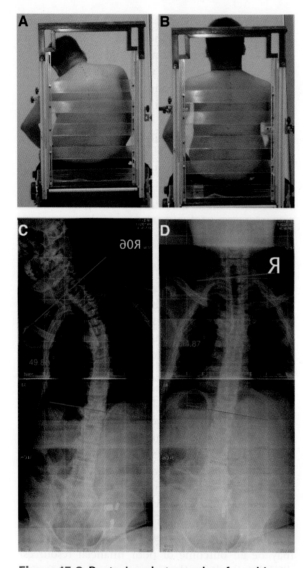

Figure 15.2 Posterior photographs of a subject with a complete C5 lesion. A, Without and B, with lateral trunk support. C, D, Corresponding mirror-imaged antero-posterior radiographs with lines indicating the calculation of the Cobb angles.

Source: Mao H.-F., Huang S.-L., et al., 2006. Effects of lateral trunk support on scoliotic spinal alignment in persons with spinal cord injury: a radiographic study. Archives of Physical Medicine and Rehabilitation 87 (6), 764–771.

osteoarthritis, sarcopenia[40] and frailty.[41] The ageing population of people with an SCI undergoes similar elderly changes as those seen in the general population; however, often the results are more deleterious.

The majority of chronic SCIs are associated with muscle atrophy and changes in muscle fibre type below the level of injury. Due to a reduction in loading, regional bone mineral density in the lower limbs is reduced and central and regional adiposity will increase post-injury. Adverse changes in muscle and bone health in individuals with an SCI contribute to an increased risk of osteoporosis, fragility fractures and endocrine-metabolic disease (e.g. diabetes, dyslipidaemia, heart disease).[42,43]

- *Osteoporosis:* SCI-induced bone loss may be described in two phases: (1) the rapid acute bone loss that plateaus approximately 2 years post-injury; and (2) chronic ongoing bone loss that is slower, but often continues for decades post-injury. The majority of individuals with long-term SCI are osteoporotic with a very high risk of fracture, the incidence of fracture risk increasing in persons more than 10 years post-injury.[44] (For further information on osteoporosis see Chapter 4.)
- *Heterotopic ossification (HO):* Following a traumatic SCI, HO in the form of neurogenic heterotopic ossification (NHO) (Fig. 15.3) may occur in any joint or muscle below the level of the lesion. NHO has a prevalence of between 10% and 53% in this population; this wide discrepancy is most likely due to the various screening protocols in place at different units. It usually occurs around the large synovial joints, the hip being the most common site.[45] (See Chapter 18 for more information on heterotropic ossification.)

Specific joint problems

- *Shoulder injuries:* Many persons with an SCI are permanent wheelchair users; this necessitates

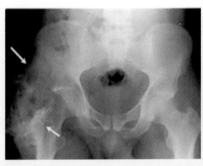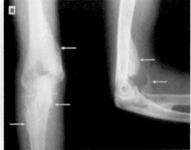

Figure 15.3 NHO usually develops around the larger synovial joints, with the hip being the most common site, followed by the knees and elbows.

Source: Reznik J.E., Biros E., et al., 2014. Prevalence and risk factors of neurogenic heterotopic ossification in traumatic spinal cord and traumatic brain injured patients admitted to specialised units in Australia. Journal of Musculoskeletal and Neuronal Interactions 14 (1), 19–28.

heavy reliance on the upper extremities to facilitate mobility and independence (see Chapters 4, 5, 6 and 8). Unfortunately, the anatomy of the shoulder does not fully protect underlying soft tissues from the joint loading that occurs during wheelchair use.[46] The resulting overuse initiates a host of degenerative factors on specific tendons around the shoulders that can weaken these tissues and induce pain.[47] Consequently, long-term manual wheelchair users are at risk of developing shoulder pain and shoulder joint injury, which can compromise their independence and QoL.[48]

- Treatment of shoulder injuries may include conservative options such as physiotherapy/ occupational therapy and/or more aggressive medical options such as injectable medications and/or surgery.[49] Initial treatment should include exercise therapy, as studies have shown that high quality home-based exercise programs (STOMPS) can be extremely effective in minimising shoulder pain.[50] If exercise programs prove inadequate in relieving the signs and symptoms of shoulder pain, then injectable medications, such as corticosteroids, may be the next level of treatment option. It is important that the patient reduce their arm use for a few days following injection therapy. This may not always be possible for the patient with an SCI. Surgical repair is an option, but one that must be considered with great caution in this patient group, as following a surgical repair the shoulder must be rested completely for 6–8 weeks. Following this complete rest, only limited use is allowed for a further 6–8 weeks. These restrictions will prevent the patient from doing independent transfers and other ADLs for more than 3 months.

- For some long-term paraplegic patients where shoulder pathology is extreme, total shoulder arthroplasty (TSA) may need to be considered. A recent systematic review[51] revealed that wheelchair-dependent patients had increased benefit long-term from the reverse total shoulder arthroplasty (RTSA). The RTSA has proven itself to sustain increased loads during transfers better than the TSA. The patient will generally require 6–12 weeks in a rehabilitation facility, but a successful RTSA may restore pain-free independent transfer and reach. Unfortunately, the postoperative period is longer and often much more complicated for the SCI population than for the general population treated with RTSA.[51]

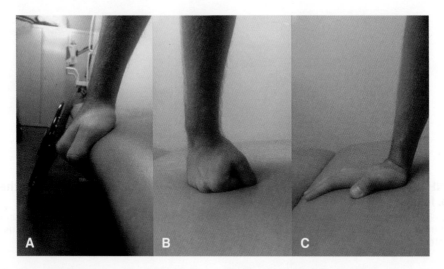

Figure 15.4 Proper and improper hand positions and use of handgrips. A, The safest position is closest to neutral with a firm grip on the surface. Unsafe positions are B, less stable or C, facilitate wrist extension and median nerve excursion under the transverse carpal ligament and over the carpal bones.
Source: Hogaboom N.S., Huang B.L., et al. 2016. Cross-sectional investigation of acute changes in ultrasonographic markers for biceps and supraspinatus tendon degeneration after repeated wheelchair transfers in people with spinal cord injury. American Journal of Physical Medicine and Rehabilitation 95 (11), 818–830.

- *Wrist injuries:* Carpal tunnel syndrome (CTS) is a compressive mononeuropathy caused by compression of the median nerve as it passes through the carpal tunnel beneath the flexor retinaculum. Due to the forceful and repetitive hand and wrist movements required for all activities of daily living (ADLs), people with an SCI are at a higher risk of developing CTS.[52] Studies by Hogaboom and colleagues[53] showed that repeated transfers are associated with a marked increase in the cross-sectional area (CSA) of the median nerve at the carpal tunnel outlet. This increase in CSA is a marker for CTS indicating compression. Furthermore, relationships were found between injury markers, specific transfer techniques and body weight. Changes were more marked in persons with higher body weight and those who performed certain transfer skills incorrectly.[53]
- The authors suggest proper hand positioning and utilisation of handgrips by the leading arm

are associated with less nerve swelling, and better overall transfer quality seemed to alleviate the negative consequences of higher body weight on the median nerve (Fig. 15.4).[53] (For further detail on management of the tetraplegic upper limb, please refer to Chapter 17.)

Pain

Pain is an extremely common complication following an SCI. A summary of the implications associated with pain following SCIs is covered in detail in Chapter 18.

EXERCISE GUIDELINES FOR THE AGEING POPULATION WITH AN SCI

Due to the extreme physical, psychosocial and environmental barriers to physical activity, the ageing population with an SCI are perhaps less active than any other section of society.[54] Dunlop and colleagues[55] associated a sedentary lifestyle in the older population with increased incidence of diabetes, cardiovascular disease and obesity. Over the past decade physical activity guidelines have been developed from systematic reviews of dose-response evidence regarding the amount of exercise required to reduce morbidity or mortality rates.[56] The World Health Organization (WHO) recommends at least 150 min/week of moderate intensity aerobic activity (or 75 min/week of vigorous intensity aerobic activity), plus muscle-strengthening activities twice weekly.

In an already at-risk population, it is therefore important that the ageing community of people with an SCI are strongly advised to commit to a regular exercise program. Based upon a recent review paper, Exercise and Sports Science Australia (ESSA) issued their position statement that exercise can improve cardiorespiratory fitness and muscular strength in people with an SCI.[57] Evidence is also emerging that these long-term exercise regimens can produce benefits such as a reduced risk of cardiometabolic disease, depression and shoulder pain, improved respiratory function, QoL and functional independence.

Specific exercise recommendations for people with SCIs as recommended by ESSA:

- ≥ 30 minutes of moderate aerobic exercise on ≥ 5 days/week or ≥ 20 minutes of vigorous aerobic ≥ 3 days/week
- strength training on ≥ 2 days/week, including scapula stabilisers and posterior shoulder girdle ≥ 2 days/week flexibility training, including shoulder internal and external rotators.

In 2018, using Appraisal of Guidelines, Research and Evaluation (AGREE II), an international panel of experts produced a new exercise guideline for cardiometabolic health benefits for adults with an SCI. Their results suggested that for cardiorespiratory fitness and muscle strength benefits, adults with an SCI should engage in at least 20 minutes of moderate-to-vigorous intensity aerobic exercise two times per week <u>AND</u> three sets of strength exercises for each major functioning muscle group, at a moderate-to-vigorous intensity, two times per week (strong recommendation). For cardiometabolic health benefits, adults with an SCI are suggested to engage in at least 30 minutes of moderate-to-vigorous intensity aerobic exercise three times per week (conditional recommendation).[58] For a more detailed explanation on the effects of activity-based therapies (active exercises) refer to Chapter 3.

CASE STUDY COPING STRATEGIES ASSOCIATED WITH CHANGING FUNCTIONAL ABILITIES

From the patient's perspective

As discussed earlier in this chapter, functional abilities of the person with an SCI decrease with age for the reasons outlined above. Although there are major physical, psychological and social implications following an SCI, there is very limited research regarding the experiences of these persons.[59] Within the ageing community of persons with an SCI, even for those who adjusted well to their initial injury and subsequent disabilities, the additional difficulties associated with the complication of ageing may prove extremely challenging (see also Chapter 21). Many older people with an SCI have great difficulty in accepting the use of assistive devices and technologies which they have never needed before (see Chapters 5 and 6).[60]

Continued

CASE STUDY COPING STRATEGIES ASSOCIATED WITH CHANGING FUNCTIONAL ABILITIES—cont'd

Mr. V. is a 67-year-old man who suffered an SCI 47 years ago. Mr. V. married nine years post-injury and has two children and five grandchildren. He describes how 'postural changes and restricted range of motion started showing probably a decade after my injury. If earlier, I did not notice as physical therapy helped to postpone it'. He goes on to describe how 'pain showed up in my shoulders only after three decades. Back pain was there before, but treatments helped to control it'. He now describes himself as having 'serious mobility issues' and objectively he has bilateral shoulder replacements (discussed earlier in this chapter) with one having a recent revision, tissue viability issues with resultant pressure sores and respiratory issues (partly due to pre-morbid asthma). Mr. V. feels that his medical problems are undoubtedly a direct result of his SCI, but he is able to cope because of his supportive family. He also feels that although socially active, he is 'less socially active than I would have been without my SCI. Many restrictions, both psychological and physical, apply'. Interestingly, although he had a car accident five years ago which had devastating results on his wellbeing and mobility, he does not refer to this in his questionnaire. Many of the issues occurring after this time are age-related, but other issues, particularly the musculoskeletal problems occurring in the upper limbs, are related to overuse injuries as a direct result of his SCI.

From the caregiver's perspective

A recent systematic review confirmed previously published estimates that the majority of caregivers for people with an SCI were made up of family and friends.[61] These figures differed for veterans, two-thirds of whom reported that they had paid caregivers. This difference is most likely to be due to the additional pension funding received by veterans.[62] A study by Bushnik and colleagues[63] reported that far fewer of the participants (16–24%) mentioned relying on a spouse, relative or friend as a caregiver. Since the study was conducted on people with an SCI 20+ years post-injury, the authors suggested that these respondents might have been required to hire caregivers because their own friends and family were no longer available to help them, possibly because of ageing of the caregiver or burnout. They also reported that there was a link between level of impairment and the reliance on paid care.

In an interview with Mr V.'s wife of 36 years, she very clearly describes that since they were married only after his SCI 'any adaptation on my part to his needs was part of our lives from the beginning and did not seem a sacrifice or strain in the least'. It was only after a recent car accident that rendered him bed-ridden for almost two years that she felt a strain on their relationship. In her own words, 'it was the first time I had ever seen him virtually helpless, and I began to understand what I had read about relationships becoming so strained as frequently to fail when one partner suffers a catastrophic injury. I dealt with this, as advised by our social worker, by "making a new contract". This meant realigning my expectations to meet his new needs on the one hand, but on the other, setting boundaries of acceptable levels of civility and responses (mine and his), even in the midst of the crisis, so we could weather the storm, which we did; I feel I am a stronger person as a result of this experience'. Not all spouses and carers may have the same level of insight or access to professionals to provide the same degree of

CASE STUDY   COPING STRATEGIES ASSOCIATED WITH CHANGING FUNCTIONAL ABILITIES—cont'd

help and advice. This further strengthens the argument for ongoing clinics, and contact with experienced healthcare professionals for the ageing communities of people with an SCI. As Mr. V. is a veteran, he has access to paid carers and they have resolved their situation by now employing a paid caregiver for the majority of the time.

With respect to the question regarding ongoing training, Mrs V. did not feel that this was necessary in the early days. However, following the accident, this changed and Mrs V. goes on to describe, 'after the accident my husband was unable to be in touch with his doctors and other professionals by himself regarding his care. It became extremely important for me to stay in touch with these professionals, ask the right questions, insist on receiving full answers, seek out additional opinions and develop my own expertise. That took a great deal of time, effort, patience and persistence. And if something didn't seem right to me in an answer I was given by medical professionals – as I found it often wasn't – I learned to rely on my gut feeling so I could insist on the best possible care'.

In response to the question of increasing time demands, this did in fact become the case, hence the importance of the paid caregiver. Mrs V. noted the toll taken on her physical health by the demands of caring for Mr V. after the accident. In addition to a variety of physical ailments, stress-related symptoms appeared; including a persistent sleep and anxiety disorder that continued even after the main crisis was over. Emanating from her own experiences, Mrs V. suggests that other family members and health professionals caring for a person with an SCI long term may be required at times to intervene in order to ensure that carers who are relatives are able to maintain good mental and physical health. This is for the benefit of both the carer and the person with the SCI.

Finally, Mrs V. makes an important statement in regards to their family: 'Children and grandchildren are not and should not be involved in caregiving. Their involvement is in helping keep morale up by regular, hearty and loving visits.'

From the professional's perspective

It is important that allied health professionals who understand the ageing process be involved in the regular check-ups of clients with an SCI. If feasible, it would be advantageous if these professionals know the clients and are up to date on innovative treatments, but since this might not always be possible, excellent records and recent research outcomes should be available. Technical developments and changing attitudes in society combined with a growing knowledge of the ageing effect on people with an SCI[1,64] have led to many changes in rehabilitation. Continuing education must be readily available for all personnel involved in the ongoing care of a person with an SCI.

Evidence-based practice points

- The secondary complications arising in the ageing population with an SCI are consistent with many of the issues in the general ageing population. It has been suggested that in the absence of compelling evidence to the contrary, exercise guidelines for people with an SCI (young or elderly) should comply with those of the general population.

- Since CVD is considered the primary risk factor for mortality in the ageing population of people with an SCI, it is important that this patient group have routine analysis of blood lipids and glucose levels. They should also have regular monitoring of weight, blood pressure, diet, physical activity, smoking and alcohol consumption.

- Concerning the musculoskeletal ageing problems – osteoporosis, osteoarthritis, sarcopenia and frailty – many of the proven strategies for the elderly can be applied to the people with an SCI. For management and prevention of these problems, regular education/exercise programs should be put in place for people with an SCI. These include weight-bearing exercises and pharmacological interventions.

- The importance of adequate nutrition has been demonstrated to have a positive effect on reducing the effects of ageing, in particular with preservation of muscle mass.

- Periodical assessment of respiratory function and lung capacity is recommended to prevent respiratory complications, particularly in the tetraplegic or high thoracic lesions where abdominals are absent and coughing may be problematic.

- Prevention of pressure injuries by the continued use of pressure mattresses and cushions, as well as pressure relief manoeuvres, is recommended.

SUMMARY

Ageing with or without an SCI is not for the 'faint-hearted', and the numerous additional problems associated with a long-term SCI cannot be overlooked. Physiological problems exist in the form of compromised tissue viability and a variety of musculoskeletal problems, often leading to chronic pain. Psychological problems associated with long-term disability and chronic pain may lead to depression, and social problems associated with accessibility concerns may lead to an increased loss of wellbeing.

It is important therefore that all professionals involved in the care of people with an SCI are made aware of these exacerbated changes associated with ageing so they can be dealt with promptly and efficiently. It is also advisable that persons with an SCI who require further treatment post-injury (for whatever reason) are able to consult with specialised health professionsals (i.e. GPs, nurses, physiotherapists, occupational therapists etc.) prior to any interventions.

References

1. Krause, J., Clark, J.M.R., et al., 2015. SCI Longitudinal aging study: 40 years of research. Top. Spinal Cord Inj. Rehabil. 21 (3), 189–200.

2. Groah, S.L., Charlifue, S., et al., 2012. Spinal cord injury and aging challenges and recommendations for future research. Am. J. Phys. Med. Rehabil. 91 (1), 80–93.

3. López-Otín, C., Blasco, M.A., et al., 2013. The hallmarks of aging. Cell 153 (6), 1194–1217.

4. Ohry, A., Shemesh, Y., et al., 1983. Are chronic spinal cord injured patients (SCIP) prone to premature aging? Med. Hypotheses 11 (4), 467–469.

5. Campbell, M.L., Sheets, D., et al., 1999. Secondary health conditions among middle-aged individuals with chronic physical disabilities: implications for unmet needs for services. Assist. Technol. 11 (2), 105–122.

6. Charlifue, S., Lammertse, D.P., et al., 2004. Aging with spinal cord injury: changes in selected health indices and life satisfaction. Arch. Phys. Med. Rehabil. 85 (11), 1848–1853.

7. Jörgensen, S., Iwarsson, S., et al., 2015. The Swedish Aging with Spinal Cord Injury Study (SASCIS): methodology and initial results. PM and R 8 (7), 667–677.

8. Furlan, J.C., Fehlings, M.G., 2009. The impact of age on mortality, impairment, and disability among adults with acute traumatic spinal cord injury. J. Neurotrauma 26 (10), 1707–1717.

9. Krause, J., 2010. Aging, life satisfaction, and self-reported problems among participants with spinal cord injury. Top. Spinal Cord Inj. Rehabil. 15 (3), 34–40.

10. Krause, J., Broderick, L., 2005. A 25-year longitudinal study of the natural course of aging after spinal cord injury. Spinal Cord 43 (6), 349–356.

11. Saunders, L.L., Clarke, A., et al., 2015. Lifetime prevalence of chronic health conditions among persons with spinal cord injury. Arch. Phys. Med. Rehabil. 96 (4), 673–679.

12. Saunders, L.L., Krause, J.S., 2015. Injuries and falls in an aging cohort with spinal cord injury: SCI aging study. Top. Spinal Cord Inj. Rehabil. 21 (3), 201–207.

13. Molton, I.R., Yorkston, K.M., 2017. Growing older with a physical disability: a special application of the successful aging paradigm. J. Gerontol. B Psychol. Sci. Soc. Sci. 72 (2), 290–299.

14. Lundström, U., Wahman, K., et al., 2017. Participation in activities and secondary health complications among persons aging with traumatic spinal cord injury. Spinal Cord 55 (4), 367–372.

15. Saunders, L.L., Krause, J.S., et al., 2012. A longitudinal study of depression in survivors of spinal cord injury. Spinal Cord 50 (1), 72–77.

16. Krause, J.S., Newman, J.C., et al., 2016. The natural course of spinal cord injury: changes over 40 years among those with exceptional survival. Spinal Cord 55 (5), 502–508.

17. Cotner, B.A., Ottomanelli, L., et al., 2018. Provider-identified barriers and facilitators to implementing a supported employment program in spinal cord injury. Disabil. Rehabil. 40 (11), 1273–1279.

18. Charlifue, S., Jha, A., et al., 2010. Aging with spinal cord injury. Phys. Med. Rehabil. Clin. N. Am. 21 (2), 383–402.

19. Hitzig, S.L., Eng, J.J., et al., 2011. An evidence-based review of aging of the body systems following spinal cord injury. Spinal Cord 49 (6), 684–701.

20. Bradlee, M.L., Mustafa, J., et al., 2017. High-protein foods and physical activity protect against age-related muscle loss and functional decline. J. Gerontol. A. Biol Sci. Med Sci 73 (1), 88–94.

21. Myers, J., 2009. Cardiovascular disease after SCI: prevalence, instigators, and risk clusters. Top. Spinal Cord Inj. Rehabil. 14 (3), 1–14.

22. Soden, R., Walsh, J., et al., 2000. Causes of death after spinal cord injury. Spinal Cord 38 (10), 604–610.

23. Stillman, M.D., Barber, J., et al., 2017. Complications of spinal cord injury over the first year after discharge from inpatient rehabilitation. Arch. Phys. Med. Rehabil. 98 (9), 1800–1805.

24. Azarhomayoun, A., Aghasi, M., et al., 2018. Mortality rate and predicting factors of traumatic thoracolumbar spinal cord injury; a systematic review and meta-analysis. Bull. Emerg. Trauma 6 (3), 181.

25. Van Den Berg, M.E., Castellote, J.M., et al., 2010. Survival after spinal cord injury: a systematic review. J. Neurotrauma 27 (8), 1517–1528.

26. Osterthun, R., Post, M.W.M., et al., 2014. Causes of death following spinal cord injury during inpatient rehabilitation and the first five years after discharge. A Dutch cohort study. Spinal Cord 52 (6), 483–488.

27. Seidler, R.D., Bernard, J.A., et al., 2010. Motor control and aging: links to age-related brain structural, functional, and biochemical effects. Neurosci. Biobehav. Rev. 34 (5), 721–733.

28. Inouye, S.K., Studenski, S., et al., 2007. Geriatric syndromes: clinical, research, and policy implications of a core geriatric concept. J. Am. Geriatr. Soc. 55 (5), 780–791.

29. Berlowitz, D. Clinical staging and management of pressure-induced skin and soft tissue injury. Uptodate. Onine 12 December 2019. Available: www.uptodate.com/contents/clinical-staging-and-management-of-pressure-induced-skin-and-soft-tissue-injury.

30. Coleman, S., Gorecki, C., et al., 2013. Patient risk factors for pressure ulcer development: systematic review. Int. J. Nurs. Stud. 50 (7), 974–1003.

31. de Laat, H., de Munter, A., et al., 2016. A cross-sectional study on self-management of pressure ulcer prevention in paraplegic patients. J. Tissue Viability 26 (1), 69–74.

32. Guihan, M., Sohn, M.W., et al., 2016. Difficulty in identifying factors responsible for pressure ulcer healing in veterans with spinal cord injury. Arch. Phys. Med. Rehabil. 97 (12), 2085–2094, e1.

33. Sezer, N., Akkuş, S., et al., 2015. Chronic complications of spinal cord injury. World J. Orthop. 6 (1), 24–33.

34. Krassioukov, A., Eng, J.J., et al., 2010. Neurogenic bowel management after spinal cord injury: a systematic review of the evidence. Spinal Cord 48 (10), 718–733.

35. Gerhart, K.A., Bergstrom, E., et al., 1993. Long-term spinal cord injury: functional changes over time. Arch. Phys. Med. Rehabil. 74 (10), 1030–1034.

36. Terson de Paleville, D.G., Sayenko, D.G., et al., 2014. Respiratory motor function in seated and supine positions in individuals with chronic spinal cord injury. Respir. Physiol. Neurobiol. 203, 9–14.

37. Good, C.R., Auerbach, J.D., et al., 2011. Adult spine deformity. Curr. Rev. Musculoskelet. Med. 4 (4), 159.

38. Amsters, D., Nitz, J., 2006. The consequences of increasing age and duration of injury upon the wheelchair posture of men with tetraplegia. Int. J. Rehabil. Res. 29 (4), 347–349.

39. Mao, H.F., Huang, S.L., et al., 2006. Effects of lateral trunk support on scoliotic spinal alignment in persons with spinal cord injury: a radiographic study. Arch. Phys. Med. Rehabil. 87 (6), 764–771.

40. Steffl, M., Bohannon, R.W., et al., 2017. Relationship between sarcopenia and physical activity in older people: a systematic review and meta-analysis. Clin. Interv. Aging 12, 835–845.

41. Dawson, A., Dennison, E., 2016. Measuring the musculoskeletal aging phenotype. Maturitas 93, 13–17.

42. Gibbs, J.C., Craven, C., et al., 2015. Muscle density and bone quality of the distal lower extremity among individuals with chronic spinal cord injury. Top. Spinal Cord Inj. Rehabil. 21 (4), 282–293.

43. Moore, C.D., Craven, B.C., et al., 2015. Lower-extremity muscle atrophy and fat infiltration after chronic spinal cord injury. J. Musculoskelet. Neuronal Interact. 15 (1), 32–41.

44. Troy, K.L., Morse, L.R., 2015. Measurement of bone: diagnosis of SCI-induced osteoporosis and fracture risk prediction. Top. Spinal Cord Inj. Rehabil. 21 (4), 267–274.

45. Reznik, J.E., Biros, E., et al., 2014. Prevalence and risk factors of neurogenic heterotopic ossification in traumatic spinal cord and traumatic brain injured patients admitted to specialised units in Australia. J. Musculoskelet. Neuronal Interact. 14 (1), 19–28.

46. Nyland, J., Quigley, P., et al., 2000. Preserving transfer independence among individuals with spinal cord injury. Spinal Cord 38 (11), 649–657.

47. Lewis, J.S., 2015. Shoulder pain. In: Graven-Nielsen, T., Arendt-Nielsen, L. (Eds.), Musculoskeletal Pain: Basic Mechanisms and Implications. IASP Press, Washington.

48. Hogaboom, N.S., Huang, B.L., et al., 2016. Cross-sectional investigation of acute changes in ultrasonographic markers for biceps and supraspinatus tendon degeneration after repeated wheelchair transfers in people with spinal cord injury. Am. J. Phys. Med. Rehabil. 95 (11), 818–830.

49. Van Straaten, M.G., Cloud, B.A., et al., 2017. Maintaining shoulder health after spinal cord injury: a guide to understanding treatments for shoulder pain. Arch. Phys. Med. Rehabil. 98 (5), 1061–1063.

50. Mulroy, S.J., Thompson, L., et al., 2011. Strengthening and optimal movements for painful shoulders (STOMPS) in chronic spinal cord injury: a randomized controlled trial. Phys. Ther. 91 (3), 305–324.

51. Kemp, A.L., King, J.J., et al., 2016. Reverse total shoulder arthroplasty in wheelchair-dependent patients. J. Shoulder Elbow Surg. 25 (7), 1138–1145.

52. Ibrahim, I., Khan, W., et al., 2012. Carpal tunnel syndrome: a review of the recent literature. Open Orthop. J. 6 (1), 69–76.

53. Hogaboom, N.S., Diehl, J.A., et al., 2016. Ultrasonographic median nerve changes after repeated wheelchair transfers in persons with paraplegia: relationship with subject characteristics and transfer skills. PM and R 8 (4), 305–313.

54. Carr, J.J., Kendall, M.B., et al., 2017. Community participation for individuals with spinal cord injury living in Queensland, Australia. Spinal Cord 55 (2), 192–197.

55. Dunlop, D.D., Song, J., et al., 2015. Sedentary time in US older adults associated with disability in activities of daily living independent of physical activity. J. Phys. Act. Health 12 (1), 93–101.

56. Arrieta, H., Rezola-Pardo, C., et al., 2018. A multicomponent exercise program improves physical function in long-term nursing home residents: a randomized controlled trial. Exp. Gerontol. 103, 94–100.

57. Tweedy, S.M., Beckman, E.M., et al., 2017. Exercise and Sports Science Australia (ESSA) position statement on exercise and spinal cord injury. J. Sci. Med. Sport 20 (2), 108–115.

58. Martin Ginis, K.A., van der Scheer, J.W., et al., 2018. Evidence-based scientific exercise guidelines for adults with spinal cord injury: an update and a new guideline. Spinal Cord 56 (4), 308–321.

59. Chen, H.Y., Boore, J.R., 2008. Living with a spinal cord injury: a grounded theory approach. J. Clin. Nurs. 17 (5), 116–124.

60. Bergström, E., 2006. Ageing with spinal cord injury. In: Tetraplegia and Paraplegia. Elsevier, pp. 345–352.

61. Smith, E.M., Boucher, N., et al., 2016. Caregiving services in spinal cord injury: a systematic review of the literature. Spinal Cord 54 (8), 562–569.

62. Robinson-Whelen, S., Rintala, D.H., 2003. Informal care providers for veterans with SCI: who are they and how are they doing? J. Rehabil. Res. Dev. 40 (6), 511–516.

63. Bushnik, T., Wright, J., et al., 2007. Personal attendant turnover: association with level of injury, burden of care, and psychosocial outcome. Top. Spinal Cord Inj. Rehabil. 12 (3), 66–76.

64. Rodakowski, J., Skidmore, E.R., et al., 2014. Additive effect of age on disability for individuals with spinal cord injuries. Arch. Phys. Med. Rehabil. 95 (6), 1076–1082.

CHAPTER 16

High cervical lesions

Jacqueline Ross

INTRODUCTION

Spinal cord injury (SCI), although a significant public health issue,[1] is relatively rare, and complete high cervical spinal cord injury (CSCI) even more so. It is estimated that only 4% of SCI patients require long-term ventilation with a tracheostomy or diaphragm pacing.[2] As a result, clinicians do not often have the opportunity to care for someone with a high CSCI leading to ventilator dependence. In a 50-year review of SCI in New South Wales, Australia, C1–4 complete tetraplegia, first-year mortality dropped from 32.4% in 1955 to 13.5% in 2006.[3] This most likely signifies an improvement in emergency management, acute care and rehabilitation of high CSCI and indicates that this condition may become more prevalent in the future (for more detail see Chapter 2).[4]

In high-income countries the main causes of death for people with tetraplegia have changed over recent decades from urological complications to respiratory complications, including pneumonia and influenza.[1] However, for those who survive the first year post-CSCI, mortality rates continue to be at least twice that of the general population,[3] indicating that there is a need to focus on the respiratory wellbeing of people living with high CSCI.

This chapter will explore the needs of individuals with a high cervical lesion who require ventilation and discuss some of the challenges, treatment options and lifestyle changes this presents.

Terminology

Many people prefer the terms 'ventilator-associated person' or 'ventilator user' rather than patient, particularly when referring to those living in the community with the need for ventilation. As this text is intended primarily for health professionals and describes hospital and community environments, the term patient will be respectfully used at times.

Aetiology

The International Standards for Neurological Classification of Spinal Cord Injury (ISNCSCI) published by the American Spinal Injury Association (ASIA) is a well-established international communication tool for researchers and clinicians to quantify the neurological impairment resulting from an SCI.[5] An injury at the level of C1–3 on the ASIA Impairment Scale (AIS) A and B will almost certainly lead to complete ventilator dependence or the requirement for ventilator usage for a substantive part of the 24-hour cycle.[4] According to data from the United States, the most common cause of C1–4 SCI is diving (25%), followed closely by falls (20.3%) and car accidents (17.9%).[6] High cervical lesions may also occur as a result of medical or surgical complications, including vascular ischaemia, intraspinal haemorrhage, cord compression secondary to stenosis, tumour, epidural abscess or disc herniation, vertebral artery dissection or vascular malformation causing compression.[7] Traumatic complete high cervical injuries resulting in immediate paralysis of the respiratory muscles occurring in an out of hospital location can only be survived if immediate resuscitation is available on site (see Chapter 2).

INITIAL MANAGEMENT

On initial presentation, patients with high cervical lesions will be cared for in the intensive care unit (ICU), preferably at a specialist spinal cord injury centre in order to receive optimal care and maximise outcomes.[8] The general principles of management are largely the same as those for management of lower cervical injuries, with some specific differences. For incomplete and lower cervical injuries, there is a decision around when or even whether to perform a tracheostomy. In the patient with a high cervical lesion, it is evident soon after injury that ventilation will be required for a long period of time or permanently, so a tracheostomy may be performed early post-admission.[9,10] Early tracheostomy has many benefits, including the possibility of ventilator-associated speech[11] and makes lip-reading easier by removing the endotracheal tube from the mouth to facilitate communication. A tracheostomy also provides a more secure airway than an endotracheal tube, so that early mobilisation to a wheelchair is safer.

Other elements of early management of SCI, such as respiratory management, immobilisation and surgical fixation, are dealt with in Chapter 4.

Airway management

Establishing a secure airway in any individual requiring ventilation is important. For the person with high CSCI, who will potentially require invasive ventilation for the rest of their life, a well-fitted and secure airway has even more significance. The diameter, angle of curvature and length of both the horizontal and the vertical sections of the tracheostomy tube are components that differ in various readily available off-the-shelf tracheostomy tubes. In cases where a standard tracheostomy tube cannot be identified to fit a patient with unusual anatomy, a customised tube may be required to achieve the correct fit. Optimal fit of the tracheostomy tube (TT) will avoid issues of cuff and/or stoma leak, decrease the occurrence of stoma breakdown and tracheomalacia and, in the most serious instances, protect against loss of the airway by dislodgement or severe malalignment of the tube. A tracheoscopy should be performed after initial tube insertion or when tube size or type is changed in order to confirm adequate positioning,[12] including appropriate distance from the carina and central placement in the trachea to avoid tube occlusion against the tracheal wall. Tracheoscopy is important, as up to 10% of TTs are malpositioned (defined as at least 50% occluded by tissue), and this is rarely detected without direct visualisation.[13] Tracheostomy teams are becoming more common in healthcare settings, and have been shown to improve outcomes for spinal patients, including enabling earlier use of speaking valves.[14] Consulting such a team can be helpful if TT customisation is required.

Inner cannula use with TTs is standard in most healthcare settings.[15] Use of an inner cannula allows for prompt and easy clearance of a TT that is blocked by secretions and this added level of safety is desirable in a patient where airway security is paramount. The reduction in airway diameter (which accompanies inner cannula use) should be taken into account in spontaneously ventilating or weaning patients, as it can increase the work of breathing.[16] In patients who do not breathe spontaneously, this consideration is less important as the ventilator delivers the breaths.

Autonomic instability

Autonomic instability will be more severe in those with a higher and more complete cervical lesion.[17]

Bradycardia and hypotension can present acute challenges early on after injury. Simple procedures, such as turning the patient, can lead to movement of respiratory secretions and sputum plugging, resulting in acute and severe desaturation. Close attention to heart rate, blood pressure and oxygenation are particularly important for the physiotherapist during treatment. In order to maintain clear lung fields, regular volume restoration and secretion clearance treatments are recommended,[18] but the risks of suctioning and moving patients needs to be anticipated in order to manage dangerous side effects, such as marked bradycardia or asystolic arrest.[19] Close medical liaison is recommended in these patients, as pharmacological management is required, including the use of agents such as aminophylline, theophylline, atropine and adrenaline (epinephrine). Use of temporary pacing wires or insertion of a cardiac pacemaker may occur in patients where pharmacological management is not successful in controlling their symptoms.[20,21]

Communication on a ventilator including speech

Strategies for communication in the ICU when on a ventilator often involve writing down/typing or pointing to letters or words on a communication board. In the setting of upper limb paralysis, lip-reading, eye-blinking, facial expression and eye gaze can be used. Eye-gaze boards are time-consuming, but can provide a high degree of accuracy. Lip-reading tends to be dependent on the person doing the lip-reading, but encouraging patients to over-enunciate and slow down can be helpful. Essentially, all these strategies are slow and prone to error and frustration. Restoration of voice as early as possible is hugely important to patients, their families and the care team. Patients frequently speak of their early frustration and anxiety in ICU and subsequent relief once ventilator-associated speech is established.

> I can't overstate how important speech is to me. Before I learnt to use leak speech my communication consisted of facial expressions, clicks made with my tongue and using an alphabet board. The alphabet board required someone to hold a board with the alphabet on it and laboriously spell out what I was trying to say letter by letter with me clicking when they arrived at the right letter.
>
> I use voice-activated software to email, research on the web and publish a blog. I would never have been able to make this contribution if I didn't have a voice. I have a voice-activated mobile phone so that I can text and converse with family and friends.
>
> Most of all, I can freely join in conversation with family, friends and visitors. I can tell a joke. How good is that!
>
> (Gerard, 67-year-old man with C1 AIS A tetraplegia)
>
> Being able to use my voice, especially after being deprived of speech for months, taught me the importance of speech as part of my identity, expressing who I am as a person. Being completely deprived of voice is degrading and frustrating at best; it feels like a whole part of personality is quietened. The first time my voice came back, I had the biggest beaming smile because even a squeak represented 'a bit of Daisy is still alive', that I have the opportunity to scream when I'm in pain or cry when I am frustrated, or laugh when I feel joy; that to me is the essence of life.
>
> (Daisy, 28-year-old woman with C1 AIS A tetraplegia)

It is possible to safely achieve speech on a ventilator by deflating the tracheostomy tube cuff and allowing air to flow over the vocal cords.[22] It is important to work in a multidisciplinary way to optimise the safety and efficacy of this technique. Aspiration is a clear risk of cuff deflation and a speech pathologist's input is recommended. A clinician with sufficient experience in ventilation assessment and adjustment needs to ensure adequate gas exchange for the patient (this is generally the role of the physiotherapist), and senior medical personnel need to be aware of the procedure in order to offer support during the first few trials. An increase in suctioning requirements is usual when the cuff is first deflated and this increases the risk of inducing bradycardia from vagal stimulation.[17] Tidal volume can be increased in order to ensure adequate ventilation and inspiratory time lengthened to improve speech.[11,23] The increase in tidal volume can be large, so that 500 mL becomes 700–800 mL, for example, during initial trials, as patients learn to control ventilation leak with their vocal cords.[22] Once control of leak is achieved, the volume can be lessened to reduce the flow through the upper airway, which is generally reported as being more comfortable. An increase in positive end expiratory pressure (PEEP) levels has also been associated with improved speech during the expiratory phase of the ventilatory cycle.[11,23] Monitoring is required to ensure adequate maintenance of blood pressure throughout the procedure as increased tidal volumes and PEEP increase intra-thoracic pressure and decrease cardiac filling.

When facilitating speech in this way, the patient achieves the best voice during the inspiratory cycle of the ventilator, which is opposite to our usual way of speaking. Some patients will find the experience of air leaking through their upper airway irritating or distressing and may benefit from partial cuff deflation to control the flow during early trials. A period of training is required, with early sessions being as brief as 5–10 minutes, as patients can tire easily when learning this technique. Most people are eventually able to progress to being ventilated with their cuff fully deflated during waking hours to enable speech.[11,23]

It is the practice of some centres to change their patients to cuffless tracheostomy tubes once they are stabilised on ventilation with periods of cuff deflation to allow vocalisation. This allows speech overnight without adjustments to the cuff or ventilator. It is proposed that one mechanism for the reduction of leak and maintenance of adequate ventilation overnight in patients with cuffless tubes is a reduction in the cross-sectional area of the pharynx in the supine position. In this position the velum and tongue fall back towards the posterior pharyngeal wall. Morning arterial blood gases will assist clinicians to monitor the adequacy of overnight ventilation. The accepted normal range of arterial blood gas CO_2 is 35–45 mmHg with a pH of 7.35–7.45. A pH below this range may indicate an acute rise in CO_2, resulting in respiratory acidosis and indicating to the clinician that the patient is potentially under-ventilated.[24]

Speech can also be achieved by using a one-way speaking valve in line with the ventilator circuit. The valve is placed to prevent loss of expired air into the expiratory limb of the circuit and all exhaled air passes up over the vocal cords to enable speech, improving phrase length and volume.[11] Using a one-way valve in line with the circuit involves an extra step in the set-up of ventilator-associated speech and also introduces the risk of the valve being used in the presence of an inflated cuff. It is important to note that the use of a one-way speaking valve in the presence of an inflated tracheostomy cuff prevents expiration while continuing to allow inspiration and is a serious adverse event that puts the patient at high risk of pneumothorax or potentially death.[22] The choice between cuff deflation alone or use of a valve in line with the ventilator circuit should be based on patient performance, preference and risk management, as assessed by the treating team.

Daisy learned to sing while on ventilation. Achieving the phrasing and consistency of voice required was extremely challenging and a great achievement for her.

> Music has always been something that has been important in my life, it's my therapy, it's my hobby, it's my passion, it's almost who I am. Before my injury, I would listen to music when I woke up and when I go to sleep. After my injury, music became an even more integral part of my life. It represented my emotions for me, it would relax me when I felt anxious, it would scream for me when I felt frustrated, I would meditate to it through pain, I would celebrate with it through accomplishments. After my injury I had music therapy and sang to improve my breathing. During this time, I was able to

use music to improve my breathing while I was on a ventilator and attempt to activate my diaphragm. It definitely contributed psychologically and physically to my overall rehabilitation and recovery. Without music, I think a huge chunk of me would be lost. (Daisy)

Speech during the use of diaphragm pacing is generally less fluent than speech on ventilation. Voicing occurs only during expiration, similar to spontaneous breathing, however, the mandatory nature of the rate and depth of the breathing cycle on pacing can make for rather stilted speech. Some skilled users can use glossopharyngeal breathing (described later in this chapter) to augment their volumes and improve fluency under these conditions. Use of an abdominal binder may improve voice quality, volume and phrase length during diaphragm pacing, by improving diaphragm positioning in the same way as it can in the spontaneously breathing, seated tetraplegic person.[22]

Early speech trials in the ICU will also improve assessment of cognition and orientation. The incidence of delirium in ICU is associated with poorer outcomes, including long-term cognitive impairment.[25] The ability to assess a patient's mental state is severely impaired if communication is limited to non-verbal means, such as eye blinking and lip-reading. It is also vital to establish orientation and competence in the setting of discussions around future directions of care for patients with high CSCI. Options for discontinuation of care may be presented to patients or their surrogate decision-makers in the early days following such an injury, and it can be argued that in the absence of clear verbal communication, informed consent is not possible.

Assessment of weaning potential

Evaluation of potential for weaning is a multifactorial process that evolves over the weeks and months following injury. In general, patients with C1–4 AIS A or AIS B are considered at risk of failure to wean from ventilation, but reduction of oedema and recovery over time may alter that outcome.[26] There

is evidence that some patients presenting with high CSCI will remain completely ventilator dependent, while others achieve partial or even complete weaning. Recent studies on patients with CSCI[26,27] have suggested the best predictors of weaning to be negative inspiratory force diaphragm needle electromyography (EMG) and bedside spirometry (negative inspiratory force and forced vital capacity). They also suggest that EMG may detect motor unit activity that is missed by fluoroscopy and is therefore a more sensitive measure.

In the clinical setting, prior to conducting diaphragm EMG or imaging of the diaphragm, evaluation of suitability for weaning should involve assessment of arterial gases, chest X-ray and bedside spirometry. Patients should be medically stable, have minimal oxygen requirements, have a manageable secretion load and be psychologically ready to participate in the process.[28–30]

As previously noted, an important sign that weaning from ventilation is possible in the high CSCI person is the presence of diaphragm activity. Prior to employing EMG, fluoroscopy or ultrasound, the diaphragm can also be assessed by direct visualisation of the patient in supine position during a trial of ventilator-free time. The patient is instructed to sniff (as this selectively recruits the diaphragm) and is observed from the end of the bed. The clinician is able to see if there is some outward movement of the upper abdominal wall on inspiration with a corresponding fall on expiration. This is an indication that the diaphragm is actively contracting and moving inferiorly, displacing the abdominal contents as it does so, resulting in abdominal distension. A paralysed diaphragm will be drawn in a cephalad direction on inspiration if intercostal muscles or strong neck accessory muscles are actively expanding the thoracic cavity, and this will result in the abdomen being drawn inwards. In cases of complete inspiratory muscle impairment, no chest or abdominal wall movement will be seen. When performing a bedside assessment of diaphragm movement, the clinician can also look at symmetry as unilateral diaphragm paralysis may exist and can then be assessed more thoroughly using EMG or other methods.

Failure to identify patients with the potential to wean can lead to them being discharged on long-term respiratory support to care facilities or home where the capacity to wean may not be recognised. Expert follow-up could uncover the potential for weaning many months after injury, leading to markedly reduced care needs and improved quality of life.[31] Referral to a dedicated weaning unit in a tertiary or quaternary healthcare service is recommended for patients with uncertain weaning potential.

Diaphragm pacing

Diaphragm pacing has been available for many years to restore function to the diaphragm with the aim of reducing dependence on or replacing mechanical ventilation.[32] The pacing device itself is smaller and less obtrusive than a portable ventilator and will require less maintenance, but in many cases the pacer will not completely replace the ventilator and so both devices will need to be maintained (Table 16.1).

> I prefer diaphragm pacing to ventilation via tracheostomy for a variety of reasons. The pacer is much safer when I'm manoeuvring through crowds. There are no tubes that can be disconnected. Not that it worries me, but it's less obvious to anyone seeing me that I am actually connected to some sort of device to breathe. (Gerard)

Pacing of the diaphragm can be achieved by direct phrenic nerve stimulation, direct diaphragm

Table 16.1 Comparison of diaphragm pacing and invasive ventilation via tracheostomy

Diaphragm pacing	Invasive ventilation via tracheostomy
Pacer is silent	Ventilators have the sound of the exhalation valve and turbine
External pacer box is quite small and can be carried attached to the torso unobtrusively.	Portable ventilators are quite large and need to be mounted to the wheelchair or carried in a bag.
Pacer box weighs approximately 500 gm.	Weight of ventilator 3–4 kg.
Alarm of pacer box is very quiet and not easily compatible with call bell systems.	Alarm of ventilator is loud enough to hear from next room and can be connected into 'call bell' systems.
Battery life of pacer box 500-hour lithium battery without back-up.	2–8 hours of internal battery life without back-up.
Speech can only occur on expiration. Speech may be less fluent.	Speech can occur on expiration and inspiration and breath rate can be increased on demand.
Fixed respiratory rate.	Respiratory rate can be altered by user depending on settings.
Minimal risk of accidental disconnection from pacer box.	Risk of accidental disconnection if tubing is pulled inadvertently or tracheostomy hub connection not secure.
Negative pressure ventilation is more physiological and may improve ventilation to basal lung segments.[11]	Positive pressure ventilation favours ventilation of areas of low resistance in the lungs.
Surgical procedure required.	No surgery required.

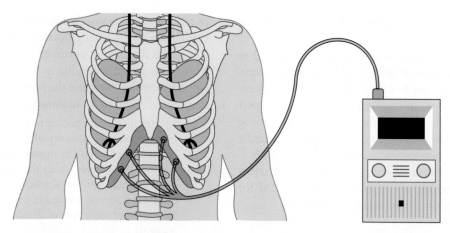

Figure 16.1 Direct diaphragm pacing system showing external pacing box and representation of positioning of internal electrodes (pacing wires) implanted directly on to the diaphragm.

stimulation or following reconstructive surgery to the phrenic nerve plus diaphragm pacing. The basic requirements for successful pacing of the diaphragm are an intact phrenic nerve and a diaphragm that has sufficient muscle integrity to allow stimulation. In the setting of high CSCI, damage to the anterior horn cells can lead to Wallerian degeneration of the phrenic nerves (for more detail see Chapter 1). This can be seen after severe haemorrhage in the cord or a large area of severe cord compression. Previously, patients with either peripheral damage to the phrenic nerve or axonal degeneration secondary to anterior horn cell damage were not considered to be candidates for diaphragm pacing; however, since 2000 there have been reports of reconstructive surgery to the phrenic nerve in order to facilitate diaphragm pacing.[33] This procedure has only recently been trialled for the first time in Australia in a candidate with high CSCI, and the functional outcome of the procedure is pending at the time of writing.

The results of both diaphragm pacing and phrenic nerve grafting following CSCI in order to facilitate pacing are more promising if performed in the early weeks and months following injury, and are also more successful in younger patients.[34] Positive pressure ventilation has been shown to lead to deterioration of the diaphragm after only 18 hours,[35] with the potential for rehabilitation of this muscle not yet quantified. Long-term ventilation can lead to degeneration of both the nerve and muscle such that pacing may not be possible, with a timeframe of 18–24 months being identified as a period at which there will be a substantially reduced success rate (Fig. 16.1).[35]

After insertion of a pacing device, a period of rehabilitation of the diaphragm muscle is required. Initial periods of training may be as brief as 5 minutes occurring hourly, and can even be performed with the patient still on mechanical ventilation to maintain adequate ventilation. Achieving a goal of 4 hours off invasive ventilation can take from 2 weeks to many months.[32]

Glossopharyngeal breathing

Glossopharyngeal breathing (GPB), also referred to as 'frog-breathing', is a technique which involves using the mouth and tongue to piston air into the lungs to either augment a small lung volume or replace the activity of paralysed inspiratory muscles. The technique was first described in the literature in 1951 when patients with poliomyelitis who were using negative pressure ventilators (iron lungs) that did not require a tracheostomy were noted to be gulping air when out of the ventilator.[36] GPB has been shown to improve pulmonary function and chest expansion in a group of individuals with CSCI after an 8-week training period.[37] In order to perform the technique, oropharyngeal musculature needs to be intact and in the presence of a tracheostomy, use of a valve or cap is required to prevent the pistoned air from escaping through the tracheostomy tube. The technique can be learned by watching videos (see Online resources at end of chapter), having face-to-face coaching with a person skilled in the technique and by studying diagrams explaining the technique.

By using a gulping motion it is possible to push air into the lower airway, and multiple gulps can deliver total volumes of up to 1–2 litres into the lungs prior to exhalation. Novices performing the technique will need to exaggerate the movement, but with practice GPB can be performed in a way that is barely noticeable to the observer. Individuals with some inspiratory capacity can use GPB to augment voice volume or cough strength. For those with no inspiratory capacity, GPB can be used to permit brief periods of separation from the ventilator to facilitate transfers or enable circuit changes. It should be noted that GPB does not improve safety in the case of accidental ventilator disconnection in a person with a tracheostomy as the pistoned air will escape via the tracheostomy tube. GPB is a difficult concept to grasp and some individuals will be unable to perform the manoeuvre despite instruction.

Neck accessory muscle breathing

Neck accessory muscle breathing (NAMB) uses muscles, such as the scalenes and sternocleidomastoid, to act as respiratory muscles. In contrast to GPB, NAMB is easier to learn and is able to be used to ventilate independently in case of accidental disconnection from the ventilator. The success of the technique is related to the preservation of neck accessory muscles (Fig. 16.2).[38]

Larger and heavier individuals[38] may experience less success with NAMB, as they need a higher tidal volume to breathe comfortably off the ventilator. This is presumably related to the fact that these patients have higher minute volume requirements

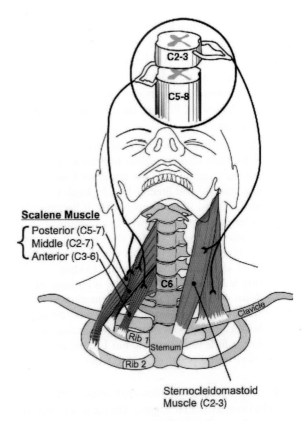

Figure 16.2 Muscles innervated for patients with high CSCI for use in neck accessory muscle breathing (NAMB).
Source: © 2002 American Physical Therapy Association

and a larger dead space through which inspired air must pass before reaching the areas of the lungs where gas exchange can occur.

Training in the use of NAMB consists of short periods of ventilator-free time under close supervision to ensure that oxygen saturations do not fall below a safe level (generally set at 92%), and that sufficient accessory muscle activity is present to enable drawing of air into the lungs via generation of upper and anterior chest wall movement. Tidal volumes should be monitored during training to provide an objective measure of progress and to contribute to the assessment of whether adequate ventilation is occurring.

Use of biofeedback during the ventilator-free training sessions may be employed to improve muscle activation. Strengthening of the accessory muscles can be achieved while on the ventilator by providing manual resistance to the neck muscles during neck forward flexion, lateral flexion, rotation and extension.[38]

> One does not know how hard breathing actually is until one loses the ability to breathe. To practise weaning from the ventilator I am disconnected and literally breathe hard; I meditate and listen to my breath. It became easier each time and slowly, I can breathe 2 minutes by myself, then 4, then 7, then 11, then 15, now 20 minutes. In between, when I feel like I am running out of breath, I engage frog-breathing – frog-breathing is pushing air down the windpipe in a similar motion to swallowing. This helps me regain some air in between NAMB breathing. It was strange at first, a little bit unnatural, but I found it effective and practice helps. (Daisy)

During weaning sessions, individuals can receive breaths from a manual bagging circuit when they are short of breath instead of being reconnected to the ventilator circuit, which takes a little longer. Some practitioners use a mouthpiece on the ventilator to allow the person performing the weaning to lean across and access resting breaths from the mouthpiece more autonomously. See Online resources for an online video guide to the technique.[39]

In order to set up a ventilator to deliver on demand breaths, assist volume control mode is used to allow for breaths to be triggered intermittently without the ventilator alarming during breaks.[40]

POSTURAL CONSIDERATIONS IN HIGH CSCI

All patients with paralysis resulting from cervical spine injuries will face postural challenges. As this is an upper motor neuron lesion, spasticity will have an effect and at times this can be severe (see Chapters 1 and 4). Maintaining symmetrical posture with good alignment in the sagittal and coronal planes will improve balance and function, including the ability to drive and use assistive technology. As with all seated clients, good posture begins at the pelvis and is supported by adequate control of the torso and finally shoulders, head and neck. For the purposes of this chapter, the focus will be on the upper body. (For more information on posture and seating related to function please see Chapters 8, Modes of transport, Part 1.)

Simple positioning measures as part of the daily routine can be helpful. A designated period of time during the day for lying supine flat without a pillow can help to maintain thoracic extension and good neck posture. Where there is sufficient activity in the neck musculature, chin tucking and rotation exercises can also be performed during the period of supine flat positioning.

As flexibility of the thoracic spine allows, a rolled towel can be placed behind the back in line with the spine to increase the amount of extension achieved. In the presence of a fixed kyphosis this may not be appropriate as excessive pressure will be put on the neck and adjustments should be made to avoid this. In very high cervical lesions, shoulder range need only be sufficient to allow for ease of dressing and hygiene and trying to achieve larger ranges of motion of shoulders not supported by active musculature can result in unnecessary discomfort.

Many patients will experience asymmetrical neck tone after a CSCI and require assistance to maintain a symmetrical head position in bed. Pillows and towels can be helpful, but sometimes are not sufficiently firm to achieve lasting effects. Sandbags can be hard and difficult to tolerate, while bags filled with other grains such as wheat or even salt are more comfortable and still provide firm support for positioning.

The surgical technique of occipital fixation, where the base of the skull is secured via a plate and screws to the cervical spine, can give rise to positioning challenges. This procedure is performed in response to congenital, traumatic, neoplastic, infective or inflammatory pathologies which compromise the stability of the cranio-vertebral junction. After this procedure it is not possible to move the head with respect to the neck and the position the surgeon has achieved intraoperatively will be the permanent position of the head and neck. In this instance, compensation for malalignment with seating and positioning can protect against the development of further deformity of the trunk over time. Excessive flexion of the neck can be compensated for by using a combination of tilt and recline in the wheelchair to allow the patient to look forwards without straining their eyes, but this will come at the cost of impaired pressure distribution at the pelvis. Occipital fixation will also limit driving and environmental control options for patients. Head movement can be used to trigger controllers in the headrest and to access controllers in front of the face. An immobile head

will limit the user to controllers that are sensitive to facial, voice and breath control (Fig. 16.3).

Types of switches/controllers suitable for use with high CSCI

Mini-joy controllers: as the name suggests, these are smaller versions of the familiar joystick controller. They sit in front of the patient's chin or lower lip and can be set so they are sensitive to pressure as well as movement (Fig. 16.4).

Headrest sensors: these are pressure sensors located in the headrest that respond to pressure from the head to, for example, drive or tilt the chair.

Sip and puff controllers: this is a flexible straw attachment, which sits in the side of

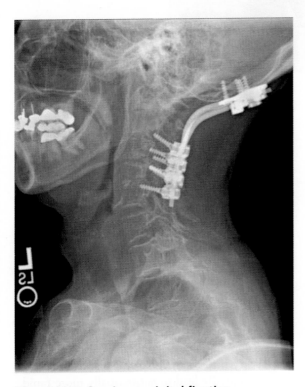

Figure 16.3 Cervico-occipital fixation.
Source: Image courtesy of Kee D Kim MC and SpineUniverse.com. https://www.spineuniverse.com/professional/case-studies/kim/basilar-invagination

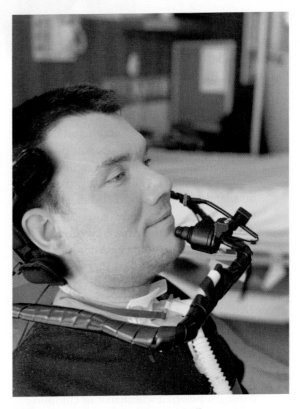

Figure 16.4 Mini joystick controller.

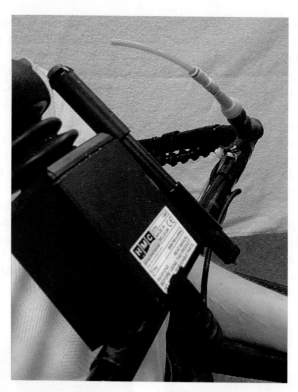

Figure 16.5 Sip and puff controller.

the mouth. These controllers are sensitive to pressure changes in the mouth and can be adjusted to soft sip, hard sip, soft puff and hard puff, to execute four different commands. Perhaps surprisingly, patients on mandatory ventilation and diaphragm pacing can use these quite successfully. A downside is that the straw and tubing require regular cleaning and can block if not well maintained (Fig. 16.5).

Tongue drive systems (TDS): this system operates by placing a magnetic tracer device embedded in a barbell or adhesive device on the tongue, which communicates with sensors located near the cheeks mounted on a headset that communicates wirelessly to a mobile device or computer. It can be used to control a powered wheelchair or computer with a high degree of accuracy. The tongue is capable of moving quickly and accurately and is not particularly susceptible to fatigue. The TDS has been shown to be faster and more accurate after five training sessions in a group of tetraplegic users in comparison to the sip and puff system.[41] Downsides for some users may be the headgear, which is quite obvious and the requirement for tongue piercing.

Voice control: voice control is now widely used for home, vehicle and mobile phone controls. The cost of voice-controlled systems has decreased dramatically as this technology has become more available. Its entry into the mainstream market will potentially lead to substantially more rapid improvements in its utility and application. Its application as a power chair control is limited mainly by the problem of interference from ambient noise, making it unsuitable for community use or even shared home environment use.

QUALITY OF LIFE

Studies evaluating people's perception of their quality of life (QoL) following an SCI are readily available, but there is a scarcity of recent work on QoL for ventilator users following SCI. In her 2011 review, Charlifue[42] hypothesised that adjustment to injury over time may be slower in the group of people with an SCI who require ventilation and that this would explain the difference in QoL scores at one year post-injury compared to the quite consistent findings many years later of improved QoL among the ventilation user (VU) group as compared to the non-ventilation user (NVU) group.

Healthcare workers have been found to have markedly negative perceptions of the potential for a good QoL when living with a ventilator and to overestimate the level of emotional distress experienced by people who live in this situation. When emergency care providers were asked if they would be 'glad to live' with a severe SCI, only 18% responded that they would. When people with an SCI in the same study were asked this question 92% responded in the affirmative.[43] Charlifue notes that this dichotomy of opinion is concerning as it may influence the willingness of healthcare providers to provide life-saving treatment to people with high CSCI.[42]

Gerard is married with two young adult sons. He sustained his injury 3 years ago, and when asked what matters to him as a person with a high CSCI, he responded:

> Family has always been important to me, but its importance has now taken a sharper focus. Remaining in contact with friends and having frequent visitors matters a lot. I am particularly lucky because I have my own wheelchair accessible van. I get to see my son play basketball, go to the cinema and live shows. Most days we get out to a cafe or shopping; I never feel like I

am isolated. It is also critically important that I feel that I still have something to offer, that I have a purpose in life. I retain that strong belief.

Daisy sustained her injury 1 year ago. In her words:

> I definitely believe I have changed as a person mentally, emotionally, physically and spiritually from before my injury. Before my injury, I was a confident, adventurous daredevil and thrill seeker, I felt indestructible in the world and I definitely acted that way. I could be described as impatient, a fast learner, bubbly and a daredevil. After my injury, I learnt how to meditate, how to accept the quietness, how to be patient, how to accept the situation as is. I started to search for happiness from the inside and because of that, the meaning of life is much simpler. The thing I have learned most from this setback is how strong I am, and how miraculous the human mind and willpower is.

SAFETY CONSIDERATIONS

Awareness among healthcare providers and members of the community of risk management and the promotion of safety in healthcare settings has increased over recent years. Quality improvement initiatives, mortality audits and root cause analyses of adverse events are routinely practised in hospitals. Patients requiring ventilation via tracheostomy are one of the highest risk groups in healthcare and require special attention.[44] Disconnection from ventilation is perhaps the most acute risk and various strategies can be used to minimise the possibility of this event.

As previously mentioned, appropriate choice of TT will ensure the best and most secure individual fit.[12,13] In addition to this, correct tension of the TT tapes, where 1–2 fingers can be inserted inside the tapes, will keep the airway safely in place. Adopting a policy of having two people perform stoma cleaning and tracheostomy dressing/tape changes will ensure that whenever TT tapes are undone one person will be holding the TT to prevent dislodgement. Additional securing devices are available, which have

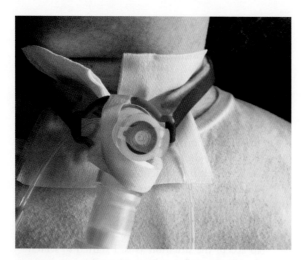

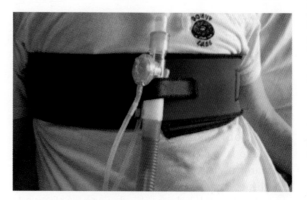

Figure 16.7 Chest strap for securing ventilation tubing.

Figure 16.6 Ventilator connection securing device.

small Velcro loops to hold the ventilator connection onto the TT hub and prevent disconnection. A similar level of security can be achieved by using additional tracheal tapes to tie the connector onto the hub (Fig. 16.6).

A strap around the chest, which can be used to hold the ventilator tubing in the midline, fulfils two purposes. The midline position of the tubing promotes a good position of the TT and prevents movement that can promote the formation of undesirable granulation tissue at the stoma. A chest strap also provides an extra level of security during turns and other transfers helping to prevent disconnection of the ventilator tubing. Leaving ventilator tubing hanging free puts a moderate amount of force on the stoma and upper trachea and, as the ventilator is almost always positioned on the same side of the bed or wheelchair, can lead to asymmetrical distortion of the tracheostoma and airway (Fig. 16.7).

Emergency procedures

During their initial hospital admission post-injury, patients on long-term ventilation will be discharged from the ICU, where invasive ventilation is a relatively routine procedure, to a non-critical care

environment. Lower staffing levels and reduced familiarity among staff with invasive ventilation requires a high degree of planning. Staff training, set-up of the necessary equipment, alarm systems and preparation of the patient and family for the move are central elements. Consideration may be given to increasing the staffing profile of the step-down unit for the first few shifts in order to accommodate a period of adjustment. Similarly, strategies for an emergency response need to be reviewed if a patient is moving to another campus or different hospital. Most hospitals have a medical emergency team (MET) response or Code Blue (cardiac or respiratory arrest) response procedure. In centres that have multiple types of emergency response teams, it is important to establish that if a call is made for an invasively ventilated patient, a team with appropriate airway management skills will respond to this call.

As well as planning for suitable emergency assistance responses, healthcare providers working directly with a VU patient need to feel confident that they can respond to an emergency. Clear emergency response procedures need to be part of the training for all staff before they are left alone on shift. Posters with flow chart instructions can be provided to staff and mounted on the wall behind the bed to assist (Figs 16.8 and 16.9). Management of invasively ventilated patients in ICU and ward settings is associated with a high level of adverse events, with

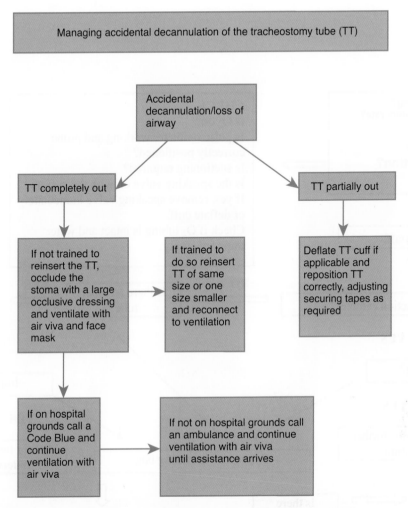

Figure 16.8 **Flow chart for emergency response to accidental decannulation.**
Source: Adapted from Victorian Spinal Cord Service Document with permission.

a recent report identifying 19% of these resulted in residual disability or death. The authors identified what they described as human factor issues to be the most common cause of adverse events, followed by knowledge-based errors.[44]

A 'Go bag' of mandatory safety equipment for invasively ventilated patients can be put together and kept with them at all times. The 'Go bag' should be portable, so that it accompanies the patient at all times inside or outside the hospital with all necessary equipment close at hand (Box 16.1).

Alarm systems

Alarm systems need to be audible from a distance as soon as a patient moves from the ICU to a ward or rehabilitation setting. In the ICU, one-to-one nursing ratios allow for alarms to be audible at a relatively close distance, but on wards where staffing ratios are less, alarms need to be heard throughout the whole work area. This can generally be achieved by connecting the ventilator's alarm system into the wider emergency alarm system of the unit. This can be disruptive for other patients, but the consequences

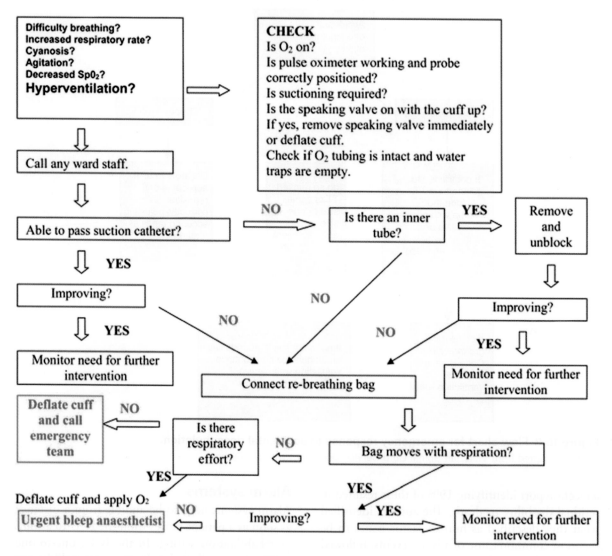

Figure 16.9 Example of emergency protocol flow diagram
Source: S. McGown, K Hunt 2015 Tracheostomy management BJA Education 15(3):149–153.

Box 16.1 Equipment required for outings

Equipment required for mobilising around the centre, e.g. going to the cafe or therapy

- Spare ventilator (internal battery fully charged) or diaphragm pacing unit
- Mobile phone (battery fully charged)
- Air Viva, swivel connector for tracheostomy and face mask
- Portable suction unit (fully charged)
- Medications as necessary
- 'Go Bag' of tracheostomy emergency equipment:
  - Suction catheters
  - Clean gloves
  - Spare tracheostomy tube of same size and another one size smaller
  - 10 mL syringe for cuff inflation/deflation
  - Piece of combine (in case of accidental tracheostomy dislodgement)
  - Tracheal dilators (in patients with new tracheostomas < 3 months)
  - Spare tracheostomy tapes/Velcro ties
  - Protective eyewear (for carer/staff member)

Box 16.2 Basic guide to troubleshooting ventilator alarms

High-pressure alarm, potential causes

- Sputum plug/secretion retention
- Malpositioned TT
- Bronchospasm
- Kinked/obstructed ventilator tubing
- Malfunction of exhalation valve

Low pressure alarm, potential causes

- Disconnection from the ventilator
- TT cuff leak
- Leak in the ventilator cicuit
- Drowsiness and consequent inability to control upper airway leak in the presence of a cuffless TT or cuffed TT with deflated cuff to allow for leak speech

High frequency alarm

- Sputum plug
- Tachypnoea secondary to hypoxia/anxiety/fever
- Condensation in the ventilator circuit

of missing an alarm can be life-threatening. Adapted call bell systems need to be sourced, so that patients with limited movement can trigger them easily. Tongue or lip trigger buzzers can be used or pressure sensitive buzzers placed next to the head. The ability to reliably call for assistance overnight is reported by patients as one of their primary safety concerns in a ward setting.

Troubleshooting ventilation

Ventilator malfunction or persistent alarming of the ventilator can be stressful for staff and patients. Having clear guidelines for troubleshooting can substantially decrease this stress. The adult manual resuscitation device can be used as a quick, reliable and almost fail-safe strategy for any situation where the stability of ventilation is in doubt. Transferring the patient from an alarming ventilator that may not be delivering sufficient ventilation to a manual bagging circuit helps gain control of a situation and allow for a 'time-out' period to calmly evaluate what the problem might be. If the problem with the ventilator cannot be identified and rectified, changing to the back-up ventilator should then be tried (Box 16.2).

LONG-TERM RESPIRATORY HEALTH

Although the risk of death from CSCI has decreased over the last 50 years, it appears that the long-term survival of those who require ventilation is still markedly decreased. Schavelle found the risk of death in VU people with an SCI to be 3.6 times that of NVU people with an SCI after the first year post-injury.[4] Of those deaths, 31% could be attributed to pneumonia and other respiratory problems, with the second most common cause being cardiac problems, at 15%. Maintaining good respiratory health over a lifetime is therefore paramount. There is moderate evidence to suggest that an intensive program of regularly applied treatments consisting of volume restoration and secretion clearance is associated with better respiratory outcomes in the first 6 weeks following injury.[18] The evidence surrounding long-term management of respiratory health is less clear and so we are reliant on extrapolation of the early evidence and consensus expert opinion.

Some patients requiring long-term ventilation will progress from acute care to rehabilitation and not require any active respiratory physiotherapy treatments. This group will generally have a low level of sputum production, no supplemental oxygen requirements and a stable level of peak inspiratory pressure, indicating consistent lung compliance. It is a decision for the VU person and their clinicians whether or not to institute a program of prophylactic respiratory care. Others, however, will continue to produce large amounts of sputum either daily or inconsistently, with intermittent episodes of lung consolidation and/or collapse. For these patients, there is anecdotal evidence that ongoing maintenance treatments improve their respiratory stability and decrease hospital re-admissions.

A program of treatment that can be incorporated into the daily routine will help compliance and present a lower burden of care. Reducing the complexity and time required to deliver treatment is important. Care hours present a substantial financial cost to patients and funding agencies, particularly

when viewed over a lifetime, and minimising these is of clear benefit. Utilising ventilator hyperinflation as a mode of treatment can also reduce costs, as it decreases the need for additional equipment purchase. Carers in the home can safely deliver ventilator hyperinflation if sufficient training is in place and good systems exist. Setting up a second or third program on the ventilator with hyperinflation settings allows for easy switching to the treatment program. Maintaining a similar minute volume during periods of ventilator hyperinflation decreases the risk of hyperventilation and resultant reductions in CO_2.

The American Congress of Rehabilitation Medicine has a useful education page on maintenance of respiratory health for people with an SCI which includes advice on use of a cough assist machine (mechanical in/exsufflation), manually assisted coughing, getting annual flu and pneumonia shots, maintenance of a healthy weight and avoidance of smoking, second-hand smoke and staying away from people with colds or flu (Figs 16.10 and 16.11) (see Online resources).[45]

Using postural drainage positions, including a head-down tip if tolerated, can augment secretion clearance.[28] Optimally, the use of mechanical exsufflation should be included in a treatment regimen for high CSCI patients as this has been shown to augment secretion clearance and is almost universally preferred to deep suctioning by patients.[28,46,47] Exsufflation units unfortunately remain a substantial expense for individuals living in the community. If a funding body is available it can be argued that the potential benefit of an exsufflator used routinely will pay for itself if it prevents even one hospital stay.

Manually assisted coughing techniques are well described in the literature,[48] and have been shown to improve the effectiveness of secretion clearance, particularly when combined with mechanical in/exsufflation.[46] This technique can be performed by most carers and family members, but not all as it requires some physical exertion (for more detail see Chapter 4).

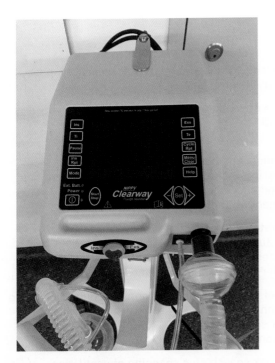

Figure 16.10 Nippy® Clearway

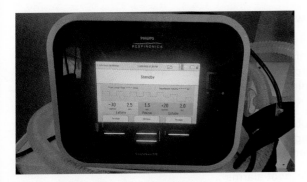

Figure 16.11 E70 Cough Assist.

TRANSITIONING TO LIFE IN THE COMMUNITY FROM HOSPITAL

Living at home with a mechanical ventilator has been demonstrated to improve quality of life and community access,[47] as well as being more cost effective in comparison to living in a hospital.[49]

Moving out of hospital or a rehabilitation centre to home is a time of celebration, but also uncertainty and enormous change. Challenges to providing mechanical ventilation in the home include carer training and retention, adequacy of respiratory care and funding.[50]

Training

Training of caregivers is a central part of a successful discharge strategy. The initial step of recruiting a care team is followed by the implementation of an intensive education plan. This plan ideally includes formal teaching sessions with audiovisual materials, written material and online education such as e-learning modules. Carers also need an opportunity to engage in care and get hands-on practice of how to use equipment, including mastering the skills of suctioning and other tasks such as ventilator troubleshooting and ventilator circuit changes (Table 16.2).

Instructions for emergency management need to be in place, including actions to be taken in case of ventilator failure, accidental decannulation, as well as episodes of autonomic dysreflexia (see Chapter 4). Trial day leave followed by overnight leave prior to discharge is strongly recommended. Graduated independent leave provides families, patients and carers with confidence and invaluable experience. Home equipment trials can be undertaken and the home environment tested out prior to a definitive discharge.

People with a CSCI who are ventilator dependent with no ventilator-free time are not able to safely spend time alone in case of accidental disconnection or ventilation failure. Ensuring the availability of skilled back-up 24 hours a day is an important consideration for those who are fully reliant on ventilation in the community.

Gerard spent 12 months in hospital after his injury. This extended length of stay was mainly due to the difficulty he and his healthcare team experienced finding a suitable discharge destination. Asked if he had any insights to share about this, he reflected:

> In those early months I learnt a lot that I would never have learnt had I been discharged earlier.

Table 16.2 Day leave skills checklist for carers/family

Knowledge	Skills demonstrated
SCI and respiratory function	• Able to discuss knowledge of respiratory muscle weakness, poor cough and vulnerability to infections
Why is ventilation necessary? How does ventilation work?	• Able to discuss basics of ventilation via tracheostomy and why it is required for high CSCI
Tracheostomy type, cuff management, dressing and tapes	• Removal of inner cannula and cleaning of same • Perform tracheal dressing, including changing of tapes/velcro ties • Inflate/deflate cuff and check pressure • Check correct alignment of trachea
Humidification	• Use of humidifier (heated, humidified) • Use of heat and moisture exchanger (HME) • Demonstrate use of nebuliser in line with ventilation circuit • Discuss signs of under-humidification and measures to rectify
Suctioning of tracheostomy	• Demonstrate set-up of equipment and perform suctioning, including use of portable suction unit • Explain indicators for suctioning • Identify risks of suctioning
Speaking on ventilation	• Deflation of cuff for leak speech plus changing of ventilation program if applicable • Placement of one-way speaking valve in line with ventilator if applicable • Placement of one-way speaking valve for use with diaphragm pacing if applicable
Ventilator circuit	• Identify elements of the ventilator circuit and identify purpose • Assemble clean circuit and attach to ventilator • Demonstrate cleaning of reusable parts
Ventilator controls	• Turn on/off • Record ventilator observations/settings check • Check alarm settings • Identify power sources and battery charge
Ventilator alarms	• Identify and troubleshoot alarms • Demonstrate attachment to wall alarm system
Diaphragm pacer	• Change from ventilator to pacer • Place speaking valve
Emergency management	• Use of air viva via tracheostomy and via facemask • Change to back-up vent • Knowledge of emergency procedures as per local protocol • Management of accidental decannulation of tracheostomy

Not only did these professionals give me extensive knowledge about my injuries and how to live and prosper with them, they instilled a sense of confidence and hope in me that has proved invaluable. I was extremely fortunate to have access to highly professional and accredited medical staff in my extended stay in hospital. Even so, I have learnt a lot more since then.

I have thought for some time that it would be extremely useful for people with spinal cord injuries leaving hospital, and their carers, to have a manual they could refer to. This manual would be full of practical tips, resources and information that ensure a smooth transition from hospital to community living.

This feedback points to the importance of providing resources to patients for discharge. Written materials and online resources consisting of videos and e-learning programs can support theory and practical teaching sessions in the hospital. Therapists receive consistent feedback from care staff that they value hands-on training extremely highly. Training patients in their own care and empowering them to direct their care are also vital components of a sustainable discharge.

Equipment

Provision of equipment, including a primary and back-up ventilator, humidifier, primary and back-up suction unit and consumables, needs planning. Ongoing maintenance and repair of ventilators, suction units and humidifiers may be outsourced to a ventilation company.[49] Purchasing of consumables needs to be set up in a sustainable way with systems for regular ordering put in place.

Support

Ongoing support for VU persons at home should include a strong relationship with a general practitioner, who is supported by an expert spinal team at the referring centre. A support system that includes access to telephone advice or teleconferencing, outpatient appointments and, where possible, home visits should be established.

A plan for changing the TT every 8 weeks, or as per local practice, should be scheduled. If the stoma is well formed and the airway is easily exchanged, a trained care provider can perform tube changes in the community; however, difficult airways will need a more supportive plan with appropriate risk management.[50]

The cost of living in the community with invasive ventilation will depend on many factors, but the main expense is always provision of care hours. Working on the premise that 24-hour care will be required, including parts of the day where two carers are needed to perform tasks such as transfers, in-home care can add up to around 27 hours per day. Twenty-seven hours per day × 356 days = 9855 hours of care annually. At a cost of $60 AUD per hour for specialised care provision through an agency, this leads to an annual cost of $590,000. Financial support is provided by the state in countries with universal healthcare systems, but this support is often less than adequate for ventilator users and their carers.[47,51]

In Australia, those aged 65 or younger when they first sustain their SCI are eligible for support through the National Disability Insurance Scheme (NDIS). At the time of writing, this scheme was still rolling out and entitlements may change over time, but the philosophy of the NDIS is to provide clients with sufficient support to maintain a life where independence and quality of life are maximised. There is a strong commitment to assist clients to live in the community where possible and, in partnership with healthcare providers, NDIS will provide funding for carers to assist in the home, as well as support for community access, return to work, study and leisure pursuits. Provision of healthcare services, such as ventilation equipment and consumables, is considered the domain of the healthcare system and is sourced separately. Unfortunately those aged over 65 at the time of injury are not able to access NDIS funding and are supported by the aged care sector, where funding is less available, resulting in most clients in this situation being unable to afford in-home care (Fig. 16.12).

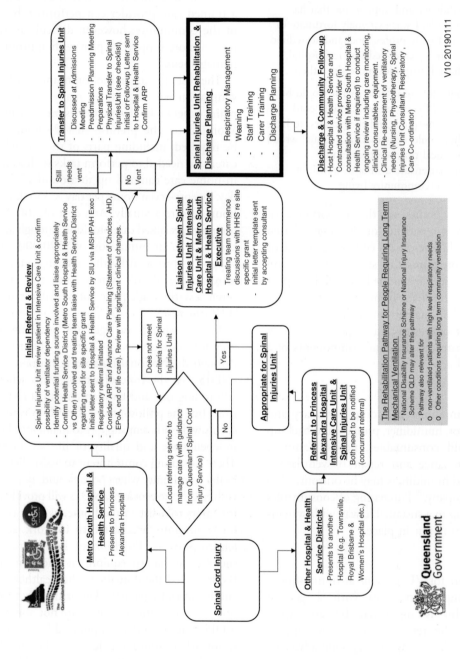

Figure 16.12 Example of a ventilator-dependent patient's journey

Source: Queensland Spinal Cord Injuries Service

Evidence-based practice points

- Facilitation of ventilator-associated speech can commence early following SCI with suitable monitoring.[11,22,23]
- After the first year post-injury VU people with an SCI report an equivalent or better QoL than their NVU SCI peers.[42] Healthcare workers have a significantly poorer perception of QoL on a ventilator to VU individuals.[43]
- Maintenance of respiratory health is important in improving survival post-CSCI.[1,3,22,28]
- Expert assessment and ongoing monitoring post CSCI is important to maximise potential for weaning from ventilation.[26,27,31,34]
- Ventilation and tracheostomy are high risk interventions in the hospital and community settings.[14,16,43,52]

SUMMARY

An injury resulting in ventilator-dependent tetraplegia is rare and carries with it an increased mortality risk that extends well beyond the first year post-injury. Maintenance of good respiratory health can contribute substantially to survival. Ventilator-associated speech is pivotal for QoL and can safely be facilitated early after injury. Healthcare workers need to be aware of the gap between their perception of life on a ventilator and the lived experience of those who are forced to do so. Tracheostomy and ventilation are associated with a high level of risk and adverse events, both in hospital and in the community, and the implementation of education, support systems and suitable care and equipment are all factors that can improve safety. Technology continues to offer improvements for ventilation, including diaphragm pacing, phrenic nerve grafting and improved controls for mobility and independence. Finally, the reduced costs of living in the community in comparison to hospital, as well as the improved QoL and community participation enjoyed by those who do, should encourage government and funding agencies to support people with an SCI and ventilation requirements to leave hospital as soon as they are safely able.

Online resources

Archives of Physical Medicine and Rehabilitation. Respiratory health and spinal cord injury. Online 10 December 2019. Available: www.archives-pmr.org/article/S0003-9993 (16)00012-5/pdf.

CANVent Ottowa. Glossopharyngeal breathing teaching session with Greg, https://www.youtube.com/watch?v=0ZgfZ01uLDQ.

References

1. World Health Organization. Disability and rehabilitation: International perspectives on spinal cord injury. Online 10 December 2019. Available: www.who.int/disabilities/policies/spinal_cord_injury/report/en.

2. Onders, R., Elmo, M., et al., 2009. Complete worldwide operative experience in laparoscopic diaphragm pacing: results and differences in spinal cord injured patients and amyotrophic lateral sclerosis patients. Surg. Endosc. 23, 1433–1440.

3. Tovell, A., 2018. Spinal cord injury, Australia 2014–15: Injury research and statistics series, no. 113, Cat. No. INJCAT 193. Canberra: AIHW.

4. Shavelle, R.M., DeVivo, M.J., et al., 2006. Long-term survival of persons ventilator dependent after spinal cord injury. J. Spinal Cord Med. 29, 511–519.

5. American Spinal Injury Association. International Standards for Neurological Classification of SCI Worksheet. Online 10 December 2019. Available: https://asia-spinalinjury.org/international-standards-neurological-classification-sci-isncsci-worksheet/.

6. Chen, Y., Tang, Y., et al., 2013. Causes of spinal cord injury. Top. Spinal Cord Inj. Rehabil. 19, 1–8.

7. Behnegar, A., Ragnarsson, K., 2010. Non-traumatic spinal cord injury. In: Bryce, T.N. (Ed.), Spinal Cord Injury: Rehabilitation Medicine Quick Reference. Demos Medical, New York.

8. Richard-Denis, A., Feldman, D., et al., 2018. The impact of a specialized spinal cord injury centre as compared with non-specialized centers on the acute respiratory management of patients with complete tetraplegia: an observational study. Spinal Cord 56, 142–150.

9. Jones, T.S., Burlew, C.C., et al., 2015. Predictors of the necessity for early tracheostomy in patients with acute cervical spinal cord injury: a 15-year experience. Am. J. Surg. 209 (2), 363–368.

10. Hou, Y.F., Lv, Y., et al., 2015. Development and validation of a risk prediction model for tracheostomy in acute traumatic cervical spinal cord injury patients. Eur. Spine J. 24, 975–984.

11. Hoit, J.D., Banzett, R.B., et al., 2003. Clinical ventilator adjustments that improve speech. Chest 124 (4), 1512–1521.

12. NCEPOD, 2014. On the right trach? A review of the care received by patients. Summary. Online 10 December 2019. Available: www.ncepod.org.uk/2014report1/downloads/OnTheRightTrach_Summary.pdf.

13. Schmidt, U., Hess, D., et al., 2008. Tracheostomy tube malposition in patients admitted to a respiratory acute care unit following prolonged ventilation. Chest 134, 288–294.

14. Cameron, T., McKinstry, A., et al., 2009. Outcomes for spinal patients before and after a tracheostomy team. Crit. Care Resusc. 11 (1), 14–19.

15. McGrath, B.A., Bates, L., et al., 2012. Multidisciplinary guidelines for the management of tracheostomy and laryngectomy airway emergencies. Anaesthesia 67 (9), 1025–1041.

16. Cowan, T., Op't Holt, T.B., et al., 2001. Effect of inner cannula removal on the work of breathing imposed by tracheostomy tubes: a bench study. Respir. Care 46, 460–465.

17. Krassioukov, A., 2009. Autonomic function following a cervical spinal cord injury. Respir. Physiol. Neurobiol. 169, 157–164.

18. Berney, S., Bragge, P., et al., 2010. The acute respiratory management of cervical spine cord injury in the first 6 weeks after injury: a systematic review. Spinal Cord 49 (1), 17–29.

19. Grigorean, V., Sandu, A., et al., 2009. Cardiac dysfunctions following spinal cord injury. J. Med. Life 2, 133–145.

20. SCIRE Professional. Interventions for cardiovascular complications during acute SCI. Online 10 December 2019. Available: https://scireproject.com/evidence/acute-evidence/cardiovascular-complications-during-acute-phase-of-spinal-cord-injury/interventions-cardiovascular-complications-during-acute-sci/.

21. Reznik, J.E., Morris, J.H., et al. (Eds.), 2016. Pharmacology for Physiotherapists. Elsevier.

22. Brown, R., DiMarco, A., et al., 2006. Respiratory dysfunction and management in spinal cord injury. Respir. Care 51 (8), 853–870.

23. Hoit, J.D., Banzett, R.B., et al., 2003. Clinical ventilator adjustments that improve speech. Chest 124, 1512–1521.

24. Main, E., Denehy, L. (Eds.), 2016. Cardiorespiratory Physiotherapy: Adults and Paediatrics, fifth ed. Elsevier.

25. Panharipande, P.P., Girard, T.D., et al., 2013. Long-term cognitive impairment after critical illness. N. Engl. J. Med. 369 (14), 1306–1316.

26. Chiodo, A.E., Scelza, W., et al., 2008. Predictors of ventilator weaning in individuals with high cervical spinal cord injury. J. Spinal Cord Med. 31, 72–77.

27. Oo, T., Watt, J.M., et al., 1999. Delayed diaphragm recovery in 12 patients after high cervical spinal cord injury. A retrospective review of the diaphragm status of 107 patients ventilated after acute spinal cord injury. Spinal Cord 37, 117–122.

28. Galeiras Vázquez, R., Rascado Sedes, P., et al., 2013. Respiratory management in the patient with spinal cord injury. Biomed Res. Int. 168757.

29. Wong, S.L., Shem, K., et al., 2012. Specialised respiratory management for acute cervical spinal cord injury: a retrospective analysis. Top. Spinal Cord Inj. Rehabil. 18, 283–290.

30. Berlly, M., Shem, K., 2007. Respiratory management during the first five days after spinal cord injury. J. Spinal Cord Med. 30, 309–318.

31. Gundogdu, I., Ozturk, E.A., et al., 2017. Implementation of a respiratory rehabilitation protocol: weaning from the ventilator and tracheostomy in difficult-to-wean patients with spinal cord injury. Disabil. Rehabil. 39, 1162–1170.

32. Di Marco, A.F., 2018. Diaphragm pacing. Clin. Chest Med. 39, 459–471.

33. Kaufman, M., Bauer, T., et al., 2017. Phrenic nerve reconstruction for diaphragmatic paralysis and ventilator dependency. In: Elkwood, A.I., Kauffman, M., et al. (Eds.), Rehabilitative Surgery. Springer, Switzerland.

34. Jarosz, R., Littlepage, M., et al., 2012. Functional electrical stimulation in spinal cord injury Respiratory Care. Top. Spinal Cord Inj. Rehabil. 18 (4), 315–321.

35. Levine, S., Nguyen, T., et al., 2008. Rapid disuse atrophy of diaphragm fibres in mechanically ventilated humans. N. Engl. J. Med. 358, 1327–1335.

36. Dail, C.W., Affeldt, J.E., et al., 1955. Clinical aspects of glossopharyngeal breathing: report of use by one hundred postpoliomyelitic patients. J. Am. Med. Assoc. 158, 445–449.

37. Nygren-Bonnier, M., Wahman, K., et al., 2009. Glossopharyngeal pistoning for lung insufflation in patients with cervical spinal cord injury. Spinal Cord 47, 418–422.

38. Warren, V., 2002. Glossopharyngeal and neck accessory muscle breathing in a young adult with C2 complete tetraplegia resulting in ventilator dependency. Phys. Ther. 82 (6), 590–600.

39. Glossopharyngeal breathing teaching session with Greg. YouTube. 2017. www.youtube.com/watch?v=0ZgfZ01u LDQ.

40. Khirani, S., Ramirez, A., et al., 2014. Evaluation of ventilators for mouthpiece ventilation in neuromuscular disease. Respir. Care 59 (9), 1329–1337.

41. Kim, J., Park, H., et al., 2013. The tongue enables computer and wheelchair control for people with spinal cord injury. Sci. Transl. Med. 5 (213), 213ra166.

42. Charlifue, S., Apple, D., et al., 2011. Mechanical ventilation, health, and quality of life following spinal cord injury. Arch. Phys. Med. Rehabil. 92 (3), 457–463.

43. Gerhart, K.A., Koziol-McLain, J., et al., 1994. Quality of life following spinal cord injury: knowledge and attitudes of emergency care providers. Ann. Emerg. Med. 23, 807–812.

44. Kamio, T., Masume, K., 2018. Mechanical ventilation – Safety incidents in general care wards and ICU settings. Respir. Care 63, 1246–1252.

45. Archives of Physical Medicine and Rehabilitation. Respiratory health and spinal cord injury. Online 10 December 2019. Available: www.archives-pmr.org/article/S0003-9993(16)00012-5/pdf.

46. Bach, J.R., 1993. Mechanical insufflation-exsufflation: comparison of peak expiratory flows with manually assisted and unassisted coughing techniques. Chest 104, 1553–1562.

47. Marchese, S., Coco, D., et al., 2008. Outcomes and attitudes toward home tracheostomy ventilation of consecutive patients: a 10 yr experience. Respir. Med. 102, 430–436.

48. Frownfelter, D., Massery, M. (Eds.), 2014. Facilitating Airway Clearance With Coughing Techniques. Elsevier Health Sciences, Amsterdam.

49. Bach, J.R., Intintola, P., et al., 1992. The ventilator-assisted individual: cost analysis of institutionalisation vs rehabilitation and in home management. Chest 101, 26–30.

50. Chatwin, M., Heather, S., et al., 2010. Analysis of home support and ventilator malfunction in 1,211 ventilator-dependent patients. Eur. Respir. J. 35, 310–316.

51. Nonoyama, M.L., McKim, D.A., et al., 2018. Healthcare utilisation and costs of home mechanical ventilation. Thorax Pii: thoraxjnl-2017-211138.

52. King, A.C., 2012. Long-term home MV in the US. Respir. Care 57, 921–932.

CHAPTER 17

Improving upper limb function

Jennifer Dunn and Johanna Wangdell

INTRODUCTION

Improved upper limb function is identified as the most important function to regain by people with tetraplegia following spinal cord injury (SCI).[1] Hand function is important not only for independence in daily life, but social and psychological factors are also improved with the ability to use the hands.[2]

The overall goal for management of the tetraplegic hand is to maximise the ability to perform daily tasks as independently as possible. To reach this goal and prevent secondary complications, interventions need to start early and should involve all members of the rehabilitation team, including the patient with the SCI and their family. Initial interventions should be aimed at maintaining a full passive range of all joints and muscles in the upper limb, free of pain, joint stiffness and contracture. A hand with no oedema, minimal stiffness in the joints and surrounding structures and balance between flexor and extensor tendons not only has the potential to be beneficial in daily use, but also minimises the risk of ongoing pain and facilitates a more attractive hand.

People with tetraplegia who have hand function surgically restored are generally satisfied following surgery and claim they can perform more daily activities, with less effort and fewer aids.[3] A number of surgical techniques are available to improve upper extremity function for people with tetraplegia, including nerve transfers and tendon transfers. These can restore lost functions, such as elbow extension, finger and thumb flexion and extension. In addition, surgical interventions can be used to improve function or positioning for the spastic upper limb when other interventions have been unsuccessful.

This chapter will provide a guideline for the management of the tetraplegic upper limb. Rehabilitation principles are described that highlight the importance of timely therapy interventions to prevent complications and develop a functional hand. Common surgical reconstruction and other interventions will be reviewed.

Abbreviations of muscles, joints and nerves used in this chapter

Abbreviation	Muscle
APL	Abductor pollicus longus
BR	Brachioradialis
ECRB	Extensor carpi radialis brevis
ECRL	Extensor carpi radialis longus
ECU	Extensor carpi ulnaris

Abbreviation	Muscle
EDC	Extensor digitorum communis
EDQ	Extensor digitorum quintii
EPL	Extensor pollicus longus
FCR	Flexor carpi radialis
FDP	Flexor digitorum profundus
FDS	Flexor digitorum superficialis
FPB	Flexor pollicus brevis
FPL	Flexor pollicus longus
PD	Posterior deltoid
PL	Palmaris longus
PQ	Pronator quadratus
PT	Pronator teres
	Joint
CMC	Carpometacarpal
DIP	Distal interphalangeal
IP	Interphalangeal
MCP	Metacarpophalangeal
PIP	Proximal interphalangeal
	Nerve
AIN	Anterior interosseous nerve
PIN	Posterior interosseous nerve

HAND FUNCTION AND PRINCIPLES OF THERAPY IN TETRAPLEGIA

The rehabilitation of the upper limb can improve activity performance, as well as life satisfaction, social interaction and quality of life. The overarching principle of rehabilitation of the upper limb in tetraplegia is to train individuals to manage functional restrictions in a manner that maximises independence. To do this, therapists use a combination of motor relearning and teaching adaptation of remaining movement or integration of alternative movements through compensation or substitution.

Function and management according to neurological level

The limitations experienced following SCI are dependent on the severity and the level of injury (Table 17.1). While individuals with the same motor level of injury will have similar muscles innervated, how they use these muscles is dependent on a number of factors, such as age, body constitution, completeness of SCI, motor planning and other injuries. Therefore, describing the expected functional capacity of a specific level of injury is difficult. What is more relevant is thorough evaluation of sensorimotor functions and impairments, task analysis and planning intervention strategies to address the activity limitations. Individuals with cervical SCI experience improvements in sensorimotor and grasping function during the first 12 months following injury, with the greatest improvement occurring in the first 3 months, and plateauing around 12–18 months.[4] Individuals with motor incomplete SCI experience greater recovery than those with complete SCI.

Following cervical SCI, upper limb function is a combination of using innervated muscles and compensatory strategies to complete a task. There are many different compensatory strategies that may be used depending on the activity being performed, the most common being *tenodesis* function of the hand. In addition, use of aids or orthoses can assist with task completion.

The tenodesis function

A balanced hand opens when the wrist is flexed and closes when the wrist is extended using passive tenodesis function (Fig. 17.1). This is used to facilitate grasp in people with tetraplegia who have wrist extension but no active finger function and is called tenodesis grip or functional hand. For people with tetraplegia, it is critical to gain tenodesis function for performance of tasks.

The process for the development of tenodesis function in a tetraplegic hand is not fully understood.

Table 17.1 Implications of motor level on function

Motor level/upper limb muscles innervated	Limitations	Functional implications
C1–4	No active movement of upper limb muscles	Unable to lift the arm and use hand High risk of subluxation of shoulder joint due to lack of innervation of shoulder girdle
C5 • Deltoid • Biceps • Brachialis • Brachioradialis	No elbow extension Supinated forearm No wrist extension No active movement of fingers or thumb	Unable to use arm above shoulder level Requires orthosis to provide wrist extension No tenodesis* grip

C6
• C5 +
• Clavicular head of Pectoralis
  Supinator
• Radial wrist extensor(s)
  (ECRL and/or ECRB)
	No elbow extension
	No active movement of fingers or thumb
		Unable to use arm above shoulder level without externally rotating
		Potential for tenodesis grip

C7 • C6 + • Sternal head of Pectoralis • Triceps • Pronator teres • Wrist flexor (FCR) • Finger extension (EDC) (possible)	May have weak finger and/or thumb extension No finger or thumb flexion	Able to use arm above head in all positions Potential for tenodesis grip
C8 • C7 + • Ulnar wrist extensor (ECU) • Finger flexors (FDP and FDS) • Thumb flexors (FPL, FPB)	May have finger and/or thumb flexors No intrinsics No thumb abduction	Some active grip function No fine movement function

*See explanation under The tenodesis function.

It is important to prevent overstretching of the finger flexors in both passive movements performed by the therapist (described more fully below) and functional activities (such as propping on extended wrists). Diverse splinting and taping strategies have been practised, but no one strategy has yet proven to be superior in providing the desired tenodesis function.[5] While SCI is commonly considered a condition of the central nervous system because of the damage to the upper motor neuron (UMN), it is not uncommon for concurrent lower motor neuron (LMN) damage to occur at the level of the injury. Recent research demonstrates LMN damage at the level of injury of finger extensors to be a strong predictor for development of tenodesis function.[6] The degree of tension in muscles, by intact reflexes, and hypertension from spasticity impacts the balance and function of the hand, and must be monitored,

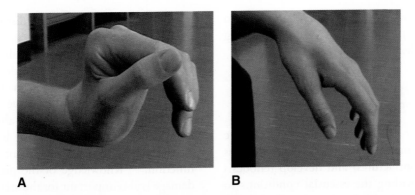

A   B

Figure 17.1 The tenodesis function driven by wrist extension.
A, Passive grip. When the wrist extends the fingers flex into the palm and the thumb flexes/adducts towards the PIP joint of the index finger. **B**, Passive opening. When the wrist flexes all fingers extend and the thumb abducts/extends.

Table 17.2 Essential conditions for a well-functioning hand

Where	What	Why
Wrist	Full extension	Motor in tenodesis grip Stable hand during transfers
	Full flexion	Secure passive opening of the hand
Digits 2–5 (MCP, PIP, DIP)	Full passive extension with wrist flexed	Secure opening of the hand.
	Full passive flexion, all joints together Observe MCP flexion	Secure closing of the hand
	No stretch of extensors when wrist extended	No stretch of tenodesis function
Thumb	Full passive motion, observe especially abduction. With exception of a slight stiffness in IP flexion No stretch of thumb flexion with wrist extended Positioned on or just distally to the PIP joint of index finger when wrist extended	Optimise pinch grip from tenodesis or active function

especially during the initial months following injury. However, there is a fine balance between maintaining as much range of motion (ROM) of the hand as possible, while achieving the balance between flexor and extensor tendons' length to achieve effective tenodesis.

There are some functions that are especially important to monitor since they are critical for future use of the hand (Table 17.2). In some situations, even a relatively small restriction in range can jeopardise efficient use of the hand. Early intervention ensures good tenodesis function and timely training of compensatory strategies for grip rather than having to focus treatments on improving ROM and addressing problems with flexor/extensor balance.

MANAGEMENT OF THE UPPER LIMB IN THE ACUTE PHASE

Management for the upper limb in the acute phase aims to prevent secondary complications (i.e. swelling, contractures) and develop tenodesis function by providing the essential conditions to develop a well-functioning hand, as described above. In the first days after injury, immobilisation results in structural changes in the muscle, characterised by shortening of muscle fibre length, disorganisation and loss of sarcomeres, increase of connective perimysium and accumulation of intramuscular collagenous connective tissue.[7] Atrophy, increased fat content and degenerative changes at the myotendinous junction are other physiological changes related to immobilisation.[8] How these changes relate to future functions is not yet fully understood, but it indicates that awareness of disuse and its treatment in the upper limb is of paramount importance and should start early following injury as muscle contractures can develop rapidly.[9] Immobilisation or disuse due to paralysis rapidly decreases cortical excitability, which may contribute to the decline in voluntary muscle activation.[10] This is important to remember when treating people with incomplete injuries and muscle recovery following spinal shock (see Chapters 1 and 4 for further information on spinal shock).

Following an SCI, damage occurs to the upper motor neurons, preserving the lower motor neurons below the level of injury (see Chapter 1). At the level of the injury, the lower motor neurons are not viable and muscle atrophy from loss of neuromuscular junctions is seen. Below the level of injury, as the anterior horn cells are viable, the neuromuscular junctions are intact, the muscle is viable and a reflex arc is present. Functional electrical stimulation (FES) stimulates these muscles by an electrical impulse directly stimulating the neuron, which then activates the muscle at the neuromuscular junction. FES can be used diagnostically to distinguish between paralysed muscles with intact versus damaged lower motor neurons. Weak or absent response to FES of a paralysed muscle recorded at least 8 days following injury indicates, with 100% certainty, that the peripheral motor nerve has undergone irrecoverable damage.[11] There is also evidence that lower motor lesions can predict both contracture development and the development of the tenodesis function.[7,12] Knowledge of the presence of LMN damage is also important for those considering nerve transfer surgery. Therefore, there may be value in the use of surface FES to assess tetraplegic upper limbs to determine functional denervation and assist in identifying appropriate interventions for maximising function.

INTERVENTIONS IN THE ACUTE PHASE

Monitoring and treatment of a well-functioning upper limb is multidimensional and a team approach is important for a successful result (Fig. 17.2).

Oedema prevention and treatment

Due to paralysis and the dependent position of the upper limb, the limited action of the muscle pump results in reduced capacity for venous and lymphatic return, which leads to oedema. Before oedema is visible the hand can contain up to 50 mL of extra volume (30% increased fluid).[13] Persistent oedema causes proteins in the fluid to increase and the fluid gradually becomes more viscous and fibrotic. If left untreated, the position of the hand can change resulting in loss of tenodesis grip; wrist in volar (palmar) flexion, hyperextension of metacarpophalangeal (MCP) joints, flexion of proximal interphalangeal nerve (PIP) and distal interphalangeal (DIP) joints, and adduction of the thumb (Fig. 17.3). Persistent oedema will restrict ROM and ultimately the ability to use the hand. It is therefore important to prevent oedema from developing and to treat existing oedema promptly. There is no consensus on how to best manage or

Observations and aims

- Maintain joint, muscle, tendon and soft tissue extensibility
- Protect weakened biomechanical structures
- Prevent, control and eliminate oedema
- Prevent, control and correct contractures
- Promote a tenodesis grip by observing and correcting the balance in the hand
- Encourage early active use of hand in daily activities
- Control spasticity and pain
- Strengthen and maintain all functioning muscles

How?

- Early interventions
- Elevate arms and hands
- Functional positioning for extended periods of time (in sitting and lying position)
- Splinting
- Education of patient, nursing staff and family
- Observe and aim for balance in the hand
- Maintain passive movement (performed by patient and/or with assistance)
- Strength training of preserved muscles
- Active use of hand in daily life as early and as much as possible
- Teaching adaptive grip and grasp strategies

Figure 17.2 Observations and interventions to maintain a balanced hand.

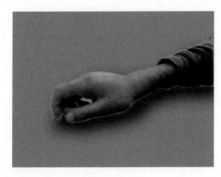

Figure 17.3 Loss of tenodesis grip due to oedema.

prevent acute oedema, but elevation, activity, orthoses and compression are commonly used.[14]

Elevation and positioning

Consistent elevation of the hand in the acute phase is particularly important to assist venous return and reduce the arterial hydrostatic pressure.[13] In bed, this can be facilitated with pillows or slings attached to the bed (Figs 17.4A and 17.4B). When sitting, positioning of the arm needs to be more flexible depending on the functional ability of the individual (Fig. 17.4C). If the shoulder is weak it is important

to provide elbow support to avoid subluxation and resultant pain. A weak wrist must be controlled to avoid extended periods of volar flexion, as this can obstruct the venous and lymphatic return on the dorsum of the hand and lead to the development of oedema (Fig. 17.5).

Hand orthoses

The use of orthoses for the management of the tetraplegic hand is an accepted and long-used treatment strategy. However, the purpose, timeframes and position of orthoses differs between clinicians. Consensus is that static splinting using an orthosis is essential and should ideally begin immediately after injury.[15] In the authors' experience, custom-made orthoses would be preferable to off-the-shelf orthoses.

The aims of splinting are to:

- facilitate good conditions for venous return
- maintain range of motion in joints, tendons and ligaments
- encourage slight shortening of the finger flexors.

This is achieved by letting the hand rest in a position of safety with capsular length and muscles in resting position for tone and length.[16] Compared to passive or active movements, orthoses aim for a low-load

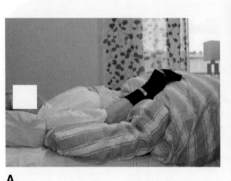
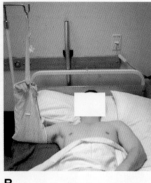
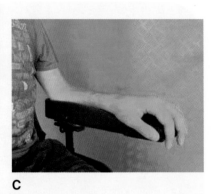

A   B   C

Figure 17.4 Recommended position of the upper limb in lying and sitting. **A,** Recommended position of the upper limb in lying, using pillows. **B,** Recommended position of the upper limb in lying, using sling. **C,** Recommended position of the upper limb in sitting.

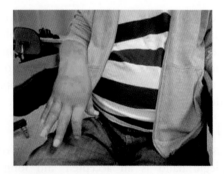

Figure 17.5 Poor positioning in sitting facilitating oedema.

prolonged stretch.[17] Recommended positioning to achieve the aims of static splinting is detailed in Table 17.3.

The orthosis should give a firm volar pressure to facilitate transport of fluid to the dorsal hand, where the majority of the venous return occurs. If oedema is significant, use of elastic bands over the dorsal hand and forearm in conjunction with the orthosis will provide additional compression (Figs 17.6A and 17.6B). Figures 17.6C and 17.6D show complete elastic compression for severe oedema.

During the bedrest stage, it is recommended that orthoses be used day and night, except for passive/ active ROM, hygiene care and holding relatives' hands. There are no specific regimens for ROM exercises; these should be personalised depending upon the risk each individual has to developing secondary complications. Once the individual becomes more active, the risk of oedema reduces as the muscle pump is activated. The need for splinting to prevent oedema decreases and can interfere with activity. Orthoses should then only be used at night.

Once the patient is mobilised, the aims of splinting changes and, as such, other types of orthoses, together with self-ranging of the hand joints, may be satisfactory, especially for the hand with no spasticity. Many orthoses have been used with the aim of providing a tenodesis grip by encouraging shortening of finger and thumb flexors. However, the use of orthoses to develop tenodesis grip by muscle shortening is not yet proven as the development of tenodesis grip appears to be multifactorial.[6,18]

For spastic hands, stretching of involved muscles using orthoses for a prolonged period is indicated. Regular, ongoing evaluation of the muscle balance in the hand is essential. It is important to rapidly adjust the treatment and the amount of use or angles of any orthosis as soon as muscle imbalance or tightness occurs (Fig. 17.7).

Table 17.3 Recommended position for splinting in the acute phase

Part of upper limb	Recommended position	Rationale
Forearm	Pronated	Functional position Prevent supinated (shortened) position
Wrist	20 degrees extension	Stabile and functional position of the wrist. Maintain long finger extensors. No full stretch of the finger flexors (some shortening possible)
MCP joints of fingers	70 degrees flexion	Balancing finger flexors/extensors and intrinsics Prevent claw hand
IP joints of fingers (DIP and PIP)	Straight	Maintains full extension of PIP joints Balancing the intrinsics Prevent claw hand
Thumb (CMC, MCP, IP)	CMC: Abducted 30 degrees, aiming for PIP of index finger. MCP: straight or slightly flexed IP: straight or slightly flexed	Position the thumb for opening without stretching thumb flexor Prevent an adducted thumb Position the thumb for a key pinch grip

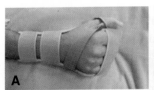 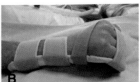 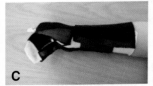 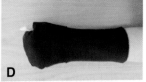

Figure 17.6 Examples of orthoses.
A, Orthosis providing volar pressure for oedema management. **B**, Orthosis with addition of elastic bands over dorsum for additional compression. **C** and **D**, Orthoses with complete elastic coverage if oedema is severe.

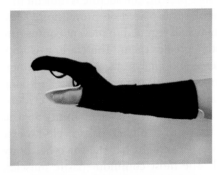

Figure 17.7 Example of orthoses for prolonged stretch of hypertoned finger and wrist flexors.

A number of orthoses are designed to compensate for lack of grip ability. Some are critical to enable function. However, the long term use of orthoses tends to be low as most people try to find ways to manage daily life with minimal equipment.[15]

Wrapping and compression gloves

If oedema is present despite the use of orthoses and elevation, wrapping or compression gloves can be effective. For wrapping, each finger should be wrapped individually (Fig. 17.8). Additionally, the hand should be placed in a position of safety using

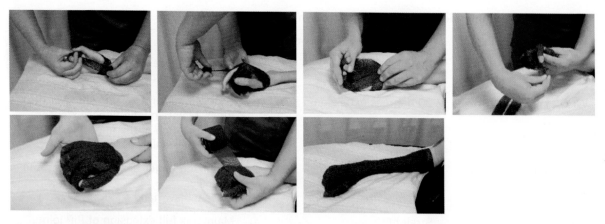

Figure 17.8 Wrapping technique for hand and forearm using Danamull Haft®.

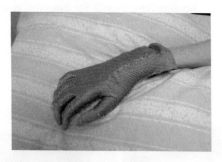

Figure 17.9 Prefabricated compression glove. The flat construction of the glove tends to position the hand in claw position.

an orthosis when the hand is not being used for functional activities. Wrapping is effective for acute oedema but, if persistent, other treatments should be considered.

The light pressure of a compression glove can be useful and easier to administer compared to wrapping. When using compression gloves it is important to observe the positioning of the hand to ensure the tenodesis position is maintained and the hand does not adopt a claw position due to the construction technique (Fig. 17.9). In addition, compression provided should be on the palmar side of the hand. There is a common risk of compression occurring mostly on the dorsum and since most of the venous return is located on this side, this type

of compression is contraindicated. If the glove or wrapping interferes with active use of the hand, the treatment should be re-evaluated, since activity is generally more effective than passive compression treatment.

Spasticity and contractures

As spasticity is related to contracture development, treatment aimed at preventing contractures should be implemented as soon as possible (see Chapters 1 and 4 for further detail on spasticity). Contracture, or loss of joint mobility, is a common complication of SCI.[12] Reported incidence of upper limb contracture varies between 41% and 85%,[19] and its presence has been shown to decrease independence in daily life.[20] Once present, contracture is difficult to reduce, thus emphasis is placed on prevention.[21] The most important skill required to prevent contractures is to accurately predict them. Therefore, it is important to observe and analyse factors such as innervation pattern, spasticity, pain, oedema and long-term position of the body.[22] There is some evidence that LMN damage at the level of injury in triceps is correlated with a higher risk of elbow extension deficits.[11] This might be true for other body parts as well. The most common spastic muscles, their effect and risk of contribution to various limitations, are listed in Table 17.4.

Table 17.4 Common spastic muscles in upper limb, effects and implications for function

Muscle	Effect	Implications for function
Pectorals	Internally rotated, adducted shoulder	Postural, breathing Difficulty/pain dressing upper body
Biceps	Elbow flexed, forearm supinated	Limit reach and grasp Unable to turn hand to use tenodesis grip
Pronator teres/quadratus	Unable to supinate arm	Compensatory strategies in shoulder for use of hand
Wrist flexors (FCR, FCU, PL)	Wrist flexed	Makes grasp difficult
Finger flexors (FDP, FDS)	Wrist flexed, fingers flexed into a fist	Difficulty opening hand to release objects Hygiene aspects
Thumb flexors	Thumb in palm	No key pinch
Thumb abductor	Thumb positioned next to index finger	Limited cylinder grasp and pinch
Intrinsics	MCP flexion	Limited hand opening

Prevention is a team approach and can include medication,[23] including pain relief, anti-spasmodics, botulinum toxin, in conjunction with passive movement and positioning throughout the day. This needs to be combined with education and empowering the person with an SCI to take responsibility for their paralysed body.

Passive movement

Daily assessment of the upper limb in the acute phase is usually combined with passive movements performed by a therapist. Passive movements are important to prevent adhesions of tendons and lubricate joints. Therefore joint-by-joint passive ranging is vital. Stretching of the joints is performed slowly and joints should never be forced. The rationale and the use of passive movement and stretching is mostly justified by old animal studies.[24] The intensity of passive movements necessary to reach therapeutic benefit is unknown, despite a strong clinical confidence in the effect. Harvey and colleagues[22] suggested that for joints with existing limited range, a therapist should perform stretching of soft tissues for long periods of time (at least 20

minutes, and perhaps for as long as 12 hours a day) to maximise the probability of attaining a clinically worthwhile effect in increasing this limited range. This prolonged stretch can be achieved with a well-fitting, individualised splint or, in some joints, plastering may be used. As it is difficult to reduce contractures once they develop, stretching is most likely to be effective if commenced before the onset of contracture, thus rehabilitation and treatments of the upper limb should be initiated as soon as possible after injury.[22] Soft tissues, such as the muscles, ligaments and joint capsules most at risk, should be targeted, particularly if contracture is likely to impose functionally important limitations (Table 17.5). Orthoses and positioning of the limbs are important complements to twice-daily passive movement.

Shoulders

Adequate ROM in the shoulders is essential for ensuring pain-free movement of the upper extremity and facilitation of function and use in daily life.[25] It is therefore important to commence early and continue to maintain full ROM in the shoulders,

Table 17.5 Critical observations and future consequences in the upper limb

Observation	Risk	Consequences
Biceps function without triceps	Elbow extension deficit	Cannot lock elbow(s) during weight bearing or transfer
	Pronation deficits	Hand turns palm-up
Supinated forearm	Wrist flexion deficits	Difficulty grasping, using active or passive grip
	MCP flexion deficits	
	Oedema in the hand (due to extended wrist blocking dorsal venous return)	
Arms internally rotated with hands resting on thighs/across body when sitting in wheelchair	Shoulder external rotation deficits	Activity limitation and pain
	MCP joint flexion deficits	Limit active/passive grip
	PIP joint extension/flexion deficits	
Pain	Increased tone in innervated muscles	Do not want to use the painful limb
Spasticity	Can work both as risk and prevention but mostly risk	See spasticity chapter
Oedema	Fluid that organises into fibrosis	Development of claw hand

particularly flexion, abduction and internal rotation. Internal and external rotation of the shoulder should be given particular attention to prevent tightness of the shoulder capsule. In addition, maintenance of scapular mobility is important as poor scapular positioning can contribute to neck and shoulder pain and loss of stability of the shoulder joint. The loss of muscle stability in the shoulder leads to a fragile joint and this joint must therefore be handled with great care. Pulling on the arms or prolonged sitting with unsupported arms can stretch or injure the structures of the shoulder joint and should be avoided. In order to maintain range of movement, and to avoid swelling and pain, the shoulders should be regularly positioned in alternating end-range positions (Fig. 17.10).

Elbow

Preservation of full elbow ROM is essential to enable a person with tetraplegia to weight-bear on their arms, especially if they have weak or absent triceps. Thus when ranging the elbow it is important to ensure that full elbow extension is combined with pronation of the forearm, so that the biceps, brachioradialis and wrist extensor muscles are stretched to prevent development of a supination contracture. Due to the imbalance of the muscles around the elbow, particularly in the C5 and C6 level injury, splinting of the elbow while in bed may be required if spasticity or contracture becomes an issue.

Hands

It is important to avoid stretching the finger and thumb flexor tendons when combined with wrist extension as this will inhibit the promotion of tenodesis function. Therefore, finger extension should only be performed with the wrist flexed (Fig. 17.11). Areas at risk and therefore needing specific attention are: flexion and extension of the wrist, flexion of the MCP joints of the fingers, extension of finger PIP joints and thumb adduction – the same positions that are lost if prolonged oedema is present. If any

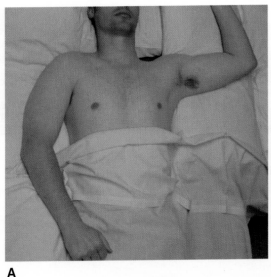
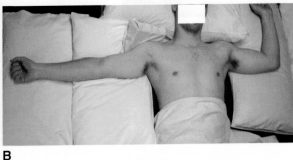

Figure 17.10 A, B Recommended positions in lying to prevent shoulder stiffness.

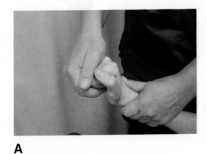
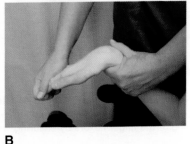

Figure 17.11 Passive movement of the hand to control for tenodesis function.
A, Extend the wrist and bend the fingers focusing on MCP joint flexion. **B**, Flex the wrist and extend the fingers.

tightness occurs, specific attention should be focused on the affected joint.

Appropriate length of the intrinsic muscles is also of importance. With intrinsic tightness, the MCP joints will not fall into extension when the wrist flexes. This will limit the passive forces to open the hand and get around objects. The intrinsic stretch, with PIP joints of the fingers in flexion and MCP joints straight, should also be performed (Fig. 17.12).

Self-management

As discussed previously, the length of time required to perform passive movements for therapeutic benefit is unknown, but could be as long as 15 minutes per joint daily, dependent upon such factors as age and presence or absence of spasticity and pain.[26] The individual should therefore be taught good habits of stretching and managing passive movements and long-term positioning as early as

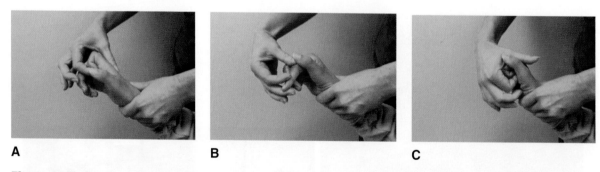

Figure 17.12 Passive movement to monitor specific joint and tendons with focus on intrinsic stretch.
A, Bend the finger with the MCP straight (intrinsic stretch). **B**, Straighten PIP and DIP joints and flex MCP to full range.
C, Flex all joints.

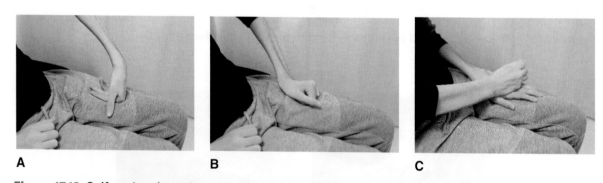

Figure 17.13 Self-assisted passive movement of the hand.
A, Start with full flexion of MCP. **B**, aim for a closed fist with extended wrist. **C**, stretch out fingers with the wrist in neutral (avoid stretching of the finger flexors by ensuring wrist in neutral).

possible. Stretching should be incorporated into everyday life activities, for example, positioning the body in front of the television or other resting positions (see Online resources at the end of the chapter). An example of a self-assisted passive movement is to push the fisted hand against the knee, focusing on MCP flexion then stretching out the fingers by dragging the hand along the leg or the other arm (Fig. 17.13). Be aware of the risk for hyperextended MCP joints and flexed wrist during the extension phase.

MANAGEMENT OF THE UPPER LIMB IN THE SUB-ACUTE PHASE

The aims of the upper limb management in the sub-acute phase are: 1) strengthening of innervated muscles; 2) education of compensatory or substitution strategies and movement patterns; and 3) translation into daily activities. As soon as possible, individuals should be encouraged and trained to use their hands in daily activities to recapture control over their life. The fundamental concept of motor learning is the

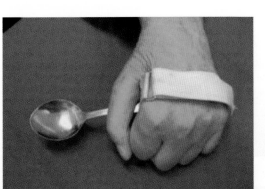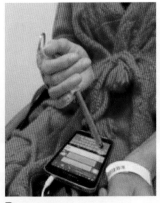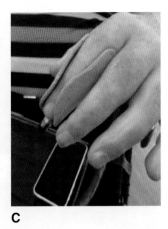

A   B   C

Figure 17.14 A–C Universal cuff or splints for substitution of hand function.

assumption that practice of task-specific movements causes plastic changes in the central nervous system and that increased frequency and duration of training are associated with improvements in performance.[27]

Strengthening of remaining innervated muscles

Strengthening of the proximal muscles of the upper limb provides stability that makes arm and hand function possible. The principles of strengthening are the same as for the able-bodied population: progressive increases in resistance aiming to increase muscle strength of innervated muscles. For those individuals with weakness of upper limb muscles resulting in inability to move the limb against gravity, active assisted or gravity eliminated exercises are initially used until the muscles strengthen. When strengthening partially innervated muscles, attention must be given to fatigue, since the muscle requires longer recovery time than a fully innervated muscle. FES can be used for treatment to strengthen weak muscles, improve hand posture/tenodesis and guiding motor relearning.[28] (See Chapter 7 for more detail on FES.)

Education of movement patterns

A person with tetraplegia has to relearn many movement patterns and most of their daily activities.

They need to learn how to move and position their upper limb despite the lack of critical functions. Compensatory strategies are movement patterns resulting from the adaptation of remaining muscles. In contrast, substitution is where functions are replaced or substituted by orthoses or assistive devices, for example, the use of a universal cuff to hold eating utensils and typing peg (Fig. 17.14).

Compensatory strategies

Frequently, individuals with an SCI are initially unable to perform tasks due to a lack of skills. Since the learning process has similarities to an able-bodied person learning an unfamiliar sport, as discussed earlier, motor skill learning is a useful treatment technique in rehabilitation. The use of technologies and adaptive aids might also be an important facilitator.

Effective motor task training should be well structured, intense and incorporate practice that is task- and context-specific.[29] In addition, effective feedback of the motor performance is an essential component and ensures correct motor patterns are reinforced during training. When the desired task is complex, it can be broken down into sub-tasks and trained individually in a similar but more simple approach.[30] There is strong evidence that repetitive activity through massed practice combined with FES

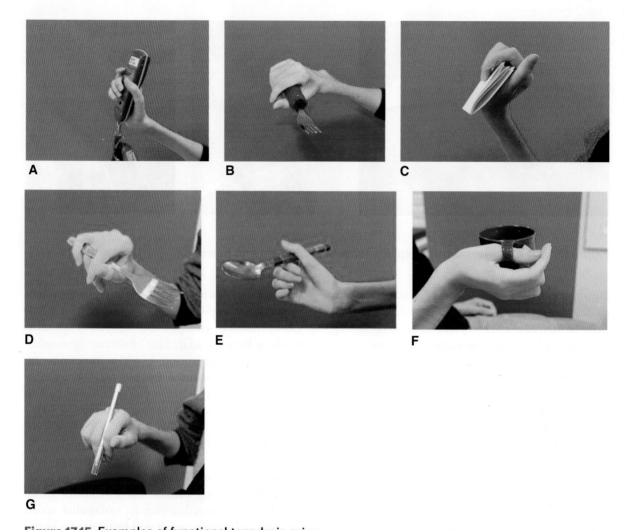

Figure 17.15 Examples of functional tenodesis grips.
A, **B**, Cylinder grip. **C**, Palmar grip. **D**, Woven grip. **E**, Key grip. **F**, Thumb hook grip. **G**, Squeeze grip.

demonstrates significant improvements in upper limb function, grip and pinch strength in people with tetraplegia.[31]

Gripping is a common sub-task the individual needs to train themselves to do in order to be able to perform various daily activities.[32] Despite lack of active grip in the hand, those with active wrist extension are able to perform several compensatory strategies, and with intense training can develop

great skills in daily activities.[33] A well-balanced tenodesis function facilitates the opportunity for several adapted grips (Fig. 17.15).

Other common grips that do not rely on strong wrist extension include balancing objects in the supinated hand and clasping an object between the wrists (Fig. 17.16). Therapists need to be familiar with the variety of possible grips to provide guidance to develop a suitable grip for optimal performance

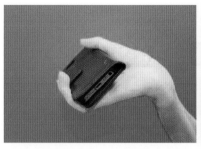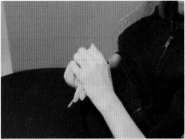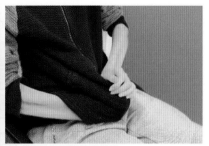

Figure 17.16 Compensatory strategies for grips without voluntary finger function.

of the task, depending on the individual and their resulting condition.

Ergonomics

Ergonomics, that is, the efficiency of these newly learned movements, is an essential aspect and should be carefully considered in this phase. Effective feedback, ensuring good movement patterns of the shoulder and shoulder girdle during functional tasks is important to reduce the risk of shoulder impingement and tendonitis. The risk of overuse and overload injuries in the upper limb is common among people with an SCI, especially when using compensatory strategies for upper limb function.

MEASUREMENT OF UPPER LIMB FUNCTION

Measurement of the upper limb in tetraplegia should follow the theoretical framework of the International Classification of Function, Disability and Health (ICF) and capture aspects from the domains of body function and structures, activity and participation.[34] Currently there is no international consensus on what measures to use.[35] Commonly used measures are detailed in Fig. 17.17 and described fully in Sinnott and colleagues.[36]

SURGICAL MANAGEMENT

For individuals with cervical SCI levels C5–C8, surgery can improve upper limb function, let

the person resume activities and reduce the need for orthoses and adaptive equipment.[2] The basic principle of surgical reconstruction of the upper limb in tetraplegia is to use a spare muscle and/or nerves to produce new movements and never jeopardise the remaining function.

Surgical reconstruction of the upper limb, using tendon transfers, for people with tetraplegia was first introduced by Eric Moberg in the 1970s.[37] However, the long immobilisation period and rehabilitation following tendon transfer surgery is a common reason why many people with tetraplegia elect to not have surgery.[38] Nerve transfers, a routine part of the surgical management of brachial plexi and peripheral nerve injuries, are now becoming a more common surgical option in the tetraplegic population as they allow direct reinnervation of muscle that is anatomically and mechanically designed to perform the desired function. This procedure avoids the technical challenges associated with tendon transfers. A single nerve transfer can reinnervate multiple muscles and allow independent movement of these muscles. For example, a transfer of the nerve to supinator to the posterior interosseous nerve (PIN) can provide active wrist extension (extensor carpi ulnaris, ECU), finger extension (extensor digitorum communis, EDC) and thumb extension (extensor pollicus longus, EPL) and thumb abduction. For tendon transfer, one donor tendon is transferred into one muscle to provide one movement. Therefore, for individuals with only one donor tendon available, they need to decide on what function they wish to

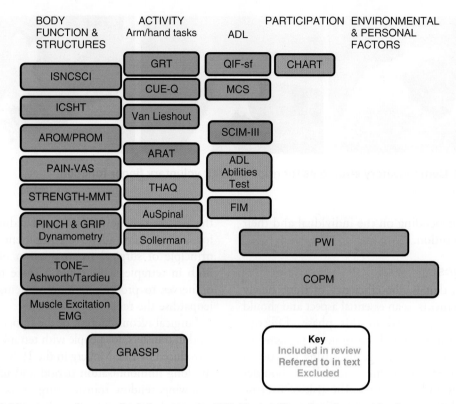

Figure 17.17 Measures of upper limb function in SCI. Variability of tools used by international centres in 2009 by ICF domain.

Abbreviations: ADL, activities of daily living; ARAT, Action research arm test; AROM, active range of motion; CHART, Craig Handicap Assessment and Reporting Technique; CUE-Q, capabilities of upper extremity questionnaire; EMG, electromyography; ICSHT, International Classification for Surgery of the Hand in Tetraplegia; ISNCSCI, International Standards for Neurological Classification of SCI; MCS, Motor capabilities scale; MMT, manual muscle test; PROM, passive range of motion; QIF-SF, Quadriplegia Index of Function – short form; SCIM III, Spinal Cord Independence Measure III; THAQ, Tetraplegia Hand Activity Questionnaire; VAS, visual analog scale.

Source: Sinnott K.A., Dunn J.A., et al., 2016. Measurement of outcomes of upper limb reconstructive surgery for tetraplegia. Archives of Physical Medicine and Rehabilitation 97 (6), S169–S181.

have restored – usually either pinch or grasp. Often in such cases, individuals choose to have different functions on each hand. The immobilisation period for nerve transfers is considerably shorter than required for tendon transfer.[39] Conversely, results from tendon transfers can be seen from day one, while reinnervation after nerve transfer can take between 4 and 9 months, depending upon the transfer.

Timing of surgery

Surgery is not usually performed until after the initial period of rehabilitation following SCI and neurological stability is achieved. In complete SCI, this may be 6 months following injury.[40] For nerve transfer, early surgery (within 1 year following SCI) is critical, as neuromuscular end-plate degeneration can occur after this time.[41] Tendon transfer surgery is not time-limited and remains an option even decades after SCI.[42] For incomplete SCI, neurological recovery takes longer and therefore any surgical intervention needs to occur after the plateau of neurological recovery has been reached to ensure natural recovery and function is not compromised by surgical options.

Assessment

As described earlier in the chapter, the residual upper extremity function following a cervical SCI depends on the level of injury. Prior to surgical reconstruction a thorough physical assessment of muscle strength, joint ROM and sensation should be performed. Pain and swelling in the upper limb are relative contraindications and management should be optimised before surgery. Tenodesis function is preferable, but is not essential. In addition, for successful rehabilitation outcomes individuals need to be psychologically stable and have good social supports.[43]

Surgical reconstruction depends on the muscle strength of the upper extremity assessed by the International Classification for Surgery of the Hand in Tetraplegia (ICSHT).[44] This characterises the most common patterns of presentation, based on the number of forearm, wrist and finger muscles that have muscle strength greater than Medical Research Council (MRC) Grade 4 and therefore considered available as a donor muscle (Fig. 17.18).

The hierarchy of surgical reconstruction of the tetraplegic upper limb consists of restoration of active elbow extension (if absent), restoration of active wrist extension (if absent), provision of active key pinch and/or grasp and restoration of opening of the hand. There are a number of surgical procedures that can be performed to provide these functions (Table 17.6 on p. 392). Individuals with more muscles available will have more options for reconstructing specific hand functions.[44]

REHABILITATION

Rehabilitation aims, immobilisation timeframes and rehabilitation timeframes differ between nerve and tendon transfers (Table 17.7, on p. 393).

Rehabilitation principles following nerve and tendon transfer surgery

Rehabilitation following nerve transfer surgery aims to maintain the integrity of the nerve transfer coadaptation while minimising scar tissue, oedema and pain. In the initial immobilisation period, attention is given to avoiding loss of passive range of joints and minimising the loss of function. Following this, Hahn and colleagues[45] have advocated early motor re-education through activation of the nerve to the recipient muscle through the activation of the donor nerve movement. Rationale for these exercises includes increasing the amount of cortical representation; however, outcomes have not been specifically studied.

Rehabilitation following tendon transfer surgery involves maintaining and regaining active and passive ROM after immobilisation, re-education of the new muscle activity and learning/practice of functional tasks and reintegration into activities of daily living (ADLs). Use of electrical stimulation or biofeedback has also been reported to be useful.[46]

The motor learning process following both nerve and tendon transfer surgery is performed using the hands-on/hands-off principle,[47] in combination with repetitive task-orientated exercise. Motor learning consists of three stages:[30]

1. *Cognitive stage:* the individual is introduced to the requirements of the motor task, but is unsure of how to do it. This requires a hands-on role for the therapist to facilitate the new muscle action and support the relearning process.

2. *Associative stage:* the individual begins to refine their skill. The hands-on facilitation is decreased as the individual begins to form appropriate associations between the movement plan and the consequence; that is, the individual learns what feels right.

3. *Autonomous stage:* the skill becomes automatic, requiring little, if any, cognitive processing and does not require facilitation by the therapist.

ISNCSCI	Level of SCI		ICSHT
Elbow Flexors	C5		**Group 0** – No muscles for transfer
Wrist Extensors			**Group 1** – Brachioradialis
	C6		**Group 2** – Extensor Carpi Radialis Longus
			Group 3 – Extensor Carpi Radialis Brevis
Elbow Extensors		C7	**Group 4** – Pronator Teres
			Group 5 – Flexor Carpi Radialis
			Group 6 – Extensor Digitorum Communis
Finger Flexors			**Group 7** – Extensor Pollicis Longus
	C8		**Group 8** – Partial Digital Flexors
			Group 9 – Lacks only intrinsics
			Group X – Exceptions

Figure 17.18 Comparison of ISNCSCI and ICSHT key muscles.

Key: ISNCSCI International Standards for Neurological Classification of Spinal Cord Injury; ICSHT International Classification for Surgery of the Hand in Tetraplegia

Source: McDowell C.L., Moberg E., et al., 1986. The second international conference on surgical rehabilitation of the upper limb in tetraplegia (quadriplegia). J Hand Surg. 11 (A), 604–608.

The autonomous stage of motor learning is usually reached between 3 and 10 weeks following tendon transfer, but can take up to 12 months to achieve following nerve transfer. This relearning process is time-consuming, demanding and unfamiliar to the patient, involving specific therapist knowledge in the skills that are attainable. It also requires training in self-efficacy and self-belief to improve the confidence of the person with tetraplegia and enable them to translate the new skills gained from surgery into daily function.[48]

Surgery for spasticity

Following an SCI, spasticity is a common complication, with spasticity limiting function reported in 87–96% of cervical SCI, and more frequent in incomplete injuries.[49] For individuals with spasticity that affects functional use of the hand, without major contracture, surgical techniques have been successful with improving function, care and hygiene.[50] Several techniques are available, although as yet no one technique has been proven to be superior

Table 17.6 Common surgical procedures

ISNCSC[a] motor level	ICSHT[b] group	Desired function	Possible procedures	
			Tendon transfer	Nerve transfer
C5	0	No muscles available for tendon transfer, possible nerve transfer. Individualised assessment required.		
	1	Elbow extension	PD to triceps TT _or_ Biceps to triceps TT	Axillary Nerve to Radial Nerve NT _or_ Musculocutaneous Nerve to Radial Nerve NT
		Wrist extension	BR to ECRB TT	Nerve to Supinator to ECRB NT
		Key pinch	FPL tenodesis _and_ Split distal FPL tenodesis	
C6	1–3	Elbow extension	PD to triceps TT _or_ Biceps to triceps TT	Axillary Nerve to Radial Nerve NT _or_ Musculocutaneous Nerve to Radial Nerve NT
		Finger/thumb extension		Nerve to Supinator to PIN NT
		Key pinch	BR to FPL TT _or_ FPL tenodesis and Split distal FPL tenodesis	Nerve to Brachialis to AIN NT
		Gross grasp	BR to FDP TT _or_ ECRL to FDP TT	
		Thumb abduction	EDQ to APL TT	
C7[c]	4–7	Finger/thumb extension	PT to EDC TT	Nerve to Supinator to PIN NT
		Key pinch	BR to FPL _and_ Split distal FPL tenodesis	Nerve to Brachialis to AIN NT
		Gross grasp	ECRL to FDP TT _or_ PT to FDP TT	
C8	8 and 9	Active intrinsics	FDS II and III to Interossei	

a. ISNCSCI, International Standards of Neurological Classification of Spinal Cord Injury

b. ISCHT, International Classification for Surgery of the Hand in Tetraplegia

c. There are many surgical options for ICSHT classes 4–7, and depending on surgeon's choice, a number of different motors may be transferred to provide the function required.

Sources: McDowell C.L., Moberg E., et al., 1986. The second international conference on surgical rehabilitation of the upper limb in tetraplegia (quadriplegia). J Hand Surg. 11A (4), 604–608; Dunn J.A., Hay-Smith E.J., et al., 2016. Decision-making about upper limb tendon transfer surgery by people with tetraplegia for more than 10 Years. Arch Phys Med Rehabil. 97 (6, Supplement), S88–S96.

Table 17.7 **Rehabilitation aims and timeframes**

	Desired function	Tendon transfer	Nerve transfer
Elbow extension:	Aims to stabilise the elbow for controlled hand use and improves activation of forearm tendon transfers by providing an antagonist	Immobilisation/rehabilitation period: 6–12 weeks for both biceps to triceps and posterior deltoid to triceps transfer	Immobilisation period: sling for up to 3 weeks to protect nerve transfer
Wrist extension	Aims to restore active wrist extension to allow tenodesis grasp	Immobilisation period: plaster cast or removable thermoplastic splint for 4 weeks. Rehabilitation: 1–2 weeks following immobilisation period.	Rehabilitation: commences once flickers of recipient muscle function is seen (usually 6–9 months following surgery).
Pinch and grasp	Aims to provide pinch and/or grasp		
Finger /thumb extension	Aims to restore active finger and thumb extension	No TT available to provide this function.	

Sources: Cain S.A., Gohritz A., et al., 2015. Review of upper extremity nerve transfer in cervical spinal cord injury. J Brachial Plex Peripher Nerve Inj. 10 (1), e34; Dunn J.A., Hay-Smith E.J., et al., 2016. Decision-making about upper limb tendon transfer surgery by people with tetraplegia for more than 10 Years. Arch Phys Med Rehabil. 97 (6, Supplement), S88–S96; Koch-Borner S., Dunn J.A., et al., 2016. Rehabilitation after Posterior Deltoid to Triceps transfer in tetraplegia. Arch Phys Med Rehab. 97 (6, Supplement), S126–S135; Kozin S.H., D'Addesi L., et al., 2010. Biceps-to-triceps transfer for elbow extension in persons with tetraplegia. J Hand Surg. 35 (6), 968–975; McDowell C.L., Moberg E., et al., 1986. The second international conference on surgical rehabilitation of the upper limb in tetraplegia (quadriplegia). J Hand Surg. 11A (4), 604–608.

to another. These include tendon lengthening/tenotomy and fractional myotendinous lengthening.

Tendon lengthening surgery primarily aims to reduce the resistance of the spastic muscle through range in order for remaining functioning synergists and antagonists to increase the use in daily life. Tendon-lengthening surgery can be performed on both well-functioning hands with partial spasticity and non-functional hands with relative stable hypertonia. Rehabilitation following tendon lengthening consists of early active rehabilitation, maintenance of ADLs and splinting.[51]

OUTCOMES FOLLOWING SURGICAL RECONSTRUCTION

Elbow extension

Outcomes following reconstruction of elbow extension are similar between tendon and nerve transfer. Reported outcomes for both deltoid to triceps and biceps to triceps tendon transfers demonstrate an increase in strength from MRC Grade 0 to Grade 3. Reported outcomes following nerve transfers are MRC Grade 3 to Grade 4 strength. Functionally this means that individuals are able to reach above their head to perform functional tasks, and have an increase in their available horizontal workspace. Common identified goals after deltoid to triceps surgery include propelling a manual wheelchair, body-weight transfers, self-care, dressing, driving a vehicle and positioning arms when lying down.[52]

Pinch and grasp

Gains in pinch and grip strength following both nerve and tendon transfer surgery are small but significant for people with tetraplegia. This improvement in strength means they can perform ADLs using one hand rather than two and without the need for orthoses or adaptive equipment (Fig. 17.19).[2] Additionally, many tasks that were impossible to perform before surgery are able to be performed

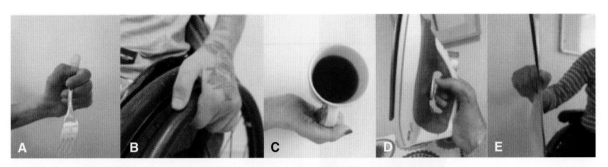

Figure 17.19 Changes in hand function following tendon transfer surgery.
A, Pinch reconstruction to hold a fork. **B**, Grasp reconstruction for wheelchair manoeuvring. **C**, Grasp reconstruction for holding cup. **D**, Grasp reconstruction for holding iron. **E**, Pinch reconstruction for holding papers.

after surgery, such as cutting food, using a remote, accessing an ATM, using a key and zippers.

To date, direct comparisons of the outcomes in tendon and nerve transfer surgery have not been made. However, nerve transfers show promise as an additional reconstructive option for the upper extremity in people with tetraplegia. In addition, there are nerve transfers that provide options for reconstruction in cases not amenable to tendon transfers such as the supinator to PIN nerve transfer for finger and thumb opening. Thus combining nerve and tendon transfers into new algorithms should further maximise outcomes in people with tetraplegia.

Spasticity corrective surgery

Reported outcomes in both the severe and the mild spasticity group following spasticity corrective surgery is limited but do demonstrate improvements in use of the hand for grasp and release, especially for activities such as holding walking aids and improvements in wheelchair propulsion and most ADLs (Fig. 17.20).[51]

TETRAPLEGIC UPPER LIMB FUNCTION FROM THE PATIENT'S PERSPECTIVE

Upper limb function is highly prioritised by people with tetraplegia since it is crucial in daily activities, social activities and participation. Effective management of the upper limb in the acute phase is fundamental for optimising rehabilitation time, preventing often painful complications and ultimately improving quality of life. Long-term use of orthoses to compensate for lost upper limb function is poor. Many people with tetraplegia learn to compensate for lost function.

> I had gotten used to the way that my hands were and I had learnt a whole lot of new tricks … I was able to hold my own cup and feed myself. I was fine, I was happy with that – that was enough for me.[53]

However, there are surgical options to provide improvements in arm and hand function and decrease the need for orthoses and decrease the effort in activities. Satisfaction for these procedures are high and have evoked comments such as:

> 'Having the surgery is the best thing I have ever done'; 'my hand appears more natural after the surgery'; 'there is a long rehabilitation time but given the improvements that I have experienced, it is really worth it'; 'I am grateful that I had the surgery.'[54]

Improvements in upper limb function have been shown to be maintained for many years following surgery.[55] These improvements are translated into both physical and psychological functioning.[2]

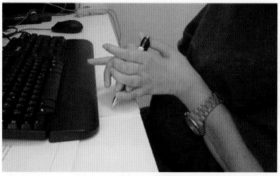

A *Pre-operative grasp*

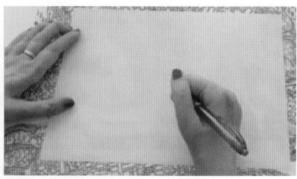

Post-operative grasp

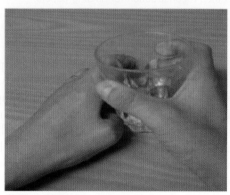

B *Pre-operative grasp*

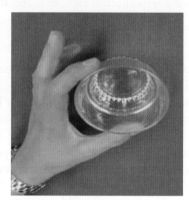

Post-operative grasp

Figure 17.20 A, B, Changes in hand function following spasticity surgery.

I hated going out to dinner … being in public to eat was a no-no for me because someone would feed me or I would have this spoon tied to my hand that I could not put down … whereas now, I can go out to a restaurant and … you are sitting there eating alongside everyone else, being able to pick up a wine glass, a beer mug whatever and it is amazing. Someone not feeding you with a straw or a spoon. So that is a huge psychological improvement.[38]

The decision to have surgical reconstruction is multi-faceted and depends on an individual's goals and priorities at that time of offer for surgery.[53] Therefore ongoing offers of surgery are recommended throughout the life of the person with tetraplegia.[53]

Evidence-based practice points

- Intervention aiming to prevent secondary complications to the upper limb must start early and is of paramount importance.
- Splinting in the acute phase following SCI aims to prevent oedema, maintain ROM in joints, tendons and ligaments and encourage slight shortening of the finger flexors.
- Promotion of tenodesis function and maintaining a balance between flexors and extensors is a presumption for optimal use in daily life for a person with tetraplegia.
- The algorithm for surgical restoration of upper limb functions is complex and requires a specialised team approach.
- Tendon transfer is a reliable technique with high patient satisfaction, whereas nerve transfer is a newer option and its use and outcome have not been fully explored.
- The combination of tendon and nerve transfer has the potential to further improve upper limb function more than using a single approach.
- Rehabilitation after surgical interventions is highly specialised and requires experienced therapists to optimise outcomes following surgery.

SUMMARY

A comprehensive program for management of the upper limb following cervical SCI will result in improved function, enriched independence and enhanced quality of life. Early management of the upper limb is essential and should begin as soon as practical following injury. Management includes: oedema treatment, prevention of secondary complications such as spasticity, contractures, overload and pain, strengthening of remaining muscles, relearning motor functions and most importantly translation into daily life including compensatory strategies.

Upper limb reconstructive surgery has been proven to be reliable in improving critical function of the upper limb following cervical SCI. A comprehensive assessment by specialised surgeons is essential to develop an individualised surgical plan that may include combinations of nerve and tendon transfer procedures. Improvements in not only physical but also psychological functioning have been demonstrated following upper limb reconstructive surgery.

Online resources

Compensatory strategies in ADL, www.spinalistips.se/en
Stretching exercises, www.physiotherapy.com

References

1. Anderson, K.D., 2004. Targeting recovery: priorities of the spinal cord-injured population. J. Neurotrauma 21 (10), 1371–1383.

2. Wangdell, J., Carlsson, G., et al., 2013. Enhanced independence: experiences after regaining grip function in people with tetraplegia. Disabil. Rehabil. 35 (23), 1968–1974.

3. Wangdell, J., Friden, J., 2010. Satisfaction and performance in patient selected goals after grip reconstruction in tetraplegia. J. Hand Surg. Eur. 35 (7), 563–568.

4. Kirshblum, S.C., O'Connor, K.C., 1998. Predicting neurologic recovery in traumatic cervical spinal cord injury. Arch. Phys. Med. Rehab. 79 (11), 1456–1466.

5. Harvey, L., 1996. Principles of conservative management for a non-orthotic tenodesis grip in tetraplegics. J. Hand Ther. 9 (3), 238–242.

6. Bersch, I., Koch-Borner, S., et al., 2018. Electrical stimulation – a mapping system for hand dysfunction in tetraplegia. Spinal Cord 56 (5), 516–522.

7. Lieber, R.L., Ward, S.R., 2013. Cellular mechanisms of tissue fibrosis. 4. Structural and functional consequences of skeletal muscle fibrosis. Am. J. Physiol. Cell Physiol. 305 (3), C241–C252.

8. Williams, P.E., Goldspink, G., 1984. Connective tissue changes in immobilised muscle. J. Anat. 138 (Pt 2), 343–350.

9. McLachlan, E.M., 1983. Atrophic effects of proximal tendon transection with and without denervation on mouse soleus muscles. Exp. Neurol. 81 (3), 651–668.

10. Ramachandran, V.S., 1993. Behavioral and magnetoencephalographic correlates of plasticity in the adult human brain. Proc. Natl. Acad. Sci. U.S.A. 90 (22), 10413–10420.

11. Bryden, A.M., Hoyen, H.A., et al., 2016. Upper extremity assessment in tetraplegia: the importance of differentiating between upper and lower motor neuron paralysis. Arch. Phys. Med. Rehabil. 97 (6 Suppl.), S97–S104.

12. Bryden, A.M., Kilgore, K.L., et al., 2004. Triceps denervation as a predictor of elbow flexion contractures in C5 and C6 tetraplegia. Arch. Phys. Med. Rehab. 85 (11), 1880–1885.

13. Vasudevan, S.V., Melvin, J.L., 1979. Upper extremity edema control: rationale of the techniques. Am. J. Occup. Ther. 33 (8), 520–523.

14. Miller, L.K., Jerosch-Herold, C., et al., 2017. Effectiveness of edema management techniques for subacute hand edema: a systematic review. J. Hand Ther. 30 (4), 432–446.

15. Krajnik, S.R., Bridle, M.J., 1992. Hand splinting in quadriplegia: current practice. Am. J. Occup. Ther. 46 (2), 149–156.

16. Wilton, J. Hand splinting/orthotic intervention: principles of design and fabrication. Vivid Publishing; 2014.

17. Glasgow, C., Tooth, L.R., et al., 2010. Mobilizing the stiff hand: combining theory and evidence to improve clinical outcomes. J. Hand Ther. 23 (4), 392–400, quiz 401.

18. Harvey, L., Baillie, R., et al., 2007. Does three months of nightly splinting reduce the extensibility of the flexor pollicis longus muscle in people with tetraplegia? Physiother. Res. Int. 12 (1), 5–13.

19. Diong, J., Harvey, L.A., et al., 2012. Incidence and predictors of contracture after spinal cord injury—a prospective cohort study. Spinal Cord 50 (8), 579–584.

20. Hardwick, D., Bryden, A., et al., 2018. Factors associated with upper extremity contractures after cervical spinal cord injury: a pilot study. J. Spinal Cord Med. 41 (3), 337–346.

21. Harvey, L., Herbert, R., et al., 2002. Does stretching induce lasting increases in joint ROM? A systematic review. Physiother. Res. Int. 7 (1), 1–13.

22. Harvey, L.A., Herbert, R.D., 2002. Muscle stretching for treatment and prevention of contracture in people with spinal cord injury. Spinal Cord 40 (1), 1–9.

23. Reznik, J., Keren, O., et al., 2016. Pharmacology Handbook for Physiotherapists. Elsevier, Sydney.

24. Tabary, J.C., Tabary, C., et al., 1972. Physiological and structural changes in the cat's soleus muscle due to immobilization at different lengths by plaster casts. J. Physiol. 224 (1), 231–244.

25. Welch, R.D., Lobley, S.J., et al., 1986. Functional independence in quadriplegia: critical levels. Arch. Phys. Med. Rehabil. 67 (4), 235–240.

26. Harvey, L., 2008. Management of Spinal Cord Injuries. A Guide for Physiotherapists. Elsevier Ltd, Sydney.

27. Carr, J.H., Shepherd, R.B., 2000. Movement Science: Foundations for Physical Therapy in Rehabilitation, second ed. Aspen Publishers, Gaithersburg, Md.

28. Bryden, A.M., Peljovich, A.E., et al., 2012. Surgical restoration of arm and hand function in people with tetraplegia. Top. Spinal Cord Inj. Rehabil. 18 (1), 43–49.

29. Shumway-Cook, A., Woollacott, M.H., 2012. Motor Control: Translating Research Into Clinical Practice, fourth ed. Wolters Kluwer Health/Lippincott Williams & Wilkins, Philadelphia.

30. Carr, J.H., Shepherd, R.B., 2010. Neurological Rehabilitation: Optimizing Motor Performance, second ed. Churchill Livingstone, Edinburgh, New York.

31. Rice, D., Faltynek, P., et al., 2016. Upper limb rehabilitation following spinal cord injury. In: Eng, J.J., Teasell, R.W., et al. (Eds.), Spinal Cord Injury Evidence. Vol Version 6.02016. pp. 1–121.

32. Johanson, M.E., Murray, W.M., 2002. The unoperated hand: the role of passive forces in hand function after tetraplegia. Hand Clin. 18 (3), 391–398.

33. Harvey, L.A., Batty, J., et al., 2001. Hand function of C6 and C7 tetraplegics 1 – 16 years following injury. Spinal Cord 39 (1), 37–43.

34. World Health Organization, 2002. International Classification of Functioning, Disability and Health. World Health Organization, Geneva.

35. Velstra, I.M., Ballert, C.S., et al., 2011. A systematic literature review of outcome measures for upper extremity function using the International Classification of Functioning, Disability, and Health as reference. Phys. Med. Rehabil. 3 (9), 846–860.

36. Sinnott, K.A., Dunn, J.A., et al., 2016. Measurement of outcomes of upper limb reconstructive surgery for tetraplegia. Arch. Phys. Med. Rehabil. 97 (6, Suppl.), S169–S181.

37. Moberg, E., 1975. Surgical treatment for absent single-hand grip and elbow extension in quadriplegia. Principles and preliminary experience. J. Bone Joint Surg. Am. 57A (196–206).

38. Dunn, J., Hay-Smith, E., et al., 2012. Issues influencing the decision to have upper limb surgery for people with tetraplegia. Spinal Cord 50 (11), 844–847.

39. Brown, J.M., 2011. Nerve transfers in tetraplegia I: background and technique. Surg. Neurol. Int. 2, 121.

40. Simcock, J.W., Dunn, J.A., et al., 2017. Identification of patients with cervical SCI suitable for early nerve transfer to achieve hand opening. Spinal Cord 55 (2), 131–134.

41. Bertelli, J.A., Ghizoni, M.F., 2015. Nerve transfers for elbow and finger extension reconstruction in midcervical spinal cord injuries. J. Neurosurg. 122 (1), 121–127.

42. Mohammed, K.D., Rothwell, A.G., et al., 1992. Upper limb surgery in tetraplegia. J. Bone Joint Surg. Br. 74B (6), 873–879.

43. Fridén, J., Gohritz, A., 2015. Tetraplegia management update. J. Hand Surg. 40 (12), 2489–2500.

44. McDowell, C.L., Moberg, E., et al., 1986. The second international conference on surgical rehabilitation of the upper limb in tetraplegia (quadriplegia). J. Hand Surg. 11A (4), 604–608.

45. Hahn, J., Cooper, C., et al., 2016. Rehabilitation of Supinator Nerve to Posterior Interosseous Nerve transfer in individuals with tetraplegia. Arch. Phys. Med. Rehab. 97 (6, Suppl.), S160–S168.

46. Bersch, I., Fridén, J., 2016. Role of functional electrical stimulation in tetraplegia hand surgery. Arch. Phys. Med. Rehabil. 97 (6, Suppl.), S154–S159.

47. Carr, J.H., Shepherd, R.B., 2011. Enhancing physical activity and brain reorganization after stroke. Neurol. Res. Int. 2011.

48. Wangdell, J., Carlsson, G., et al., 2014. From regained function to daily use: experiences of surgical reconstruction of grip in people with tetraplegia. Dis. Rehabil. 36 (8), 678–684.

49. Adams, M.M., Hicks, A.L., 2005. Spasticity after spinal cord injury. Spinal Cord 43 (10), 577.

50. Pidgeon, T.S., Ramirez, J.M., et al., 2015. Orthopaedic management of spasticity. RI Med. J. 98 (12), 26–31.

51. Wangdell, J., Fridén, J., 2016. Rehabilitation after spasticity-correcting upper limb surgery in tetraplegia. Arch. Phys. Med. Rehab. 97 (6, Suppl.), S136–S143.

52. Wangdell, J., Friden, J., 2012. Activity gains after reconstruction of elbow extension in patients with tetraplegia. J. Hand Surg. 37 (5), 1003–1010.

53. Dunn, J.A., Hay-Smith, E.J.C., et al., 2013. Liminality and decision making for upper limb surgery in tetraplegia: a grounded theory. Dis. Rehabil. 35 (15), 1293–1301.

54. Bunketorp-Kall, L., Wangdell, J., et al., 2017. Satisfaction with upper limb reconstructive surgery in individuals with tetraplegia: the development and reliability of a Swedish self-reported satisfaction questionnaire. Spinal Cord 55 (7), 664.

55. Dunn, J.A., Rothwell, A.G., et al., 2014. The effects of aging on upper limb tendon transfers in patients with tetraplegia. J. Hand Surg. 39 (2), 317–323.

CHAPTER 18

Common complications of spinal cord injury

Jacqueline Reznik, Marnie Graco, David Berlowitz and Anthony Wright

Acute complications following spinal cord injury (SCI) are dealt with in earlier chapters of this book. They include motor and sensory deficits, and instabilities of the cardiovascular, thermoregulatory and bronchopulmonary systems.

In this chapter, four of the most common complications associated with chronic SCI will be discussed. These include: neurogenic bladder and bowel, sleep apnoea, pain and neurogenic heterotopic ossification.

1. NEUROGENIC BLADDER AND BOWEL

Jacqueline Reznik

NEUROGENIC BLADDER

Neurogenic bladder (NGB) is a term applied to urinary bladder malfunction due to neurological dysfunction arising from internal or external trauma, disease or injury,[1] and is a common complication following SCI. In the United States it has been reported that more than 80% of patients with an SCI exhibit bladder dysfunction.[2] NGB negatively impacts on functional recovery, health-related quality of life (QoL), length of stay and healthcare costs due to the loss of voluntary bladder control and increased risk of urinary tract infection (UTI).[3,4]

Urological management is a primary care priority for both inpatient and community-based persons with an SCI. Urological management includes a broad range of interventions, including catheterisation approaches, for example, indwelling, intermittent and suprapubic; assisted bladder emptying; electrical stimulation; pharmacological agents; and surgery.[2]

Pathophysiology

Normal micturition requires the coordination of a neuronal circuit between the brain and spinal cord, and the bladder and urethra. The sacral micturition centre (S2–S4), pontine micturition centre and cerebral cortex are responsible for the facilitation and inhibition of voiding. Parasympathetic efferents from the sacral cord at S2–S4 via the pelvic nerves provide excitatory input to the bladder. Bladder contraction results from muscarinic receptor stimulation. The external sphincter is inhibited through somatic nerves via the pudendal nerve. The sympathetic efferents originate from the intermediolateral grey column T11–L2 and supply the bladder and urethra. These nerves provide inhibitory input to the bladder through the hypogastric nerve. Sympathetic stimulation causes relaxation of the bladder through beta receptor stimulation and contraction of the sphincter through alpha receptor stimulation (Fig. 18.1).[2]

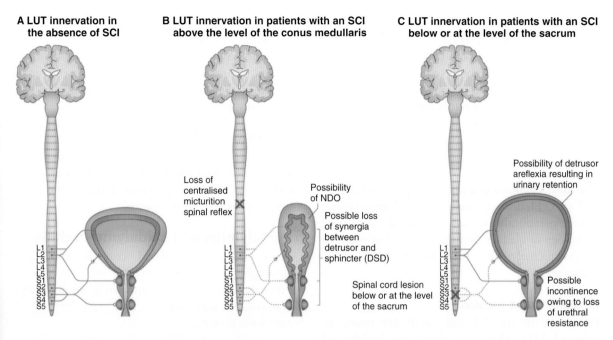

A LUT innervation in the absence of SCI

B LUT innervation in patients with an SCI above the level of the conus medullaris

Loss of centralised micturition spinal reflex

Possibility of NDO

Possible loss of synergia between detrusor and sphincter (DSD)

Spinal cord lesion below or at the level of the sacrum

C LUT innervation in patients with an SCI below or at the level of the sacrum

Possibility of detrusor areflexia resulting in urinary retention

Possible incontinence owing to loss of urethral resistance

Figure 18.1 Types of bladder dysfunction typically observed after SCI.

Key: LUT lower urinary tract; NDO neurogenic detrusor overactivity; DSD detrusor sphinter dyssynergia

Source: Wyndaele J.-J., 2016. The management of neurogenic lower urinary tract dysfunction after spinal cord injury. Nat. Rev. Urol. 13 (12), 705–714.

Spinal shock

Spinal shock occurs following an acute SCI and can last for up to 3 months (see Chapter 4 for further information on spinal shock). Autonomic activation of the bladder by the parasympathetic nerves is rendered inactive. The bladder becomes atonic, and there is no conscious awareness of bladder filling. Interruption of the neuraxis below the pons due to SCI eliminates the micturition reflex, which causes urine retention. Initial urodynamic studies should be performed after the patient is beyond the spinal shock phase, and urine retention should be managed initially with an indwelling catheter (IDC), transitioning to intermittent catheterisation (IC) as soon as possible.[5] After spinal shock, involuntary and uncoordinated bladder contraction might occur and result in reflex bladder function.[6]

Suprasacral lesion

Reflex bladder function will occur following spinal shock, in lesions above S1. Consciousness of bladder-filling might not be totally absent; however, voluntary inhibition of the micturition reflex is lost. Typical urodynamic findings include neurogenic detrusor overactivity (NDO) and detrusor sphincter dyssynergia (DSD). Dis-coordinated contraction will result in high voiding pressure, residual urine volume and urinary incontinence, which, if not treated, will result in upper tract deterioration and renal failure.[2]

Sacral lesion

Spinal cord lesions at the sacral level result in parasympathetic decentralisation of the bladder and denervation of the sphincter. In cases of complete lesion, conscious awareness of bladder filling is lost, and the micturition reflex is absent.

Patients will have acontractile bladders with competent but non-relaxing smooth and striated sphincters that retain some fixed tone. The classic outlet findings are a competent but non-relaxing smooth sphincter and a striated sphincter that retains some fixed tone but is not under voluntary control.[2]

COMPLICATIONS OF NGB

The most common complications of NGB due to SCI are UTI, urinary stones and renal impairment. These complications are associated with the pathology of bladder dysfunction itself or occur as a consequence of the use of urinary catheters for drainage.

Urinary tract infection

Patients with an SCI and NGB are prone to repeated UTIs that pose significant health and wellbeing problems. They also have a substantial effect on healthcare costs, being a frequent cause of re-admission to hospital for this patient group.[7] Symptomatic UTIs might include fever, foul smelling urine and/or haematuria. Other more complex symptoms of UTIs in persons with an SCI include increased hypertonicity or in severe cases autonomic dysreflexia (see Chapter 4 on spasticity and autonomic dysreflexia).

Bladder catheterisation practices following acute SCI also influence bladder health. Prolonged use of an indwelling catheter (IDC) increases the risk of UTIs and resulting re-admissions and health effects. Transitioning from IDC to IC – where the bladder is emptied at a specified frequency by inserting a catheter and then removing it after complete drainage – reduces the incidence of bladder problems such as UTIs.[7]

Management/treatment of UTIs

Prophylaxis does not appear to significantly decrease symptomatic infections but may be associated with a reduction in asymptomatic bacteriuria.[2] Importantly, prophylaxis results in a two-fold increase in antimicrobial-resistant bacteria. Modification of antibiotic treatment regimens might reduce drug resistance. SCI-neurogenic bladder dysfunction on IC and recurrent UTIs requires multiple courses of antibiotic therapy which increases the incidence of multidrug-resistant bacteria.[2]

Urethritis and prostatitis

In order to decrease the possibility of urethritis, patients are recommended to use IC and avoid indwelling catheters. *Escherichia coli* is the most frequent bacteria in prostatitis.

Epididymitis and epididymo-orchitis

These are catheter-related complications, and although patients with an SCI will not usually experience pain, they might exhibit swelling and occasionally skin redness. Treatment consists of antibiotic therapy.

Bladder and renal stones

High residual urine levels and IDCs are the main two reasons for bladder stone formation. Stone formation can cause severe irritative symptoms and haematuria. Weekly catheter changes may reduce the possibility of bladder stone formation.[2]

Renal stones have an overall incidence of 3.5% in patients with NGB. Successful treatment depends upon complete elimination of the calculus and eradication of the infection.[8] Depending upon stone location, size and the extent of the symptoms, lithotripsy may be a treatment option for both bladder and renal stones. Renal stones will only be removed if they are in a problematic location or are causing problems, otherwise they will just be monitored.[8,9]

Reflux and renal insufficiency

Vesicoureteral reflux occurs in more than 20% of patients with NGB and is more common in suprasacral lesions. High detrusor pressure and reflux are responsible for renal damage and renal failure. The best treatment for reflux is to normalise the detrusor pressure.

Bladder cancer

The risk of bladder cancer is 20 times higher in persons with an SCI compared to the general population, with squamous cell cancer occurring more commonly than transitional cell cancer. The risk factors are UTI, bladder stones and indwelling catheters. Unfortunately, the diagnosis is usually made in the more advanced stages.

EVALUATION OF PATIENTS WITH NEUROGENIC BLADDER

This is covered during the initial assessment of the patient, as outlined in Chapter 4. The initial evaluation includes history-taking and a voiding diary. The examiner should determine the level of the spinal motor lesion, the extent of injury, i.e. whether it is complete or incomplete, limb tone, rectal tone and the bulbocavernosus reflex.[10] In their review, Al Taweel and Seyam[2] strongly recommend video urodynamics as the most comprehensive assessment procedure for all patients with NGB.

Conservative management

Factors that need to be considered when choosing an appropriate method of bladder management in patients with an SCI include: age, gender, comorbidities, level and completeness of injury, upper extremity function, availability and compliance of caregiver assistance, body habits, spasticity and, in developing countries, access to running water, sanitation and catheter supplies.

Intermittent catheterisation is the most effective method of bladder management in patients with NGB, and is now considered to be the 'gold-standard' approach to treatment.[11] Following this, a suprapubic catheter is preferred if IC is not possible. Other management options might include timed voiding, the Valsalva and Credé manoeuvre (executed by exerting manual pressure on the abdomen at the location of the bladder, just below the navel) and triggered reflex voiding with and without sphincterotomy. These options are now generally discouraged due to the risk of high detrusor pressures

and subsequent upper tract damage. Patients with an SCI are most likely to choose treatments that they regard as most convenient to their lifestyle (Fig. 18.2).

Pharmacological interventions

Romo and colleagues presented their conclusions on oral drug therapy with relevant levels of evidence, as shown in Table 18.1.[5]

The use of Botulinum neurotoxin (in the form of onabotulinumtoxinA, or BoNTA) has changed the rate of bladder augmentations over the past 20 years. Conclusions reached by Roma and colleagues[5] are listed below, followed by levels of evidence (LOEs):

- BoNTA bladder injections are effective in the treatment of SCI neurogenic bladder related DO and incontinence. BoNTA also improves urodynamic detrusor storage pressure, compliance and cystometric capacity, as well as patient quality of life (LOE-I).

- In NGB patients, 200 U has excellent clinical effectiveness with only slightly better results with 300 U; however, both doses are safe (LOE-I).

- Limited data suggest that BoNTA injections into the external urethral sphincter can be effective in some male patients with an SCI. The optimal patient for this treatment would be: (1) someone without bladder neck obstruction; (2) someone with some ability to void; and (3) someone who is unsure of their ability to maintain a condom catheter and who is interested in a reversible treatment option, whether it is because they may not want to manage their bladders chronically this way and/or their hope of neuro-recovery in the future (LOE-III).

- Repeat bladder injections of BoNTA are safe and the effects sustainable (LOE-III).

- There is a high risk of urinary retention with bladder injection of BoNTA, particularly in patients with neurogenic bladder who are voiding (LOE-I).

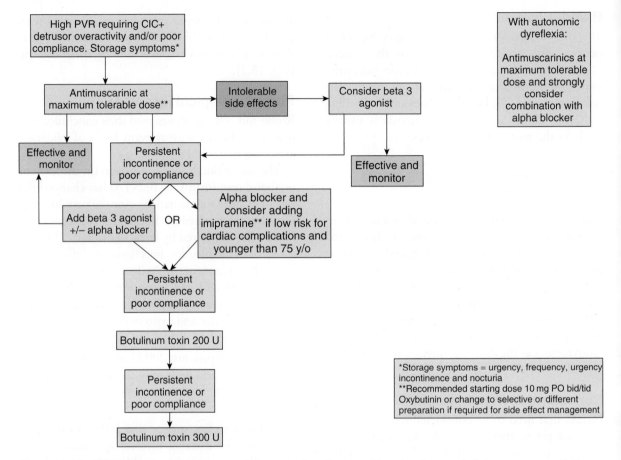

Figure 18.2 Algorithm for bladder management of patients with retention and detrusor overactivity or poor bladder compliance due to neurogenic bladder.
Source: Roma P.G.B., Smith C.P., et al., 2018. Non-surgical urologic management of neurogenic bladder after spinal cord injury. World Journal of Urology 36 (10), 1555–1568.

- BoNTA antibodies can occur due to prior exposure to the drug, but can resolve over time (LOE-III).

Surgical management

A number of surgical options are possible for those patients who fail conservative or pharmacological treatments. These surgical options vary from simple to complex, i.e. non-invasive to highly invasive, and include surgery to promote urine storage, facilitation of bladder emptying or even circumventing the problem. Wyndaele and colleagues published a comprehensive literature search on a variety of surgical techniques which have been applied to patients with an SCI for NGB.[12] They concluded that the choice of techniques proposed to the patients depends upon the exact functional pathology in bladder, bladder neck and urethral sphincter. The final informed choice is to be made by the patient.

Other treatment options

- Neuromodulation/electrical stimulation
- Nerve grafting/nerve transfer

Table 18.1 Oral drug therapy of the injured bladder after SCI

Drug	Effects	LOE
Anticholinergics (oxybutynin is the most studied of this class)	Improve bladder capacity, incontinence, lower urinary tract symptoms and bladder compliance and reduce upper tract complications in patients with an SCI who manage their bladder with either IC or indwelling catheters	I
Mirabegron either as an alternative or an addition to anticholinergics It is an agonist of beta 3 adrenergic receptors	Activates beta 3 adrenergic receptors in the detrusor muscle of the bladder Shows promising positive effects but requires validation	III
Alpha adrenergic blockers	Facilitates voiding and increases the capacity and compliance in combination with anticholinergics	III
Desmopressin Synthetic form of vasopressin	Successful treatment of nocturnal polyuria	III

LOE – Level of Evidence; SCI – Spinal Cord Injury; IC – Intermittent Catheterisation

Source: Adapted from Roma P.G.B., Smith C.P., et al., 2018. Non-surgical urologic management of neurogenic bladder after spinal cord injury. World Journal of Urology 36 (10), 1555–1568.

- Muscle grafts
- Urethral stents
- Bladder tissue engineering.

NEUROGENIC BOWEL

Neurogenic bowel disorder (NBD), particularly constipation and faecal incontinence, is highly prevalent in patients with an SCI, estimates sometimes being as high as 75% of all patients.[13] NBD and NGB disorders are strong predictors for mortality, occurrence of complications and re-admission to hospital,[14] causing significant impact on QoL.[15]

NBD due to SCI has been traditionally categorised according to the neurological level of injury, with implications for bowel symptoms, pathophysiology and approach to management. Injury to the cauda equina with resulting bowel dysfunction is also common. Although NBD is more likely to develop in patients with a complete SCI, it is also highly prevalent in patients with an incomplete SCI, having a substantial effect on the patient's lifestyle, medication use and QoL.[16]

Neurogenic bowel physiology

NBD in patients with an SCI shows up as changes in colon motility and/or loss of anorectal sphincter function. Patients with injuries above the conus medullaris (above approximately L1–L2) generally have symptoms of increased bowel motility and poor anorectal sphincter relaxation. Patients with injuries below the conus medullaris (below approximately L2) are more likely to have an areflexic colon and low anal sphincter tone (Fig. 18.3).[16]

Assessment tools

As with the NGB, no specific assessment tool has been universally accepted. In their recent review, Stoffel and colleagues[16] suggest that different conclusions may be drawn, depending upon which assessment tool is used.

Treatment

Treatment plans for SCI-related neurogenic bowel are directed to timely, predictable evacuation of the bowels. It is important to recognise that the achievement of successful treatment regimens

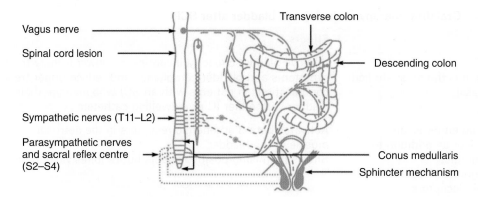

Figure 18.3 **Innervation of the colon, anal sphincters and pelvic floor.**
Source: Pryor, J., Fisher, M., Middleton, J., 2014. Management of the Neurogenic bowel for adults with spinal cord injuries. NSW Agency for Clinical Innovation, Chatswood.

require the appropriate level of caregiver support and resources for the patient with an SCI.

Management of neurogenic bowel can be summarised as follows:[16]

- High-fibre diet may increase colon transit time, resulting in more constipation in patients with an SCI.[17]
- Transanal irrigation is an effective, low-morbidity intervention for refractory neurogenic bowel in patients with an SCI.[16]

- Neurostimulation and neuromodulation have shown positive results, but to date numbers are small and these interventions are still considered to be experimental in the management of NBD for patients with an SCI.[13]
- Colostomy may significantly reduce stool transit time in patients with an SCI compared to conservative bowel management plans.[18]
- Colostomy may offer better QoL compared to ileostomy.[19]

Evidence-based practice points

- NGB and NBD disorders are strong predictors for mortality, occurrence of complications and re-admission to hospital, causing significant impact on QoL.
- Urological management is a primary care priority for both inpatient and community-based persons with an SCI.
- Urological management includes a broad range of interventions, including catheterisation approaches, for example, indwelling, intermittent and suprapubic; assisted bladder emptying; electrical stimulation; pharmacological agents; and surgery.
- The most common complications of neurogenic bladder due to SCI are UTI, urinary stones and renal impairment.

Evidence-based practice points—cont'd

- The most frequently applied treatment option for NGB is conservative management. This approach to treatment relies upon patient education and might include timed voiding, the Credé manoeuvres, medications, intermittent catheterisation or an IDC.
- A number of surgical options varying from simple to complex is possible for those patients who fail conservative or pharmacological treatments.
- NBD, particularly constipation and faecal incontinence, may be as high as 75% of all patients with an SCI.
- Patients with injuries above the conus medullaris (above approximately L1–L2) generally have symptoms of increased bowel motility and poor anorectal sphincter relaxation. Patients with injuries below the conus medullaris (below approximately L2) are more likely to have an areflexic colon and low anal sphincter tone.
- Treatment plans for SCI-related neurogenic bowel are directed to timely, predictable evacuation of the bowels.
- No universally accepted assessment tools are available for NGB and NBD, hence it is difficult to develop useful clinical practice guidelines.

SUMMARY

The importance of good bladder and bowel management cannot be overemphasised in the acute phase in order to reduce long-term complications and increase QoL for the individual with an SCI. The opportunities arise for both physiotherapists and occupational therapists to be imaginative and potentially build devices that can assist with ICs when there is poor hand function.

It is also important to build universally accepted assessment tools for both NGB and NBD in order to develop useful clinical practice guidelines.

2. SLEEP DISORDERED BREATHING

Marnie Graco and David Berlowitz

INTRODUCTION

Sleep disorders are highly prevalent in SCI with a demonstrated negative impact on quality of life (QoL).[20,21] The literature demonstrates that individuals with an SCI are more likely than the general population to experience greater levels of sleep disturbance and daytime sleepiness, use sleeping pills and snore than a normative population.[22] Although the causes of poor sleep in people with an SCI are not clear, a tendency towards obesity, sleeping in supine position, nasal congestion, disruption of the melatonin pathway, pain, spasm and medications are all thought to contribute to the increased prevalence of sleep disorders in this population.[23]

This portion of the chapter on common complications of an SCI focuses on obstructive sleep apnoea (OSA) in tetraplegia because it is the most prevalent sleep disorder in persons with an SCI and provides an overview of the epidemiology, pathophysiology, morbidity and recommended management of OSA. It discusses the current clinical management of OSA, including issues with access to services, and provides insights from people with tetraplegia who have been diagnosed with, and treated for, OSA.

WHAT IS SLEEP DISORDERED BREATHING?

Sleep disordered breathing is characterised by repetitive periods of total cessation in breathing (apnoeas) or reductions in breathing (hypopnoeas) that occur during sleep. These events are typically associated with a reduction in oxygen saturation and an arousal from sleep. Sleep disordered breathing is an umbrella term representing a group of sleep disorders involving the respiratory system. According to the International Classification of Sleep Disorders, sleep disordered breathing consists of three main categories of disorders: OSA, central sleep apnoea (CSA) disorders and sleep-related hypoventilation disorders. All of these are known to affect people with an SCI, particularly those with tetraplegia.[24]

The pathophysiological mechanisms underpinning the breathing disruption define the different groups of disorders. OSA is characterised by complete or partial obstruction of the upper airway resulting in complete or reduced airflow. In contrast, CSA is primarily due to a reduced chemical and/or neural drive to breathe. While the reduction in airflow may be essentially the same, it is the absence of respiratory effort at the time of reduced airflow that distinguishes CSA from OSA. Sleep-related hypoventilation disorders are characterised by reduced ventilation and gas exchange during sleep.

OBSTRUCTIVE SLEEP APNOEA

Epidemiology of OSA in persons with an SCI

OSA is the most common sleep disorder in persons with an SCI. Population surveys published in the last decade suggest that the prevalence of OSA in individuals with tetraplegia lies somewhere between 53% and 97%.[23,25] In contrast, a recent meta-analysis of OSA prevalence among the non-disabled estimated rates of between 9% and 38%.[26]

Characteristics significantly associated with OSA have included: higher (cervical) lesions, complete injuries, larger neck circumference, obesity, supine sleeping position, increasing age, increasing time since injury, male gender, cardiac and antispasmodic medications, daytime sleepiness, self-reported snoring and awakenings.[23]

A seminal study by Berlowitz and colleagues[27] investigated incidence of OSA in acute tetraplegia by following a cohort of people with new tetraplegic injuries for 12 months. Within 2 weeks of injury, 60% of the sample had developed OSA and prevalence peaked at 83% 3 months after injury. Only three (10% of the sample) were predicted to have had OSA prior to their injury. As a result of this study, OSA is considered to be a direct consequence of tetraplegia. While there is less published data in paraplegia, it is generally considered that risk factors in paraplegia are overall more similar to those in the non-disabled community rather than 'SCI specific'.

Morbidity of OSA in tetraplegia

People living with OSA and tetraplegia have a substantially lower health utility value than their tetraplegic peers without OSA. This would suggest that effectively treating OSA might substantially improve health and QoL for these individuals.[20]

OSA is also associated with impaired cognition in people with chronic tetraplegia, particularly in the areas of attention, concentration, memory and learning skills.[28] Analysis of neuropsychological function in people with OSA following acute tetraplegia (approximately 2–3 months after injury) found that more severe OSA was associated with poorer attention, information processing and immediate recall.[29] Impairment in neuropsychological function is likely to affect vocational outcomes, particularly for people with tetraplegia, whose physical disabilities usually limit engagement in physical jobs.

Diagnosis of OSA

Sleep disordered breathing is usually assessed by a combination of clinical presentations and an objective sleep study. Sleep studies can be divided into four categories, from Level I to Level IV. They can be supervised or unattended, and their duration can be full night, split night (diagnostic followed by treatment) or restricted.[30]

The 'gold-standard' sleep study is a Level I, overnight, attended polysomnography (PSG). Level I studies involve an overnight stay in a sleep laboratory where the individual is connected to a multichannel device, which takes a comprehensive recording of the biophysiological changes that occur during sleep. It is a highly specialised test, which requires a sleep scientist and sleep physician for analysis and reporting. Level I studies are often accompanied by arterial blood gas analysis and/or transcutaneous monitoring of CO_2 pressure for detection of hypoventilation. The signals required for a Level I PSG are illustrated in Fig. 18.4 and include electroencephalogram (EEG), electromyogram (EMG), electrooculogram (EOG), airflow sensor (nasal pressure and oronasal thermistor), respiratory effort sensors, pulse oximetry (SpO_2), electrocardiograph (ECG), body position, leg movement and snoring sensor.[24,30]

A staged and scored Level I PSG will produce a metric known as the apnoea hypopnoea index (AHI). This is the number of apnoeas and hypopnoeas per hour of sleep. Different thresholds for the AHI are used to diagnose OSA and its severity (Fig. 18.5).

By contrast, Level II sleep studies are conducted with a portable PSG device and are 'unattended' by staff, enabling them to be performed at home rather than in a sleep laboratory. Level II studies must still include EEG, EOG, EMG, ECG, oxygen saturation, airflow and respiratory effort recordings.

However, due to financial, logistical and failure rate issues, they may not be commonly used in clinical practice.[30]

Level III and IV sleep studies record fewer signals and are frequently referred to as 'limited channel studies'. These studies typically do not measure EEG, rendering sleep staging impossible. Oximetry has been suggested as the single most important signal for the diagnosis of sleep disordered breathing. Overnight oximetry (Level IV studies) and partial channel/partial time devices (Level III studies) have been studied as cheaper and more accessible alternatives to full PSG.[30]

As alternatives to full PSG, few screening tools developed for non-disabled populations have been tested in people with an SCI. Questionnaires commonly used to identify OSA in non-disabled populations have performed poorly when applied to people with an SCI.[20,31]

Treatment for OSA

Applying positive airway pressure (PAP) via a mask to stabilise the upper airway is the primary respiratory treatment for sleep disordered breathing, including OSA, CSA and sleep-related hypoventilation. Continuous Positive Airway Pressure (CPAP) and bi-level PAP are the most widely known and prescribed forms of PAP (see Chapter 16 for further information on respiratory management of high cervical lesions).

CPAP

CPAP remains the first-line treatment for OSA. CPAP maintains a continuous PAP, typically 4 to 20 cmH_2O, throughout inspiration and expiration during sleep to prevent upper airway collapse. Overnight manual or automatic pressure titration determines the optimal level that abolishes hypopnoeas and apnoeas. Typically, patients attend a sleep laboratory for manual titration and initiation of CPAP, whereas automatic titration may potentially be undertaken at home. Fixed CPAP prescription can be based on the 90th percentile pressures provided from up to 1 week of automatic PAP.[32] Fixed CPAP

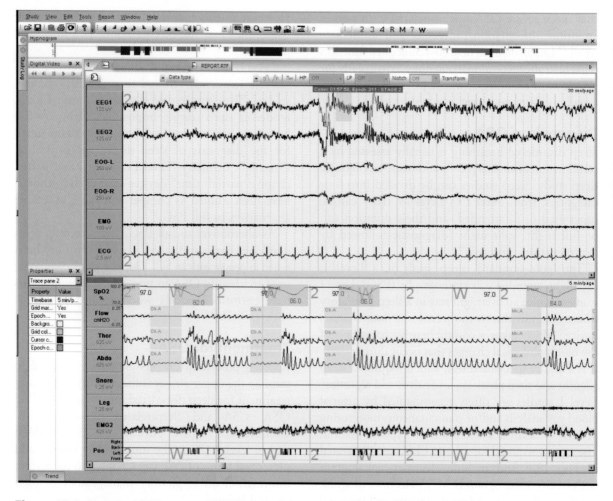

Figure 18.4 A typical PSG montage, showing 30 seconds of EEG recording and 5 minutes of respiratory data recording.

The signals included are (from top to bottom):

- two electroencephalograms to record brain waves, required for analysis of sleep and its stages (EEG1 and EEG2)
- bilateral electrooculogram to record eye movements in sleep, required for detection of REM sleep (EOG-L and EOG-R)
- electromyogram to record muscle activity (e.g masseter muscle), required for detection of REM sleep (EMG)
- electrocardiograph (ECG) to detect heart rate and rhythm
- pulse oximeter, to detect oxygen saturation and pulse
- airflow sensor (nasal pressure and oronasal thermistor)
- respiratory effort sensors (thorax and abdomen). These are bands around the thorax and abdomen to detect movement of the chest wall and abdomen
- snoring sensor, usually by microphone
- leg movement sensors, usually EMG of tibialis anterior to detect periodic leg movements during sleep (Leg)
- an additional sensor (option EMG2) for this research study is a surface diaphragm EMG sensor to detect respiratory activity
- body position sensor (Pos), which detects whether the patient is lying on their back, front, right or left side.

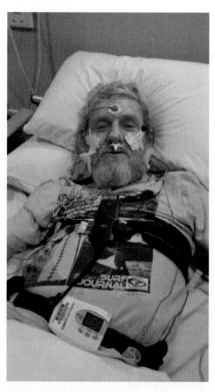

Figure 18.5 Example of patient set-up for Level 1 PSG.

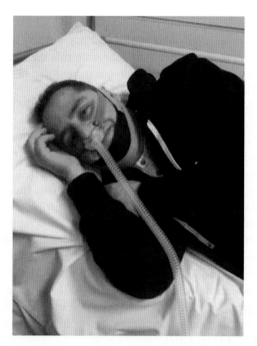

Figure 18.6 An individual with an SCI receiving CPAP.

in tetraplegia appears lower than in the non-disabled for any given degree of OSA severity (Fig. 18.6).[33]

CPAP has been shown to improve daytime sleepiness, measures of sleep quality, health-related QoL and mood in people without disability.[24] A meta-review of neurocognitive function in OSA concluded that CPAP appears to improve executive function, memory, attention and global cognitive function.

To date, only one clinical trial has examined the effect of CPAP in persons with an SCI. This international multi-site randomised controlled trial examined the effect of CPAP on neuropsychological function, sleepiness, QoL, anxiety and depression and found that while CPAP significantly improved sleepiness after acute tetraplegia, it did not improve the neurocognitive function beyond that seen with post-injury, spontaneous recovery.[34]

Despite the known benefits of CPAP, its effectiveness is limited by poor adherence to the therapy. When defined as an average of at least 4 hours per night, adherence to CPAP in the non-disabled population is reported to range between 30% and 60%.[35] Recent studies have estimated CPAP adherence in people with tetraplegia to be around 25%.[34,36]

A significant limitation of CPAP effectiveness is poor adherence and acceptance of the therapy. When adherence is defined as greater than 4 hours per night, rates of 30–60% are reported in the non-disabled population with OSA.[37]

Other treatments

Bi-level PAP may also be used to treat OSA, although it is more commonly used to provide respiratory support to treat hypoventilation disorders. Bi-level PAP provides a higher pressure during inspiration and lower pressure during expiration, which increases overall minute ventilation and is suggested to be more comfortable for the individual. Bi-level PAP is often trialled clinically after the patient has 'failed CPAP'; however, clinical trials investigating this method in non-disabled populations do not suggest that bi-level PAP is better tolerated.[38]

Mandibular advancement splints have been prescribed as an alternative to CPAP or as a first-line treatment for mild OSA. These mouthguard-like devices pull the lower jaw forwards to open up the upper airway posteriorly and increase the tension in the soft tissues and muscles of the throat, thereby making it less likely to collapse during sleep. Similar improvements to sleepiness, neurocognitive performance and functional outcomes have been observed in non-disabled populations with a mandibular advancement splint compared to CPAP, although they do not reduce the AHI to the same degree.[24] As yet, there have been no published trials of mandibular advancement splints in people with an SCI (Fig. 18.7).

Positional therapy to prevent supine sleeping may be effective for patients whose respiratory events occur predominantly when they are in the supine position; however, clinical practice in many spinal units is to 'train' supine sleep in an attempt to manage pressure injury risk. Weight loss and bariatric surgery reduce OSA severity in obese patients. Surgery on the upper airway (e.g. tonsillectomy, nasal septoplasty) may be effective for patients whose upper airway anatomy has been assessed as contributing to OSA

and is suitable for the procedure.[24] None of these alternatives has been systematically trialled in people with an SCI.

Patient experiences

Poor sleep quality and quantity, including frequent disturbances, and poor sleep patterns were identified as major issues for people with an SCI.[21] The factors contributing to poor sleep included:

- SCI dysfunction and care – such as bladder management, medications and positioning
- sleep environment – particularly for those in institutions such as hospitals or care homes
- pain and mental health issues
- occupational disengagement, daytime fatigue and impaired cognitive functioning.

The barriers and enablers to CPAP use among people with tetraplegia have also been investigated qualitatively.[36] This study found the burdens of CPAP to be substantial in this population, and included mask discomfort, skin breakdown, dry eyes/mouth and psychosocial problems such as guilt about partner burden, frustration, fear and claustrophobia.

The following are quotes from people taking part in this study:

> 'My eyes are very sore of a morning, and my mouth gets very dry.' (65-year-old female, C6 AIS-C)

> 'I finished up with pressure marks on the inside of my septum and then I think I had a scab under my nose, which has gone now.' (71-year-old male, C6 AIS-A)

> 'It makes me feel like I'm a nuisance. Waking up my husband once a night is fine, but four to five times, I think that's a bit unfair. It's a big ask.' (65-year-old female, C6 AIS-C)

> 'I also found that lying down flat, and I couldn't move, that anything could have happened to me. I had no control over it, and being claustrophobic, that made it worse as well.' (65-year-old female, C6 AIS-C)

These problems were frequently being managed alongside other secondary complications of an

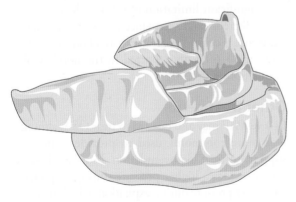

Figure 18.7 Mandibular advancement device.

SCI, and some individuals felt that CPAP added a substantial burden to an already difficult routine.

> 'I guess it's just another thing you have to do. Just another thing that you need to worry about, to annoy you.' (43-year-old male, C6 AIS-A)

Significant trial and error was required and participants of this study reported making active decisions about whether the benefits outweighed the burdens.

Common benefits included improvements to sleep quality, less daytime sleepiness and napping, fewer leg spasms and improvements to mood, energy levels, concentration and productivity.

> 'On days where I do use CPAP and I sleep fine with it, I feel like I can just fly out of bed.' (23-year-old male, C7 AIS-A)

> 'With the CPAP I'm finding that I'm more alert and I don't need a nap. I can stay awake in the afternoon.' (65-year-old female, C6 AIS-C)

> 'I feel so refreshed. I've got more energy, more get up and go.' (71-year-old male, C6 AIS-A)

> 'My family notice that I'm not as short and as sharp.' (75-year-old male, C6 AIS-B)

Participants were motivated by their immediate daytime benefits of CPAP, and were less concerned with long-term consequences of untreated OSA.

> 'The main reason I am using CPAP is so I'll have better days, physically and mentally.' (65-year-old female, C6 AIS-C)

Patient-reported barriers to diagnosis of sleep disordered breathing were also described in this study. Daytime sleepiness is commonly not recognised by people with tetraplegia, or it is incorrectly attributed to ageing with an SCI.

> 'I didn't realise I had sleep apnoea, I just took it for granted that this is what happens as you get old with tetraplegia. I thought, 'well, just suck it up'. But now I realise what I've been missing out on.' (71-year-old male, C6 AIS-A)

Many people with tetraplegia reported reluctance to attend a sleep laboratory for an overnight sleep study, because of the potential disruption to their healthcare routines, and the inability of these services to meet the care needs of people with an SCI.

> 'And being in a wheelchair, the thought of having to travel somewhere to go and do a sleep study and stay overnight, it's not very appealing.' (49-year-old male, C5 AIS-B)

CLINICAL PRACTICE GUIDELINES FOR THE MANAGEMENT OF OSA IN PEOPLE WITH AN SCI

Although the evidence supporting treatments for OSA in people with an SCI is limited, current guidelines developed by the Consortium for Spinal Cord Medicine recommend PSG evaluation for all people with an SCI with excessive daytime sleepiness or other symptoms for sleep disordered breathing.[39] These guidelines also recommend the prescription of PAP therapy, starting with CPAP, for those with a positive diagnosis of OSA. Similar recommendations have been published by the Spinal Cord Injury Rehabilitation Evidence (SCIRE) project.[40] The SCIRE recommendations include vigilance for suggestive signs and symptoms and further testing with oximetry or PSG when these signs are present. Both guidelines are underpinned by evidence from non-controlled studies, and based on strong clinical opinion.

Both guidelines recommend diagnosis of OSA with PSG; however, access to PSG is limited. While the true proportion of people with tetraplegia and undiagnosed OSA is unknown, available data suggest that it is high. Two separate audit studies of spinal units have estimated that only 15–20% of patients are diagnosed with OSA.[41,42] Given OSA prevalence estimates of 53–97% in people with tetraplegia, this represents an enormous burden of disease that is overlooked. If these data are accurate, the proportion of those with undetected OSA lies between 45% and 82%. The usual model of care for people with an SCI and symptoms of OSA is referral from the GP or spinal rehabilitation doctor to a specialist sleep or respiratory physician for further investigation and management.

Evidence-based practice points

Screening and diagnosis

- Most people with tetraplegia have sleep disordered breathing, and, as such, should be screened.
- Witnessed apnoeas and snoring during sleep are highly likely to be associated with OSA.
- Daytime sleepiness is often poorly recognised by people with an SCI and their health professionals. Sleepiness and fatigue may be wrongly attributed to ageing, medication and other comorbidities.
- Risk factors for sleep disordered breathing in paraplegia have not been well described, but are likely to be similar to those in the non-disabled population.
- Diagnosis is typically made following referral for a sleep specialist review.

Treatment

- Positive airway pressure (PAP) therapy is the mainstay treatment for sleep disordered breathing.
- For those who use PAP therapy well, the benefits are substantial.
- Adherence with PAP therapy can be challenging in tetraplegia because of the additional physiological, physical and psychosocial challenges of living with an SCI.
- People with tetraplegia require more support for longer to overcome these challenges when compared to their non-disabled peers with sleep disordered breathing.

SUMMARY

Sleep disorders are highly prevalent in people with an SCI. Obstructive sleep apnoea is the most prevalent of these, particularly in tetraplegia. The mainstay of treatment is CPAP, however adherence to therapy appears more challenging in tetraplegia than for the non-disabled. In those able to tolerate treatment, the benefits can be profound and as such, there is an urgent need to develop new, perhaps combinations of therapies that work synergistically to reduce OSA severity to a level that confers demonstrable benefit.

For further insight into these issues please watch the 4-minute video (located in Online resources section at the end of the chapter), which looks at four patients with an SCI discussing the importance of being tested for sleep apnoea and the positive effects of the use of a CPAP machine.

3. PAIN

Anthony Wright

INTRODUCTION

One of the most common and disabling features of SCI is the development of chronic pain. While it may not be the first issue that would be commonly associated with SCI, patients have rated pain as the third most difficult problem they face following SCI, behind reduced mobility and reduced sexual function.[43] Those people with an SCI who experience pain also rate their global health as being significantly worse than those who do not experience pain, and it has been shown to have a significant impact on their mood.[43] Chronic pain is therefore an important and sometimes unrecognised and underestimated complication of an SCI. It has the capacity to negatively impact quality of life (QoL), social functioning, employment, mood and participation in rehabilitation and treatment.[44]

Management of chronic pain is often challenging and made more complex by the effects of an SCI.

Therefore, many people with an SCI experience sub-optimal pain management.[45]

PAIN PRESENTATIONS

Many people with an SCI will have a mixed pain presentation,[46] presenting with different types of pain, in different bodily locations. The International Spinal Cord Injury Pain (ISCIP) Classification has been developed and supported by international SCI organisations (Table 18.2).[47] The revised classification of spinal cord injury pain was put together by an

Table 18.2 International spinal cord injury pain (ISCIP) classification

Tier 1: Pain type	Tier 2: Pain subtype	Tier 3: Primary pain source and/or pathology (write or type in)
☐ Nociceptive pain	☐ Musculoskeletal pain	☐_____ e.g. glenohumeral arthritis, lateral epicondylitis, comminuted femur fracture, quadratus lumborum muscle spasm
	☐ Visceral pain	☐_____ e.g. myocardial infarction, abdominal pain due to bowel impaction, cholecystitis
	☐ Other nociceptive pain	☐_____ e.g. autonomic dysreflexia headache, migraine headache, surgical skin incision
☐ Neuropathic pain	☐ At level SCI pain	☐_____ e.g. spinal cord compression, nerve root compression, cauda equina compression
	☐ Below level SCI pain	☐_____ e.g. spinal cord ischaemia, spinal cord compression
	☐ Other neuropathic pain	☐_____ e.g. carpal tunnel syndrome, trigeminal neuralgia, diabetic polyneuropathy
☐ Other pain		☐_____ e.g. fibromyalgia, Complex Regional Pain Syndrome type I, intersititial cystitis, irritable bowel syndrome
☐ Unknown pain		☐_____

Source: Bryce T.N., Biering-Sorensen F., et al., 2012. International Spinal Cord Injury Pain Classification: part I Background and description. March 6–7, 2009. Spinal Cord. 50 (6), 413–417.

international group of SCI and pain experts and reviewed by all the major SCI and pain organisations. The classification was tested for utility and reliability by random sample members of the American Spinal Injury Association (ASIA) and the International Spinal Cord Society (ISCoS). The authors hoped that the format and definitions presented in the table would help both experienced and non-experienced clinicians, as well as clinical researchers classifying pain after SCI.[47]

This classification recognises that people with an SCI may experience both nociceptive and neuropathic pain, hence the concept of a mixed pain presentation.[46] Nociceptive pain refers to pain that originates in the peripheral tissues and in which the nociceptive input is conveyed by an intact nervous system.[48] Neuropathic pain refers to pain that arises because of damage to the somatosensory system itself and in which there is evidence of nervous system dysfunction.[49] Disease or injury may affect both the peripheral nervous system and/or the central nervous system (CNS).

Nociceptive pain

Nociceptive pain after SCI is recognised as occurring primarily either from musculoskeletal tissues or from visceral organs.[43,47] Musculoskeletal pain may arise from tissues such as bone or ligament that might be injured at the time of SCI or due to phenomena such as heterotopic ossification (discussed in Part 4 of this chapter). Pain can also arise as a result of overuse of musculoskeletal tissues or alterations in posture following SCI.[50] This is particularly the case with upper limb pain related to increased use of the upper extremity for weight-bearing, and back pain resulting from altered sitting postures.[50] It is possible that some people will also experience somatic referred pain because of excessive central sensitisation in response to nociceptive input from musculoskeletal structures.[51] For example, pain may be perceived in the shoulder or upper back region due to injury of the cervical spine.[52] Visceral pain may also arise as a consequence of injury to abdominal organs concurrent with the SCI or it may occur

spontaneously at some time after the SCI, possibly related to long-term alterations in gut function.[43]

Neuropathic pain

Neuropathic pain is classified as either 'at-level neuropathic pain' or 'below-level neuropathic pain'.[47] At-level neuropathic pain may involve damage to both peripheral and CNS structures and may include radicular referred pain.[52] At-level neuropathic pain is likely to occur as a result of damage to nerve roots and elements of the peripheral nervous system, resulting in ectopic discharge and the development of evoked pain and allodynia.[50] Below-level neuropathic pain is likely to arise primarily as a result of disease, injury or neuronal plasticity affecting the CNS.[43,47] Below-level neuropathic pain can also be considered a form of referred pain, but in this case the mechanism relates more to processes of cortical and sub-cortical plasticity that occur as a result of deafferentation, in a similar manner to phantom limb pain.[53]

Neurological damage and disease will often affect myelinated afferent neurons, as well as the thinly myelinated and unmyelinated nociceptive afferents (see Chapter 1 for more detail on neurological damage). Ectopic neuronal activity arising at some point along the axon rather than at the peripheral receptor seems to be one of the key mechanisms triggering neuropathic pain.[54] This tends to result in a very distinctive pattern of pain and dysaesthesia that is not easily modulated. This aberrant neuronal activity may also initiate central sensitisation and will often trigger some degree of neuroanatomical reorganisation within the CNS.[55,56] These changes, which may be triggered by SCI, often mean that the capacity for the nervous system to modulate neuropathic pain is also significantly impaired.[56] An SCI may further impact upon the ability to effectively modulate pain since descending neurons modulating nociceptive input may be directly affected by the SCI.

People with an SCI may also have pre-existing pain problems that continue following SCI.[43] For example, a person might suffer from migraine and continue to experience episodes of migraine in addition to other pain problems occurring as a direct result of the SCI.

PREVALENCE OF PAIN

The exact prevalence of pain following an SCI remains a matter of some conjecture, with reported prevalence rates ranging from 19% to 96%.[57,58] This wide disparity seems to be related to a number of research-related factors including: definitions of pain, whether studies were primarily designed to assess pain, whether the study was prospective or not and the response rate for surveys.[57] In summary, it appears that two out of three people with an SCI are likely to experience some degree of ongoing pain, and approximately two out of five are likely to report more severe pain.[43,57] The period of time following the SCI is important because some people may experience more musculoskeletal pain in the period immediately following injury, while the development of below-level neuropathic pain and visceral pain may be delayed for a significant period of time following injury.

In a prospective study, 59% of patients with an SCI experienced musculoskeletal pain, 41% experienced at-level neuropathic pain, 34% experienced below-level neuropathic pain and only 5% reported visceral pain.[43] The average onset of at-level neuropathic pain occurred after 1.2 years (SD ± 1.5 years), whereas below-level neuropathic pain occurred later (average onset 1.8 years ± 1.7 years) and visceral pain had a much later onset (4.2 years ± 0.8 years).[43]

Cardenas and Felix reviewed the prevalence of different types of musculoskeletal pain in people with an SCI, without specific limitations on the duration of pain.[50] They concluded that shoulder pain was the most common form of musculoskeletal pain, with reported prevalence ranging from 30–78% compared to 32% for elbow pain, 53–64% for wrist pain and 48% for hand pain. These figures are likely to reflect the much greater use of the upper extremity for weight-bearing in people with an SCI (see Chapter 15 for further detail on the problems and long-term treatments of shoulder pain). Approximately 60% of participants reported back pain.[50]

Below-level neuropathic pain appears to be more common in people with tetraplegia (50%) compared to those with paraplegia (18%).[43] Whether the SCI is complete or incomplete does not seem to influence the development of most forms of pain although there was a positive correlation between the presence of an anterior cord lesion and the development of below-level neuropathic pain.[43]

One potential area of overlap between neuropathic and musculoskeletal pain is the development of pain associated with spasticity. The pathophysiological mechanisms that contribute to the development of neuropathic pain also contribute to the development of spasticity.[59] For example, the loss of descending inhibition, axonal sprouting and neuronal reorganisation may all contribute to developing both neuropathic pain and spasticity (see Chapter 1 on the pathophysiology and possible management of spasticity).[59] Hence, it could be anticipated that spasticity-related pain would be predominantly neuropathic. However, excessive muscle contraction, increased stress on ligamentous tissues and the possibility of local ischaemia might also contribute to the development of musculoskeletal pain in areas affected by spasticity. This highlights the complexity of pain presentation that may be present in some patients with an SCI.

In summary, pain is a common feature of SCI; it can vary in type and severity, and it can be present in multiple different locations. Effective management of pain is therefore an important aspect of the ongoing management of patients following SCI.

MANAGEMENT OF PAIN FOLLOWING SCI

Management of pain following SCI should be based on a comprehensive clinical examination. As mentioned earlier, patients can present with pain in multiple locations with a mixed pain presentation.[46] A detailed pain diagram, identifying pain and other sensations in different body areas, is valuable in identifying different sources of pain. There are a number of screening tools that can be used to evaluate the presence of neuropathic pain. The most commonly used and validated tools include PainDETECT, the Leeds Assessment of Neuropathic Symptoms and Signs (LANSS), the Neuropathic Pain Questionnaire (NPQ) and Doleur Neuropathique (DN4).[60] These questionnaires are largely based on the characteristics of the pain report. A diagnosis of neuropathic pain also requires a clinical examination that identifies sensory deficits associated with the area of pain and imaging or other diagnostic information that identifies a particular pathology likely to have caused the pain.[49]

MANAGEMENT OF MUSCULOSKELETAL PAIN

Musculoskeletal pain should be managed using commonly applied strategies for the joints or muscles involved. This would include strategies for activity modification and activity pacing to manage the stresses imposed on the tissue.[61] It might also include the use of splints, supports or adaptive equipment (e.g. wrist supports) to control the stresses on particular structures. Consideration needs to be given to the fact that muscular control of specific joints may be impaired as a result of the SCI and the fact that weight-bearing through the upper limbs may impose significantly greater stress on areas such as the shoulders. Consideration should be given to transfer technique and techniques for wheelchair use or aspects of wheelchair design (see Chapters 5, 6 and 8). Spinal support and spinal posture may also be important considerations for patients reporting back pain.

The use of pharmacological treatments would normally be based on procedures and guidelines for the management of similar painful conditions in the general population.[37] Such guidelines are likely to emphasise the use of simple analgesics, such as paracetamol or non-steroidal anti-inflammatory drugs (NSAIDs) if the pain is more severe.[50] Caution is required to avoid excessive dosing with paracetamol or long-term use of NSAIDs. In some cases where pain is fairly localised, topical NSAID treatments may be useful.[62] While opiate medications may be utilised in the management of acute musculoskeletal pain at the time of SCI, the use of opiates to manage ongoing pain is not recommended, particularly due to the risk of respiratory depression, problems with constipation and risk of addiction.[50] Interventional treatments such as hydrocortisone injections under ultrasound imaging may be of some value for particular musculoskeletal problems (e.g. rotator cuff tendinopathy), but the effect may be relatively short-lasting and guideline recommendations should be considered, depending on the particular musculoskeletal structures affected.

Exercise may also be effective for reducing pain associated with some musculoskeletal conditions in people with an SCI, but this will be heavily dependent on the level of injury and the degree of voluntary movement present.[50] In some cases, it may be possible to utilise graduated eccentric loading to address pain associated with some forms of tendinopathy.[63] This approach has demonstrated value in the reduction of pain associated with lateral elbow tendinopathy for example.[63] While most of the research has focused on sporting populations, the approach could also be of value to people with an SCI who experience tendinopathy in the upper limb.

Physical treatments such as massage, acupuncture and joint mobilisation or manipulation may be beneficial in reducing musculoskeletal pain in some patients with an SCI. Specific studies in this population are limited and the effectiveness of these interventions may be reduced, depending on the site of pain and the level of SCI, because many of these treatments act through descending pain modulatory systems,[64] which are likely to be impaired following SCI. For example, Nayak and colleagues suggested that acupuncture was mainly effective for patients with pain above the level of their SCI and that people with an incomplete lesion may show a better treatment response than those with a complete spinal cord lesion.[44,65] However, massage is recognised as a popular treatment option for many people with an SCI.[66] In a survey of 117 people with an SCI, massage was the most commonly used alternative therapy for pain management and it produced good pain relief, although the duration of pain relief was relatively short.[67] It is important that patients have a well-structured and individualised treatment plan to assist in managing ongoing musculoskeletal pain.

MANAGEMENT OF NEUROPATHIC PAIN

While neuropathic pain is less common than musculoskeletal pain, the prevalence of neuropathic pain in people with an SCI is still very high.[57] This form of pain may also be particularly severe and difficult to manage,[68] particularly when there is significant central sensitisation and neuroanatomical reorganisation.[69]

Management of neuropathic pain should also be based on available evidence and appropriate guidelines.[56] Pharmacological management will generally utilise gabapentinoids (gabapentin and pregabalin) as first-line treatment for neuropathic pain.[37] Gabapentin and pregabalin have been shown to have a moderate to large effect size for improving neuropathic pain in people with an SCI,[70] including incomplete SCI.[71] Treatment with pregabalin will generally involve careful titration of the dose to ensure effective treatment with minimisation of side effects. In a systematic review of clinical trials in patients with an SCI, Teasell and colleagues concluded that there is Level 1 evidence to support the use of pregabalin and gabapentin in the management of neuropathic pain post-SCI.[72] They also reported that lamotrigine may be effective in reducing pain for people with incomplete SCI.[73] These anticonvulsant medications act through GABA inhibition and sodium channel modulation to produce a suppression of neuronal excitability.[70]

Tricyclic antidepressant medications are also used as a first-line approach in the management of neuropathic pain; in particular, serotonin and norepinephrine re-uptake inhibitors (SNRI), such as amitriptyline and duloxetine. These medications act by enhancing the effect of descending pain modulatory systems, so they may be effective in the management of at-level neuropathic pain, but are unlikely to be effective in managing below-level neuropathic pain. There is Level 1 evidence to support the use of amitriptyline in the management of pain post-SCI, but primarily in people who are also experiencing depression.[72] There is limited evidence to support the use of duloxetine,[74] although the location of the pain and the nature of the SCI lesion are likely to significantly impact the effectiveness of this medication. It does appear to have an effect on allodynia, which suggests that it may be more effective in treating at-level neuropathic pain.[75]

There is evidence to support the use of lidocaine (lignocaine) via intravenous injection or intrathecal infusion in the management of neuropathic pain in patients with an SCI, at least over short timeframes.[72] Intrathecal injection or infusion of baclofen is another commonly used treatment for spasticity and research suggests that it has a positive influence in reducing pain as well as reducing spasticity.[76]

An alternative approach to the management of at-level neuropathic pain when there is evidence of cauda equina or nerve root lesions is the use of surgical stimulation or ablation techniques. The most common approach is dorsal root entry zone (DREZ) lesioning. This type of procedure carries considerable risk, but it may be effective in managing some forms of intractable pain, with low level evidence to support the use of DREZ in the treatment of neuropathic pain in individuals for whom other less invasive treatments were ineffective.[77]

Below-level neuropathic pain is less likely to respond to local treatments such as DREZ or nerve root stimulation. The mainstay of treatment is likely to be pharmacological, particularly with treatments such as gabapentin or pregabalin.

Many physical and behavioural treatments have been suggested to have some benefit in the management of neuropathic pain post-SCI. A relatively recent development in the management of neuropathic pain post-SCI has been the use of transcranial electrical and magnetic stimulation (TES and TMS).[78] Level 1 evidence provides good support for the use of TES, and more limited support for the use of TMS, in the management of SCI pain.[79] This form of treatment likely influences cortical reorganisation occurring as a result of deafferentation post-SCI. Transcutaneous electrical nerve stimulation (TENS) has been available as a treatment option for a much longer period of time, but the evidence to support its effectiveness is more equivocal.[79] Similarly, there is limited evidence to support the use of acupuncture in the treatment of neuropathic pain post-SCI.[79] Regarding the use of acupuncture and/or TENS for pain management, the location of the pain and the possibility that the descending pain modulating systems have remained intact must be taken into account.

Behavioural treatments include cognitive behavioural therapy (CBT), mindfulness training and visual imagery. CBT may be useful in improving mood, coping behaviour and function in people with neuropathic pain post-SCI, but evidence suggests that it has limited effects on pain intensity.[79] Mental imagery appears to have some value for motor recovery, but it has been suggested that it has limited value for pain management in the person with an SCI,[80] although Moseley has reported substantial reductions in pain in a small group of people with an SCI who engaged in an activity where they visualised themselves walking pain-free on a daily basis.[81] The varied ability of individuals to effectively visualise may be an important factor influencing the effectiveness of this type of intervention. Mindfulness training has been increasingly utilised in the management of chronic pain,[82] although further research is required to determine its value in the management of neuropathic pain post-SCI. Effective pain management clearly needs to be adapted to the particular presentation of individual patients with careful consideration of an effective mechanisms-based approach.

Evidence-based practice points

Prevalence

- Pain is a more common complication after SCI than is generally recognised.
- Two out of three people may experience some ongoing pain.
- Two out of five people may experience more severe chronic pain.

Classification

- Many people will have a mixed pain presentation, including both nociceptive and neuropathic pain.
- Nociceptive pain may include both musculoskeletal and visceral pain.
- Neuropathic pain is often distinguished as at-level neuropathic pain and below-level neuropathic pain.

Treatment

- Musculoskeletal pain may be treated with simple analgesics, NSAIDs and activity modification.
- Neuropathic pain is normally treated with anticonvulsant and antidepressant medications.
- Physical and psychological treatments may also be effective for some people.

SUMMARY

Pain is a more common and more disabling problem following SCI than is generally recognised. Two out of three people with an SCI may experience some degree of ongoing pain. Effective management of pain depends on a comprehensive assessment with the expectation that many patients will have a mixed pain presentation. Appropriate pharmacological treatments are available to manage both musculoskeletal and neuropathic pain and in addition there are a range of physical and psychological treatments that may be of value for individual patients. It is important to consider the neurophysiological processes likely to be initiating the pain and to utilise treatments with a mechanism of action that is likely to be effective for the specific individual. This mechanisms-based approach is particularly important for this population of people with an SCI. A comprehensive treatment plan should result in reduced pain, improved function and better QoL.

4. HETEROTOPIC OSSIFICATION
Jacqueline Reznik

INTRODUCTION

Riedel, a German physician, first identified heterotopic ossification (HO) in 1883. HO has been given multiple names, including paraosteoarthropathy, myositis ossificans, periarticular new bone formation, periarticular ectopic ossification, neurogenic osteoma, neurogenic ossifying fibromyopathy and heterotopic calcification.[83] Neurogenic heterotopic ossification (NHO) mainly occurs following spinal trauma and head injuries.[84,85]

In patients with traumatic spinal cord injury (TSCI) the prevalence of NHO has been reported as ranging between 10% and 53%.[86–88] These high discrepancies in the prevalence of NHO would appear to be because the majority of centres confirm the presence of NHO only when it becomes clinically significant, i.e. causes pain, interferes with movement and/or restricts function. These inconsistencies are further highlighted in a study describing the incidence of NHO at a Level-1 trauma centre as being 21.9% in patients with traumatic SCI.[89] It should be noted that in this study all patients with an SCI were screened for the development of NHO with ultra-sonography every two weeks. Interestingly, the prevalence of NHO after TSCI is lower in paediatric patients than in adults, and spontaneous resorption of NHO has been reported exclusively in children.[90]

Localisation of neurogenic heterotopic ossification

NHO is always found below the level of the TSCI lesion[85] and is usually found around the major joints, the hip being the most common site of occurrence following traumatic spinal cord injury.[84]

A variety of risk factors have been identified associated with the development of NHO in TSCI patients (Table 18.3), although the biological basis of these risk factors is often unclear.

POSSIBLE PATHOPHYSIOLOGICAL MECHANISMS

The pathophysiological mechanisms associated with NHO formation seems to be more complex than simply inappropriate differentiation of fibroblasts

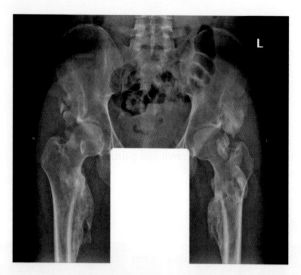

Figure 18.8 Bilateral NHO in male tetraplegic patient.

Table 18.3 Risk factors for developing NHO following traumatic SCI

Risk factors	Goldman, 1980	Coelho & Beraldo, 2009
Gender	M	M
Age	20–40	Not documented
Level of injury	Thoracic lesion	Thoracic lesion
Complete/ incomplete	Complete	Complete
Spasticity	Absent/mild	Absent/mild
Pressure injuries	Present	Present
VTE	No	No
Length of stay	>6 weeks	Not documented
Type of injury	MVC	Not documented
Smoking	Not documented	No
Urinary complications	Not documented	Present

M = male; F = female; VTE = venous thromboembolism; MVC = motor vehicle collision

into bone-forming cells, as originally thought.[87] In the patient with a TSCI, NHO originates from the connective tissue lying between the muscles, outside of the joint capsule, and the joint space and capsule are preserved.[91,92] A widely accepted theory suggests that NHO begins as an oedematous inflammatory reaction with an increased blood flow in the affected soft tissue area. First, exudative cell infiltration takes place; then fibroblastic cell proliferation occurs, followed by osteoid formation and, finally, bone matrix development.[93] Within the first 2 weeks, primitive bone foci are observed as small masses in the fibroblastic mesenchymal reaction area, primarily in the periphery. Osteoblasts produce tropocollagen, which is a polymerised form of collagen, and synthesise alkaline phosphatase (AP).[94] AP degrades pyrophosphate, which is a compound that prevents calcium deposition. The newly developing ectopic bone matrix inactivates nearby pyrophosphate. Therefore, AP allows precipitation of calcium and mineralisation of bone matrix (Fig. 18.9).[92,95]

Recent animal studies have identified new signalling pathways within the muscles of affected mice, which may act as a potential therapeutic target to reduce NHO development following SCI.[96]

CLINICAL DIAGNOSIS

Early diagnosis of NHO is based predominantly on clinical signs and symptoms. These early symptoms, which include fever, swelling, erythema and decreased joint range of motion (ROM), are typically seen in early NHO, but may also be easily confused with venous thromboembolism (VTE), infection and trauma.[97] NHO usually presents about 2 months post-neurological injury, but has been described in the literature as early as 2 weeks and as late as 12 months post-injury.[95] In the author's experience, the decreased ROM is typically accompanied by a hard

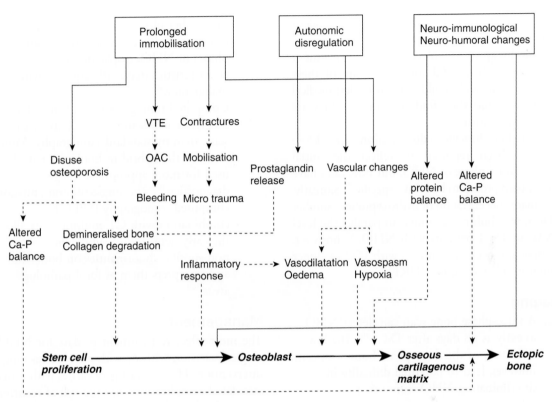

Figure 18.9 Suggested pathophysiological mechanisms of NHO in patients with an SCI.
VTE: venous thromboembolism; OAC: oral anti-coagulant
Source: Van Kuijk A.A., Geurts A.C.H., 2002. Neurogenic heterotopic ossification in spinal cord injury. Spinal Cord 40 (7), 313–326.

end feel or block at the end of range and therefore it is most often the treating physiotherapist who is the first person to suspect the development of NHO in the patient. Since the physiotherapist may be the first to recognise these signs and symptoms, it is important that they are aware of this possible complication.

LABORATORY INVESTIGATIONS

Serum alkaline phosphatase (SAP) levels have been reported to parallel the activity of ossification.[98] AP levels start to rise about 7 weeks before the first clinical signs of NHO become apparent, exceed normal levels 1 week later and reach peak levels 3 weeks after the first clinical signs.[99] Subsequently, the AP levels gradually decline to normal. However, in a more recent retrospective study Citak and colleagues concluded that assessment of bone alkaline phosphatase (BAP), SAP or C-reactive protein (CRP) is not a reliable method for diagnosing early HO in patients with an SCI.[100]

The normative value for alkaline phosphatase (ALP) is 53–128 units per litre (U/L) in a 20- to 50-year-old male and 42–98 U/L in a 20- to 50-year-old female. Adults over 61 years have normative values of ALP of 51–153 U/L (ALP is equivalent to the SAP values).[101]

Physiotherapists involved in the treatment of patients with an SCI must be aware of these normative values and should be ready to alert medical personnel should they find that these values are exceeding the norm.

Elevated erythrocyte sedimentation rates (ESR) have also been reported to reflect the initial 'inflammatory' phase of NHO, but ESR rates have also not been proven to be NHO-specific.[95] Similarly, the urinary concentration of hydroxyproline, another collagen metabolite, was found to parallel the level of SAP in TSCI patients with NHO;[102] however, this may also occur in patients with UTI or upper respiratory tract infection (URTI).[95]

Imaging

1. A three-phase bone scan can detect NHO as early as 18 days after TSCI.[103] The low specificity of the three-phase bone scan can, however, lead to potential difficulty in discriminating NHO from other inflammatory, traumatic or degenerative processes of the skeleton. In addition, bone scanning requires expensive specialist equipment and involves the use of ionising radiation.[104]

2. The use of sonography as an early diagnostic tool for NHO has been shown to be both convenient and cost-effective.[105] It may also be of use as a simultaneous screening tool for NHO and VTE in TSCI patients.[95]

3. Radiographs are quick, inexpensive and allow detection of HO approximately 4–5 weeks after the initial neurological trauma.[98] Standard radiography is therefore often the first imaging modality to confirm clinically suspected HO.[106]

4. Magnetic resonance imaging (MRI) is not routinely used for the evaluation of heterotopic ossification.[103] MRI is more technically demanding and expensive than either ultrasound or radiography and lacks specificity, especially in the early phases of NHO, displaying MRI characteristics frequently equated with malignancy.[107]

5. Computed tomography (CT) may detect soft tissue ossification at a relatively earlier stage than by standard radiography. More recently, the hybrid technologies have been used for more appropriate image diagnostics.[108] The single-photon emission computed tomography (SPECT) in combination with CT multiple cuts allows the early detection of subtle and non-specific abnormalities on bone scan and interprets them as focal pathology areas.[109]

Management

The most effective treatment to date for NHO is surgical excision with or without pharmacological intervention. However, surgery carries with it many associated complications and the risk of recurrence is considerable.[110]

Prophylactic methods such as pharmacotherapy or radiotherapy are not effective in reducing the symptoms of established NHO and may carry high-risk side effects. Investigation of non-invasive treatment options with minimal associated side effects is urgently needed; a well-planned prospective study with extracorporeal shock wave therapy (ESWT) is one such alternative. A series of single case studies on the effects of ESWT on NHO in traumatic brain injured patients has shown efficacy in reducing pain and improving function.[111,112]

Once NHO has been confirmed, irrespective of the type of treatment or management that may be implemented, it is important that the physiotherapist continue with passive and active ranges of motion to the affected joints in order to maintain maximum joint range. Continuous passive motion (CPM) may also prove a useful adjunct to treatment as well as exercises in water (hydrotherapy) (see Chapter 10 on hydrotherapy).

Evidence-based practice points

- NHO in patients with an SCI is always found below the level of the lesion; the hip joint is the most common site of occurrence.
- Multiple risk factors have been identified; the most common include vascular stenosis, oedema and prolonged swelling in the affected limb.
- Demographic factors such as age, gender and ethnicity have also been suggested to increase the risk of the development of NHO.
- Early diagnosis depends predominantly on clinical signs and symptoms; these include fever, swelling, erythema and decreased joint motion around the affected joint(s).
- NHO usually presents approximately 2 months post-injury.
- Laboratory investigations have not been shown to be reliable for early diagnosis.
- CT/SPECT is the most useful diagnostic imaging technique.
- To date, the only management is surgical excision, although newer non-invasive techniques such as ESWT are being investigated.

SUMMARY

NHO is a relatively common complication of neurological trauma in general and, in particular, TSCI. If it remains undiagnosed and untreated, NHO may prove to be an extremely debilitating complication in an already functionally compromised individual, as they cause pain, partial or total joint ankylosis and vascular and nerve compression. As the possible first-liner in the detection of NHO, if the treating physiotherapist suspects that NHO is developing or has developed they must request the appropriate laboratory and imaging investigations in order to confirm or refute the diagnosis, in order that the appropriate management and/or treatment be implemented. The physiotherapist must also continue to encourage the patient to perform both active and passive movements to the affected limb(s) to maintain the optimal joint range. The physiotherapist must also be aware of all new treatment paradigms as they become available.

Online resources

Neurogenic bladder and bowel

Clinical practice guidelines. https://www.aci.health.nsw.gov.au/__data/assets/pdf_file/0019/155215/Management-Neurogenic-Bowel.pdf.

Sleep disordered breathing

Four patients with an SCI discussing the importance of being tested for sleep apnoea and the positive effects of the use of a CPAP machine. https://ibas.org.au/blog/read/77/do-you-have-spinal-cord-injury-tired-get-treated.

References

1. Dorsher, P.T., McIntosh, P.M., 2012. Neurogenic bladder. Adv. Urol. 816274.

2. Al Taweel, W., Seyam, R., 2015. Neurogenic bladder in spinal cord injury patients. Res. Rep. Urol. 7, 85.

3. Bragge, P., Guy, S., et al., 2019. A systematic review of the content and quality of clinical practice guidelines for management of the neurogenic bladder following spinal cord injury. Spinal Cord 57 (7), 540–549.

4. Skelton, F., Salemi, J.L., et al., 2019. Genitourinary complications are a leading and expensive cause of emergency department and inpatient encounters for persons with spinal cord injury. Arch. Phys. Med. Rehabil. 100 (9), 1614–1621.

5. Roma, P.G.B., Smith, C.P., et al., 2018. Non-surgical urologic management of neurogenic bladder after spinal cord injury. World J. Urol. 36 (10), 1555–1568.

6. Hiersemenzel, L.P., Curt, A., et al., 2000. From spinal shock to spasticity: neuronal adaptations to a spinal cord injury. Neurology 54 (8), 1574–1582.

7. May Goodwin, D., Brock, J., et al., 2018. Optimal bladder management following spinal cord injury: evidence, practice and a cooperative approach driving future directions in Australia. Arch. Phys. Med. Rehabil. 99 (10), 2118–2121.

8. Welk, B., Fuller, A., et al., 2012. Renal stone disease in spinal-cord–injured patients. J. Endourol. 26 (8), 954–959.

9. Welk, B., Schneider, M.P., et al., 2018. Early urological care of patients with spinal cord injury. World J. Urol. 36 (10), 1537–1544.

10. Panicker, J.N., de Sèze, M., et al., 2010. Rehabilitation in practice: neurogenic lower urinary tract dysfunction and its management. Clin. Rehabil. 24 (7), 579–589.

11. Wolfe, D.L., Ethans, K., et al., 2010. Bladder Health and Function Following Spinal Cord Injury, vol. 3. Spinal Cord Injury Rehabilitation Evidence Version, pp. 1–19.

12. Wyndaele, J.J., Birch, B., et al., 2018. Surgical management of the neurogenic bladder after spinal cord injury. World J. Urol. 36 (10), 1569–1576.

13. Mazor, Y., Jones, M., et al., 2016. Anorectal biofeedback for neurogenic bowel dysfunction in incomplete spinal cord injury. Spinal Cord 54 (12), 1132–1138.

14. Pagliacci, M., Franceschini, M., et al., 2007. A multicentre follow-up of clinical aspects of traumatic spinal cord injury. Spinal Cord 45 (6), 404.

15. Liu, C., Attar, K.H., et al., 2010. The relationship between bladder management and health-related quality of life in patients with spinal cord injury in the UK. Spinal Cord 48 (4), 319.

16. Stoffel, J.T., Van der Aa, F., et al., 2018. Neurogenic bowel management for the adult spinal cord injury patient. World J. Urol. 36 (10), 1587–1592.

17. Yeung, H.Y., Iyer, P., et al., 2019. Dietary management of neurogenic bowel in adults with spinal cord injury: an integrative review of literature. Disabil. Rehabil. 15, 1–12. (EPUB ahead of print).

18. Hughes, M., 2014. Bowel management in spinal cord injury patients. Clin. Colon Rectal Surg. 27 (3), 113–115.

19. Boucher, M., Dukes, S., et al., 2019. Early colostomy formation can improve independence following spinal cord injury and increase acceptability of bowel management. Top. Spinal Cord Inj. Rehabil. 25 (1), 23–30.

20. Berlowitz, D.J., Spong, J., et al., 2012. Relationships between objective sleep indices and symptoms in a community sample of people with tetraplegia. Arch. Phys. Med. Rehabil. 93 (7), 1246–1252.

21. Fogelberg, D.J., Leland, N.E., et al., 2017. Qualitative experience of sleep in individuals with spinal cord injury. OTJR (Thorofare N J) 37 (2), 89–97.

22. Biering-Sorensen, F., Biering-Sorensen, M., 2001. Sleep disturbances in the spinal cord injured: an epidemiological questionnaire investigation, including a normal population. Spinal Cord 39 (10), 505–513.

23. Giannoccaro, M.P., Moghadam, K.K., et al., 2013. Sleep disorders in patients with spinal cord injury. Sleep Med. Rev. 17 (6), 399–409.

24. Kryger, M.H., Roth, T., et al., 2017. Principles and Practice of Sleep Medicine. Elsevier, Philadelphia, PA.

25. Graco, M., Schembri, R., et al., 2018. Diagnostic accuracy of a two-stage model for detecting obstructive sleep apnoea in chronic tetraplegia. Thorax thoraxjnl-2017-211131.

26. Senaratna, C.V., Perret, J.L., et al., 2017. Prevalence of obstructive sleep apnea in the general population: a systematic review. Sleep Med. Rev. 34, 70–81.

27. Berlowitz, D.J., Brown, D.J., et al., 2005. A longitudinal evaluation of sleep and breathing in the first year after cervical spinal cord injury. Arch. Phys. Med. Rehabil. 86 (6), 1193–1199.

28. Sajkov, D., Marshall, R., et al., 1998. Sleep apnoea related hypoxia is associated with cognitive disturbances in patients with tetraplegia. Spinal Cord 36 (4), 231–239.

29. Schembri, R., Spong, J., et al., 2017. Neuropsychological function in patients with acute tetraplegia and sleep disordered breathing. Sleep 40 (2).

30. Chai-Coetzer, C., Douglas, J., et al., 2014. Guidelines for sleep studies in adults. Prepared for the Australasian Sleep Association.

31. Sankari, A., Martin, J., et al., 2015. Identification and treatment of sleep-disordered breathing in chronic spinal cord injury. Spinal Cord 53 (2), 145–149.

32. Rosen, C.L., Auckley, D., et al., 2012. A multisite randomized trial of portable sleep studies and positive airway pressure autotitration versus laboratory-based polysomnography for the diagnosis and treatment of obstructive sleep apnea: the HomePAP study. Sleep 35 (6), 757–767.

33. Le Guen, M., Cistulli, P., et al., 2012. Continuous positive airway pressure requirements in patients with tetraplegia and obstructive sleep apnoea. Spinal Cord 50 (11), 832–835.

34. Berlowitz, D.J., Schembri, R., et al., 2018. Positive airway pressure for sleep-disordered breathing in acute quadriplegia: a randomised controlled trial. Thorax thoraxjnl-2018-212319.

35. Weaver, T.E., Sawyer, A.M., 2010. Adherence to continuous positive airway pressure treatment for obstructive sleep apnea: implications for future interventions. Indian J. Med. Res. 131, 245–258.

36. Graco, M., Green, S.E., et al., 2019. Worth the effort? Weighing up the benefit and burden of continuous positive airway pressure therapy for the treatment of obstructive sleep apnoea in chronic tetraplegia. Spinal Cord 57 (3), 247–254.

37. Wright, A., Benson, H.A.E., et al., 2016. Pain and analgesia. In: Reznik, J., Keren, O., et al. (Eds.), Pharmacology Handbook for Physiotherapists. Elsevier, Sydney, pp. 199–225.

38. Antonescu-Turcu, A., Parthasarathy, S., 2010. CPAP and bi-level PAP therapy: new and established roles. Respir. Care 55 (9), 1216–1229.

39. Consortium for Spinal Cord Medicine, 2005. Respiratory management following spinal cord injury: a clinical practice guideline for health-care professionals. J. Spinal Cord Med. 28 (3), 259–293.

40. Sheel, A.W., Welch, J.F., et al., 2014. Respiratory management following spinal cord injury. In: Spinal Cord Injury Rehabilitation Evidence, fifth ed. Vancouver.

41. Burns, S., Kapur, V., et al., 2001. Factors associated with sleep apnea in men with spinal cord injury: a population-based case-control study. Spinal Cord 39 (1), 15–22.

42. Sankari, A., Martin, J., et al., 2015. A retrospective review of sleep-disordered breathing, hypertenstion and cardiovascular diseases in spinal cord injury patients. Spinal Cord 53 (6), 496.

43. Siddall, P.J., McClelland, J.M., et al., 2003. A longitudinal study of the prevalence and characteristics of pain in the first 5 years following spinal cord injury. Pain 103 (3), 249–257.

44. Nayak, S., Matheis, R.J., et al., 2001. The use of complementary and alternative therapies for chronic pain following spinal cord injury: a pilot survey. J. Spinal Cord Med. 24 (1), 54–62.

45. Finnerup, N.B., Baastrup, C., 2012. Spinal cord injury pain: mechanisms and management. Curr. Pain Headache Rep. 16 (3), 207–216.

46. Freynhagen, R., Arevalo Parada, H., et al., 2019. Current understanding of the mixed pain concept: a brief narrative review. Curr. Med. Res. Opin. 35 (6), 1011–1018.

47. Bryce, T.N., Biering-Sorensen, F., et al., 2012. International Spinal Cord Injury Pain Classification: part I Background and description. March 6–7, 2009. Spinal Cord 50 (6), 413–417.

48. Merskey, H., Bogduk, N., 1994. Classification of Chronic Pain: Descriptions of Chronic Pain Syndromes and Definitions of Pain Terms. IASP Press, Seattle.

49. Treede, R.D., Jensen, T.S., et al., 2008. Neuropathic pain: redefinition and a grading system for clinical and research purposes. Neurology 70 (18), 1630–1635.

50. Cardenas, D.D., Felix, E.R., 2009. Pain after spinal cord injury: a review of classification, treatment approaches, and treatment assessment. PM R 1 (12), 1077–1090.

51. Graven-Nielsen, T., 2006. Fundamentals of muscle pain, referred pain, and deep tissue hyperalgesia. Scand. J. Rheumatol. Suppl. 122, 1–43.

52. Bogduk, N., 2011. The anatomy and pathophysiology of neck pain. Phys. Med. Rehabil. Clin. N. Am. 22 (3), 367–382, vii.

53. Ramachandran, V.S., Hirstein, W., 1998. The perception of phantom limbs. The D. O. Hebb lecture. Brain 121 (Pt 9), 1603–1630.

54. Devor, M., 1991. Neuropathic pain and injured nerve: peripheral mechanisms. Br. Med. Bull. 47 (3), 619–630.

55. Woolf, C.J., Mannion, R.J., 1999. Neuropathic pain: aetiology, symptoms, mechanisms, and management. Lancet 353 (9168), 1959–1964.

56. Wright, A., 2002. Neuropathic pain. In: Strong, J.S., Unruh, A.M., et al. (Eds.), Pain: A Textbook for Occupational Therapists and Physiotherapists. Churchill Livingstone, Edinburgh, pp. 351–377.

57. van Gorp, S., Kessels, A.G., et al., 2015. Pain prevalence and its determinants after spinal cord injury: a systematic review. Eur. J. Pain 19 (1), 5–14.

58. Dijkers, M., Bryce, T., et al., 2009. Prevalence of chronic pain after traumatic spinal cord injury: a systematic review. J. Rehabil. Res. Dev. 46 (1), 13–29.

59. Finnerup, N.B., 2017. Neuropathic pain and spasticity: intricate consequences of spinal cord injury. Spinal Cord 55 (12), 1046–1050.

60. Hallstrom, H., Norrbrink, C., 2011. Screening tools for neuropathic pain: can they be of use in individuals with spinal cord injury? Pain 152 (4), 772–779.

61. Nielson, W.R., Jensen, M.P., et al., 2013. Activity pacing in chronic pain: concepts, evidence, and future directions. Clin. J. Pain 29 (5), 461–468.

62. Derry, S., Conaghan, P., et al., 2016. Topical NSAIDs for chronic musculoskeletal pain in adults. Cochrane Database Syst. Rev. (4), CD007400.

63. Woodley, B.L., Newsham-West, R.J., et al., 2007. Chronic tendinopathy: effectiveness of eccentric exercise. Br. J. Sports Med. 41 (4), 188–198, discussion 199.

64. Wright, A., Zusman, M., 2004. Neurophysiology of pain and pain modulation. In: Boyling, J.D., Jull, G.A. (Eds.), Grieve's Modern Manual Therapy: The Vertebral Column. Churchill Livingstone, Edinburgh, pp. 155–171.

65. Nayak, S., Shiflett, S.C., et al., 2001. Is acupuncture effective in treating chronic pain after spinal cord injury? Arch. Phys. Med. Rehabil. 82 (11), 1578–1586.

66. Dalyan, M., Cardenas, D.D., et al., 1999. Upper extremity pain after spinal cord injury. Spinal Cord 37 (3), 191–195.

67. Cardenas, D.D., Jensen, M.P., 2006. Treatments for chronic pain in persons with spinal cord injury: a survey study. J. Spinal Cord Med. 29 (2), 109–117.

68. MacFarlane, B.V., Wright, A., et al., 1997. Chronic neuropathic pain and its control by drugs. Pharmacol. Ther. 75 (1), 1–19.

69. Wright, A., 1999. Recent concepts in the neurophysiology of pain. Man. Ther. 4 (4), 196–202.

70. Guy, S., Mehta, S., et al., 2014. Anticonvulsant medication use for the management of pain following spinal cord injury: systematic review and effectiveness analysis. Spinal Cord 52 (2), 89–96.

71. Yu, X., Liu, T., et al., 2019. Efficacy and safety of pregabalin in neuropathic pain followed spinal cord injury: a review and meta-analysis of randomized controlled trials. Clin. J. Pain 35 (3), 272–278.

72. Teasell, R.W., Mehta, S., et al., 2010. A systematic review of pharmacologic treatments of pain after spinal cord injury. Arch. Phys. Med. Rehabil. 91 (5), 816–831.

73. Finnerup, N.B., Sindrup, S.H., et al., 2002. Lamotrigine in spinal cord injury pain: a randomized controlled trial. Pain 96 (3), 375–383.

74. Hagen, E.M., Rekand, T., 2015. Management of neuropathic pain associated with spinal cord injury. Pain Ther. 4 (1), 51–65.

75. Vranken, J.H., Hollmann, M.W., et al., 2011. Duloxetine in patients with central neuropathic pain caused by spinal cord injury or stroke: a randomized, double-blind, placebo-controlled trial. Pain 152 (2), 267–273.

76. Kumru, H., Benito-Penalva, J., et al., 2018. Analgesic effect of intrathecal baclofen bolus on neuropathic pain in spinal cord injury patients. Brain Res. Bull. 140, 205–211.

77. Mehta, S., Orenczuk, K., et al., 2013. Neuropathic pain post spinal cord injury part 2: systematic review of dorsal root entry zone procedure. Top. Spinal Cord Inj. Rehabil. 19 (1), 78–86.

78. Nardone, R., Holler, Y., et al., 2014. Invasive and non-invasive brain stimulation for treatment of neuropathic pain in patients with spinal cord injury: a review. J. Spinal Cord Med. 37 (1), 19–31.

79. Mehta, S., Orenczuk, K., et al., 2013. Neuropathic pain post spinal cord injury part 1: systematic review of physical and behavioral treatment. Top. Spinal Cord Inj. Rehabil. 19 (1), 61–77.

80. Aikat, R., Dua, V., 2016. Mental imagery in spinal cord injury: a systematic review. J. Spine 5 (3), 1–8.

81. Moseley, G.L., 2007. Using visual illusion to reduce at-level neuropathic pain in paraplegia. Pain 130 (3), 294–298.

82. Hilton, L., Hempel, S., et al., 2017. Mindfulness meditation for chronic pain: systematic review and meta-analysis. Anns Behav. Med. 51 (2), 199–213.

83. Balboni, T.A., Gobezie, R., et al., 2006. Heterotopic ossification: pathophysiology, clinical features, and the role of radiotherapy for prophylaxis. Int. J. Radiat. Oncol. Biol. Phys. 65 (5), 1289–1299.

84. Cipriano, C.A., Pill, S.G., et al., 2009. Heterotopic ossification following traumatic brain injury and spinal cord injury. J. Am. Acad. Orthop. Surg. 17 (11), 689–697.

85. Teasell, R.W., Mehta, S., et al., 2010. A systematic review of the therapeutic interventions for heterotopic ossification after spinal cord injury. Spinal Cord 48 (7), 512–521.

86. Alexander, M.S., Biering-Sorensen, F., et al., 2009. International standards to document remaining autonomic function after spinal cord injury. Spinal Cord 47 (1), 36–43.

87. Sakellariou, V.I., Grigoriou, E., et al., 2012. Heterotopic ossification following traumatic brain injury and spinal cord injury: insight into the Etiology and Pathophysiology. J. Musculoskelet. Neuronal Interact. 12 (4), 230–240.

88. Emami Razavi, S.Z., Aryan, A., et al., 2015. Prevalence of hip ossification and related clinical factors in cases with spinal cord injury. Arch. Neurosci. 2 (4), e25395.

89. Citak, M., Suero, E.M., et al., 2012. Risk factors for heterotopic ossification in patients with spinal cord injury. Spine 37 (23), 1953–1957.

90. Hitzig, S.L., Tonack, M., et al., 2008. Secondary health complications in an aging Canadian spinal cord injury sample. Am. J. Phys. Med. Rehabil. 87 (7), 545–555.

91. Ohlmeier, M., Suero, E.M., et al., 2017. Muscle localization of heterotopic ossification following spinal cord injury. Spine J. 17 (10), 1519–1522.

92. Yildiz, N., Ardiç, F., 2010. Pathophysiology and etiology of neurogenic heterotopic ossification. Turk. J. Phys. Med. Rehab. 56 (2), 81–87. (original in Turkish with English translation)

93. Rossier, A., Bussat, P., et al., 1973. Current facts on para-osteo-arthropathy (POA). Spinal Cord 11 (1), 36–78.

94. Bolger, J., 1975. Heterotopic bone formation and alkaline phosphatase. Arch. Phys. Med. Rehabil. 56 (1), 36–39.

95. Van Kuijk, A.A., Geurts, A.C.H., et al., 2002. Neurogenic heterotopic ossification in spinal cord injury. Spinal Cord 40 (7), 313–326.

96. Alexander, K.A., Tseng, H.W., et al., 2019. Inhibition of JAK1/2 Tyrosine kinases reduces neurogenic heterotopic ossification after spinal cord injury. Front. Immunol. 10, 377.

97. Shehab, D., Elgazzar, A.H., et al., 2002. Heterotopic ossification. J. Nucl. Med. 43 (3), 346–353.

98. Furman, R., Nicholas, J.J., et al., 1970. Elevation of the serum alkaline phosphatase coincident with ectopic-bone formation in paraplegic patients. J. Bone Joint Surg. Am. 52 (6), 1131–1137.

99. Orzel, J.A., Rudd, T.G., 1985. Heterotopic bone formation: clinical, laboratory, and imaging correlation. J. Nucl. Med. 26 (2), 125–132.

100. Citak, M., Grasmucke, D., et al., 2016. The roles of serum alkaline and bone alkaline phosphatase levels in predicting heterotopic ossification following spinal cord injury. Spinal Cord 54 (5), 368–370.

101. Burtis, C.A., Ashwood, E.R., et al., 2012. Tietz Textbook of Clinical Chemistry and Molecular Diagnostics, fifth ed. Elsevier Health Sciences.

102. Chantraine, A., Nusgens, B., et al., 1995. Biochemical analysis of heterotopic ossification in spinal cord injury patients. Paraplegia 33 (7), 398–401.

103. Freed, J.H., Hahn, H., et al., 1982. The use of the three-phase bone scan in the early diagnosis of heterotopic ossification (HO) and in the evaluation of Didronel therapy. Paraplegia 20 (4), 208–216.

104. Mavrogenis, A.F., Soucacos, P.N., et al., 2011. Heterotopic ossification revisited. Orthopedics 34 (3), 177.

105. Lin, S.H., Chou, C.L., et al., 2014. Ultrasonography in early diagnosis of heterotopic ossification. J. Med. Ultrasound 22 (4), 222–227.

106. Seipel, R., Langner, S., et al., 2012. Neurogenic heterotopic ossification: epidemiology and morphology on conventional radiographs in an early neurological rehabilitation population. Skeletal Radiol. 41 (1), 61–66.

107. De Smet, A.A., Norris, M.A., et al., 1992. Magnetic resonance imaging of myositis ossificans: analysis of seven cases. Skeletal Radiol. 21 (8), 503–507.

108. Lima, M.C., Passarelli, M.C., et al., 2014. The use of SPECT/CT in the evaluation of heterotopic ossification in para/tetraplegics. Acta Ortop. Bras. 22 (1), 12–16.

109. Scharf, S., 2009. SPECT/CT imaging in general orthopedic practice. Semin. Nucl. Med. 39 (5), 293–307.

110. Melamed, E., Robinson, D., et al., 2002. Brain injury-related heterotopic bone formation: treatment strategy and results. Am. J. Phys. Med. Rehabil. 81 (9), 670–674.

111. Reznik, J.E., Biros, E., et al., 2017. A preliminary investigation on the effect of extracorporeal shock wave therapy as a treatment for neurogenic heterotopic ossification following traumatic brain injury. Part II: effects on function. Brain Inj. 31 (4), 533–541.

112. Reznik, J.E., Biros, E., et al., 2017. A preliminary investigation on the effect of extracorporeal shock wave therapy as a treatment for neurogenic heterotopic ossification following traumatic brain injury. Part I: effects on pain. Brain Inj. 31 (4), 526–532.

CHAPTER 19

Psychological sequelae of spinal cord injuries

Iftah Biran and Jacqueline Reznik

INTRODUCTION

This chapter describes in detail spinal and vertebral somatoform disorders, including the more common conversion disorders. These disorders resemble various neurological presentations; however, no organic explanation can be found. The chapter first places spinal cord injury (SCI) conversion in an historical context. This is followed by a general description of conversion and somatic symptom disorder, the various clinical presentations and the clinical approach. The remainder of the chapter is devoted to the psychiatric and psychological sequela of genuine spinal cord injury.

HISTORICAL PERSPECTIVE OF CONVERSION DISORDERS

Hysteria has been known about since ancient times and its protean chameleon-like presentations have intrigued medical practitioners both then and now. In essence, hysteria is the appearance of medically unexplained syndromes, which were originally described in Babylon, Assyria, ancient Egypt, Greece and Rome, as well as throughout the medieval ages and modern times. The multiple diagnostic terms given to these disorders include, among others, hysteria, conversion disorders, dissociative disorders, functional neurological disorders and psychogenic disorders – testimony to the difficulty of defining and understanding this condition.[1]

Although epileptic-like seizures were, and still are, one of the major manifestations of conversion disorders,[1,2] hysteria and conversion disorders can mimic almost any neurological deficit and presentation, among them spinal-like presentations. These spinal presentations have an important role in the modern formulations of hysteria. In the middle of the nineteenth century the emergence of 'railway spine' (clinical complaints and physical somatic ailments related to train accidents) opened a discussion on the relative contribution of somatic versus physical factors to this syndrome. Railway spine, which was first regarded as a physical disorder, gradually lost its physical stand and was eventually regarded as a psycho-neurosis. In a way, this process paved the road for Charcot and Freud in creating modern formulations of hysteria.[3]

This inconclusive boundary between the physical and the psychological is still observed nowadays in multiple disorders.[4] Spinal disorders, although not the leading presentations of conversion functional morbidity, still take a prominent place in this controversy. For example, whiplash injury is a condition associated with an acceleration–deceleration injury to the spine. The ongoing debate regarding the relative contribution of the physical and psychological factors to this condition follow the debates of the nineteenth century and, as such, whiplash injury could be regarded as the modern offspring of railway spine.[5]

CONVERSION AND SOMATIC SYMPTOM DISORDER

SCI disorders related to psychological mechanisms and mental disorders are usually attributed, according to the 5th edition of the Diagnostic and Statistical Manual of Mental Disorders (DSM-5), to the category of somatic symptom and related disorders. The mainstay of this group of disorders is the emergence of somatic symptoms, or the exaggerated concern regarding these symptoms without an explanatory neurological or other medical aetiology. These symptoms might be related to psychological factors; hence, their inclusion in DSM-5.[6] Those who work with patients who suffer from spinal complaints commonly encounter two disorders within this category:

- Somatic symptom disorder:

  Patients who suffer from this disorder manifest with at least one distressing somatic symptom and are excessively occupied with it. This is manifested by disproportionately thinking about the symptom and its severity, exaggerated anxiety related to the symptom and overly immersing one's self in behaviours related to the symptom (e.g. multiple doctor visits and consultations). The duration of the disorder must be at least 6 months. Some of these patients present with a significant pain component. Many of the patients with back pain can be diagnosed with this disorder.[7]

- Conversion disorder or functional neurological symptom disorder:

  Patients with this disorder suffer from a neurological deficit or symptom, which is incompatible with a neurological or medical condition and cannot be explained by an organic cause. In the context of spinal disorders, these would be the patients who suffer from awkward gait deficit, unexplained tetra-paresis or tetraplegia, peculiar sensory deficits involving the limbs or the trunk, as well as urinary or bowel incontinence.

People who suffer from the above two disorders have at least, by their opinion, a genuine and authentic deficit. However, at times when the patient seems to be producing the deficit actively and consciously, two other disorders should be considered. The first is factitious disorder, in which the patient falsifies the spinal complaints for a primary psychologically motivated gain (adopting the sick role). The second is malingering, in which the patient actively falsifies the complaints and the clinical presentation, not only for a primary gain, but also for a secondary gain (i.e. for an obvious external reward). While factitious disorder is included in the somatic symptom and related disorders sections of DSM-5, malingering is not regarded as such, and so is no longer included.[6]

The interaction between psychological symptomatology and spinal impairments is bi-directional; not only can psychological conditions present with spinal symptomatology, but spinal symptoms can lead to psychological stress. Therefore, it is not surprising that a large percentage of those who suffer from spinal disorders present with psychological co-morbidities, such as depression and anxiety.[8] This connection will be discussed later in the chapter.

Spinal symptoms

Psychological-related spinal symptomatology mimics and follows known medical and neurological spinal

Box 19.1 Presentation of spinal cord conversion

- Presentations that follow 'regular' syndromes:
  - tetraplegia
  - paraplegia
  - central cord-like syndrome
  - Brown-Séquard-like syndrome
  - anterior cord-like syndrome
  - conus cauda-like syndromes
- Unique presentations:
  - astasia-abasia
  - camptocormia
  - opisthotonus

and vertebral syndromes, although incompletely and aberrantly (Box 19.1). The various SCI symptomatologies are extensively described elsewhere in this book. However, in order to orientate the reader of this chapter, a brief description of spinal symptomatology is included here.

Spinal syndromes following organic anatomical damage and pathological processes are classified according to the American Spinal Injury Association into five distinct syndromes.

1. Central cord syndrome – incomplete cervical injury leading to loss of sensation and motion in the upper limbs.
2. Brown-Séquard syndrome – an asymmetric damage to the cord leading to hemi-sensory loss of motor and proprioception sensation below the level of the injury and contralateral loss of pain and temperature sensation.
3. Anterior cord syndrome – loss of motor and all sensory sensations aside from preserved proprioception.

4. Cauda equina syndrome – injury to the lower nerve roots leading to flaccid paralysis of the legs, as well as sensory impairment across all modalities and areflexic bowel and bladder.
5. Conus medullaris syndrome – similar to cauda equina syndrome; however, as the cord is also involved there is a combination of upper and lower motor deficit (see Chapters 1 and 11 for further information on spinal syndromes).[9]

Psychogenic spinal symptomatology can thus manifest with any combination of these syndromes, including sensory impairments, pain, weakness and paresis (e.g. tetra-paresis, para-paresis), urinary and bowel complaints and gait impairments.

Specific and unique presentations are astasia-abasia and camptocormia. Astasia-abasia is a term for hysterical gait disorders that can take various forms. In clinical practice, whenever a patient presents with an awkward gait that does not fit the known neurological and orthopaedic gait impairments, the term astasia-abasia is used (Fig. 19.1).[10–12]

Camptocormia, or bent spine, is a condition whereby subjects present with marked flexion of the thoraco-lumbar spine (in Greek, *campto* means bent and *kormos* means trunk). The flexion increases during walking and recedes while lying down. Among the multiple aetiologies of this condition, there are also psychogenic cases, some of which are related to post-traumatic stress disorder (PTSD). During World Wars I and II it was described in soldiers and recruits who were unable to cope with the stress of battle (Fig. 19.2).[13–15]

Another unique psychogenic manifestation that appears prima facie as involving the spine is psychogenic opisthotonus. Opisthotonus is characterised by severe spastic hyperextension of the head, neck and spine forming an arc-like posture. It can follow neurological conditions (e.g. tetanus, brain stem damage). Decerebrate posturing (opisthatonus) indicates brain stem damage, specifically damage below the level of the red nucleus, as well as psychological conditions (e.g. psychogenic seizures)

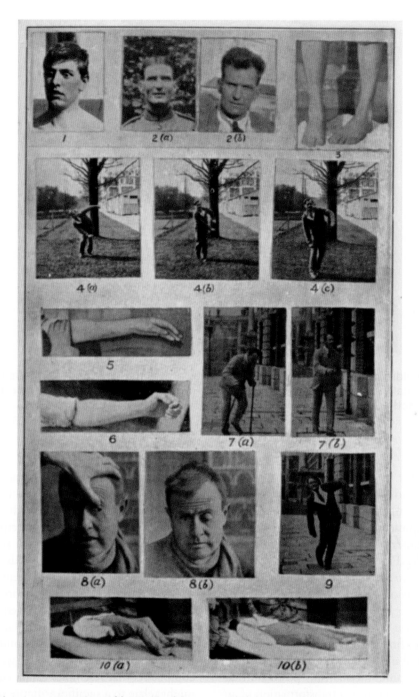

Figure 19.1 Various presentation of hysterical (conversion) impairments.
Figs 4(a–c), 7(a–b) and 9 depict hysterical gait disorders, including astasia-abasia
Source: Hurst A.F., 1918. Medical diseases of the war. London, UK: Edward Arnold; Fig II, p. 38.

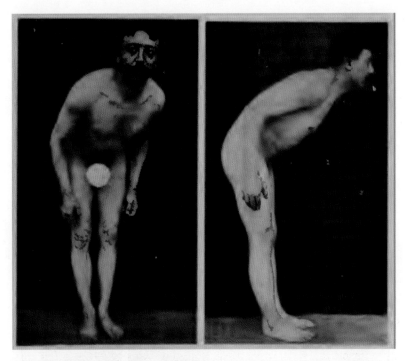

Figure 19.2 A soldier who was buried alive in debris by a shell during World War I. His trunk was flexed symmetrically and was impossible to correct. However, on a bed or on the floor he was completely relaxed and could be straightened, suggesting a psychological aetiology.

Source: Roussy G., Lhermitte J., 1918. The psychoneuroses of war: University of London Press; pp. 28–9.

(see Chapter 1 for further detail on red nucleus). This disturbing and disquieting posture presents as a genuine spine injury. It is no wonder that the artistic visual representations of a woman with this condition is at times referred to as 'The nymph with the broken back' (Figs 19.3, 19.4).[16–18]

Despite extensive research and emerging academic interest in conversion disorders, the mechanism of conversion disorders in general, and spinal conversion disorders in particular, is far from understood. Suggested mechanisms range from psychodynamic-based models to more biological models.

The psychodynamic mechanisms postulate that the neurological symptom is a transformation of an emotional unconscious conflict. According to this explanation, the symptom has an inner symbolic meaning that has to be deciphered. (For example,

a patient who walks in a peculiar way with a bent posture describes his fear of confronting his employer and assertively demanding an increase in his salary; the therapist would interpret his bent gait as a manifestation of his fear to stand in front of authoritative figures in his life.) This disorder can also be related to past adverse life events and trauma.[19]

Cognitive and learning theories suggest that the bodily symptom is a learned symptom that follows early exposure to similar manifestations and their impact on the environment and other family members. A patient with psychogenic urinary complaints that resembles cauda equina syndrome might relate to a significant figure in his childhood that suffered from similar organic manifestation, stressing its impact on getting the attention of other family members.

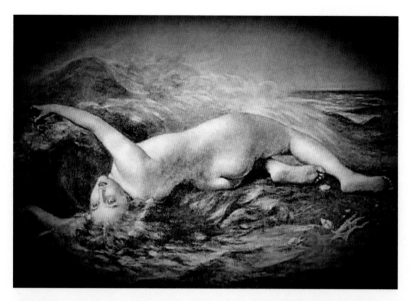

Figure 19.3 Pierre Dupuis, 'An Ondine Playing on the Waves' (circa 1896), depicting the concept of the 'nymph with the broken back' and illustrating an opsthotonus-like posture.

Source: Dijkstra B., 1986. The weightless woman; the nymph with the broken back; and the mythology of therapeutic rape. Idols of perversity; fantasies of feminine evil in *fin-de-siècle* culture. New York, NY: Oxford University Press; pp. 83–118.

Evolutionary models suggest that conversion symptoms might be a manifestation of various ways of coping with stress, such as the fight, flight or freeze response. In this regard, a patient who has a psychogenic magnetic gait, during which it appears as though his legs are stuck to the floor, might be demonstrating a derivative of the freeze response.

Functional studies suggest that the generation of conversion disorders, especially those with motor involvement, are related to an impaired network involved in motor programming by the prefrontal cortex. The role of limbic structures, as well as structures related to body schema, has also been implicated in spinal conversion.[20]

Regardless of all the above mechanisms, conversion spinal symptoms can follow various triggers and predisposing conditions without a clear cause and effect mechanism. These triggers can be spinal surgery,[21] as well as spinal anaesthesia for various disorders, including disorders and conditions that are not related to the spine, such as caesarean section[22] and arthroscopic surgery of a knee.[23] This is in accordance with the notion that conversion disorders 'use' a somatic predilection of the bodily organs.[24] A similar occurrence is that of subjects with low back pain with clear structural aetiology, who can present with hysterical paralysis that is not related to the structural lesion.[25]

Diagnosis

Diagnosis of a conversion disorder is based on a combination of three factors:

1. Clinical presentation that is not typical for an organic neurological syndrome (e.g. astasia-abasia).
2. Neurological examination that does not show the expected findings (e.g. lack of signs for motor pyramidal impairment in a subject suffering from what seems like spastic paraplegia; anaesthesia not following an expected dermatomal pattern).

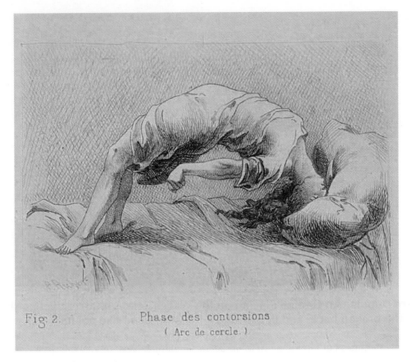

Figure 19.4 A female patient during an attack of hysteria with an arc-like opsthotonic posture of the spine and body.

Source: Richer P., Charcot J.-M., 1885. Etudes cliniques sur l'hystéro-épilepsie ou grande hystérie. 2nd ed. Paris: A. Delahaye et E. Lecrosnier; Plate III, p. 68.

3. Lack of an organic neurological pathology in laboratory tests (e.g. imaging studies, nerve conduction studies) or an organic impairment which, according to the discretion of the clinician, has an impact beyond what would be expected.

At times, the clinical picture is not straightforward and the clinician has to weigh these three factors.

The diagnosis can be supported by both the psychiatric and the psychological evaluation. As described above, subjects with somatic symptom disorders tend to show exaggerated cognitive preoccupation with the symptoms, as well as an increase in behaviours related to the symptoms (e.g. multiple consults and laboratory tests). Their emotional reaction might be amplified or blunted to the extent of being oblivious to the deficit. At the extreme end, this is called 'la belle indifférence'

– a lack of concern related to the impairment.[26] Previous editions of the DSM (i.e. up to DSM-IV TR) required a psychological trigger for the diagnosis of conversion disorder. However, the most recent edition (DSM-5) discarded this requirement and psychological factors are recorded only as specifiers.[6]

Another clinical task in the diagnosis of such conditions is the elimination of factitious disorders and malingering. While in conversion disorders and somatic symptom disorders the sufferer is genuinely impaired and does not fake any of their complaints, in factitious disorders and malingering the patient is faking the deficit for a primary (e.g. taking the patient role) or secondary gain (e.g. monetary compensation) respectively. It is important to note the diagnosis of all these conditions is not mutually exclusive; therefore the clinician has to weigh up the various contribution of each component.[6]

Epidemiology

In general, conversion disorders and somatic symptom disorders are relatively common. The prevalence of somatic symptom disorders is 7% in the general population and conversion disorders are found in up to 5% of all referrals to neurology clinics.[6]

SCI-like conversion symptoms, however, are relatively rare. In a series of 1144 patients with symptoms unexplained by neurological disease, out of which 209 patients had conversion symptoms, only 58 could be clear mimics of SCI disorders presenting with functional gait impairment.

The analysis of the patients' presentations was not according to a neurological localising approach and therefore extracting this data is not conclusive.[2] In a large retrospective study looking at the incidence of psychogenic paraplegia among referrals to spinal injury centres, there were only 20 referrals with conversion paraplegia out of 7000 referrals (less than 0.3%).[27] However, SCI-like symptoms can account for approximately from one-fifth up to two-thirds of subjects with motor conversion.[28,29]

Interventions

The approach to the patient with SCI conversion disorders should be an integrative multidisciplinary approach encompassing psychiatric therapy, psychological interventions and behavioural modification, as well as occupational therapy, speech therapy and physical rehabilitation.[28,30,31]

- *Psychiatric therapy:* there are no medications approved specifically for conversion disorders and there is only minimal data regarding the use of antidepressants for somatic symptom and related disorders. Therefore, the psychiatric interventions are usually aimed at psychiatric co-morbidity such as depression or anxiety. However, in somatic symptom disorders with prominent pain component, it is advisable to use antidepressants with nociceptive function.[32,33]

- *Psychological interventions:* these can be directed at exposing and solving the conflict that lies beneath the spinal symptom. This is in accordance with the classic notion that hysteria and conversion disorders stem from 'conversion' of an unconscious conflict into a bodily symptom. However, currently most accepted protocols for the treatment of motor conversion are based on cognitive behavioural therapy (CBT).[31] CBT-based interventions include, among other things, psychoeducation aiming at building insight into the psychological basis of the symptom, challenging cognitive distortions and regarding, among others, the ability of the patient to cope with the disability. Relaxation techniques, as well as behavioural modifications, are taught, aimed at encouraging adaptive functional behaviours, while unwanted behaviours are discouraged, usually by using positive reinforcements.[31,34]

- *Physiotherapy:* physiotherapists stand in the frontline of treating these patients (Box 19.2). However, they face multiple

Box 19.2 Practice highlights for the physiotherapist

- Adopt a bio-psycho-social work model
- Work in a multidisciplinary team including, among others, social workers, psychologists and psychiatrists
- De-emphasise the deficit; emphasise the function
- Avoid mobility aids
- Structured programs are of benefit (structured session etc.)
- Accepting attitude
- Using non-derogatory terms to convey the diagnosis, such as 'functional disorder'
- Use the patient's preserved function as a tool for empowerment rather than as a way to confront them.

obstacles in providing adequate care to this population, such as lack of structured services and non-optimal communication with the referring doctors, usually neurologists.[35] A recent consensus recommendation stressed that the physiotherapist should approach the patient through a bio-psycho-social aetiological framework and use specific techniques tailored for the patient with conversion disorder, such as de-emphasising the deficit and focusing on the function and avoiding mobility aids. In the context of gait impairments, as observed in spinal conversion, the physiotherapist can use specific techniques such as walking backwards or sideways or walking to a rhythm.[36]

A more recent study suggests that specialist neuro-physiotherapy intervention may demonstrate even greater efficacy. The specific program consisted of eight sessions over five consecutive days, each lasting 45–90 minutes. Each session consisted of an education segment, a movement-retraining segment and the development of a management plan.[37]

Some of the interventions have a distinct placebo effect. A single case study demonstrated a dramatic improvement in a patient with flaccid paraplegia following transcranial magnetic stimulation (TMS), which was used as a diagnostic tool, demonstrating normal motor-evoked potentials.[38] Motor-evoked potentials can be effective due to both neuro-physiological changes and to a placebo effect. Faradic current therapy can also be used as a placebo alongside regular rehabilitation.[39] Above all, the approach should be accepting and not blaming, and communication with the patient should aim at trying to put the neurological deficit in the appropriate context, emphasising the therapeutic options available.[40]

Accordingly, the terms used to deliver the diagnosis are crucial, as some might be offensive to the patient and therefore less acceptable. A preferred term for delivering the diagnosis is 'functional disorder', while terms found to be rather insulting, even after a detailed explanation, are 'psychogenic' and

'medically unexplained'.[41] Similarly, the characteristic inconsistencies observed throughout the evaluation should be used to show the patient their preserved capabilities and intact neurological system, stressing the reversibility of the deficit (i.e. the ability to move the legs in the bed while the inability to walk), rather than as a tool to 'catch' the patient out.[42]

Outcome and prognosis

The data regarding prognosis in conversion SCI disorders is inconclusive. The outcome for spinal motor conversion (patients with tetraplegia or paraplegia) is variable, ranging from full recovery in all patients to around one-third reaching full recovery or partial recovery.[27,28,43]

Specific prognostic factors for spinal conversion are not well documented. However, according to a systematic review, prognostic factors for motor conversion are as follows:

- Positive prognostic factors are short duration of symptoms, early diagnosis and high satisfaction with care.
- Negative prognostic factors were delayed diagnosis and personality disorder.

Factors with unclear prognostic influence are age, comorbid anxiety and depression, IQ, educational status, marital status and pending litigation.[44]

PSYCHOLOGICAL ADAPTATION TO SPINAL CORD INJURY

Although this chapter primarily examines conditions in which psychological factors present as bodily symptoms, in particular SCI symptoms, 'genuine' SCI impairments can lead to psychological stress and co-morbidity. This is of no surprise. As described elsewhere in this book, SCI brings havoc to people's lives and the person with an SCI has to face issues of disability, pain syndromes, medical complications, loss of work and much more (see Chapters 20 and 21 for more detail).

An ongoing debate in the literature is differentiating between normal adjustment processes to such a loss versus psychological morbidity that is beyond what would be expected in normal adaptation,[8,45,46] and there is an effort to understand how a person adapts to such a severe injury (the Spinal Cord Injury Adjustment Model (SCIAM)).[47]

Regardless of this debate, recent studies, including prospective studies[48] and reviews,[8] suggest that following SCI an individual is prone to developing severe psychological morbidities, including depression (probably the most prevalent psychiatric morbidity), anxiety, PTSD, suicidality, alcohol dependence and abuse disorder, drug dependence and abuse disorder, bipolar disorders, as well as rare cases of psychosis. The proportion of subjects with mental disorders in this population can reach 22% at the beginning of a rehabilitation program; it falls to 17% upon discharge from rehabilitation; although it can rise as high as 25% after the 6-month period following discharge (see Chapter 15).[48]

The treating physiotherapist is often best placed to manage patients with suspected psychiatric disorders because of their daily routine with the patient. In cases where the physiotherapist suspects that further evaluation is required or that the patient may pose a risk to themselves (e.g. depression, severe anxiety, suicidality, exacerbation of substance abuse or acute deterioration due to exacerbation of PTSD following the trauma that caused the spinal injury), it is important that they are aware of the following issues.

Firstly, the physiotherapist should be familiar with these conditions. It is beyond the scope of this chapter to address all these conditions; however there are many useful resources available.[49,50] Secondly, the physiotherapist should adopt a well-informed clinical approach that will enable him to direct the patient to the appropriate caregiver and therapy in a gentle non-coercive manner.[51]

When considering the best approach to managing the psychiatric co-morbidity of this population, especially depression, it is important to note that there are many features that herald poor prognosis to drug therapy such as chronic pain, chronic medical conditions, unemployment and dependence on activities of daily living. However, regardless of these features, interventions with anti-depressants can decrease depression levels; Psychotherapy may also be of benefit in these conditions.[52–54]

Specific considerations regarding the management of depression, anxiety, PTSD and suicidality are given here.

Depression

Although, as stated above, depression is the leading manifestation of psychopathology following SCI and up to 30% of this population might suffer from depression,[8] it should be remembered that most subjects with an SCI do not suffer depression.[55] Diagnosing depression is based on documenting its core features, such as depressed mood, anhedonia (the inability to feel pleasure in normally pleasurable activities), feelings of guilt, suicidality, impaired concentration, low self-esteem and changes in psychomotor activity, sleep and weight.[56] As some of these are also directly related to the physical effects of the spinal injury (e.g. decreased motor activity or sleepiness secondary to medications or sleep apnoea (see Chapter 18)), the clinician should try to weigh up the relevance of each of the symptoms.

Another important distinction is between depression and grief reaction, as the latter requires different interventions.[45] Screening self-questionnaires for depression can be of benefit in the diagnosis and PHQ-9 and PHQ-2 are the recommended questionnaires to use.[57] The caregiver should also beware of the high prevalence of co-morbidity with other psychiatric disorders, such as anxiety, PTSD, substance abuse, alcohol abuse and bipolar disorder.[58] Treatment can follow classical interventions, such as the use of selective serotonin reuptake inhibitors (SSRIs), serotonin and norepinephrine reuptake inhibitors (SNRIs), psychotherapy, as well as a physical training program, and all of these can be of benefit.[52,53,59,60]

Anxiety

Anxiety is not a single disorder, but encompasses multiple conditions such as general anxiety disorder, panic disorder and simple phobias. Its prevalence following SCI is high and up to 45% of subjects with an SCI might report various symptoms of anxiety on self-report measures. However, there is a lack of consensus regarding the diagnosis and screening of anxiety in the population with an SCI and therefore there is a wide range of reported prevalence of anxiety and its related conditions. When using a clinical diagnostic interview, the prevalence of general anxiety disorder can reach 5.4% and that of panic disorder 5%.[61] Subjects can benefit from cognitive behavioural therapy,[62] as well as from pharmacotherapy. There are no specific guidelines as to specific interventions; however, it is possible that many individuals with an SCI are treated with anxiolytics.[58]

Post-traumatic stress disorder (PTSD)

PTSD occurs following an exposure to a stressful and traumatic event and is characterised by a psychological distress that encompasses symptoms from four domains, including: 1) avoidance of memories or reminders of the event, 2) re-experiencing the trauma, 3) increased arousal and reactivity, and 4) negative cognitions and mood. It is only diagnosed at least 30 days following the event. Earlier symptoms can be diagnosed as acute stress disorder.[63] PTSD is common in subjects with an SCI, and its reported prevalence ranges from 7% to 60%.[64] Psychological

interventions, such as prolonged exposure therapy, which includes imaginal and in-vivo exposure to the traumatic memory, can be of benefit. However, to date there has been no published data regarding prolonged exposure therapy in subjects with an SCI,[60] as well as specific evidence-proofed guidelines for pharmacological interventions.

Suicidality

Suicide is one of the three leading causes of death post-SCI (alongside cardiovascular disease and systemic infections). It is responsible for 6.3% of total deaths in this population, 8.6% in tetraplegics and 2.8% in paraplegics.[65] Some patients refuse life-sustaining treatment or ask for the removal of such treatment and this should be discussed in the context of euthanasia.[66]

CLINICAL CASE PRESENTATIONS

This section illustrates some of the issues that were described above through two clinical illustrations. The clinical illustrations are based on the stories of real patients and follow typical clinical presentations' and management course; however, in order to maintain patient confidentiality, extensive changes including combining clinical stories of different patients have been made.

THE LITTLE MERMAID

M. was a 21-year-old woman who presented with a one-week history of gait impairment and urinary retention. On admission she was paraplegic and asked to be catheterised in order to relieve her urinary retention. She described a normal upbringing, completed all her developmental milestones in time and was a high school graduate. She was currently in her first year of college. She was recently married

and the paraplegia started a few days after she returned from her honeymoon trip abroad. On her neurological examination there was a complete paralysis of the legs with normal tone, normal to slightly increased deep tendon reflexes and a questionable up-going toe while checking for Babinski sign. Sensory-wise, there was an inconsistent sensory level at the level of her scapulae and a saddle-like anaesthesia

THE LITTLE MERMAID—cont'd

involving her genitalia. She could move from lying in bed to sitting without any assistance, suggesting preserved function of her abdominal muscles. There were no other findings in her neurological examination. A urinary catheter was inserted, demonstrating no urinary retention. The lack of significant pyramidal signs and the atypical anaesthesia suggested a non-neurological aetiology. A psychiatric consult was not suggestive for any psychiatric disorder.

In the following days a physiotherapist, who encouraged any sign of movement in the lower limb, treated her. Following this, she started to walk with a peculiar gait. It looked as though her legs were fused together and there was no space between her thighs, thus resembling a mermaid. While talking about that with the psychiatrist she expressed her ambivalence towards having sex with her husband, attributing the ambivalence to recollections of a sexual assault years ago. Following an extensive period in rehabilitation with both physiotherapy and CBT-inspired psychotherapy she returned to her normal life with normal gait (see earlier in this chapter for a fuller description of these interventions).

This case illustrates the psychogenic traumatic aetiology and the role of multidisciplinary assessment and treatment.

THE SHIVERING PARAPLEGIC

R. was a 45-year-old man who worked as a manual labourer. Following an accident in his workplace where he was trapped under collapsing scaffolding, he developed a peculiar gait typified by shaking, shivering and staggering, as well as episodic stuttering exacerbated when he was stressed, and diffuse pains and aching all over his body. The aches soon localised to his legs and lower back, and the gait disorder worsened and he became wheelchair bound. Neurological examination was inconclusive. Extensive medical workup, including brain MRI, total spine MRI and nerve conduction studies, were negative for any abnormality.

His psychiatric examination, 6 months following the accident, was notable for symptoms of PTSD related to the accident, as well as profound dissociative signs, such as depersonalisation, dis-ownership of his legs and minimal de-realisation.

He was treated for more than 6 months in a rehabilitation ward with multiple interventions and therapies, including physiotherapy, speech therapy and psychotherapy, as well as anti-depressants. Regardless of all these interventions, there was minimal change in his condition and he remained with these disabilities for the next couple of years.

This case demonstrates that psychiatric co-morbidity is detrimental for a patient's outcome.

Evidence-based practice points

Unfortunately, there are no established evidence-based practice recommendations for conversion disorders, particularly for those with SCI disorder presentations. Similarly, there are no specific guidelines for the psychological and psychiatric manifestations of SCI. However, there are some points that should be taken into consideration when treating these patients:

- Work with a multidisciplinary team to address both the neurological manifestations and the psychological co-morbidities.
- Adopt a respectful attitude, both in the delivery of the diagnosis, by using the appropriate terms and labels (i.e. functional disorders), and in giving psychoeducation.
- Treat both neurological and psychiatric co-morbidities.
- In physiotherapy, emphasise function and not deficits.
- Avoid using medical rehabilitation devices that can aggravate disability.
- If needed, allow a long-term rehabilitation program, working and using the interpersonal connection as a tool for therapeutic alliance.
- Address, with the multidisciplinary team, psychiatric co-morbidities, especially for depression, suicidality, post-trauma and substance abuse.

SUMMARY

Somatic symptoms and related disorders in general, and SCI conversion disorders in particular, stand in a unique place in the medical nosological model, where an organic bodily-based explanation is not readily available. Therefore, diagnosing and treating patients with such conditions is a challenging task that requires the simultaneous use of both medical–pathophysiological knowledge and psychological insight and understanding. This can be achieved through the coordinated work of a multidisciplinary team, including the treating physiotherapists, neurologists, orthopaedists, neurosurgeons, as well as psychiatrists and psychologists.

Physiotherapists are in a unique and important position in the team, as they are the caregivers who see these patients for the most amount of time. Accordingly, their input for diagnosis and therapy is of paramount value and a deep understanding of these conditions is highly warranted. Therapeutic interventions are both bodily- and psychology-based and at times are intertwined together.

The physiotherapist should also be aware of the high prevalence of psychiatric co-morbidity in all spinal presentations, both in conversion disorders and in spinal injury following an illness or trauma. Treatment for al psychiatric co-morbidities requires a multidisciplinary approach with psychological as well as pharmacological interventions, as necessitated.

References

1. Trimble, M., Reynolds, E., 2016. A brief history of hysteria: from the ancient to the modern. Handb. Clin. Neurol. 139, 3–10. Elsevier.

2. Carson, A., Lehn, A., 2016. Epidemiology. Handb. Clin. Neurol. 139, Elsevier.

3. Harrington, R., 2003. On the tracks of trauma: railway spine reconsidered. Soc. Hist. Med. 16 (2), 209–223.

4. Showalter, E., 1998. Hystories: Hysterical Epidemics and Modern Media. Columbia University Press.

5. Pearce, J., 1999. A Critical Appraisal of the Chronic Whiplash Syndrome. BMJ Publishing Group Ltd.

6. American Psychiatric Association, 2013. Somatic Symptoms and Related Disorders. Diagnostic and Statistical Manual of Mental Disorders: DSM-5, fifth ed. American Psychiatric Publishing, Washington, DC, pp. 309–327.

7. Robertson, D., Kumbhare, D., et al., 2017. Associations between low back pain and depression and somatization in a Canadian emerging adult population. J. Can. Chiropr. Assoc. 61 (2), 96.

8. Craig, A., Tran, Y., et al., 2009. Psychological morbidity and spinal cord injury: a systematic review. Spinal Cord 47 (2), 108.

9. Kirshblum, S.C., Burns, S.P., et al., 2011. International standards for neurological classification of spinal cord injury (revised 2011). J. Spinal Cord Med. 34 (6), 535–546.

10. Keane, J.R., 1989. Hysterical gait disorders: 60 cases. Neurology 39 (4), 586–589.

11. Roussy, G., Lhermitte, J., 1918. The Psychoneuroses of War. University of London Press.

12. Hurst, A.F., 1918. Medical Diseases of the War. Edward Arnold, London, UK.

13. Pérez-Sales, P., 1990. Camptocormia. Br. J. Psychiatry 157 (5), 765–767.

14. Azher, S.N., Jankovic, J., 2005. Camptocormia pathogenesis, classification, and response to therapy. Neurology 65 (3), 355–359.

15. Skidmore, F., Anderson, K., et al., 2007. Psychogenic camptocormia. Mov. Disord. 22 (13), 1974–1975.

16. Dijkstra, B., 1986. The Weightless Woman; the Nymph With the Broken Back; and the Mythology of Therapeutic Rape. Idols of Perversity; Fantasies of Feminine Evil in Fin-De-Siècle Culture. Oxford University Press, New York, NY.

17. Didi-Huberman, G., 2003. Invention of Hysteria. MIT Press, Cambridge, MA, USA.

18. Richer, P., Charcot, J.M., 1885. Etudes Cliniques Sur L'hystéro-Épilepsie Ou Grande Hystérie, second ed. A. Delahaye et E. Lecrosnier, Paris.

19. Nicholson, T., Aybek, S., et al., 2016. Life events and escape in conversion disorder. Psychol. Med. 46 (12), 2617–2626.

20. Saj, A., Raz, N., et al., 2014. Disturbed mental imagery of affected body-parts in patients with hysterical conversion paraplegia correlates with pathological limbic activity. Brain Sci. 4 (2), 396–404.

21. Boudissa, M., Castelain, J., et al., 2015. Conversion paralysis after cervical spine arthroplasty: a case report and literature review. Orthop. Traumatol. Surg. Res. 101 (5), 637–641.

22. Attri, J., Khetarpal, R., et al., 2015. Hysterical paraplegia. Karnataka Anaesth. J. 1 (4), 208–209.

23. Tsetsou, A., Karageorgou, E., et al., 2017. Conversion disorder: Tetraplegia after spinal anesthesia. The Greek E-Journal of Perioperative Medicine 16 (a), 71–77.

24. Freud, S., 1905. Fragment of an analysis of a case of hysteria. In: Strachey, J. (Ed.), The Standard Edition of the Complete Psychological Works of Sigmund Freud, Volume VII (1901–1905): A Case of Hysteria, Three Essays on Sexuality and Other Works. pp. 3–122. 1901.

25. Higuchi, T., Tonogai, I., et al., 2016. Hysterical conversion paralysis in an adolescent boy with lumbar spondylolysis. J. Pediatr. Orthop. B 25 (3), 271–274.

26. Stone, J., Smyth, R., et al., 2006. La belle indifférence in conversion symptoms and hysteria: systematic review. Br. J. Psychiatry 188, 204–209.

27. Baker, J.H., Silver, J.R., 1987. Hysterical paraplegia. J. Neurol. Neurosurg. Psychiatry 50 (4), 375–382.

28. Heruti, R.J., Reznik, J., et al., 2002. Conversion motor paralysis disorder: analysis of 34 consecutive referrals. Spinal Cord 40 (7), 335–340.

29. Stone, J., Warlow, C., et al., 2010. The symptom of functional weakness: a controlled study of 107 patients. Brain 133, 1537–1551.

30. Heruti, R.J., Levy, A., et al., 2002. Conversion motor paralysis disorder: overview and rehabilitation model. Spinal Cord 40, 327.

31. McCormack, R., Moriarty, J., et al., 2014. Specialist inpatient treatment for severe motor conversion disorder: a retrospective comparative study. J. Neurol. Neurosurg. Psychiatry 85 (8), 895–900.

32. Somashekar, B., Jainer, A., et al., 2013. Psychopharmaco-therapy of somatic symptoms disorders. Int. Rev. Psychiatry 25 (1), 107–115.

33. Kleinstauber, M., Witthoft, M., et al., 2014. Pharmacological interventions for somatoform disorders in adults. Cochrane Database Syst. Rev. (11), CD010628.

34. Guenther, R.T., Frank, R.G., et al., 1993. Management of behavior on a spinal cord injury unit. Neurorehabilitation 3 (2), 50–59.

35. Edwards, M.J., Stone, J., et al., 2012. Physiotherapists and patients with functional (psychogenic) motor symptoms: a survey of attitudes and interest. J. Neurol. Neurosurg. Psychiatry 83 (6), 655–658.

36. Nielsen, G., Stone, J., et al., 2015. Physiotherapy for functional motor disorders: a consensus recommendation. J. Neurol. Neurosurg. Psychiatry 86, 1113–1119.

37. Nielsen, G., Buszewicz, M., et al., 2017. Randomised feasibility study of physiotherapy for patients with functional motor symptoms. J. Neurol. Neurosurg. Psychiatry 88 (6), 484–490.

38. Jellinek, D.A., Bradford, R., et al., 1992. The role of motor evoked potentials in the management of hysterical paraplegia: case report. Paraplegia 30, 300.

39. Karaahmet, O.Z., Gurcay, E., et al., 2017. Beneficial effect of faradic stimulation treatment on the rehabilitation of hysterical paraplegia. J. Back Musculoskeletal Rehabil. 30 (5), 1117–1119.

40. Roper, B.L., Martelli, M.F., 2002. Providing useful diagnostic feedback to patients with functional medical disorders and making referral for psychological treatment. Phy. Med. Rehabil. 16 (1), 163–166.

41. Ding, J.M., Kanaan, R.A.A., 2016. What should we say to patients with unexplained neurological symptoms? How explanation affects offence. J. Psychosom. Res. 91, 55–60.

42. Stone, J., Edwards, M., 2012. Trick or treat? Showing patients with functional (psychogenic) motor symptoms their physical signs. Neurology 79 (3), 282–284.

43. Apple, D., 1989. Hysterical spinal paralysis. Spinal Cord 27 (6), 428.

44. Gelauff, J., Stone, J., et al., 2014. The prognosis of functional (psychogenic) motor symptoms: a systematic review. J. Neurol. Neurosurg. Psychiatry 85 (2), 220–226.

45. Klyce, D.W., Bombardier, C.H., et al., 2015. Distinguishing grief from depression during acute recovery from spinal cord injury. Arch. Phys. Med. Rehabil. 96 (8), 1419–1425.

46. Bracken, M.B., Shepard, M.J., 1980. Coping and adaptation following acute spinal cord injury: a theoretical analysis. Spinal Cord 18 (2), 74.

47. Craig, A., Tran, Y., et al. Theory of adjustment following severe neurological injury: evidence supporting the spinal cord injury adjustment model. 2017.

48. Craig, A., Perry, K.N., et al., 2015. Prospective study of the occurrence of psychological disorders and comorbidities after spinal cord injury. Arch. Phys. Med. Rehabil. 96 (8), 1426–1434.

49. Biran, I., Reznik, J., 2017. Mental health. In: Morris, J., Perera, C., et al. (Eds.), Pharmacology Handbook for Physiotherapists. Chatswood. Elsevier, Australia, pp. 276–314.

50. Probst, M., Skjaerven, L.H., 2017. Physiotherapy in Mental Health and Psychiatry: A Scientific and Clinical Based Approach. Elsevier Health Sciences.

51. Physiotherapy Alberta College & Association. Managing challenging situations – a resource guide for physiotherapists. 2016. Online 17 December 2019. Available: https://www.physiotherapyalberta.ca/files/guide_managing_challenging_situations.pdf.

52. Fann, J.R., Bombardier, C.H., et al., 2011. Depression after spinal cord injury: comorbidities, mental health service use, and adequacy of treatment. Arch. Phys. Med. Rehabil. 92 (3), 352–360.

53. Fann, J.R., Bombardier, C.H., et al., 2015. Venlafaxine extended-release for depression following spinal cord injury: a randomized clinical trial. JAMA Psychiatry 72 (3), 247–258.

54. Elliott, T.R., Kennedy, P., 2004. Treatment of depression following spinal cord injury: an evidence-based review. Rehabil. Psychol. 49 (2), 134.

55. Dixon, T.M., Budd, M.A., 2017. Spinal Cord Injury. Practical Psychology in Medical Rehabilitation. Springer.

56. American Psychiatric Association, 2013. Depressive Disorders. Diagnostic and Statistical Manual of Mental Disorders: DSM-5, fifth ed. American Psychiatric Publishing, Washington, DC, pp. 155–188.

57. Poritz, J.M.P., Mignogna, J., et al., 2018. The patient health questionnaire depression screener in spinal cord injury. J. Spinal Cord Med. 41 (2), 238–244.

58. Ullrich, P.M., Smith, B.M., et al., 2014. Depression, healthcare utilization, and comorbid psychiatric disorders after spinal cord injury. J. Spinal Cord Med. 37 (1), 40–45.

59. Fann, J.R., Crane, D.A., et al., 2013. Depression treatment preferences after acute traumatic spinal cord injury. Arch. Phys. Med. Rehabil. 94 (12), 2389–2395.

60. Poritz, J.M., Warren, A.M., 2018. Psychosocial factors in spinal cord injury. In: Kirshblum, S., Lin, V.W. (Eds.), Spinal Cord Medicine. Springer Publishing Company, pp. 857–869.

61. Le, J., Dorstyn, D., 2016. Anxiety prevalence following spinal cord injury: a meta-analysis. Spinal Cord 54 (8), 570–578.

62. Mehta, S., Orenczuk, S., et al., 2011. An evidence-based review of the effectiveness of cognitive behavioral therapy for psychosocial issues post-spinal cord injury. Rehabil. Psychol. 56 (1), 15–25.

63. American Psychiatric Association, 2013. Trauma and Stressor-Related Disorders. DSM-5 Diagnostic and Statistical Manual of Mental Disorders, fifth ed. American Psychiatric Association, Washington, DC, pp. 265–290.

64. Cao, Y., Li, C., et al., 2017. Posttraumatic stress disorder after spinal cord injury. Rehabil. Psychol. 62 (2), 178.

65. Chamberlain, J.D., Buzzell, A., et al., 2019. Comparison of all-cause and cause-specific mortality of persons with traumatic spinal cord injuries to the general Swiss population: results from a national cohort study. Neuroepidemiology 52 (3–4), 205–213.

66. Waals, E.M.F., Post, M.W.M., et al., 2018. Experiences with euthanasia requests of persons with SCI in Belgium. Spinal Cord Ser. Cases 4, 62.

CHAPTER 20

Sociological issues associated with spinal cord injury – a personal journey

Dan Buckingham

INTRODUCTION

This chapter is based more on anecdotes and conjecture rather than academic studies and research-based facts because my background involves a significant amount of lived experience of spinal cord injury (SCI). I broke my neck in 1999. Back then I was an 18-year-old university student absolutely loving life, playing a bit of club rugby amid a very active social life and studying. It was while playing rugby that I fractured and dislocated my 6th and 7th cervical vertebrae. The nature of my injury has meant that, while I do not have any muscle function from the chest down, I have good arm and hand function with finger movement, which has allowed me to live as a high functioning tetraplegic and able to do most things independently. As I was leaving hospital after my initial rehabilitation, my doctor's parting words were that I would 'wave the flag high for people who live with disability'. While I did not exactly know what he meant, it was something I held on to, and it is an expectation that I hope I am living up to. Over the past 19 years, I have had significant involvement with the disability community through sport, work and my social life.

In my first year following discharge from the Burwood Spinal Injury Unit (the year 2000) I returned to the University of Otago to be back around my friends and my old life. However, it was a relatively isolating year as I tried to work out this new way of life with no one to use as a sounding board or reference point. The redeeming feature was travelling to Christchurch to practise and play wheelchair rugby. I loved the scene and the sport so much I moved to Christchurch the following year to immerse myself in it.

Sport became a huge, at times, all-encompassing part of my life. The focus of my sporting career has been representing New Zealand in wheelchair rugby, as part of the 'Wheel Blacks' for 16 years. I was first selected for the Wheel Blacks in 2001. That period of my life, up until I moved to Auckland at the end of 2007, was very much focused on playing wheelchair rugby. However, during this time I also completed a BA in Mass Communications at the University of Canterbury. The degree took an extended amount of time to complete as I took semesters off to travel and play wheelchair rugby for club teams overseas, including stints in Australia, USA and Canada. This I did in addition to playing

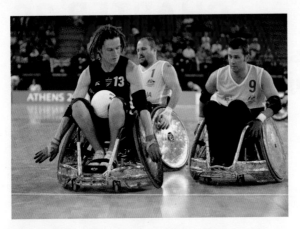

Figure 20.1 Playing for the Wheel Blacks at the Athens 2004 Paralympic Games.

for Canterbury and New Zealand. I also became active in sports administration, taking roles with ParaFed Canterbury, Canterbury Wheelchair Rugby and New Zealand Wheelchair Rugby (see Online resources for contact details).

By default, my circle of friends and social life throughout this period revolved around this world

of sport for people with disabilities. During this time, I also tried many other sports from sit-skiing to wheelchair tennis.

In 2008, while continuing to be heavily involved in wheelchair rugby, I moved to Auckland and began working with Attitude Pictures Ltd. An opportunity to work with the company was the catalyst for moving cities, although after seven years of being based in Christchurch, I was generally ready for change. The main focus of Attitude Pictures is to produce a television series focusing on disability and, more recently, other content that may be published directly to online portals. Our stories cover all forms of disability, including physical, intellectual and sensory disabilities, as well as mental health issues. Although disability is unique for all experiences and the disability sector is fragmented in many ways, I believe there are common themes, such as access to the physical environment, education, employment and transport; as well as social issues such as parenting and relationships. My time with the company began as a researcher and presenter. Now, 10 years later, I am the general manager of the company, second in charge to the CEO.

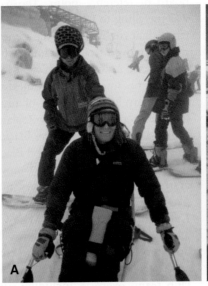
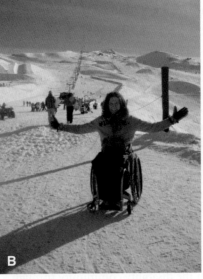

Figure 20.2 A, B, Snow sports.

In the political arena, since 2014, I have been part of a disability advisory panel for Auckland City Council. Similar to Attitude Pictures, this panel's work covers the whole spectrum of disability, with a focus on advocating and advising the council on behalf of Aucklanders who live with disability.

I still play wheelchair rugby occasionally, but wheelchair racing is my latest focus. Highlights to date in this fledgling career have included completing the New York and Auckland marathons, and breaking the New Zealand half-marathon record (for athletes with a T52 classification) (see Chapter 13 for more details on classification in para-sport). Sport has connected me to many people who live with an SCI from many walks of life and from many places. I have been privileged enough to travel the world, meet with royalty and be part of a Paralympic gold medal winning team. Through my sporting connections, I have also been able to learn from and be mentored by many great people on how to live a full life with a disability.

Using this background, I will explore some of the sociological issues associated with having an SCI, drawing heavily from my own lived experiences, while referencing evidence and discussion from others more qualified than me who have researched the topic. Specifically, I will be touching on employment, leisure time, relationships/partnerships and changing family relationships.

EMPLOYMENT

I see employment as one of the great challenges for people who live with a spinal injury, as well as being one of the greatest opportunities to help live a full and better life, and lead to social change. My personal point of view is backed by a 40-year longitudinal study by Krause and colleagues:[1]

> One of the most important findings has been the survivor effect, whereby those individuals who were more active, employed, and had better overall psychosocial adjustment were more likely to live to subsequent follow-ups. The first longitudinal analysis indicated that those who had greater psychosocial and vocational adjustment, more so than medical adjustment, were more likely to have survived over the 11-year interval. This trend continued in subsequent analyses. Participation in social activities outside the home and sitting tolerance were important protective factors for mortality, whereas self-reported physical and psychological health problems, dependency, and economic barriers represented significant risk factors.

To put the current situation simply, statistics relating to employment for people living with disability are appalling. Statistics New Zealand shows that disabled people in New Zealand are three times less likely to be employed. In the June

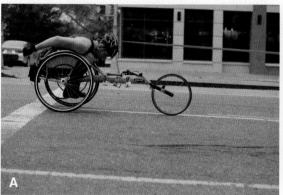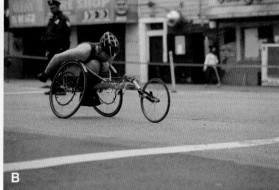

Figure 20.3 A, B, Road-racing.

2018 quarter, just 22.3% of disabled people were working, compared to 70% of non-disabled people, putting the disability employment gap at 47.7%. The median weekly income for disabled people was $358, less than half that of non-disabled people.[2]

I believe that turning these statistics around is vital for improvement of quality of life for individuals, as well as feeling it has the potential to be a vital factor in shifting perceptions of all people with disability and effecting social change. Again, my personal experience is supported by evidence in the literature:[1,3]

> Without question, there is pressure to maintain employment and financial resources among persons who have worked into later adulthood. It will be important for further research to evaluate whether the pressure to maintain employment may affect an individual's ability to sustain other aspects of life, including health, participation, and subjective well-being (SWB).

On an individual and personal level, the benefits of employment are in line with any able-bodied person. This includes an increased sense of self-worth, fulfilment, interaction with peers, personal growth and accumulation of wealth. Work is a major factor in how we develop interpersonal relationships. Beyond the individual, I believe the visibility and presence of having people who live with an SCI in the workplace and climbing their respective corporate ladders has the potential to be the greatest catalyst for social change. When it becomes commonplace for people who live with an SCI to have regular interactions with colleagues, clients and other professionals, on expectations of what can be achieved, then, I believe, the sociological barriers to leading a full and productive life for all persons with an SCI will be removed. There are some seemingly obvious barriers to employment, including physical access and bias – both unconscious and conscious. In my experience, one of the greatest sociological barriers is low expectations, which comes from both sides of the equation. People living with little or no connection to disability may have low expectations of what a person who lives with an SCI can achieve. However, I have found repeatedly that it is people who live with an SCI themselves who also have low expectations of what they are indeed capable of achieving.

An example of the situation described above occurred several years ago when I ran into an acquaintance who lives with a low-level SCI and uses a wheelchair. She had trained as a teacher and had been working part-time as a teacher's aide. I had heard that she had gained full-time employment and I excitedly congratulated her as soon as I saw her. It turns out I had heard incorrectly – she was not working full-time. However, not only was she not working full-time, she quickly waved off even the idea of it, saying words to the effect of, 'I would never be able to work full-time'. I was dumbstruck. Here was someone sitting in front of me who has significantly more functional potential ability than I have (she lives with a lower level SCI lesion, resulting in more muscles innervated … effectively, she is less disabled than I am). She knew what my work involved, since both her parents worked in the television and film industry. She knew the hours and amount of work I was doing in my role. Yet, even with me, as an example of someone living with an SCI and successfully working full-time (as well as playing high-level international sport at that time), her mindset was that she would never be able to 'handle' full-time employment due to her disability. This was a watershed moment for me when I realised it was not just society holding back people who live with an SCI, it had become embedded and engrained in our psyche that we ourselves are not capable.

It is important to note that coupled with low expectation for employment is the ease of assured income that can come from large insurance payouts or disability pensions, which may affect a person's motivation to return to the workforce. Australian state and territory governments previously implemented a scheme to assist in the financial management of catastrophic injuries, although these schemes are slowly being replaced by the National Disability Insurance Scheme (NDIS), which aims to spread the cost of an individual's current and future needs across the broader community.[4]

Similarly, New Zealand has the Accident Compensation Corporation (ACC), which is effectively compulsory insurance, whereby everyone who earns a wage pays ACC levies, so that if anyone has an injury as a result of an accident of any kind, they receive cover from the ACC.[5] As a result, someone who sustains an SCI falls under a team that focuses specifically on serious injuries and the ACC will pay for things such as wheelchairs, cars (including modifications), house modifications and carer support. The ACC also pays a living wage that is managed through a system called Loss of Potential Earnings (LOPE). The recipient receives a percentage of what they were earning at the time of their injury (there is a base threshold rate if a person was not earning a wage at the time or was a minimum wage earner). While it is a very comprehensive and effective scheme, despite best efforts to add programs and incentives for vocational rehabilitation, it can be said that it creates a culture and environment where there is a lack of motivation to get back to work.

There is, of course, the issue of how to kick-start the employment drive when the expectation is not yet there. I have witnessed a recurring theme of many people wanting to create disability-specific employment job sites, mentoring and internship programs. While there may be a case for helping to get a foot in the door, I believe that ultimately, potential employees want to be part of where everyone else is going. If I was looking for a job, I believe I would follow a similar pathway to any other person looking for a job. My first port of call would be Seek (a New Zealand-based employment site for job seekers), as well as leveraging contacts and networks, and pushing my CV in front of as many places as possible.

While not every individual who sustains an SCI might possess the confidence, skills, personality, opportunities or support to put themselves forward, if those of us who can, do, then we will create pathways and become role-models for others to follow. In short, I feel simply by doing and becoming, this will create a snowball effect of bringing others with us.

LEISURE TIME

There can be no argument that leisure time is significantly affected by an SCI. For me, the essence of leisure is based on physical activity. Growing up in rural New Zealand, imagery that springs to mind about leisure is time spent near waterways – our rivers, lakes and beaches – as well as generally exploring and appreciating the great outdoors. Typical sport and recreational activities include skiing, surfing and playing rugby. From hiking to fishing to trail running we have an abundance of activities to enjoy. Urban elements further the range with less physical pursuits, such as exploring museums and art galleries, but there are still the urbanised versions of all that comes from the countryside, such as parks and beaches.

What does one do when they live with a spinal injury? Well, all of the above are options as it turns out … but they all come with caveats. The built environment is generally designed for able-bodied people, with accommodations created to allow subsequent access. The movement towards universal design is progressing, but it is still in its relative infancy, particularly in third world countries. Mobility aids have been created to help facilitate access, but ultimately these solutions are add-ons and work-arounds. For example, the Great Walks of New Zealand could not be accessed by someone with an SCI without a significant amount of aid and support from others. Accessible beaches can be created, but they are rare and Auckland is only now in the throes of creating their first wheelchair accessible beach, and even then there is again a significant amount of aid and/or support from others required to access these beaches.

However, it is not all doom and gloom; the first significant point that is useful to acknowledge is that while a person who lives with an SCI may not be able to do a three-day hike, how often would they have ever done this if they were able-bodied? How often do their peers do it? How often do the majority of New Zealanders do it? If the answer to these questions is few to none, then is the person

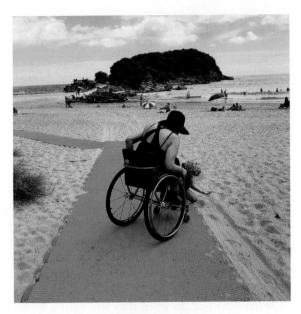

Figure 20.4 **Accessible beaches.**

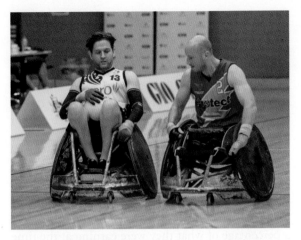

Figure 20.5 **Playing wheelchair rugby at the Australian Nationals, 2016.**

really missing out on what they cannot do when they would not have done it anyway?

Another point that may help to maintain a certain level of sanity is acknowledging that yes, it is unfortunate one cannot partake in certain activities, but there are an ever-increasing number of activities that the person with an SCI can participate in. In fact, in terms of high-performance sport, the number of para-sports on offer is significant to the point that there can be too many to choose from to fit into life and do well at. From personal experience, I have been involved with wheelchair rugby, wheelchair tennis, wheelchair basketball, sit-skiing, track racing and field events for athletics (for further detail see Chapter 13). However, similar to an able-bodied athlete, to do well at any of these means zeroing in on that specific sport, which has meant only focusing on one and forsaking many of the other para-sports available.

There are clear pathways for people to achieve and reach elite status, with 31 para-sports recognised by the International Paralympic Committee for people to compete in (see Chapter 13). However, it should be noted that only 209 New Zealanders can call themselves Paralympians – this is how many people have attended a Paralympic Games since New Zealand sent their first team to the Tel Aviv Games in 1968. Not all people want to compete, and certainly not all people will end up competing, on the world stage.

On a personal note – which I believe many other people with an SCI may relate to – when my injury has felt like it has hindered me is when it has precluded me from being able to undertake shared experiences with able-bodied people who I love and want to spend time with. An example of this is that my fiancée is an avid hiker, and we would love to be able to travel and experience hikes together. However, our experience is limited to short bushwalks, and even then I require a different set of wheels for my wheelchair (mountain bike wheels), an add-on to the front of my chair (I use a product called a free wheel) and still I require assistance (see Chapter 8 on wheelchair modifications).

My strategy for dealing with situations like these is to first acknowledge that, yes, life does not always seem to be fair. The next step is to ask if there is anything that can be done about it. If the answer is

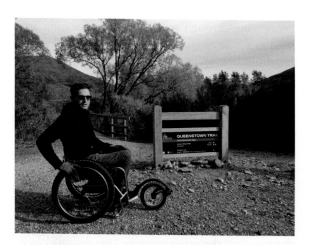

Figure 20.6 Rough terrain wheelchair modifications (Mountain bike tyres and Freewheel™).

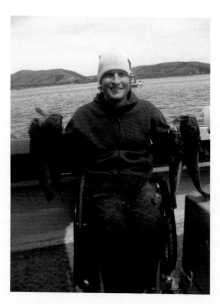

Figure 20.7 Fishing for blue cod off the Southern Coast of New Zealand.

that a similar but alternative activity is possible, or perhaps the same activity with aids or adaptations which will still provide fulfilment and/or joy, then it is easy to forge ahead with an altered option. However, if there is no way to partake in the activity in a joyful, meaningful way, then I have found that it is best to say, 'I am going to do this instead'. There are too many other options of pursuits I can follow to dwell on those that I cannot. This strategy follows a sports psychology theory learned early on in my wheelchair rugby career that I often refer back to, which is 'control the controllable'. Seek out the things that are within your control to influence or change. For those things that you cannot change, accept they are what they are and do not waste brain space dwelling or ruminating on them – they are out of your control. The hardest part to following this strategy is when it affects others or, more aptly, when it means one cannot share the experience with a significant other.

For sports that can be accessed, such as wheelchair rugby, one of the great things I find is how much learning for life can be acquired off-court. Playing any wheelchair sport brings together many people in a similar situation, creating an environment for sharing knowledge about everything from how to transfer into a car most effectively to what adaptive aids are available for accessing the environment. I found out about wheelchair rugby while I was still in the spinal unit post-injury and was able to go along to a training session at a nearby gym. While I may not have consciously registered it in as many words at the time, I believe I was very quick to recognise the team I was watching train was made up of a group of guys who had gone through a similar experience to me and were obviously thriving. Here was a group of people I could learn from; I did not need to reinvent the wheel myself. I also remember thinking that regardless of disability, here were some very cool guys who all seemed to be either working or studying; they all had girlfriends, wives or partners, and they were travelling the world playing a sport they loved. Expectations were set high for what my life could become. In this regard, I am the product of the aspirations of Sir Ludwig Guttman – the German-born British neurologist who established the forerunner to the Paralympic Games. He believed sport was a major method of therapy for injured military personnel, helping them build up physical strength and self-respect (for further detail see Chapter 13).

Anecdotally, health professionals working in this field report that it is those tetraplegics who become involved in wheelchair rugby (or indeed any other high level sport) who tend towards being the most independent. The knowledge gained from being around others who have found solutions for challenges that come through living with an SCI, the sheer physical fitness needed to play the game well and the self-help attitude that seems to be prevalent in sport will inevitably lead to greater independence. This peer pressure to be as self-reliant as possible or receive jest from other players is a great catalyst for doing more for yourself. For example, it quickly becomes obvious that things such as armrests and anti-tips on your chairs are not cool, unless absolutely necessary.

PARTNERS/RELATIONSHIPS

In the hope of helping friends who are going through a relationship breakup, I have often related that living through breaking my neck and all the pain and angst that came with it was, in fact, a less difficult experience than the pain of a relationship breakup. Regardless of disability, some things cut through all barriers, and this is one. Whether disability is in the mix or not, relationships are full of the highest of highs and the lowest of lows in terms of life experience (see Chapter 12 for further detail on relationships).

How does one who lives with an SCI meet and get to know someone they want to enter into a relationship with? From my experience, in a broad sense people who live with disability connect with someone else in similar ways to anybody else. For instance, there are shared experiences or interests, such as work or sport, or a mutual friend that facilitates a connection. There can be the instant attraction of meeting someone at a party or at a bar and working up the courage to say hello. More recently, of course, there has been the option of

connecting through social media or a dating app, such as Tinder. Living with an SCI may add a filter for those that are available. A friend of mine who lives with an SCI has said that while she meets people to date through the same means and ways as before her injury, using a wheelchair does add what she calls an 'asshole filter'. Her take is that anyone who would see a person they are interested in but not want to date them because of their disability is someone she would not want to date regardless of living with a disability.

Once a connection has been made, I would say that this is where things start to differ, depending in the main on the other person's knowledge of SCI. This may include anything from how one drives (who will pick who up for the date), to (depending on how upfront one is) how sex works and what positions are the best, to what your disability means in terms of the muscles that are still within your control and where you still have feeling or sensation (for further information on sexual rehabilitation, see Chapter 12). Most people are genuinely intrigued, and it makes for an interesting way to connect and get to know each other quickly and in a deeper, more meaningful way. By front-footing some details about one's injury, it will potentially help a new partner be open to asking more questions that may arise which, in my experience, leads to a more open relationship.

While there are many positive things to focus on in terms of how well a relationship can work when one, or both, people live with an SCI, I feel it is important to understand those aspects that may be more challenging. The small things are often the most difficult; for example, not being able to walk down the street holding hands. Then there are practical standpoints that can be very challenging, such as dating someone who lives in a two-storey house. The seemingly simple solution here is that you may have to meet at your place, or other accessible places. The more challenging solution (but one that can be completely worth it) is to be open and willing to learn how to traverse a flight of stairs by getting out of your wheelchair and transferring up the stairs on your bottom, one step at a time. Whatever the solution, I have found that it is best to at least acknowledge that it is not ideal, and then work towards the best resolution.

PHYSICAL INTIMACY

From my experience, I have found the topic of sex is of specific intrigue for all, from the person who has sustained an injury, to their friends and family, the public at large and, of course, potential partners. It was, of course, of great importance for me to find out what it would mean following my spinal cord injury as an 18-year-old.

Unfortunately, some members of the public at large feel that it is acceptable to launch into asking intimate questions of someone who lives with spinal injury, regardless of how well they know them. I have heard many anecdotes of strangers asking very direct questions about a person's sexual function out of the blue. While I wholeheartedly agree it is not OK to question a stranger about their life, I do understand that people are genuinely intrigued. Given the right situation and the right timing, I feel very comfortable sharing what my SCI means for me. Without this sharing of information there is the potential alternative of exacerbating misconceptions, such as a person with an SCI being asexual, that they may not be able to have sex, or they are not interested in sex. (See Chapter 12 for more detail on physical intimacy and sexual rehabilitation.)

A contrary view to the perception that people may not be interested in sex is that men who have had spinal injuries are better lovers than their able-bodied counterparts. Obviously, whether this is true or not depends very much on the individual, as with the able-bodied population. However, the reasoning behind this theory is that with reduced function and/or feeling the man discovers that there is much more to sex than the male orgasm. Extreme pleasure can be found by being more attentive and more in tune with what their partner wants. Through openness, as in being open-minded about trying new things and open to conversation with their partner, either a dawning or gradual realisation will be found that the psychological aspect of sex can be far more pleasurable than the physical aspect.

However, the physical aspects should not be discounted. Again, through openness and experimentation there are many ways for people to keep the physical side inventive and interesting. There are specific aids that can be purchased to help, as well as toys used by the public that can be co-opted and adapted to enhance the sex life of a person who lives with an SCI (see Chapter 12).

It is important to note, as with all things to do with SCI, the caveat in any conversation should be 'depending on the individual'. While there are general themes and issues that cut across the population, due to the difference in function that can occur from one person to the next I believe it is very dangerous to assume that by being familiar with what one person can do you could assume another to be the same. For example, on the topic of sexual function, there seems to be a wide variety of circumstances as to whether a male who lives with an SCI can ejaculate or not.

While I have focused on what living with an SCI means in terms of how sexual intimacy fits in with a relationship, other aspects that are true of any relationship should not be ignored. Namely, regardless of living with an SCI, a shared life with someone you love, someone you want to build a future with, someone you look forward to spending time with and want to be around always, is one of the greatest things life has to offer. To be open about your SCI and what it means to be in a relationship with someone who has an SCI, to be open to adapting and making it work, to be vulnerable and open to the fear of failure or rejection, is all worth it for the potential for happiness and sense of fulfilment it can bring (see Chapters 15 and 21 for further detail on the personal issues of SCI).

A relationship may also grow, in terms of growing into a family by creating a new human to bring into the world. I know many people, both male and female, who either had children before sustaining an SCI, or who conceived after their injury. Like so

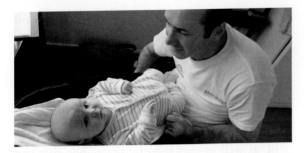

Figure 20.8 Tetraplegic Jai Waite, with his daughter on a baby carrier attached to his wheelchair.

many things to do with SCI it is difficult to make blanket statements about how it all works, due to individual injuries and individual personalities … but, needless to say, it does work.

It seems that similar to so many other things in life, solutions are found out of necessity. An example of a mobility aid that I have heard is of huge benefit initially is a baby carrier that attaches to a wheelchair and acts as a platform directly in front of the person using the wheelchair, with the baby facing them. This is where baby can be changed, fed or simply able to enjoy quality time with their parent.

Like many other things to do with SCI, it seems as though strong communication is key with both the child's other parent (if they are raising the child together or co-parenting) and with the child throughout its various ages and stages and all the various complications that come with each phase (see Chapter 15 for some further anecdotal evidence of raising a family when one parent has an SCI).

CHANGING FAMILY RELATIONSHIPS

There is a saying, 'disability does not discriminate'. I believe it is meant to be in the context that disability can cut through any demographic, including class, gender, age and ethnicity. In the context of how an SCI may impact upon family relationships I feel that it does not discriminate in terms of the person it may immediately affect. It could be a parent, child, sibling, partner, or any combination

of these, each having their own dynamics to take into consideration, depending on that specific relationship and those specific individuals.

At the risk of zeroing in on a broad generalisation and neglecting to give other family relationships the justice they deserve, there is a saying, 'the narrower the focus, the stronger the portrait'. With this in mind, it can be noted that statistics for the demographic population most prone to sustain an SCI are males aged 18 to 25.[6] Effectively the risk-takers of our society, this is the group that has a burgeoning physical prowess they are champing at the bit to push to the limit and show off.

To paint a picture of the potential family relationships this person may have, they could be a young man entering into the autonomy of living his own life, while still having the support and safety net of a parent or parents available as a backstop. On the cusp of adulthood, he is on one hand fiercely independent while remaining relatively reliant on parental guidance, advice and support. Moving forwards, the pathway set up may be the notion of being the one who will be strong and supportive (physically and financially) for his parents, as well as potentially his own family. In this over-simplified theoretical family vignette, siblings will be of a similar age and seen as their peer/s. Following a spinal injury, these dynamics may quickly change to one where parental instinct returns to the mother and/or father, with a need to nurture and look after their child. Going from independence (or at least being on the cusp of it) to needing support and care may lead to resentment as the person comes to grips with such a large upheaval in their existence.

There are many 'ifs', 'mights' and 'coulds' in the above scenario. I would like therefore to provide a case study using my own personal experience as a way of sharing insight of how one person's family relationships changed, albeit from my perspective only.

I am the youngest of three siblings and at the time of my injury I was 18 (turning 19 while in rehabilitation in the spinal unit), celebrating with a keg of beer in the hospital grounds with some friends). I was halfway through second semester of my first year at Otago University where I was studying surveying, when I fractured and dislocated my cervical vertebrae 6 and 7 in a rugby injury. I was playing the position of hooker in the front row of the scrum. When a scrum in the later stages of the game went to engage it was not set properly and my head was in the wrong place. The weight of the opposing scrum went through my head, and my neck was the weak point that gave way to the pressure that was being exerted through my body. The result is an incomplete ASI B spinal injury (see Appendix 1, the ISNCSCI, for details on the assessment of SCIs), where I exhibit good hand and arm function (minor loss of finger dexterity and strength) for my level of injury, but I am paralysed from the chest down and also exhibit expected loss of function of autonomic nervous system relative to this level of injury.

Up until this incident, I was having the time of my life during that first year of university. I was staying at a Hall of Residence, I was achieving well enough academically, while prioritising a very full social life. I went from a relatively carefree existence to undergoing surgery, then three and a half months in the Burwood Spinal Unit in Christchurch, before returning home to the family farm for summer.

My parents are open-minded and broadly intelligent. However, they were both born in the 1940s and grew up in an era where the medicalised model of disability was the prominent school of thought. This model focuses on disability being something to be cured or managed. Prior to the changes introduced by Sir Ludwig Guttman in the 1950s,[7] people with significant disabilities were not expected to survive, let alone live full lives. While significant change is underway regarding the perspective of what a catastrophic injury means in today's society for quality of life, unless a family has previously come into contact with someone with a significant disability (which is less common in rural and remote settings), it is hard to know intuitively how to respond to someone who has experienced a major life-changing injury. The following two stories

can help illustrate where their mindset was at when I sustained my injury, and how my parents' world was opened as I forged ahead with my life.

The first story begins when I left hospital three and a half months after breaking my neck. By that stage I was ready to live independently. With funding from the ACC (as explained earlier in the chapter), I had bought a car, had it adapted and when it came time to be discharged I drove the 7-hour trip home to my parents farm with my brother and sister. We were all home for the first time in a long time and planned to be there for summer. While I had been in hospital, Mum and Dad had organised for the house to be adapted, with a ramp in the garage and an en-suite added to my room. They also had Sky TV (New Zealand's pay TV service) installed – a great novelty!

Fast forward several years and I was visiting Mum and Dad again at their home. I was living in Auckland at the time, and had been working for a television production company for some time. While home at the farm we were seeing if there was anything decent on TV when my father reflected why they had got Sky installed:

> You know we got Sky installed because we weren't sure what you'd do with your life and thought you might want distraction … but the only thing we ever watch on it now is 'Attitude' (the TV program produced by the company I work for).

The second story involves another reflective moment from my father. It came after a recent episode from the series we produce, featuring my primary physician from my time in rehabilitation at Burwood Hospital. Dad said that during those initial days they had no reference point of what to expect. I imagine they would have been extremely distraught, but handling it in a very unwavering way. They found a moment with the doctor to ask for some clarity, as to what they could expect for my future. This particular doctor had already garnered their respect and they trusted him, but what he said next confounded them: 'I don't believe he will walk out of here; he will need to use a wheelchair, but he will lead a very full life'. To them, this was putting two juxtaposing thoughts – using a wheelchair and living a full life – together.

I use these two stories to illustrate how hard it is to know intuitively how to respond to what is a catastrophic life-changing event for parents. I believe awareness and exposure are increasing in the digital age as we increase representation of people with disabilities; however, growing up in a rural area where physicality is a key resource means that for my parents there would have been little contact with people living with significant disability. Through myself, and others around me, they quickly got up to speed with what was possible; however, it shows the lens many parents initially may look through when their son or daughter is injured.

Growing up I was always the annoying little brother to my older 'cool' sibling. My older brother and I were both at Otago University and we had just got to the point where it was relatively OK for me to hang out with him and his friends when I broke my neck. As steadfast, rural Southerners, we were not prone to expressing emotion, but he did enough to let me know he was there for me, and it felt like (and still does) that he has my back if I ever need anything. We have never spoken much about my injury, or what it meant to either of us. It has felt like for him it was something that happened, I was still me, and he was my older brother who was ready to be there for me if I ever needed him.

My sister was travelling through South East Asia and happened to be in Vietnam when my injury occurred. In 1999, it was still very difficult to make a phone call out of the Communist-run country. It involved a convoluted system where she would have to call a New Zealand landline and recite a number to call her back on, then hang up before the charges got out of control. She had been trying to get through for a few days when she finally got my father on the other end. She recited the number, then hung up, waiting for a call back that never came. She tried again, and impatiently tried to recite the number again when Dad stopped her: 'Don't worry about the cost; I need to tell you something'. She

wrote a short story of the time and place, trying to give words to the shock she felt, of how life can suddenly be turned upside down.

'Daniel … rugby accident … hospital … Christchurch …'

The words are barely registering, I am panicking inwardly and need to know what is happening, what has happened.

'His neck is broken. At the moment he is paralysed from the armpits down.'

I feel the wind knocked out of me. I am aware of the Vietnamese clerks and customers outside the glass booth. They are staring at me. Am I calm? Hysterical? Screaming? Crying? I don't know.

'You mustn't come home; he doesn't want you to come home. We're not accepting he will remain paralysed. We have no intention of accepting that.'

'Bad news?' The pronunciation soft, like 'bat nuuse?' Her face soft also.

'Brother.'

The effort of talking produces sobs. I take a tissue.

'Little brother', gesturing as if placing my hand on the head of a little person, though Dan is 6 foot tall.

I don't sleep all night. When I stop crying I lie and stare blankly at the ceiling. I wiggle my toes. In the morning I am exhausted.

I talked to her soon after. In the early stages of my rehabilitation, I told her to carry on with her travels, that I would rather (naively) focus on walking again. She arrived in New Zealand late in my rehab and joined my brother as a network of support that was never really articulated, but always felt.

For me, the family dynamics stayed exactly how I wanted them to, insofar as someone who appreciated the privileged position I had come from, by being part of such an awesome family, while also being fiercely independent and wanting to carve my own path in the world. One of the biggest shifts was that as I went back to university, got into sport and started to travel the world it became a little bittersweet visiting the family farm. It was, and still is, a part of the world I absolutely love. When I used to drive down there while I was living in Dunedin, then later Christchurch, the closer I would get to home the greater the connection I would feel with the land. To be clichéd about it, it felt warming to the soul. However, it also represented what I could no longer do. The Catlins is a rugged part of the world, where physicality reigns supreme. The weather is fierce, making you feel alive … however, it is also brutal when you live with an SCI and struggle to regulate your temperature. When I was 17 I had talked with my father about whether I would want to take over the farm. At that stage, I wanted to go to university, get my degree and then see the world. 'Give me 10 years,' I had said. I was 18 when I broke my neck, and in the years that came after I realised taking over the farm, while technically possible, was not meant to be for me.

Our family dynamics are probably better now than they have ever been. I think it would be egocentric for me to think that having an SCI has anything to do with it. It was a formative time for all of us as individuals and as a family. No doubt, we all learned from it in a variety of seen and unseen ways, and it still lives with us all to a degree. Family dynamics, however, are a reflection of lived experiences and as we mature and add new experiences they will inevitably change. Children become parents and parents become grandparents, all contributing to the inescapable alterations in family dynamics.

The concerns for my siblings and me are now the same as what I imagine many others have. How will we care for our parents as they get older? How do I make time when I live so far away in another city, with my own family, home, career? How do we ever give back to the people who have given so much to us?

The conclusion drawn from this section is that while sustaining an SCI had a significant impact on us as individuals and as a family, and it was a formative experience at the time, it is now but a bit-part in the ever-changing nature of a family dynamic that is forever weaving its way through the fabric of life.

SUMMARY

In 2017, I passed the line of having lived my life with a disability longer than being able-bodied. I marked the year by doing the New York Marathon, while raising money for the CatWalk Trust, whose remit is to provide funding for finding a cure for SCI. It was a fine line to tread. On one hand, I live a full life, including working for a TV company whose flagship program is about raising expectations for people who live with disability and to show people that being able-bodied is not the be-all and end-all of life. However, here I was supporting an organisation whose mission is to focus on getting people to walk again. A complicated question to be asked is, 'would I like to be able to walk again?' At the risk of oversimplifying it, the answer is yes. I am mindful that, as much as I do live a full life, there would have been a lot less heartache for my family and friends, a lot less money spent by ACC, my life would be a lot easier now and getting old would not come with as many complications, if I could have regained the function lost from fracturing and dislocating my 6th and 7th vertebrae 18 years ago.

I would like to finish the chapter with extracts from my fundraising page for the New York Marathon, which I believe sum up, to a large degree, the journey of where I have come from since breaking my neck during a game of rugby to where I am now.

WHAT HAPPENED?

14 August 1999: that was the last time I could walk. I was 18, in my first year at Otago University, and having the time of my life. I remember lying on the ground waiting for the ambulance. I wasn't in any pain. My legs felt like they were there, but it was almost like they were floating – I couldn't feel the ground beneath them.

Partial memories endure. A plane ride to Christchurch. Being in a room waiting for surgery. Knowing Mum and Dad were there, but not being able to communicate with them. The next thing I really recall is waking up in the Burwood Hospital Spinal Injury Unit, a place with an eclectic bunch of people who had somehow found themselves seriously injured. No one was really sick though; we were all working towards learning how to live life again.

The lasting memories I have of my 3 months in Burwood are my visitors. They came from everywhere. Mum and Dad basically lived on the hospital grounds. Then there were my friends from school and university – some would hitchhike up for the weekends. My rugby team hired mini-vans to visit. There were friends of friends, friends of family, people from outside my circles of friends … and even those I didn't particularly get along with.

It was overwhelming at times. All these people who came simply to wish me well. People who took time out of their lives to think of me in some way, drop me a note or pay their respects. It was humbling, and the experience is something I still carry with me.

And now here I am, raising money for a cause that some would say devalues people who live with disability. It is a fine line to tread.

Why would helping to find the cure to SCI devalue the lives of people who live with disabilities?
It's all in the framing. If you want to get someone to buy into anything, to invest financially, then a quick and sure-fire way to get people to dig deep is to get them to invest emotionally. Don't get me wrong – it is a real thing – that when someone acquires a disability through illness or injury then the pathway of life takes a massive deviation. There is a great sense of loss.

However, when we frame disability as a tragedy, it can create an environment where it's OK to treat disabled people as invalids, which in turn sometimes encourages an environment that is patronising and overly sympathetic and actually curtails the ability to deal with disability. I've been treated like this many times, and it's not productive.

If we widen the frame, we also see that those who live with an SCI sit alongside people who may live with cerebral palsy or spina bifida, or amputations; disability comes in many shapes and forms. While disabilities are all different, there are common challenges that cut through and bind us together.

But here's the sticking point – not all disabilities have the potential to be 'cured'. So, while it might be seen to be disempowering for people with disabilities if an organisation focuses purely on getting people back to being 'normal', there is the potential here to fix something that is broken.

Somewhere along the way, we learned how to fix a broken leg, and though healing an SCI is chalk and cheese compared to lining up a fractured tibia and putting a cast on it for 6 weeks, if we cut to the chase, I broke my neck, and the researchers funded by the CatWalk Trust are trying to find a way to fix it.

I'm mindful that, as much as I do live a full life, there would have been a lot less heartache and complications if I could have regained the function lost from popping out and fracturing my 6th and 7th vertebrae. Later this year I will surpass the length of time in my life that I was able-bodied. I will have spent more time living life with an SCI than not. I raise money for CatWalk knowing I may never experience the benefit of the proceeds, but another fresh-faced 18-year-old boy from Invercargill and his family might.

Online resources

Accident Compensation Corporation (ACC). www.acc.co.nz/.

Attitude Pictures. www.attitudepictures.com.

Canterbury Wheelchair Rugby (FB page only). https://Catwalk Trust: https://catwalk.org.nz/.

New Zealand Wheelchair Rugby: www.wheelblacks.com/.

Parafed Canterbury: www.parafedcanterbury.co.nz/.

References

1. Krause, J., Clark, J.M.R., et al., 2015. SCI Longitudinal Aging Study: 40 years of research. Top. Spinal Cord Inj. Rehabil. 21 (3), 189–200.

2. Macfarlane, A. Disabled people three times less likely to be employed. 1 News. Online 18 December 2019. Available: www.tvnz.co.nz/one-news/new-zealand/disabled -people-three-times-less-likely-employed.

3. Groah, S.L., Charlifue, S., et al., 2012. Spinal cord injury and aging challenges and recommendations for future research. Am. J. Phys. Med. Rehabil. 91 (1), 80–93.

4. National Disability Insurance Scheme (NDIS), 2019. About us. Online 23 December 2019. Available: www.ndis.gov.au/about-us.

5. Accident Compensation Corporation. Online 23 December 2019. Available: www.acc.co.nz.

6. Lee, B.B., 2014. The global map for traumatic spinal cord injury epidemiology: update 2011, global incidence rate. Spinal Cord 52 (2), 110–116.

7. Buckinghamshire County Council. Mandeville legacy. Online 18 December 2019. Available: www.mandevillelegacy.org.uk.

CHAPTER 21

The hazards of living with a spinal cord injury

Arik Vamosh, Col Mackereth and Katie Hammond

INTRODUCTION

This chapter will present three case studies written by individuals who have sustained a traumatic spinal cord injury (TSCI). The number of years since their injury, the epidemiology, type and level of injury, their age at injury and their social circumstances are all very different. However, certain recurrent themes are apparent, as well as some obvious differences.

CASE STUDY 1

The first case study is based on Arik Vamosh, who is a complete paraplegic with an ISNCSCI classification of T11 AIS A.

In the almost 44 years since I suffered my SCI and became a wheelchair user I have been exposed to and suffered much damage. My initial injury was caused by an army vehicle I was driving being blown up. Injuries I have since suffered have included fractures, burns, a variety of musculoskeletal injuries, neck problems and more. Although many warnings are given when preparing for discharge from the initial rehabilitation, it is quite impossible to even begin to visualise the hazards that will ensue.

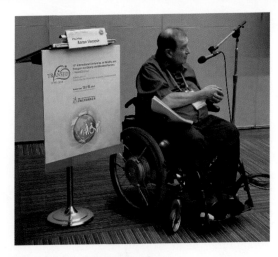

Figure 21.1 Arik Vamosh

CASE STUDY 1—cont'd

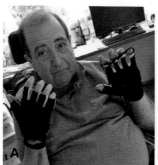 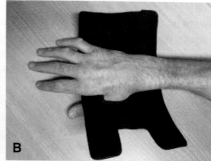

Figure 21.2 A, Push gloves for paraplegic. B, Push gloves for tetraplegic.
Source: A Courtesy Arik Vamosh. B © The Active Hands

Damage to joints

Firstly, let me describe the damage that may occur in a variety of joints. Fingers are frequently injured, particularly in manual chairs. Where the brakes are located too high, when pushing hard, fingers catch in the brakes and in the worst scenario, fractures may occur. My suggestion would be to relocate the brakes so that they do not interfere when pushing the chair. If you are a very active wheelchair user and are pushing for long distances, or on hard surfaces such as hills, grass fields etc, the wrist is easily hurt. Using push gloves may help somewhat (Fig. 21.2A and B), but over a prolonged period of time the pain may eventually be so great that you will need to switch to a power or power-assisted wheelchair. Early use of power-assisted chairs may slow down the onset of wrist problems.

Relying totally on one's shoulder for transfers and wheelchair pushing tends to cause damage to the shoulder joint – a joint not specifically designed for weight-bearing, but rather for mobility. On a personal note, I damaged my shoulders pushing many kilometres on grass fields during archery competitions while serving as an international judge. I now have bilateral shoulder replacements

(these procedures are described in more detail in Chapters 15 and 17).

Lack of muscle tone, or increased muscle tone in the form of spasticity, around the joints, particularly the hips, may cause dislocation or worse in various situations. I will describe injuries I have experienced around the hips in more detail when I discuss flight injuries.

Burn injuries

The type and level of injury sustained and the degree of sensory disturbance will influence whether or not the person with an SCI will be susceptible to suffering from burns. An example of an early burn injury I experienced was when, fairly soon after my discharge from hospital, I made myself a big mug of boiling hot tea. While attempting to take the mug to another room, I tried to steer the chair with one hand, but as I was turning in circles, I placed the mug between my legs and pushed back to the other room. I developed huge blisters on both thighs, although to my good fortune they were painless! Another example is when I was visiting overseas during winter and my hosts kindly put a rubber hot-water bottle in my bed. As I was not aware of

Continued

CASE STUDY 1—cont'd

it – I could not feel it – I awoke with large blisters on my heels. Be aware that burns can occur with either hot or cold substances; ice burns can also cause severe blisters. It is therefore not advisable to place anything on, under or between one's legs, or indeed any paralysed limbs, if there are sensory disturbances.

Pressure injuries

As described in Chapters 4 and 15, there are many causes of pressure injuries (PIs). Apart from the obvious ones such as poor seating, inadequate cushions and so on, there are hazards of specific items of clothing, particularly denims with double seams and metal studs. A person with an SCI must choose his/her clothing with great care.

Fractures

Apart from finger fractures described earlier in this chapter, other fractures may occur due to osteopenia or osteoporosis (see Chapter 15 for more details on these conditions). Additional fractures post-injury may be due to the position of the hand controls on the vehicle being used by the person with an SCI. Most hand controls have a horizontal bar fitted at knee level. In a collision, the driver may be pushed forwards and their knees hit the horizontal bar causing severe comminuted fractures in both femurs, an injury I once sustained, which initiated a prolonged period of incapacitation. A clavicular fracture may also be sustained when applying the brake with great force.

Falls with or from the wheelchair when navigating kerbs or high steps may also result in fractures.

Travelling, cruise and flight injuries

While travelling or flying to different places it is often necessary to rely on help from untrained helpers. Unfortunately, flight staff on aeroplanes are not trained on how to assist or transfer patients with an SCI. Too often I have experienced this on flights, and inadequate transfer techniques can result in serious injuries, such as dislocated shoulders and hips.

Sports injuries

As with any sporting venture, injuries will occur. Again, because we are using our shoulders for many weight-bearing activities for which they were not designed, shoulder injuries are by far the most prevalent. As seen in Chapter 13, sport is an integral part of rehabilitation and socialisation for the person with an SCI. Where possible, however, precautions should be taken to avoid unnecessary injuries.

Neck problems

Being seated constantly in a standing person's world means that the person with an SCI is forced to look up for most of the time. As a result, many individuals suffer long-term damage to their neck muscles, ligaments and joints. The newer wheelchairs, which allow the seated person to raise him/herself to standing height, may be useful in some cases, but wherever possible it is useful to ask the people around you to sit and converse with you at eye level.

Weight control

Obesity is a global problem, but for those of us in wheelchairs it is even more difficult. If we gain weight, it is extremely difficult to lose it. We need to adopt a lifestyle that will ensure we maintain an ideal weight. Dietitians are usually available to assist in developing the optimum plan.

Secondary damage

Secondary damage from over-enthusiastic or poorly trained therapists is my final word of warning. Having been rehabilitated in specialised units and treated by highly trained doctors, nurses and therapists, many people with an SCI assume that this is the general level of knowledge. This is not necessarily so, and it is therefore up to the individual him/herself to guide and teach others if we find ourselves in a situation where the professional is less well-trained in our needs than we are.

Raising pets and children

Many households would consider themselves incomplete without the family pets. As people with an SCI, we are no different, but it is important that we choose the pet that is right for our abilities. Indeed today, there are helper dogs trained to ease our burden of living.

My wife (of 36 years) and I have two daughters and four grandchildren. We were adamant from the beginning that neither the children nor the grandchildren would ever be involved in my care-giving.

I have studied and worked in communications ever since my injury (I was a student at the time of injury). As a retired war veteran, I am still involved giving lectures in international forums on SCIs.

A final word on how many people speak to us when we are sitting in wheelchairs. It is uncanny how often people speak over our heads or address our carers as to our needs or wants. It has often been overheard that people describe us as 'the wheelchair' rather than 'the person in the wheelchair'. As professionals, I would like to say that the wrong choice of words can hurt and cause people to lose confidence and self-esteem. Education is the key and part of the therapist's job – and mine – is to educate those people who have not had the same exposure as we have to our situation. We would hope that through knowledge we could change people's attitude to all wheelchair users, giving them the dignity and respect they deserve.

CASE STUDY **2**

The second case study is based on Col Mackereth, who is a sensory incomplete tetraplegic with an ISNCSCI classification of C6 AIS B.

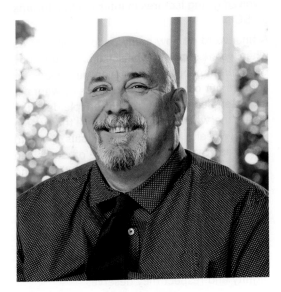

Figure 21.3 Col Mackereth

It is now 40 years since my spinal cord injury (SCI), which I sustained as a result of a diving accident. I have experienced many complications in life due to this injury. These include fractures, burns, pressure injuries, shoulder damage, skeletal changes, fertility and other medically related issues.

It is my belief that many of these complications are a result of not heeding the advice and information that I received during my rehabilitation, although I also believe that some are the result of living a full, active and independent lifestyle. It was my choice as a young man to choose function over form and by that I mean using equipment and techniques that afforded me greater independence in exchange for long-term health benefits.

Now as I approach my 60s I wonder about those choices.

Fractures post-injury

As a younger person I was quite flexible post-injury, to the point where I was able to put on my own shoes and socks. I would do this by getting my wrist under my knee and lifting my leg up over the other knee. This method served me well for about 15 years until the time it went pear-shaped. Without having true sensation in my legs, I was unaware of the force I was placing on my bones and subsequently I broke my femur during this process. What followed was not a good experience and only after throwing a tantrum after a week without any attempt to fix the fracture did I go to surgery. After that the recovery process was long and clumsy.

On another occasion, after a big night on the rum, for some unknown reason I decided to go for a wander through my goat paddock in the dark. The inevitable happened, I can only assume because I woke up next morning on the ground with three broken ribs from falling out of my wheelchair. I don't remember getting any medical treatment other than going to the emergency department. I do remember being in a lot of pain and a lot of spasm, which in turn caused more pain for a few weeks.

Skin management and pressure injuries

My first seven or eight wheelchairs were set up with 26-inch wheels, which I found easier to push and better to get around my 20-acre property. The down side was that I would lean on the wheels for balance and developed a hard callus on my elbows. This callus on my right elbow cracked and became an ongoing issue for several years. Without having sensation in

CASE STUDY **2**—cont'd

that area and not being able to see it, the 'issue' soon developed into a pressure injury. I treated the injury for several more years with various dressings and medications, unconventional methods and protective devices. The actual cause (the 26-inch wheels) was never addressed, so the injury continued to get worse to the point where I needed surgery to repair it. A flap rotation surgery and a 6-week hospital stay followed. The cause was eliminated and now my elbow is holding up OK. Following this surgery in 2005, my manual wheelchair use was restricted to eliminate any further pressure on my elbows and I got my first power chair to use as well as the manual chair.

I now exclusively use a power chair to reduce wear and tear on my elbows and shoulder muscles. This change has brought about a new skin issue on my *bum*. Because I'm now a lot more active and move around a lot faster I experience a lot more stress through friction and shearing between my bum and seating. For the last 4–5 years the skin on my bum has broken down many times and I have been trying to find a transfer technique that doesn't cause damage, especially the car transfer. I now use a transfer board and slide sheets, but still need to be very careful.

Using a power chair for most of my mobility meant that I also had to change vehicles as I couldn't lift a power chair into the car. I bought my first ute and was using ramps and someone to help load the chair into the back. I now have a light crane fitted to my ute, but still require some assistance to position the chair on the tray.

In total I would have spent 80–100 days in bed to repair these skin breakdowns. After trialling a range of pressure-relieving cushions I am now using a ROHO Quattro and enjoying better results.

Burns

I have had numerous burns ranging from sunburn to third degree burns.

Without having sensation, it is very easy to forget that you are getting burned and I have burned the skin on my belly several times from carrying hot food or beverages on my lap. Just a few weeks ago I bought a coffee and carried it in my hand so that it would not burn my belly. Not long afterwards I noticed a huge blister on the tip of my finger. There was no sensation in my fingertips. This one took about a month to heal completely.

The most serious burn occurred one morning while I was making boiled eggs for breakfast. I had gotten up early and not had my shower or got dressed. I was just wearing a shaving jacket. The eggs had just boiled, and I was taking them off the hotplate to place on a breadboard on my lap. The edge of the saucepan touched my belly causing my legs to spasm and tip the contents into my lap. Oops! I immediately went into the shower, but the damage was already done. Everything got cooked. The hot water ran straight down my groin and pooled there between my bum and cushion. The resulting burns were very severe. I spent 6 weeks in hospital and I don't know how long afterwards to recover from that one. The scarring is now breaking down regularly and is a major contributing factor to my ongoing skin issues.

Musculoskeletal injuries, including shoulder injuries and carpal tunnel syndrome

Where do I start with shoulder injuries? I used to do up to seven transfers before breakfast: bed – chair, chair – toilet, toilet – chair, chair – shower chair, shower chair – chair, chair – bed, bed – chair; that's a lot of work for

Continued

CASE STUDY 2—cont'd

your shoulders. Then there was the transfer into the car and lifting the wheelchair into the car. I would often feel sharp, intense pain while lifting my chair into the car. With a busy lifestyle and work commitments there was never time to rest the injuries. After a few days of struggling with the pain I would usually find a way to carry on and the pain would decrease. Usually though, another part of my shoulder would tear, and the same process would continue. Tear, repair, tear, repair, to the point where my strength was so compromised that I could no longer transfer; well, not easily, anyway. I now rely on carers to hoist me out of bed into a shower chair. I can still manage my transfer into my wheelchair, but I am no longer as independent as I was. While it is nowhere near as frequent as before, I still experience shoulder injuries from time to time and still lead too busy a lifestyle to be able to rest completely enough to fully recover.

Contractures

My posture is very poor, and I have developed a significant pelvic obliquity. This has caused a lot of issues over the years, such as neck pain and tightness from trying to maintain balance. Ribs rubbing on the back canes of a manual wheelchair have caused skin damage. The most significant, longstanding issue is that my left foot is now rolled over and fixed in a bent position (inverted and plantar flexed). The result is that my foot now rests on the lateral border and a pressure injury has developed on it.

Fertility

When I discharged from hospital I believed that I would not be able to have children of my own. It was not until about 6 years later that I found out that there may be a way. My wife and I were very keen to try. The fertility program was quite complicated, especially as we lived in North Queensland and the procedure needed to be done in Brisbane. Altogether we did 10–12 fertility programs and eventually had two sons (twins). Each procedure started with my wife having a series of injections, a 1500 km drive to Brisbane, a procedure at one hospital to extract semen, another procedure at a different hospital to implant the eggs. Then the wait. It was not the way either of us pictured starting a family, but the end result was worth it.

Having babies in the house meant lots of changes to my routine and my role in the family. Working full-time, I now had to fit in time to wash, dry and fold 40 nappies a day (luckily, I do not have the dexterity to change them).

I have been fortunate to have had many occupations throughout my career and have now relocated to Brisbane, where I am currently working as a peer support officer for Spinal Life Australia while also developing my professional speaking career. The boys are now in their mid-twenties and have young children of their own.

CASE STUDY 3

The third case study is based on Katie Hammond, who is a complete paraplegic with an ISNCSCI classification of T12 AIS A with Zones of Partial Preservation to L3.

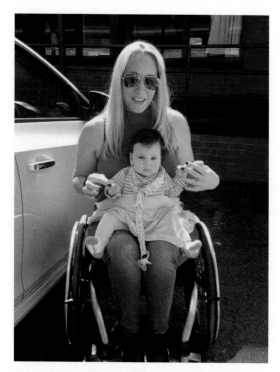

Figure 21.4 Katie Hammond

Obstetric/gynaecological issues

My first pregnancy was in 2001 when I was 21 years old and had been living with my SCI for 5 years. I fell pregnant naturally and went through the first 18 weeks without incident.

It was around the 18-week mark that I started developing excessively swollen feet. Each appointment with my obstetrician would cause concern that my condition would quickly turn into pre-eclampsia (a condition during pregnancy where there is a sudden rise in blood pressure and swelling, mostly in the face, hands and feet. If preeclampsia is untreated, it can develop into eclampsia, a potentially life-threatening condition in which the mother can experience convulsions, or even coma). Every appointment would prove that it was not an issue and my swollen feet were in fact due to my SCI. The weight of my growing baby was putting pressure on the arteries in my legs, slowing down the blood flow in my legs, which has been compromised since my injury.

At around the same time I found that my chosen bladder management (self-catheterising) was becoming difficult during pregnancy. I discovered the weight of my growing baby meant my bladder did not hold as much fluid. In addition, when I did do a catheter, the flow would be considerably slower than normal, and it would take a very long time for what little fluid was in my bladder to empty. As a result, from 18 weeks on I wore a pad to keep dry. With so many bladder changes, I was concerned I might have bladder infections, but most of the time that was not the case; it was just my bladder under too much pressure.

Weight gain was another complication during my first pregnancy. Like many pregnant women, I succumbed to most of my food cravings and rapidly gained a total of 20 kg on top of my baby's weight. This weight gain made it incredibly difficult to safely transfer in and out of bed or the shower bench and I found myself on the floor on more than one occasion.

From an obstetric point of view, I was medically quite uncomplicated until it came time for the baby to be born. In 2001, doctors could not find a lot of information about vaginal birth for people who had an SCI and from all the information I could find, the biggest warning sign was autonomic dysreflexia (see Chapter

Continued

CASE STUDY 3—cont'd

4). Considering my injury was around L1/T12, it meant this was not a complication that I had. Nonetheless, the idea of it scared the doctor enough to convince me to have a caesarean. My first baby was born full-term healthy with no complications by caesarean section in September 2001.

My second pregnancy was in 2004 and because I had learnt a lot about weight gain during my first pregnancy, I did everything I possibly could to make sure that I kept my weight in check and remained active and eating healthy throughout the pregnancy. I had no complications with my second pregnancy until 28 weeks when my feet started to swell up, and my bladder became hard to manage. At 32 weeks I was having difficulty transferring, but was still remaining safe and confident.

Again, this pregnancy remained uncomplicated until it was time for the baby to be born, when my obstetrician explained that normal labour and a vaginal birth would have been an option for me, but now because I had previously had a caesarean section it complicated my birthing plan and I had no choice but to have another caesarean section. My second baby was born healthy via caesarean section full term with no complications in August 2004.

I am now in a new relationship and my present partner also has an SCI (T4 AIS A). We decided to do a full round of IVF. My third pregnancy occurred in 2017 as a result of a fresh embryo transfer. This time, the swelling in my feet started at 22 weeks, as did the issues with my bladder. I remained as active as I possibly could and at 32 weeks I was still climbing into a four-wheel-drive.

There were some complications towards the end of gestation where the baby had stopped growing, was failing to thrive and measured in the third percentile. This resulted in a planned early caesarean section delivery at 37 weeks. Fortunately, the birth itself was uncomplicated and the baby was born healthy.

Following all three caesarean sections, I remained in bed for three days without moving. I had an indwelling catheter for 5 days to minimise my transfers and my bed mobility was easy as I remained on a foam mattress instead of an air mattress. The biggest difficulty I found in the maternity ward was not being able to get my baby in an out of the bassinet that they provide. For my first two pregnancies I had to buzz the nurse every time I wanted to feed or hold my baby.

For my third pregnancy I arranged with the nurse prior to the birth for a large single room. The rooms in the hospital are smaller and shared rooms don't leave much room for wheelchairs. Nurses sometimes insist the wheelchair be left in the corridor to allow better access to their patients. The larger room was requested so it could also accommodate my husband and ensure that we had a better chance to manage everything while living outside of our comfort zone and ability. By that, I mean that our home is set up with everything within reach, and nobody moves or interferes with our system. The change table is the perfect height at home, with wipes, creams, towels and nappies all within reach. In hospital, we didn't have this. There is no place to change the baby except for on your lap. Furthermore, because of my husband's level of injury, his balance does not allow for this. On top of this, my new C-section wouldn't allow me to sit up without a huge amount of pain, we were unable to lift the baby in and out

CASE STUDY 3—cont'd

of the mandatory cribs used on the ward and co-sleeping was frowned upon.

In November 2018 and April 2019, we attempted to have another child and tried IVF using a frozen embryo transfer. Each attempt included an 8-week cycle of hormones with a frozen embryo transfer at the 6-week mark and a 2-week wait to confirm a pregnancy. The first attempt was an automatic fail and left us feeling upset at how unfair it was. The second time resulted in a pregnancy; however, I miscarried at 8 weeks. The reason for using IVF was due to my partner's type of SCI. The emotional turmoil and mentally destructive thought processes that comes from spending over $22,000, putting up with injections, mood- and cycle-altering medications, weight gain and coming out with empty arms can be unbearable. Although this is talked about in the spinal injuries unit, what is missed is the guilt the male goes through watching his partner experience something so physically, emotionally and mentally taxing because of his SCI. (See Chapter 12 for further detail on sexual rehabilitation and obstetrics following SCI.)

Breastfeeding in the very early days was complicated by the increased possibility of shearing on my tailbone. I very quickly realised for myself that it was easier to stay in my chair and use pillows or to sit on a comfy couch at home. The difficulty that arises from this is once you're on the couch breastfeeding your baby you can't get up to grab something else, so for my first baby I spent a lot of time on the couch. However, because I had to get up and chase after other kids for my second and third baby, I spent a lot of time breastfeeding in my wheelchair.

Finding the right equipment can be a challenge. I found a pram that I could push around the shopping centre confidently and folded into a manageable size and was light enough to get to

the car. Also, trying to get the right carseat for a baby is a problem that any parent will come across. However, as somebody with an SCI can discover, getting your baby into that car seat is incredibly tricky. Balance and reach are issues, although this constantly changes. I use my abdominal muscles to stabilise myself when I get the baby in and out of the car, whereas my husband relies mainly on one arm to lift and position the baby and uses the other arm to steady himself. Babies grow and change very quickly as does the way you negotiate each task with your baby; for example, now that my youngest daughter is two years old, my husband now relies more on bribery to get her in and out of the car.

Burns

I really enjoying spending time outdoors, including riding motorbikes. I had been riding a 250 cc motorbike with a friend who was doing the gears for me, when later that night I got undressed to have a shower and found a very large blister on the inside of my calf that hung down to my ankle. I went to emergency and it was assessed as a large third-degree burn about the same size as your hand; it required surgery and a skin graft. The skin graft was taken from the top of my thigh and I spent a week in hospital with my leg healing. I swore from that day on that while I was riding motorbikes I would always wear my riding boots.

One lunch break I thought I'd duck over to the takeaway food shop and grab some hot chips. The ones in the hotbox looked disgusting so I asked for some new chips to be made and said that I was happy to wait for them. However, by the time I finished waiting for them I was going to be late back from my lunch break, so I took the cup of hot chips and put them between my knees and pushed back to work. It was approximately

Continued

CASE STUDY 3—cont'd

a three-minute push and when I got the chips from between my knees and went to eat them I had approximately 15 little blisters on the inside of both my legs. I've been told 1 million times not to do this with hot coffee because I would burn my legs. Turns out it burns with hot chips too.

Pressure injuries

After 23 years of being in a chair I have started to notice some skin changes. My seating doesn't seem to suit me and I'm struggling to find something that meets my needs. I do not have a lot of meat sitting over my ischial tuberosities any more and for the last three years I have dealt with blackened skin and referred pain. I find most days I cannot sit for more than 8 hours. I feel that I have not had to deal very much with SCI-related issues for most of my time in a wheelchair, and I can honestly say this feels like the most debilitating, mood-altering and goal-changing concern that I have had to date.

Good seating from the beginning is an absolute necessity and maintaining your seating and skin are just as important (see Chapter 8 on seating options). I feel that this change has something to do with my hip flexor contractions. This has become steadily worse over the years as I am a busy mum, going on long drives for work and managing the financial stressors associated with being able to look after myself. Combined with my lumbar lordosis, the change in my hip flexor length is putting everything into a different position, particularly my pelvis, which impacts on my seating and preventing me from moving freely. This makes me want to point out that being able to do your stretches is also so incredibly important and a worthwhile five minutes of your day.

COMMON THEMES

As alluded to in the introduction, although these three cases are very different, the common themes that are apparent in each case are:

- musculoskeletal injuries – particularly shoulder injuries
- fractures
- pressure injuries, often as a result of poor posture and sitting
- long-term sitting issues/pain
- burns injuries as a result of poor sensation or complete lack of sensation
- excessive weight gain due to the sedentary lifestyle (or pregnancy).

On the positive side, each of these individuals has a life partner and children (and grandchildren in two cases). Each of them has maintained an independent lifestyle and a fulfilling life despite the challenges thrown at them by having sustained a TSCI.

It is important we remember that, as physiotherapists working in the field of rehabilitation of people with an SCI, it is our role to give that person back the ability to choose how they would like to live their lives.[1]

Reference

1. Ida Bromley, Head of the Physiotherapy Department at The National Spinal Injuries Centre Stoke Mandeville Hospital, UK, 1972, personal communication to Jackie Reznik.

POSTFACE

During the writing of this book, we have had the privilege of meeting some extra-ordinary people who not only turned their lives around, after what could have been a most devastating event, but went on to write themselves the most amazing success stories. Some of these people were persuaded to author chapters for us in the book, Jonathan, Dan, Arik, Col and Katie, we thank you for your contributions and for turning what could have been just another textbook on Spinal Cord Injuries into a book with a heart.

One young man, Omer, went one-step farther and turned his father's spinal cord injury into a lifetime's work. Omer's father Shmulik was injured in when his tank rolled over in the 1973 Yom Kippur War in Israel. Shmulik received burns and a complete low cervical lesion, but went on to complete his degree, take up full time work, marry and father three children. A success story in its own right, but aged 23, Omer decided that his father had been denied the trek that many young people enjoy. Since no other chairs existed that could undertake such a journey safely, Omer went on to design an all-terrain wheelchair - the Trekker- that would allow his father to embark on the trip he had never been able to experience as a young man – and Paratrek was born. Ten years later Paratrek, https://www.paratrek.org/ is a thriving company-allowing wheelchair bound young and young -at -heart individuals to experience the trip (or trips) of a lifetime. Their motto "where there's a wheel, there's a way".

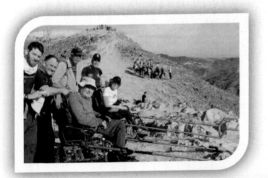

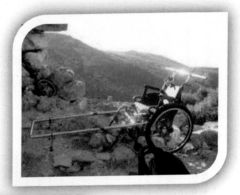

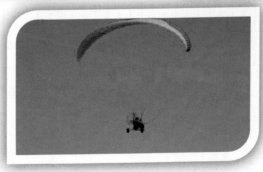

We hope that this book will inspire its readers as much as these people have inspired us.

Jackie Reznik, Josh Simmons

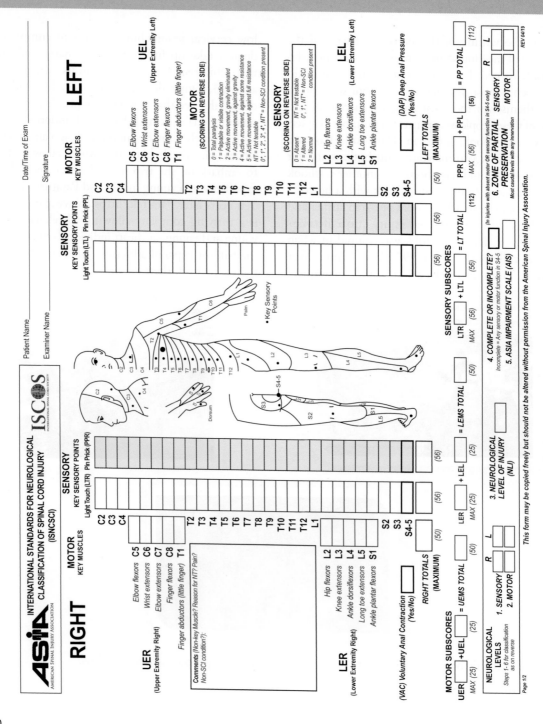

Muscle Function Grading

0 = Total paralysis

1 = Palpable or visible contraction

2 = Active movement, full range of motion (ROM) with gravity eliminated

3 = Active movement, full ROM against gravity

4 = Active movement, full ROM against gravity and moderate resistance in a muscle specific position

5 = (Normal) active movement, full ROM against gravity and full resistance in a functional muscle position expected from an otherwise unimpaired person

NT = Not testable (i.e. due to immobilization, severe pain such that the patient cannot be graded, amputation of limb, or contracture of > 50% of the normal ROM)

0*, 1*, 2*, 3*, 4*, NT* = Non-SCI condition present [a]

Sensory Grading

0 = Absent   1 = Altered, either decreased/impaired sensation or hypersensitivity

2 = Normal   NT = Not testable

0*, 1*, NT* = Non-SCI condition present [a]

[a]Note: Abnormal motor and sensory scores should be tagged with a '*' to indicate an impairment due to a non-SCI condition. The non-SCI condition should be explained in the comments box together with information about how the score is rated for classification purposes (at least normal / not normal for classification).

When to Test Non-Key Muscles:

In a patient with an apparent AIS B classification, non-key muscle functions more than 3 levels below the motor level on each side should be tested to most accurately classify the injury (differentiate between AIS B and C).

Movement	Root level
Shoulder: Flexion, extension, abduction, adduction, internal and external rotation Elbow: Supination	C5
Elbow: Pronation Wrist: Flexion	C6
Finger: Flexion at proximal joint, extension Thumb: Flexion, extension and abduction in plane of thumb	C7
Finger: Flexion at MCP joint Thumb: Opposition, adduction and abduction perpendicular to palm	C8
Finger: Abduction of the index finger	T1
Hip: Adduction	L2
Hip: External rotation	L3
Hip: Extension, abduction, internal rotation Knee: Flexion Ankle: Inversion and eversion Toe: MP and IP extension	L4
Hallux and Toe: DIP and PIP flexion and abduction	L5
Hallux: Adduction	S1

ASIA Impairment Scale (AIS)

A = Complete. No sensory or motor function is preserved in the sacral segments S4-5.

B = Sensory Incomplete. Sensory but not motor function is preserved below the neurological level and includes the sacral segments S4-5 (light touch or pin prick at S4-5 or deep anal pressure) AND no motor function is preserved more than three levels below the motor level on either side of the body.

C = Motor Incomplete. Motor function is preserved at the most caudal sacral segments for voluntary anal contraction (VAC) OR the patient meets the criteria for sensory incomplete status (sensory function preserved at the most caudal sacral segments S4-5 by LT, PP or DAP), and has some sparing of motor function more than three levels below the ipsilateral motor level on either side of the body. (This includes key or non-key muscle functions to determine motor incomplete status.) For AIS C – less than half of key muscle functions below the single NLI have a muscle grade ≥ 3.

D = Motor Incomplete. Motor incomplete status as defined above, with at least half (half or more) of key muscle functions below the single NLI having a muscle grade ≥ 3.

E = Normal. If sensation and motor function as tested with the ISNCSCI are graded as normal in all segments, and the patient had prior deficits, then the AIS grade is E. Someone without an initial SCI does not receive an AIS grade.

Using ND: To document the sensory, motor and NLI levels, the ASIA Impairment Scale grade, and/or the zone of partial preservation (ZPP) when they are unable to be determined based on the examination results.

Steps in Classification

The following order is recommended for determining the classification of individuals with SCI.

1. Determine sensory levels for right and left sides.
The sensory level is the most caudal, intact dermatome for both prick and light touch sensation.

2. Determine motor levels for right and left sides.
Defined by the lowest key muscle function that has a grade of at least 3 (on supine testing), providing the key muscle functions represented by segments above that level are judged to be intact (graded as a 5).
Note: in regions where there is no myotome to test, the motor level is presumed to be the same as the sensory level, if testable motor function above that level is also normal.

3. Determine the neurological level of injury (NLI).
This refers to the most caudal segment of the cord with intact sensation and antigravity (3 or more) muscle function strength, provided that there is normal (intact) sensory and motor function rostrally respectively.
The NLI is the most cephalad of the sensory and motor levels determined in steps 1 and 2.

4. Determine whether the injury is Complete or Incomplete.
(i.e. absence or presence of sacral sparing)
If voluntary anal contraction = **No** AND all S4-5 sensory scores = 0 AND deep anal pressure = **No**, then injury is **Complete**.
Otherwise, injury is **Incomplete**.

5. Determine ASIA Impairment Scale (AIS) Grade.

Is injury Complete?   If YES, AIS=A

   NO ↓

Is injury Motor Complete? If YES, AIS=B

   NO → (No=voluntary anal contraction OR motor function more than three levels below the <u>motor</u> level on a given side, if the patient has sensory incomplete classification)

Are at least half (half or more) of the key muscles below the neurological level of injury graded 3 or better?

  NO ↓   YES ↓

  AIS=C   AIS=D

If sensation and motor function is normal in all segments, AIS=E
Note: AIS E is used in follow-up testing when an individual with a documented SCI has recovered normal function. If at initial testing no deficits are found, the individual is neurologically intact and the ASIA Impairment Scale does not apply.

6. Determine the zone of partial preservation (ZPP).
The ZPP is used only in injuries with absent motor (no VAC) OR sensory function (no DAP, no LT and no PP sensation) in the lowest sacral segments S4-5, and refers to those dermatomes and myotomes caudal to the sensory and motor levels that remain partially innervated. With sacral sparing of sensory function, the sensory ZPP is not applicable and therefore "NA" is recorded in the block of the worksheet. Accordingly, if VAC is present, the motor ZPP is not applicable and is noted as "NA".

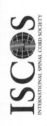

AMERICAN SPINAL INJURY ASSOCIATION

ISCOS
INTERNATIONAL SPINAL CORD SOCIETY

INTERNATIONAL STANDARDS FOR NEUROLOGICAL CLASSIFICATION OF SPINAL CORD INJURY

Page 2/2

APPENDIX 2

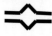

LOEWENSTEIN HOSPITAL REHABILITATION CENTER
Affiliated with the Sackler Faculty of Medicine, Tel-Aviv University

Department IV, Medical Director: Prof. Amiram Catz **Tel: 972-9-7709090 Fax: 972-9-7709986 e-mail: amiramc@clalit.org.il**

כללית

Patient Name: _____**ID:**_____ **Examiner Name:** _____
(Enter the score for each function in the adjacent square, below the date. The form may be used for up to 6 examinations.)

SCIM-SPINAL CORD INDEPENDENCE MEASURE

Version III, Sept 14, 2002

Self-Care

EXam 1   2   3   4   5   6

DATE   \ \ \ \ \ \

1. Feeding (cutting, opening containers, pouring, bringing food to mouth, holding cup with fluid)
0. Needs parenteral, gastrostomy, or fully assisted oral feeding
1. Needs partial assistance for eating and/or drinking, or for wearing adaptive devices
2. Eats independently; needs adaptive devices or assistance only for cutting food and/or pouring and/or opening containers
3. Eats and drinks independently; does not require assistance or adaptive devices

2. Bathing (soaping, washing, drying body and head, manipulating water tap). **A-upper body; B-lower body**
A. 0. Requires total assistance
   1. Requires partial assistance
   2. Washes independently with adaptive devices or in a specific setting (e.g., bars, chair)
   3. Washes independently; does not require adaptive devices or specific setting (not customary for healthy people) (adss)
B. 0. Requires total assistance
   1. Requires partial assistance
   2. Washes independently with adaptive devices or in a specific setting (adss)
   3. Washes independently; does not require adaptive devices (adss) or specific setting

3. Dressing (clothes, shoes, permanent orthoses: dressing, wearing, undressing). **A-upper body; B-lower body**
A. 0. Requires total assistance
   1. Requires partial assistance with clothes without buttons, zippers or laces (cwobzl)
   2. Independent with cwobzl; requires adaptive devices and/or specific settings (adss)
   3. Independent with cwobzl; does not require adss; needs assistance or adss only for bzl
   4. Dresses (any cloth) independently; does not require adaptive devices or specific setting
B. 0. Requires total assistance
   1. Requires partial assistancewith clothes without buttons, zipps or laces (cwobzl)
   2. Independent with cwobzl; requires adaptive devices and/or specific settings (adss)
   3. Independent with cwobzl without adss; needs assistance or adss only for bzl
   4. Dresses (any cloth) independently; does not require adaptive devices or specific setting

4. Grooming (washing hands and face, brushing teeth, combing hair, shaving, applying makeup)
0. Requires total assistance
1. Requires partial assistance
2. Grooms independently with adaptive devices
3. Grooms independently without adaptive devices

SUBTOTAL (0-20)

Respiration and Sphincter Management

5. Respiration
0. Requires tracheal tube (TT) and permanent or intermittent assisted ventilation (IAV)
2. Breathes independently with TT; requires oxygen, much assistance in coughing or TT management
4. Breathes independently with TT; requires little assistance in coughing or TT management
6. Breathes independently without TT; requires oxygen, much assistance in coughing, a mask (e.g., peep) or IAV (bipap)
8. Breathes independently without TT; requires little assistance or stimulation for coughing
10. Breathes independently without assistance or device

6. Sphincter Management - Bladder
0. Indwelling catheter
3. Residual urine volume (RUV) > 100cc; no regular catheterization or assisted intermittent catheterization
6. RUV < 100cc or intermittent self-catheterization; needs assistance for applying drainage instrument
9. Intermittent self-catheterization; uses external drainage instrument; does not need assistance for applying
11. Intermittent self-catheterization; continent between catheterizations; does not use external drainage instrument
13. RUV <100cc; needs only external urine drainage; no assistance is required for drainage
15. RUV <100cc; continent; does not use external drainage instrument

7. Sphincter Management - Bowel
0. Irregular timing or very low frequency (less than once in 3 days) of bowel movements
5. Regular timing, but requires assistance (e.g., for applying suppository); rare accidents (less than twice a month)
8. Regular bowel movements, without assistance; rare accidents (less than twice a month)
10. Regular bowel movements, without assistance; no accidents

8. Use of Toilet (perineal hygiene, adjustment of clothes before/after, use of napkins or diapers).
0. Requires total assistance
1. Requires partial assistance; does not clean self
2. Requires partial assistance; cleans self independently
4. Uses toilet independently in all tasks but needs adaptive devices or special setting (e.g., bars)
5. Uses toilet independently; does not require adaptive devices or special setting)

SUBTOTAL (0-40)

Mobility (room and toilet) DATE \ \ \ \ \ \

9. Mobility in Bed and Action to Prevent Pressure Sores

0. Needs assistance in all activities: turning upper body in bed, turning lower body in bed, sitting up in bed, doing push-ups in wheelchair, with or without adaptive devices, but not with electric aids
2. Performs one of the activities without assistance
4. Performs two or three of the activities without assistance
6. Performs all the bed mobility and pressure release activities independently

10. Transfers: bed-wheelchair (locking wheelchair, lifting footrests, removing and adjusting arm rests, transferring, lifting feet).

0. Requires total assistance
1. Needs partial assistance and/or supervision, and/or adaptive devices (e.g., sliding board)
2. Independent (or does not require wheelchair)

11. Transfers: wheelchair-toilet-tub (if uses toilet wheelchair: transfers to and from; if uses regular wheelchair: locking wheelchair, lifting footrests, removing and adjusting armrests, transferring, lifting feet)

0. Requires total assistance
1. Needs partial assistance and/or supervision, and/or adaptive devices (e.g., grab-bars)
2. Independent (or does not require wheelchair)

Mobility (indoors and outdoors, on even surface)

12. Mobility Indoors

0. Requires total assistance
1. Needs electric wheelchair or partial assistance to operate manual wheelchair
2. Moves independently in manual wheelchair
3. Requires supervision while walking (with or without devices)
4. Walks with a walking frame or crutches (swing)
5. Walks with crutches or two canes (reciprocal walking)
6. Walks with one cane
7. Needs leg orthosis only
8. Walks without walking aids

13. Mobility for Moderate Distances (10-100 meters)

0. Requires total assistance
1. Needs electric wheelchair or partial assistance to operate manual wheelchair
2. Moves independently in manual wheelchair
3. Requires supervision while walking (with or without devices)
4. Walks with a walking frame or crutches (swing)
5. Walks with crutches or two canes (reciprocal walking)
6. Walks with one cane
7. Needs leg orthosis only
8. Walks without walking aids

14. Mobility Outdoors (more than 100 meters)

0. Requires total assistance
1. Needs electric wheelchair or partial assistance to operate manual wheelchair
2. Moves independently in manual wheelchair
3. Requires supervision while walking (with or without devices)
4. Walks with a walking frame or crutches (swing)
5. Walks with crutches or two canes (reciprocal waking)
6. Walks with one cane
7. Needs leg orthosis only
8. Walks without walking aids

15. Stair Management

0. Unable to ascend or descend stairs
1. Ascends and descends at least 3 steps with support or supervision of another person
2. Ascends and descends at least 3 steps with support of handrail and/or crutch or cane
3. Ascends and descends at least 3 steps without any support or supervision

16. Transfers: wheelchair-car (approaching car, locking wheelchair, removing arm- and footrests, transferring to and from car, bringing wheelchair into and out of car)

0. Requires total assistance
1. Needs partial assistance and/or supervision and/or adaptive devices
2. Transfers independent; does not require adaptive devices (or does not require wheelchair)

17. Transfers: ground-wheelchair

0. Requires assistance
1. Transfers independent with or without adaptive devices (or does not require wheelchair)

SUBTOTAL (0-40)

TOTAL SCIM SCORE (0-100)

APPENDIX 3 MODIFIED ASHWORTH SCALE

- Measures resistance to passive movement (tone)
- Does NOT differentiate between:
  - Neural (spasticity) components and
  - Non-neural (muscle stiffness, shortening) components

EQUIPMENT REQUIRED

- Plinth

TESTING POSITION

- Supine

GRADES

0 = No increase in muscle tone
1 = Slight increase in muscle tone, manifested by a catch and release or by minimal resistance at end of range of motion when affected part(s) is moved in flexion or extension
1+ = Slight increase in muscle tone, manifested by a catch, followed by minimal resistance throughout the remainder (less than half) of the range of movement
2 = More marked increase in muscle tone through most of the range of movement, but affected parts easily moved
3 = Considerable increase in muscle tone, passive movement difficult
4 = Affected part(s) rigid in flexion or extension

EXAMPLE

- Elbow flexors
  1. Subject lies supine
  2. Person to be tested must be relaxed

3. Operator moves elbow through the full passive range of movement of elbow flexion
4. Record grade

RECORDING SHEET — Modified Ashworth Scale

	0	1	1+	2	3	4
Elbow flexion	☐	☐	☐	☐	☐	☐
Elbow extension	☐	☐	☐	☐	☐	☐
Wrist flexion	☐	☐	☐	☐	☐	☐
Wrist extension	☐	☐	☐	☐	☐	☐
Knee flexion	☐	☐	☐	☐	☐	☐
Knee extension	☐	☐	☐	☐	☐	☐
Dorsiflexion	☐	☐	☐	☐	☐	☐
Plantarflexion	☐	☐	☐	☐	☐	☐

Grades

0 = No increase in muscle tone
1 = Slight increase in muscle tone, manifested by a catch and release or by minimal resistance at end of range of motion when affected part(s) is moved in flexion or extension
1+ = Slight increase in muscle tone, manifested by a catch, followed by minimal resistance throughout the remainder (less than half) of the range of movement
2 = More marked increase in muscle tone through most of the range of movement, but affected parts easily moved
3 = Considerable increase in muscle tone, passive movement difficult
4 = Affected part(s) rigid in flexion or extension

APPENDIX 4 TARDIEU SCALE

- A measure of spasticity
- Used to provide an accurate objective measure of the effect of an intervention for spasticity e.g. Botulinum toxin, casting
- Spasticity = velocity-dependent increase in tonic stretch reflexes with exaggerated tendon jerks resulting from hyper-excitability of the stretch reflex
- Compares how a spastic muscle 'catches' at slow and high speeds
- It measures:
  - Intensity of the muscle reaction to being stretched
  - The angle at which the catch is felt
  - How angle changes as muscle is stretched slowly and quickly

EQUIPMENT REQUIRED

- Plinth – use as a bed and a table
- Goniometer – to measure joint angle at which catch occurs
- Recording sheet

TEST PROCEDURE

- Test position must be consistent for each testing session
  - UL → sitting or supine
    - Elbow flexors – shoulder adducted
    - Elbow extensors- shoulder abducted
  - LL → supine
    - Knee flexors – hip flexed to 30 degrees
    - Knee extensors – hip flexed

DEFINITIONS

- Velocity of stretch

  V1 = as slow as possible (minimising stretch reflex)

  V2 = Speed of the limb segment falling under gravity

  V3 = As fast as possible (faster than natural drop of limb segment under gravity)

NB: V1 is used to measure PROM   V2 & V3 are used to rate spasticity

- Quality of muscle reaction (X)

  0 = no resistance throughout the course of the passive movement

  1 = slight resistance throughout the course of the passive movement, with no clear catch at a precise angle

  2 = clear catch at precise angle, interrupting the passive mvt, followed by a release

  3 = fatigable clonus (<10 seconds when maintaining pressure) occurring at a precise angle

  4 = investigable clonus (>10 seconds when maintaining pressure) occurring at a precise angle

- Angle of muscle reaction (Y)

  Measured relative to the position of minimal stretch of the muscle for all joints except the hip, which is measure relative to the resting anatomic position

EXAMPLE

- Elbow flexors
  1. Subject lies supine with shoulder abducted ~ 45°

2. Flex elbow as much as possible
3. Extend elbow as slowly as possible (V1)
    1. Record quality of muscle reaction (X)
    2. Record angle if a clear catch or clonus occurs (Y)
4. Repeat for two more velocities of stretch
    1. V2 → speed of falling forearm under gravity
    2. V3 → speed as fast as you can, faster than V2

INTERPRETATION OF FINDINGS

- The difference between V1 and V3
  - Large difference indicates there's a large dynamic component in which case there's greater opportunity for change in the angle of V2 if Botulinum Toxin A is used to affect the muscle
  - Small difference indicates that there's a predominantly fixed contracture of the muscle → Botulinum toxin not indicated
- The difference between PROM and normal ROM
  - If V1 X values (PROM) near normal ROM values → pharmacological Mx of spasticity alone is likely to be effective
  - If V3 X values are present in a slightly shortened range, pharmacological Mx may need to be supplemented with casting or splinting
  - If V3 X values are present in a severely shortened range, contracture may be present and the use of Botulinum toxin should be questioned

RECORDING SHEET   Tardieu

Elbow flexion		
Shoulder _____ o _____ Hand		
V1	X =	Y =
V2	X =	Y =
V3	X =	Y =
Elbow extension		
Shoulder _____ o _____ Hand		
V1	X =	Y =
V2	X =	Y =
V3	X =	Y =
Knee flexion		
Hip _____ o _____ Foot		
V1	X =	Y =
V2	X =	Y =
V3	X =	Y =
Knee flexion		
Hip _____ o _____ Foot		
V1	X =	Y =
V2	X =	Y =
V3	X =	Y =

APPENDIX 5

1906

Queensland Government

Princess Alexandra Hospital

**Physiotherapy
Spinal Injuries Unit
Posture Assessment**

(Affix identification label here or complete if E-Form)

URN:

Family name:

Given name(s):

Address:

Date of birth: Sex: ☐ M ☐ F

MAT Evaluation

Pelvis		Comments: e.g. Fixed/ Flexible/ Corrects with difficulty
Obliquity:	☐ None	
Right lower than left by:	cm	
Left lower than right by:	cm	
Tilt:	☐ Neutral	
	☐ Anterior	
	☐ Posterior	
Rotation:	☐ None	
Right forward of left by:	cm	
Left forward by right by:	cm	

Trunk		Comments: e.g. Fixed/ Flexible/ Corrects with difficulty
Straight:	☐	
Scoliosis: Convex to	☐ R ☐ L	
Kyphosis:	☐ Mid thoracic	
	☐ Upper thoracic	
Lumbar space:	☐ Norm	
	☐ Flat	
	☐ Lordotic	
Rib cage:	☐ Even	
	Fwd on ☐ R ☐ L	

Head and Neck		Comments: e.g. Fixed/ Flexible/ Corrects with difficulty
Aligned:	☐	
Lat Flexed:	☐ R ☐ L	
Forward Flexed:	☐	
Hyperextended:	☐	
Rotated to:	☐ R ☐ L	

Range of Motion

True Hip Flexion: ....

....

Ankle Range: ....

....

Knee Range: ....

....

Upper Limb: shoulder, elbow, wrist, hands (list any concerns):

....

....

....

....

....

DO NOT WRITE IN THIS BINDING MARGIN

V1.0 04/2014
Locally Printed

00011-1906

Physiotherapy Spinal Injuries Unit PostureAssessment

Queensland Government **Princess Alexandra Hospital** **Physiotherapy** **Posture Assessment**	(Affix identification label here or complete if E-Form) URN: Family name: Given name(s): Address: Date of birth:　　　　　　　Sex: ☐ M　☐

Sitting Evaluation

Sitting balance on firm surface:	**Comments:**
☐ Hands free	
☐ Hands dependent	
☐ None	

Assistance from examiner:	**Comments:**
☐ Minimum	
☐ Moderate	
☐ Maximum	
☐ None	

Demonstrates:	**Comments:**
☐ Righting response	
☐ Equilibrium response	
☐ Protective response	

Additional Notes: Make note of any postural deformities (as per previous page) that are apparent in sitting:

....

....

....

....

....

....

....

....

....

....

....

....

Plan: (Features to consider for seating)

....

....

....

....

....

....

....

....

....

....

....

Therapist Name: ....　Signature: ....　Date: ....

2336

<table>
<tr><td>

Queensland Government

Princess Alexandra Hospital

Spinal Injuries Unit

Manual Wheelchair Set-Up

</td><td>

(Affix identification label here)

URN:

Family name:

Given name(s):

Address:

Date of birth: Sex: ☐ M ☐ F

</td></tr>
</table>

Body Dimensions

Hip width (GT to GT)		
Chest width		
Thigh depth (back of pelvis to popliteal fossa)	L:	R:
Lower leg length (popliteal fossa to heel of foot)	L:	R:

Comments:

Initial Set-Up

Front seat height	Rear seat height	Backrest height	Seat to footplate length	Centre of gravity	Backrest angle

Chair:

Backrest:

Cushion:

Date	Adjustments	Outcomes

Print name: ....   Signature:...

Designation: ....   Date:...

Queensland Government	(Affix identification label here)
Princess Alexandra Hospital **Spinal Injuries Unit** **Manual Wheelchair Set-Up**	URN: Family name: Given name(s): Address: Date of birth: Sex: ☐ M ☐ F

1. Trial Set-Up

Front seat height	Rear seat height	Backrest height	Seat to footplate length	Centre of gravity	Backrest angle

Chair:

Backrest:

Cushion:

Date	Adjustment	Outcome

2. Trial Set-Up

Front seat height	Rear seat height	Backrest height	Seat to footplate length	Centre of gravity	Backrest angle

Chair:

Backrest:

Cushion:

Date	Adjustment	Outcome

Scripted Equipment (include model and dimensions)

Chair	
Backrest	
Cushion	
Date equipment scripted	
Clinicians present during scripting	

Print name: .... Signature:...

Designation: .... Date:...

INDEX

Page numbers followed by 'f' indicate figures, 't' indicate tables, and 'b' indicate boxes.

E

M